AMERICAN PSYCHIATRIC PRESS

REVIEW OF PSYCHIATRY

VOLUME
7

**EDITED BY ALLEN J. FRANCES, MD
and ROBERT E. HALES, MD**

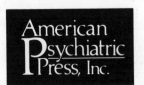

American
Psychiatric
Press, Inc.

1400 K Street, N.W.
Washington, DC
1988

American Psychiatric Press, Inc.

Note: The Editors, section editors, contributors, and publisher have worked to ensure that all information in this book concerning drug dosages, schedules, and routes of administration is accurate at the time of publication and consistent with standards set by the U.S. Food and Drug Administration and the general medical community. As medical research and practice advance, however, therapeutic standards may change. For this reason and because human and mechanical errors sometimes occur, we recommend that readers follow the advice of a physician directly involved in their care or the care of a member of their family.

The opinions or assertions contained herein are the private ones of Dr. Hales and are not to be construed as official or reflecting the views of the Department of Defense, the Uniformed Services University of the Health Sciences, Walter Reed Army Medical Center, or the Department of the Army. This book was prepared in the author's private capacity. Neither government-financed time nor supplies were used in connection with this project.

Books published by American Psychiatric Press, Inc., represent the views and opinions of the individual authors and do not necessarily reflect the policies and opinions of the Press or the American Psychiatric Association.

Typeset by VIP Systems, Alexandria, VA
Manufactured by Arcata Graphics, Fairfield, PA

Review of Psychiatry: Volume 7
ISSN 0736-1866
ISBN 0-88048-245-1 (hardbound)

To my mentors—*John Talbott and Bob Spitzer*—with admiration
and appreciation.

A.J.F.

To my wife, Dianne, who lights up my life, and to my two-year-
old daughter, Julia, who keeps me up at night.

R.E.H.

PSYCHIATRY UPDATE: THE AMERICAN PSYCHIATRIC ASSOCIATION ANNUAL REVIEW, VOLUME 4 (1985)

Robert E. Hales, M.D., and Allen J. Frances, M.D., Editors

An Introduction to the World of Neurotransmitters and Neuroreceptors
Joseph T. Coyle, M.D., Section Editor

Neuropsychiatry
Stuart C. Yudofsky, M.D., Section Editor

Sleep Disorders
David J. Kupfer, M.D., Section Editor

Eating Disorders
Joel Yager, M.D., Section Editor

The Therapeutic Alliance and Treatment Outcome
John P. Docherty, M.D., Section Editor

PSYCHIATRY UPDATE: THE AMERICAN PSYCHIATRIC ASSOCIATION ANNUAL REVIEW, VOLUME 5 (1986)

Allen J. Frances, M.D., and Robert E. Hales, M.D., Editors

Schizophrenia
Nancy C. Andreasen, M.D., Ph.D., Section Editor

Drug Abuse and Drug Dependence
Robert B. Millman, M.D., Section Editor

Personality Disorders
Robert M.A. Hirschfeld, M.D., Section Editor

Adolescent Psychiatry
Carolyn B. Robinowitz, M.D., and Jeanne Spurlock, M.D., Section Editors

Psychiatric Contributions to Medical Care
David Spiegel, M.D., and W. Stewart Agras, M.D., Section Editors

Group Psychotherapy
Irvin D. Yalom, M.D., Section Editor

PSYCHIATRY UPDATE: THE AMERICAN PSYCHIATRIC ASSOCIATION ANNUAL REVIEW, VOLUME 6 (1987)

Robert E. Hales, M.D., and Allen J. Frances, M.D., Editors

Bipolar Disorders
Frederick K. Goodwin, M.D., and Kay Redfield Jamison, Ph.D., Section Editors

Neuroscience Techniques in Clinical Psychiatry
John M. Morihisa, M.D., and Solomon H. Snyder, M.D., Section Editors

Differential Therapeutics
John F. Clarkin, Ph.D., and Samuel W. Perry, M.D., Section Editors

Violence and the Violent Patient
Kenneth Tardiff, M.D., M.P.H., Section Editor

Psychiatric Epidemiology
Myrna M. Weissman, Ph.D., Section Editor

Psychopharmacology: Drug Side Effects and Interactions
Philip Berger, M.D., and Leo Hollister, M.D., Section Editors

AMERICAN PSYCHIATRIC PRESS REVIEW OF PSYCHIATRY, VOLUME 8 (1989)

Allan Tasman, M.D., Robert E. Hales, M.D., and Allen J. Frances, M.D., Editors

Borderline Personality Disorder
John G. Gunderson, M.D., Section Editor

Child Psychiatry
Jerry Weiner, M.D., and James Egan, M.D., Section Editors

Alcoholism
Roger E. Meyer, M.D., Section Editor

Psychiatry and the Law
Paul S. Appelbaum, M.D., Section Editor

Difficult Situations in Clinical Practice
William Sledge, M.D., Section Editor

CONTENTS

Section

IV Electroconvulsive Therapy

Introduction

As the President of the American Psychiatric Association, it is a great privilege to write this Introduction to Volume 7 of the *American Psychiatric Press Review of Psychiatry*. This is the fourth volume edited by Drs. Allen J. Frances and Robert E. Hales. They have crafted a series of outstanding volumes summarizing the current state of clinical psychiatry and future directions for psychiatric research. Drs. Frances and Hales have earned the respect and admiration of psychiatrists everywhere for keeping us up-to-date on the newest developments in the field. The *Review of Psychiatry* series has become *the* annual publication which concisely yet comprehensively summarizes selected significant topical areas in psychiatry. Many eagerly await publication of each volume and especially of Volume 7, which is of the highest caliber.

The reader will note that the title of this series has now been changed to the *Review of Psychiatry*. This is in recognition of the fact that the material in this book is relevant for the year of publication and contains information which will be operational for several years—similar to current textbooks and major journals. As noted in the previous volumes of this series, the time from submission of manuscripts to their publication is less than that for many psychiatric journals. This results in keeping this series the most up-to-date summary on the subjects covered.

The topics chosen for Volume 7 focus on five major areas of interest to clinicians, researchers, and educators. The editors state in their Foreword to this volume that they have selected five topics which are timely and closely related: panic disorders, unipolar depression, suicide, electroconvulsive therapy, and cognitive therapy. The comorbidity of panic disorders and unipolar depression is being increasingly studied and better understood. The risk of suicide in patients with unipolar depression is well known and represents a preventive and therapeutic challenge for all psychiatrists. Electroconvulsive therapy remains the most effective treatment for severe unipolar depression. Finally, cognitive therapy has been shown to be quite effective in the treatment of depression and of panic disorders. The editors have succeeded in presenting these topics so that there is a minimal overlap of information, while providing appropriate recognition of where these disorders, conditions, and treatments interface.

At recent American Psychiatric Association Annual Meetings, the topic of panic disorder has attracted impressive crowds. The section editors, M. Katherine Shear, M.D., and David H. Barlow, Ph.D., have assembled prominent investigators who explore this subject. The section provides a summary of theoretical hypotheses for panic disorders and includes one of the best compendiums available on current biological, psychopathological, and epidemiological findings for this disorder. The section also provides the clinician with state of the art guidelines on the diagnosis and assessment of panic disorder and the pharmacologic and nondrug treatment of this serious and potentially disabling condition.

In the section on unipolar depression, edited by Martin B. Keller, M.D., there is a summary of the latest genetic research findings and correlative studies of biological factors found in patients with depressive illness and how these findings apply to clinical practice. Excellent chapters include the diagnosis and clinical course of depression and the latest information on both somatic and psychotherapeutic treatments. The importance of recognizing depression secondary to medical illness is highlighted. This information is particularly relevant for those psychiatrists working in consultation settings in general hospitals.

The topic of suicide has received considerable research interest and media attention. J. John Mann, M.D., and Michael Stanley, Ph.D., have assembled the works of some of the leading experts in this field of research. These scientists have summarized the latest epidemiologic studies and have outlined the major risk factors. Chapters present the biological factors associated with suicide and provide guidance to clinicians in assessing and treating such patients. Finally, chapters are included on the topics of evaluating suicidal behavior in children and young adults and on suicide prevention programs.

The section on electroconvulsive therapy was edited by Robert Rose, M.D., and Harold Alan Pincus, M.D., both of whom were involved in the recent National Institute of Mental Health Consensus Conference on this treatment. The leading clinicians and researchers in this area have contributed to this portion of Volume 7. The authors summarize in clear and clinically relevant fashion proposed mechanisms for the action of electroconvulsive therapy and outline indications for its use. Other chapters discuss details of this treatment, summarize the adverse effects of ECT, and provide the latest information on significant legal regulations and ethical issues as related to this therapeutic modality.

The final section, on cognitive therapy, is edited by the two individuals most prominently identified with this psychotherapeutic treatment: A. John Rush, M.D., and Aaron T. Beck, M.D. They have assembled one of the best reviews of this topic available to date. They provide basic information concerning the development and theory of cognitive therapy and identify ways in which a clinician would use this technique in treating patients with depression and panic disorder. Other chapters examine the use of cognitive therapy in children and adolescents and the development of group approaches in using a cognitive therapy framework. Chapters review the use of cognitive treatments to improve adherence and review empirical studies concerning the effectiveness of cognitive therapy in the treatment of depression, panic, and other psychiatric disorders.

Volume 7 promises to be one of the best and most exciting in this very useful series. The sections and chapters highlight, in a convincing fashion, my Presidential theme for 1987–1988: Opportunities and Challenges for Psychiatrists and Psychiatry: 1988–2000. This edition of the *Review of Psychiatry* is an excellent update and reference for clinicians, academicians, investigators, and residents. It is one of the books that all psychiatrists should purchase and read each year. Its level of excellence, overall comprehensiveness, and timeliness is not approached by any other book series or journal. The sections are well integrated, thought provoking, and highlight exciting and clinically relevant research findings.

Since this is the last volume for which Drs. Frances and Hales will serve as senior editors, I would like to express the deep gratitude of the American Psychiatric Association and thank them for a job well done. They have pioneered, persevered, and succeeded in establishing a tradition of publishing excellence. Being a good editor is a tedious and sometimes thankless job. Drs. Frances and Hales have dedicated themselves to the task at hand and have provided readers with an excellent product. The section editors and authors for this current volume have also made a valuable contribution to the field. They and previous section editors and authors have spent much time and energy in educating all of us on the importance of their respective research areas. We greatly appreciated their work.

I hope all of you will join me in reading, discussing, and applying the information to be found in the excellent sections and chapters contained in this year's volume.

George H. Pollock, M.D., Ph.D.

Foreword to Volume 7

by Allen J. Frances, M.D., and Robert E. Hales, M.D.

This is the fourth *Review of Psychiatry* that we have done together and, for several reasons, it has been the most enjoyable. In part, this is a consequence of our growing experience with the task and with working together as a team. We were able to anticipate and avoid many of the pitfalls that bedevil editing and that sometimes make it an exercise in small frustrations and quiet desperation. We also decided early on to take a calculated editorial gamble in Volume 7. In previous *Reviews*, we were careful to avoid redundancy by selecting topics that did not overlap to any great extent with one another. For Volume 7, we deliberately selected topics—Panic Disorder, Unipolar Depression, Suicide, Electroconvulsive Therapy, and Cognitive Therapy—that would necessarily overlap with one another in complex and multifaceted ways. Such an approach provides an opportunity to deal with these topics in much greater depth and with increased contextual richness; however, we did not want to have the same material presented over and over again in different sections. To minimize the likelihood of this latter situation, we requested and received quite detailed outlines from our section editors and contributors, plotted out points at which chapters might interact across sections, and attempted to provide a division of labor that would render the sections harmonious and complementary, rather than repetitious and dull. Readers will form their own judgements as to how well we have succeeded in this effort, but generally we found the redundancies that were included to be welcome rather than burdensome.

Aside from our desire for a degree of thematic unity in Volume 7, the topic selection was guided by recent research and clinical innovation that enriches each of the areas. Panic disorder is especially fascinating because it has engendered different, but interacting, explanatory models and treatments drawn from the somatic, cognitive, behavioral, and psychodynamic orientations in psychiatry. Unipolar depression is perhaps the most commonly encountered diagnosis in clinical practice and has been the subject of numerous advances in our understanding of epidemiology, pathogenesis, course, and treatment response. Suicide has become a major public health concern leading to an extensive research effort that has already demonstrated important clinical applications. Electroconvulsive therapy (ECT) is perhaps the most controversial of the effective treatments in psychiatry. The indications for ECT recently have been spelled out in an NIMH Consensus Conference and the accumulating research on its effectiveness demands the attention of clinicians. Cognitive therapy is one of the promising psychotherapeutic innovations of the past two decades. Many clinicians use a great deal of cognitive therapy in their practice without characterizing their treatment in this manner. We all can benefit from a more systematic incorporation of some of the newer cognitive techniques that have been developed.

Our Section Editors—Drs. Shear, Barlow, Keller, Mann, Stanley, Rose, Pincus, Rush, and Beck—have all been an absolute delight. Each is a master at integrating scientific research and clinical practice in a fashion that enhances both endeavors. Our chapter authors were carefully selected for their special expertise, and we are grateful to them for their diligence in meeting deadlines and their patience in what must have seemed like endless nagging.

We would like to acknowledge just a few of the many people who were especially helpful with this volume. First, and most important, are our able Editorial Assistants, Ms. Sandy Landfried and Joanne Mas. They have handled all the voluminous correspondence with our chapter authors and section editors and managed the many details involved in putting the book together. They have both been marvelous for us and for the book and have maintained their sense of humor through some demanding and interesting times. Our Editor at the American Psychiatric Press (APPI), Ms. Eve Shapiro, did an outstanding job with the detailed copy editing of this volume and has produced a book with readily accessible prose. Richard Farkas, APPI Production Manager, had the challenging job of turning manuscripts into finished product in less than six months. Ms. Jill Zaklow-Leepson has brought the *Review* to the attention of psychiatrists around the country. Ron McMillen, the General Manager of APPI, has overseen all aspects of publishing this book and provided sustained support and leadership. We would like to thank our Departmental Chairmen, Drs. Bob Michels and Harry C. Holloway, for their advice, consultation, and support. Finally, we are appreciative of our understanding wives, Vera Frances and Dianne Hales, who tolerated our spending holidays and weekends immersed in galleys and page proofs.

We have been working closely together for many years now, not only on the last four *Reviews* but also on the APA Annual Meetings and on other projects. Our very different personalities and academic backgrounds have made our collaboration particularly enriching to both of us, professionally as well as personally. We hope you have as much fun reading this review as we have had putting it together.

Contributors

James C. Ballenger, M.D.
Professor and Chairman, Department of Psychiatry and
Behavioral Sciences, Medical University of South Carolina,
Charleston, South Carolina

David H. Barlow, Ph.D.
Professor of Psychology; Director, Center for Stress and
Anxiety Disorders, State University of New York at Albany,
Albany, New York

Aaron T. Beck, M.D.
University Professor of Psychiatry, Center for Cognitive
Therapy, University of Pennsylvania School of Medicine,
Philadelphia, Pennsylvania

David A. Brent, M.D.
Assistant Professor of Psychiatry, Western Psychiatric Institute
and Clinic, Pittsburgh, Pennsylvania

Evelyn Bromet, Ph.D.
Professor of Psychiatry, State University of New York at Stony
Brook, Stony Brook, New York

Edwin H. Cassem, M.D.
Associate Professor of Psychiatry, Harvard Medical School;
Chief, Psychiatric Consultation Service, Department of
Psychiatry, Massachusetts General Hospital, Boston,
Massachusetts

C. Edward Coffey, M.D.
Assistant Professor of Psychiatry and Medicine (Division of
Neurology), Duke University Medical Center, Durham, North
Carolina

Lino Covi, M.D.
Clinical Associate Professor, Treatment Assessment Research
Unit, the University of Maryland at Baltimore School of
Medicine, Pikesville, Maryland

Michelle G. Craske, Ph.D.
Associate Director, Phobia and Anxiety Disorders Clinic, Center
for Stress and Anxiety Disorders, Department of Psychology,
State University of New York at Albany, Albany, New York

Lucy Davidson, M.D., Ed.S.
Clinical Assistant Professor in Psychiatry, Emory University
School of Medicine, Atlanta, Georgia

Mary Amanda Dew, Ph.D.
Assistant Professor of Psychiatry, Western Psychiatric Institute
and Clinic, Pittsburgh, Pennsylvania

Irene Elkin, Ph.D.
Coordinator, Treatment of Depression Collaborative Research
Program, Affective and Anxiety Research Branch, National
Institute of Mental Health, Rockville, Maryland

Max Fink, M.D.
Professor of Psychiatry, State University at Stony Brook School
of Medicine; Editor, *Convulsive Therapy*

Allen J. Frances, M.D.
Professor of Psychiatry, Cornell University Medical College;
Director, Outpatient Division, New York Hospital, Payne
Whitney Psychiatric Clinic, New York, New York

Abby J. Fyer, M.D.
Assistant Professor of Clinical Psychiatry, College of Physicians
and Surgeons of Columbia University; Co-Director, Anxiety
Disorders Clinic, New York State Psychiatric Institute, New
York, New York

Minna R. Fyer, M.D.
Assistant Professor of Psychiatry, Cornell University Medical
College; Director, Central Evaluation Services and Associate
Director, Anxiety Disorders Clinic, Payne Whitney Psychiatric
Clinic, New York, New York

Alan Jay Gelenberg, M.D.
Psychiatrist-in-Chief, The Arbour; Chief, Special Studies Clinic,
Massachusetts General Hospital; Associate Professor of
Psychiatry, Harvard Medical School; Editor-in-Chief, *Journal of
Clinical Psychiatry*, Boston, Massachusetts

Elliot S. Gershon, M.D.
Chief, Clinical Neurogenetics Branch, National Institute of
Mental Health, Bethesda, Maryland

Lynn R. Goldin, Ph.D.
Research Geneticist, Clinical Neurogenetics Branch, National
Institute of Mental Health, Bethesda, Maryland

Ruth L. Greenberg, Ph.D.
Center for Cognitive Therapy, University of Pennsylvania
School of Medicine, Philadelphia, Pennsylvania

Robert E. Hales, M.D.
Associate Professor of Psychiatry, Uniformed Services
University of the Health Sciences, F. Edward Hebert School of
Medicine, Bethesda, Maryland; Director of Psychiatry
Residency Training, Walter Reed Army Medical Center; Clinical
Associate Professor of Psychiatry, Georgetown University
School of Medicine, Washington, D.C.

Robert M. A. Hirschfeld, M.D.
Chief, Affective and Anxiety Disorders Research Branch,
Division of Clinical Research, National Institute of Mental
Health, Rockville, Maryland

Steven D. Hollon, Ph.D.
Associate Professor of Psychology, Vanderbilt University,
Nashville, Tennessee

Rolf G. Jacob, M.D.
Associate Professor of Psychiatry, Department of Psychiatry,
Western Psychiatric Institute and Clinic, University of
Pittsburgh School of Medicine, Pittsburgh, Pennsylvania

Martin B. Keller, M.D.
Associate Professor of Psychiatry, Harvard Medical School;
Director of Outpatient Research, Psychiatry Department,
Massachusetts General Hospital, Boston, Massachusetts

Pamela A. Kulbok, D.N.Sc.
Department of Psychiatry, Washington University School of
Medicine, St. Louis, Missouri

David J. Kupfer, M.D.
Professor and Chairman of Psychiatry, University of Pittsburgh
School of Medicine; Director of Research, Western Psychiatric
Institute and Clinic, Pittsburgh, Pennsylvania

J. John Mann, M.D.
Associate Professor of Psychiatry and Director, Laboratory of
Psychopharmacology, Cornell University Medical College, New
York, New York

George E. Murphy, M.D.
Professor of Psychiatry; Director of Psychiatric Outpatient
Services, Washington University School of Medicine, St. Louis,
Missouri

Lisa Najavits, B.A.
Department of Psychology, Vanderbilt University, Nashville,
Tennessee

Cynthia R. Pfeffer, M.D.
Associate Professor of Clinical Psychiatry, Cornell University
Medical College; Chief, Child Psychiatry, Inpatient Unit—New
York Hospital, White Plains, New York

Harold Alan Pincus, M.D.
Deputy Medical Director; Director, Office of Research,
American Psychiatric Association, Washington, D.C.

George H. Pollock, M.D., Ph.D.
President, American Psychiatric Association; President, Institute
for Psychoanalysis, Chicago; Professor of Psychiatry and the
Behavioral Sciences Northwestern University Medical and
Graduate Schools, Evanston, Illinois

Robert F. Prien, Ph.D.
Chief, Somatic Treatments Program, Affective and Anxiety
Disorders Research Branch, National Institute of Mental Health,
Rockville, Maryland

Laura Primakoff, Ph.D.
Assistant Professor, Treatment Assessment Research Unit, the
University of Maryland at Baltimore School of Medicine,
Pikesville, Maryland

Lee N. Robins, Ph.D.
Department of Psychiatry, Washington University School of
Medicine, St. Louis, Missouri

Robert M. Rose, M.D.
Professor and Chairman, Department of Psychiatry and
Behavioral Sciences, the University of Texas Medical Branch at
Galveston, Galveston, Texas

Mary Jane Rotheram-Borus, Ph.D.
Associate Clinical Professor of Medical Psychology, College of
Physicians and Surgeons of Columbia University and the New
York State Psychiatric Institute, New York, New York

A. John Rush, M.D.
Betty Jo Hay Professor of Psychiatry, Mental Health Clinical
Research Center, University of Texas Southwestern Medical
Center at Dallas, Dallas, Texas

Gary Sachs, M.D.
Instructor in Psychiatry, Harvard Medical School
Psychopharmacology Unit, Massachusetts General Hospital,
Boston, Massachusetts

Harold A. Sackeim, Ph.D.
Associate Professor of Clinical Psychology, Department of
Psychiatry, College of Physicians and Surgeons of Columbia
University; Deputy Chief, Department of Biological Psychiatry,
New York State Psychiatric Institute, New York, New York

Diana P. Sandberg, M.D.
Instructor in Clinical Psychiatry, College of Physicians and
Surgeons of Columbia University, New York, New York

Zindel V. Segal, Ph.D.
Cognitive and Behaviour Therapies Section, Clarke Institute of
Psychiatry, Toronto, Ontario, Canada

Brian F. Shaw, Ph.D.
Department of Psychology, Toronto General Hospital;
Departments of Psychiatry and Behavioural Sciences, University
of Toronto, Toronto, Ontario, Canada

M. Tracie Shea, Ph.D.
Staff Psychologist, Psychosocial Treatments Program, Affective
and Anxiety Disorders Research Branch, National Institute of
Mental Health, Rockville, Maryland

M. Katherine Shear, M.D.
Associate Professor of Clinical Psychiatry, Cornell University
Medical College; Director, Anxiety Disorders Clinic, the New
York Hospital, New York, New York

Michael Stanley, Ph.D.
Associate Professor, Departments of Psychiatry and
Pharmacology, College of Physicians and Surgeons, Columbia
University; Department of Neurochemistry, New York State
Psychiatric Institute, New York, New York

Paul D. Trautman, M.D.
Assistant Professor of Clinical Psychiatry, College of Physicians
and Surgeons of Columbia University and the New York State
Psychiatric Institute, New York, New York

Samuel M. Turner, Ph.D.
Associate Professor of Psychiatry and Psychology, Western
Psychiatric Institute and Clinic, University of Pittsburgh School
of Medicine, Pittsburgh, Pennsylvania

Richard D. Weiner, M.D., Ph.D.
Associate Professor of Psychiatry, Duke University Medical
Center; Staff Psychiatrist, Durham VA Medical Center,
Durham, North Carolina

Myrna M. Weissman, Ph.D.
Professor of Epidemiology in Psychiatry, College of Physicians
and Surgeons of Columbia University; Chief, Department of
Clinical and Genetic Epidemiology, New York State Psychiatric
Institute, New York, New York

William J. Winslade, J.D., Ph.D.
Professor of Psychiatry and Behavioral Sciences, Professor of
Preventive Medicine and Community Health, Institute for the
Medical Humanities; Director, Ethics Consultation Service,
University of Texas Medical Branch, Galveston, Texas

Jesse H. Wright, M.D., Ph.D.
Professor, Department of Psychiatry and Behavioral Sciences,
University of Louisville School of Medicine; Medical Director,
Norton Psychiatric Clinic, Louisville, Kentucky

I

Panic Disorder

Contents

Section I

Panic Disorder

Foreword

by David H. Barlow, Ph.D., and M. Katherine Shear, M.D.,
Section Editors

As recently as several years ago few people were aware of the phenomenon of panic. Now we are quickly realizing that we cannot deal effectively with the anxiety disorders, and perhaps all of the emotional disorders including depression, without a fuller understanding of panic and its consequences. For this reason, it is surprising that the pervasiveness and significance of panic has been overlooked for so long.

Once sensitized to the importance of panic, clinicians encounter it everywhere. The popular press is replete with accounts of the debilitating consequences of unexpected panic. Consider the case of John Madden, the well-known sportscaster and former professional football coach. Madden has done much to publicize the experience of panic and anxiety and uses it in a humorous way in several television commercials. While Madden has obviously overcome the stigma and embarrassment sure to be felt by a 6'4", 260-pound former football player whose business it was to be tough, he has not overcome the anxiety itself. Rather than taking a few hours to fly from New York to Los Angeles to announce the next football game, he spends the better part of his week on a train traveling across the country.

Although always tense in planes, he originally assessed his tension as a reaction to altitude, perhaps the symptom of an inner ear infection. When he realized that his anxiety began before the plane took off, but after the stewardess closed the door, he began to think otherwise. One day while flying across the country, he experienced a particularly severe panic attack, left the plane at a stop halfway across the United States, and never flew again.

John Madden and countless other individuals suffering from panic find it a devastating experience. For this reason data on the prevalence and ubiquity of panic are startling. In her chapter, Myrna Weissman reviews the very latest information on the prevalence of panic, panic disorder, and agoraphobia. She reports that 10 percent of the very large sample from the National Institute of Mental Health (NIMH) epidemiological catchment area (ECA) study reported unexpected or "spontaneous" panic attacks. These data are in substantial agreement with reports from Norton and colleagues (1986) in which a similar percentage reported unexpected panic and with recent data from Germany (Wittchen, 1986). Of course, not all of these people come in for treatment. In Chapter 1 we consider the implications of the high prevalence of panic attacks in the population for various models of panic disorder.

Weissman also draws our attention to the very unexpected finding that a minority of agoraphobics report a history of *Diagnostic and Statistical Manual of*

Mental Disorders, Third Edition, Revised (DSM-III-R) (American Psychiatric Association, 1987) panic attacks or panic symptoms. This is surprising because data from almost all clinical settings indicate that agoraphobics who come for treatment began avoiding situations because of the fear of having another unexpected panic while away from a safe place or a safe person. In this way agoraphobic avoidance was seen as a consequence of panic. Weissman admits that patients with "pure" agoraphobia probably do not come for treatment. But who are these people, and how and why do their symptoms develop? This is just one of the mysteries confronting us.

Recent findings also indicate excess mortality rates in panic disorder. For example, long term follow-up studies of both inpatients (Coryell et al, 1982) and outpatients (Coryell et al, 1986) have found a greater than expected mortality rate in patients with original diagnoses of anxiety neurosis, particularly panic disorder. This excess mortality rate can be attributed primarily to cardiovascular disease and suicide. In fact, suicide rates in anxious patients were equal to or slightly greater than a matched group of patients suffering from depression at follow-up. Interestingly, excess mortality due to cardiovascular disease was limited to males with panic disorder. Expected death rates for females with panic disorder from cardiovascular disease were normal.

Death by suicide is an event usually associated with depression. The fact that preliminary studies find an equal frequency in patients with anxiety and panic should alert clinicians to the necessity of becoming more familiar with these problems. Why would people who are anxious kill themselves? Coryell and colleagues (1986) speculate that patients diagnosed with anxiety disorders may subsequently develop major depression or alcoholism as a complication. It is possible that earlier studies overlooked the possibility of suicide in anxious patients because they noticed only the subsequent complication of alcoholism or depression. But if alcoholism or depression is a consequence of anxiety and panic, then the long road to suicide often begins with anxiety.

In her chapter, Weissman also presents the very latest data on the strong association between panic and depression. She reviews data from the ECA study demonstrating that the presence of major depression produces an 18.8-fold increased risk of panic disorder. Recent data from a study designed to look specifically at this issue reveal that 50 percent of a group of patients with a *DSM-III* depressive diagnosis presented with panic attacks (Benshoof, 1987). This seems representative of data from a number of studies. The now well-known study by Leckman and colleagues (1983) illustrated the strong relationship between major depression and panic in another way. This study demonstrated that relatives of probands with major depression plus panic disorder had higher rates of panic disorder and of major depression when compared to the relatives of other proband groups.

The consequence of substance abuse presents a more pressing problem. For example, Quitkin and associates (1972) reported in some detail on 10 patients with anxiety disorders who also suffered severe complications from drug and alcohol abuse. The important suggestion by Quitkin and colleagues was that patients presenting with substance abuse problems may well be self-medicating an anxiety disorder. While this was always a common clinical observation, a study appearing in 1979 by Mullaney and Trippett attracted new attention to this potentially severe complication. They discovered that 33 percent of 102 alcoholics also had severe, disabling agoraphobia and/or social phobia. In addition, another 35 percent had mild versions of the same phobias. Panic attacks played a prominent role in both conditions. Thus, over 60 percent of a large group of alcoholics admitted to an alcoholism treatment unit presented with identifiable anxiety disorders of varying severity in which panic attacks played a role. It is possible that any treatment program for these alcoholics may have to target anxiety to be successful as well as to prevent relapse.

Research suggests that a complex relationship exists among panic, anxiety, and substance abuse. Severe anxiety disorders may well precede substance abuse in many cases, and the use of alcohol or drugs may be utilized primarily for anxiolytic purposes by these patients. However, once addicted, the patient's use of alcohol (or drug) may have a deleterious effect on mood, creating a vicious cycle (Stockwell et al, 1984). For this reason, patients with anxiety disorders who are also alcoholic may present with more severe anxiety *because* of the use of alcohol. Thus, anxiety and panic self-medicated with alcohol (or drugs) result in an ever-increasing downward self-destructive spiral not only from the effects of alcohol (or drug) addiction, but also from the exacerbating effects of drugs on the anxiety itself. It may be this complication, along with the development of helplessness and depression, that leads to the increased risk of suicide in patients with anxiety and panic (Coryell et al, 1986).

The information presented above attests to the clinical significance of panic and panic disorder. The severity and pervasiveness of panic attacks and the strong association of panic with a number of common psychiatric disorders ensures that every clinician will have to develop the ability to recognize and deal with panic disorder and its consequences. But advances during the past several years in our study of panic have resulted in what may be a more important development. As the chapters comprising this section illustrate very clearly, the study of panic is resulting in an exciting integration of biological, psychological, and social approaches to mental illness.

In the first chapter, both biological and psychological models of panic are reviewed. But investigators and theorists are becoming increasingly aware that biological and psychological models alone are insufficient to explain the complexity of panic. This is leading to a growing rapprochement between biological and psychological investigators as each begins to realize the essential contribution of the other. Increasingly this means sharing methods, measures, and procedures in a coordinated attempt to discover new facts about panic disorder. And this collaboration is not limited to studies on the nature of panic. Recent developments in both pharmacological and cognitive-behavioral treatments of panic are posing new questions regarding the most efficient and effective integrated treatment approaches. While the answers to these questions are not yet in, the important thing is that they are being asked. Thus, while many investigators have long since speculated on the desirability of a biopsychosocial approach to mental illness, ongoing collaborative efforts in the study of panic disorder are leading the way.

The chapters in this section present the latest developments in our knowledge of panic disorder from a number of perspectives. In Chapter 1, Dr. Barlow presents a brief overview of current models of panic, both biological and psychological. The chapter concludes with an outline of a new theory of panic that attempts to integrate biological and psychological approaches.

Chapter 2, by Drs. Shear and Fyer, selectively reviews the most important research findings from both biological and psychological approaches on the nature of panic. Many of these findings emerge from a new generation of studies provoking panic in the laboratory using either biological or psychological procedures. It is in this area in particular that a psychobiological approach seems to be increasingly necessary. It will also be interesting to the reader to compare some of the recent biological and psychopathological findings in panic disorder with recent findings in unipolar depression reviewed in the second section.

In Chapter 3, Dr. Weissman presents a succinct and current review of the epidemiology of panic disorder and agoraphobia. Some of the very surprising highlights from this review have already been mentioned.

Chapters 4, 5, and 6 examine the current status of our assessment and treatment techniques for panic disorder. In Chapter 4, Drs. Jacob and Turner review the revisions to *DSM-III* definitions of panic disorder and their implications for the clinician in regard to diagnosis and assessment. Particularly important in this section is a practical guide to help the clinician to differentiate those organic conditions which resemble panic disorder from actual panic disorder.

Perhaps no area has progressed as quickly during the past two years as the treatment of panic disorder. In Chapter 5, Drs. Fyer and Sandberg review the latest developments in pharmacological treatments and describe the panoply of new drugs which seem effective for panic disorder. In addition to suggesting a specific medical workup prior to pharmacological treatment, Fyer and Sandberg make useful recommendations on the advantages and disadvantages of the variety of drugs now available for treating panic. This information, along with practical advice on implementing treatment and dealing with various problems that arise during therapy, will make this chapter very useful for all clinicians prescribing drugs for panic.

Finally, Chapter 6, by Dr. Craske, describes the newest developments in cognitive-behavioral treatments for panic. Preliminary evidence reviewed in this chapter indicates that we now have a reliable, nondrug alternative for the treatment of panic disorder, although further corroborating evidence is required. What is particularly interesting about this new treatment approach is that it focuses directly on panic attacks. Thus, it is unlike in-vivo exposure-based treatments that many clinicians associate with behavior therapy for agoraphobia. Craske also presents useful information on how clinicians can implement this rather straightforward treatment in their offices.

It will also be interesting for the clinician to compare the latest developments in pharmacological and psychosocial treatments for panic with similar developments in depressive disorders described in Section 2 of this volume. In addition, Drs. Beck and Greenberg present another variation of the psychosocial treatment of panic disorder in their chapter in Section 5, which describes cognitive therapy for panic disorder. Procedurally, this approach is very similar to the treatment approach presented by Craske, although there are distinct conceptual and strategic differences. Reading both of these chapters will enable the clinician to begin to pick and choose among nondrug strategies now available for treating panic, much as he or she can now pick and choose among various pharmacological agents. These choices will often depend on clinical considerations and individual preferences.

In the meantime, clinical research should continue to advance very quickly in identifying the important mechanisms of action in all treatments, drug and nondrug. This will lead to yet more powerful integrated treatments for panic disorder than are now available.

REFERENCES

American Psychiatric Association: Diagnostic and Statistical Manual of Mental Disorders, Third Edition, Revised (DSM-III-R). Washington, DC, American Psychiatric Association, 1987

Benshoof BG: A comparison of anxiety and depressive symptomatology in the anxiety and affective disorders. Unpublished doctoral dissertation. State University of New York at Albany, 1987

Coryell W, Noyes R, Clancy J: Excess mortality in panic disorder: a comparison with primary unipolar depression. Arch Gen Psychiatry 1982; 39:701-703

Coryell W, Noyes R, House JD: Mortality among outpatients with anxiety disorders. Am J Psychiatry 1986; 143:508-510

Leckman JF, Weissman MM, Merikangas KR, et al: Panic disorder and major depression. Arch Gen Psychiatry 1983; 40:1055-1060

Mullaney JA, Trippett CJ: Alcohol dependence and phobias: clinical description and relevance. Br J Psychiatry 1979; 135:565-573

Norton RG, Dorward J, Cox BJ: Factors associated with panic attacks in non-clinical subjects. Behavior Therapy 1986; 17:239-252

Quitkin FM, Rifkin A, Kaplan J, et al: Phobic anxiety syndrome complicated by drug dependence and addiction. Arch Gen Psychiatry 1972; 27:159-162

Stockwell R, Smail P, Hodgson R, et al: Alcohol dependence and phobic anxiety states, II: a retrospective study. Br J Psychiatry 1984; 144:58-63

Wittchen HU: Epidemiology of panic attacks and panic disorders, in Panic and Phobias. Edited by Hand I, Wittchen HU. Berlin, Springer Verlag, 1986

Chapter 1

Current Models of Panic Disorder and a View from Emotion Theory

by David H. Barlow, Ph.D.

The study of panic is in its infancy. Therefore, it is not surprising that current models of panic disorder tend to be one-dimensional. One-dimensional models attempt to account for all of the symptoms of panic disorder, both physiological and psychological, as a function of one process or operation. The cause of panic disorder is then conceptualized in a linear fashion. That is, a process, whether it is biological, cognitive, developmental, or related to conditioning, occurs and this process alone is directly linked to panic attacks and panic disorder.

The development of knowledge in any field often begins with relatively simplistic one-dimensional models before moving on to more complex multidetermined causal sequences. These multidetermined theories usually take on the structure of a system characterized by feedback loops. But these more sophisticated inter-actionist models often emerge out of grains of truth contained in the variety of one-dimensional linear models.

A number of diverse one-dimensional models of panic and panic disorder have appeared in the past several years. The purpose of this chapter will be to review briefly these models. This will be followed by an outline of a more complex and systemic theory of panic and panic disorder currently in construction, which is derived from the rich heritage of emotion theory.

ONE-DIMENSIONAL MODELS OF PANIC

Biological

Models of panic based on biological dysregulation have received by far the greatest amount of experimental attention to date. Most biological models of panic point to random biological dysregulation resulting in eruptions that we call panic. In these causal models the neurobiological eruption can account for all of the symptoms of panic, both physiological and psychological. In this way, panic is a unique event and can be distinguished from generalized anxiety.

It would seem logical that a biological dysregulation underlies panic. After all, the very nature of panic as it presents in panic disorder specifies that there is no readily identifiable antecedent or cue. For this reason, investigators have attempted to identify a biological marker in patients with panic disorder that would be associated with an underlying biological dysregulation, or at least point in the direction of a biological dysregulation. Speculations on the source of these disruptions range far and wide across a variety of central and peripheral mechanisms.

As this research advances, we are learning a great deal more about the neurobiological basis of anxiety and panic (Wambolt and Insel, in press; Ballenger, 1986). This research and the leading biological models of panic are reviewed by Drs. Shear and Fyer in Chapter 2. Among the many current possibilities mentioned are deficiencies in Alpha 2 receptors, which would tend to cause disruptions in central noradrenergic function; abnormalities in the locus coeruleus, with a resulting dysregulation of the modulation of sensory input; or, most recently, heightened central CO_2 sensitivity which would make individuals susceptible to rapid breathing and feelings of suffocation (Fyer et al, 1986; Woods et al, 1986).

However, biological researchers as of now have been unable to come up with any specific biological marker or, for that matter, any important neurobiological differences, between patients with panic disorder and patients with other anxiety disorders, as noted by Shear and Fyer. Even if a biological dysregulation is discovered, it will be difficult to determine whether this is a cause or effect of the disorder. For example, the fascinating finding of abnormalities in the symmetry of parahippocampal blood flow in some panic patients (Reiman et al, 1986) might be the result of another process associated with panic attacks such as hyperventilation (Turner et al, in press). Alternatively, as suggested by Reiman and colleagues (1986), it might be a reversible marker of anticipatory anxiety.

In fact, one finding consistently appearing in panic disorder is chronic overarousal, which seems a biological marker of sorts. However, chronic overarousal and its as yet undiscovered biological underpinnings characterize almost all anxiety disorders and would not qualify as a specific biological marker for panic. However, it may interact with other variables and contribute to the genesis of panic disorder.

For these and other reasons, many leading neurobiological researchers are eschewing one-dimensional biological models of panic in favor of more complex interactionist models (for example, Liebowitz, 1986). Nevertheless, the evidence is very strong that neurobiological processes play an important role in panic disorder.

Cognitive

An alternative one-dimensional model beginning to receive increased attention is the cognitive model of panic. These developing models are based on the creative theorizing and important clinical innovation of Aaron T. Beck (Beck and Emery, 1985). In its simplest form, this model assumes that the sharp spiral into panic is due to catastrophic misinterpretations of otherwise normal bodily sensations. Implicit in this theorizing is the notion that nothing particularly unique is occurring in the individual from a neurobiological perspective. For example, mild chest pain experienced after certain types of exercise might be interpreted in a vulnerable individual as an impending heart attack. Individuals who develop panic disorder would differ from those who don't only in their tendencies to misinterpret somatic events in a variety of ways. Thus, panic would be considered, by and large, to be a severe form of generalized anxiety. Research findings from this approach are also highlighted in Chapter 2, by Drs. Shear and Fyer.

Most recently, sophisticated investigators examining cognitive aspects of panic (Clark, 1986; Rapee, in press; Salkovskis, in press) have suggested that biological disruptions may play a role in some panic attacks. For example, they theorize that there are individual differences in respiratory response to stress. That is, in certain stressful situations, vulnerable individuals will overbreathe, resulting in a hyperventilatory episode. Hyperventilation will then produce a variety of physical sensations. In some individuals, these sensations will be misinterpreted in a catastrophic fashion. The consequence is panic. The cause of panic, then, is not seen as a hyperventilatory episode, but rather the catastrophic misinterpretation of symptoms produced by hyperventilation. As these authors themselves acknowledge, there are many pathways to panic (Barlow, 1986; Barlow, in press), and the evidence suggests that hyperventilation does not seem in any way a necessary or sufficient condition for the occurrence of panic (Gelder, 1986; Barlow, **in press**). Thus, we are left with the need to specify other minor physical disruptions or "normal" disturbances to homeostasis that are misinterpreted. This theorizing begins to move away from a one-dimensional cognitive model of panic, but the burden is still placed squarely on cognitive distortion.

Conditioning

Conditioning models of fear acquisition have changed considerably since they were introduced several decades ago. Thus, in order to comprehend a conditioning model of panic disorder, it will be necessary to review briefly contemporary conditioning models of phobia. Nevertheless, we will conclude that conditioning models, in isolation, remain one-dimensional.

For years investigators have searched the histories of phobic individuals for signs of traumatic conditioning. The primary finding is that most phobics cannot recall a traumatic conditioning event to account for the development of their fear or phobia. It is also clear that many fears and some phobias are acquired vicariously by observing someone else who is very fearful (Murray and Foote, 1979; Rimm et al, 1977). More recent information suggests that panic attacks may play a major role.

For example, McNally and Steketee (1985) interviewed 22 outpatients presenting for treatment with animal phobias. When questioned about etiology, most (15) of these patients could not remember what happened. Of the remaining seven cases, five did report a frightening encounter with an animal which might have resulted in a traumatic conditioning process. Two seemed to acquire their fear through instructional or vicarious modes. That is, they reported that a fearful parent had warned them early and often about the supposed danger of the small animal. Nevertheless, what they all dreaded now was not attack by the animal, which they had long since realized was harmless. Rather, they were afraid of uncontrollable panic and the consequence of panic following an unavoidable encounter with the animal.

Munjack (1984), in a very interesting retrospective analysis, questioned a more common type of a simple phobic about the etiology of their fear, the fear of driving. Of his 30 patients, a few (30 percent) reported some traumatic incident, such as a collision, while driving that seemed to lead to their fears. But almost one-half reported no such incident. Rather, they noted that suddenly, for no apparent reason, they "panicked" while driving and since then had been unable to drive on freeways. While these patients presented with a fear of driving, their anxiety, much as with McNally's and Steketee's patients, revolved around the possibility of having another panic attack in this very specific, limited situation. (Panic attacks did not occur in other situations.) Even in the remaining patients for whom the etiology was not clear, it seems possible that experiences similar to panic or "limited symptom attacks" might have played a role.

It is entirely possible then, that a few simple phobics experience fear or panic in response to a realistic threat to their well being, which then becomes associated with the same or similar objects or situations. Being attacked by a dog might be an example. But many simple phobics experience fear or panic for no reason. In other words, they experience a "false alarm." This panic attack or false alarm is of such intensity that learning also occurs. Specifically, false alarms are triggered by the object or situation associated with its initial onset. In this model, this association is an example of basic emotional learning (conditioned emotional response) rather than a cognitively mediated misinterpretation, although catastrophic misinterpretations would certainly be present if one searched for them. Thus, the individual would experience anxiety in the presence of the object or situation (or similar objects or situations) that were associated with the first panic attack or false alarm. But anxiety would occur primarily over the possibility of having another (unpredictable) false alarm in the presence of the cues that have become associated with this event.

The implications of this model for simple phobics are clear. An actual traumatic event, which could be characterized as a "true alarm" since real danger is present, would not be necessary. All that would be required would be a "false alarm" or unexpected panic attack in the presence of a previously benign object or situation. This would insure that anxiety and possibly another panic attack might occur the next time the object or situation were encountered.

Of course, this would not be a random event. For example, phobic development is more likely if the object or situation were "prepared" in an evolutionary sense (Ohman et al, 1985; Seligman, 1971). That is, we are more likely to develop fear of snakes than electrical outlets because the propensity to develop this fear served our ancestors well. Recent research has confirmed the importance of certain "prepared" stimuli in phobia acquisition compared to "unprepared" stimuli.

Another possible association hitherto overlooked may account for much of the nonrandom quality of phobic reactions. A common theme running through many phobic situations is the danger of being trapped. These themes are obvious in agoraphobia, in which fears of sitting far from the door in church or a movie theater, or feeling trapped in a crowded mall, are common (see below). One early name for agoraphobia—the "Barber's Chair Syndrome"—reflects the difficulty many of these individuals have with confinement to dentist, barber, or beautician chairs. Feeling "trapped" is also strongly present in phobias of driving, flying, or other forms of transportation, as well as in phobias of crossing bridges and so on. What all of these situations have in common is that the context prevents easy escape in the event of a panic attack or false alarm.

One possible explanation for this can be found in emotion theory, a topic to which we will turn later in this chapter. The purpose of intense fear is to mobilize the organism for instantaneous emergency action most usually characterized as fight or flight (Izard, 1977). Flight, or escape, in emotion theory is not a rational process but rather a compelling action tendency that has had obvious survival value down through the ages. But what if one experiences intense fear or panic in a situation where it is difficult or impossible to leave quickly? In that case, the overwhelmingly powerful ethologically ancient tendency to escape is thwarted.

At the very least this intensifies and prolongs the panic and therefore potentiates learning. This event may be crucial in "convincing" the organism not to let this happen again at any cost. And the cost is often high. For if emotions are fundamentally behavioral acts (Lang, 1985) anything that interferes with the execution of this most important of all emotional acts will have profound significance.

CONDITIONING AND PANIC DISORDER. But what of patients with panic disorder? The majority of these individuals are unable to report a clearly demarcated cue for their panics, such as small animals, airplanes, or public speaking, although agoraphobics often report a series of diffuse situations of which they are wary. Based on a conditioning model, it is possible that the major difference between agoraphobics and other phobics may be whether they have associated their panic attacks with a specific cue or not. What is learned in this case? Conditioning theorists point to an important but little known line of research conducted by Russian investigators.

For years, Russian investigators conducted a series of experiments demonstrating that fear could be conditioned to internal physiological stimuli which came to be known as "interoceptive" stimuli (Razran, 1961). To take one example which is typical of this line of research: The colon of a dog was slightly stimulated (conditioned stimulus) at the same time that an electric shock was administered to the dog. As a result of this conditioning procedure, the dog began to evidence signs of intense anxiety during the natural passage of feces. The Russians demonstrated that this type of learning was particularly resistant to extinction. That is, it would persist indefinitely despite repeated physiological sensations in the absence of the original unconditioned stimulus (shock).

The implication of this work is that it is possible to learn an association between internal cues and panic attacks or false alarms. Furthermore, these internal cues serve the same function for patients with panic disorder (with or without agoraphobia) that external cues do for simple phobics. That is, they signal the possibility of another panic attack.

The association of false alarms or panic attacks with internal or external cues results in what conditioning theorists might call a "learned alarm." Furthermore, a characteristic of any learned response is that it need not fully replicate its unlearned counterpart. For example, limited cues present in a given context might elicit only one part of the response or emotion (Lang, 1985). Thus, "learned alarms" may be only partial responses in many cases, such as cognitive representations without the marked physiological component. Physiologic monitoring of panic attacks supports the idea that panic can occur without physiologic accompaniments (Taylor et al, 1986; see Chapter 2 of this volume).

One clear consequence of this learning, in those individuals who go on to become phobic, is the rapid development of acute sensitivity and vigilance to newly acquired phobic cues. Someone recently bitten by a dog will quickly become acutely sensitive to any signs of dogs, and this vigilance will extend to unfamiliar areas where dogs might be roaming free. Someone experiencing a panic attack (or a false alarm) in an elevator will become acutely aware of any plans in the immediate future that might require entry into an elevator. And someone who has learned to associate interoceptive cues with panic attacks will become acutely sensitive to and vigilant of specific somatic cues associated with this alarm.

It is also interesting to consider, in this regard, the minority of patients with panic disorder who can clearly cite an unfavorable experience with drugs such as anesthesia or cocaine, or a first experience with marijuana as the setting event for their first panic (Aronson and Craig, 1986). Here, the "cause" in terms of a temporally associated event seems clear, and anesthesia and marijuana are avoided. However, a full panic disorder syndrome also develops, including marked sensitivity to a variety of somatic cues and repeated panic attacks in the absence of external cues. It is possible that this reflects a process of interoceptive conditioning.

Evidence that people presenting with panic disorder fear interoceptive cues is accumulating along several fronts (Rapee, 1986; van den Hout et al, 1987). This may account for the consistent clinical observation of the extreme sensitivity to somatic cues in panic patients. Data from studies provoking panic in the laboratory, as well as the interesting phenomenon of nocturnal panic, support this model (Barlow, in press; Barlow and Craske, in press). Of course, if one is "trapped" in a situation where no exit is possible while experiencing the full effects of the panic attack, then it is more likely that attention will be directed to this "trapped" situation that prevents the powerful tendency to escape (flight), as already noted.

As with biological and cognitive models, it seems likely that conditioning, particularly interoceptive conditioning, plays some role in the development of panic disorder. But conditioning, in isolation, is also a one-dimensional model that cannot begin to account for the complexity of panic disorder. For example, even in the rather oversimplified description just presented, it was necessary to introduce ethological concepts of emotion theory to account for some of the facts. Conditioning models cannot easily account for the observation that panic disorder strongly aggregates in families, without incorporating biologically based vulnerabilities to conditioning. Conditioning models also cannot account for the observation receiving increasing confirmation that many people experience occasional panic attacks, with only a few subsequently developing panic disorders (Norton et al, 1986; see below). Finally, conditioning models cannot easily account for the initial panic attack or false alarm. Thus, to the extent that conditioning models require all of the psychological and somatic symptoms of panic disorder to be caused by a traumatic conditioning experience surrounding the first panic attack, this is clearly a one-dimensional linear model.

Stress–Diathesis

A remarkably consistent observation of biological and psychological clinicians and investigators for a number of years has been the extremely high incidence of negative life events preceeding the first panic attack in patients later presenting with panic disorder. What makes this more interesting is that few of these patients can identify a precipitating event when asked a question such as, "What caused your first panic attack?" However, further systematic questioning about life events reveals that approximately 80 percent of these patients will describe very clearly a negative life event closely associated with their first panic (Buglass et al, 1977; Doctor, 1982; Finlay-Jones and Brown, 1981; Mathews et al, 1981; Roth, 1959; Snaith, 1968; Solyom et al, 1974; Uhde et al, 1985). For example, Shafar (1976) reported precipitating stressors in 83 percent of her sample, and Sheehan and colleagues (1981) reported precipitating stressors in 91 percent of their large sample.

Typical of these studies and the types of negative life events reported are results from an early series of 58 agoraphobics (53 females and 5 males) from our clinic (Last et al, 1984). The occurrence of negative life events was assessed by structured clinical interviews. Categories of life events and the frequencies with which they were reported are presented in Table 1.

Eighty-one percent of the 58 agoraphobics reported one or more of these stressful life events, while 19 percent reported no significant life event prior to the development of agoraphobia. For heuristic purposes, we collapsed life events reported by our patients into conflict events versus endocrine-physiological reactions. The results are presented in Table 2. These two major categories account

Table 1. Life Events Occurring Prior to Onset of Agoraphobia

Precipitating Events	Frequency*	%
Interpersonal conflict (marital/familial)	20	34.5
Birth/miscarriage/hysterectomy	17	29.3
Death/illness of significant other	9	15.5
Drug reaction	7	12.1
Major surgery/illness	2	3.4
Stress at work/school	2	3.4
Move	2	3.4
Total	58	

*Frequencies exceed the number of patients interviewed since many patients reported more than one significant life event occurring prior to their first panic attack.

Reprinted from Last CG, Barlow DH, O'Brien GT: Precipitants of agoraphobia: role of stressful life events. Psychological Reports 1984; 54:567-570. Copyright 1984 by Psychological Reports. Reprinted by permission.

Table 2. Conflict Events versus Endocrine/Physiological Reactions Occurring Prior to Onset of Agoraphobia

	Number	Frequency	%
Conflict Situations		29	50.0
Marital/familial	20		
Death/illness significant other	9		
Endocrine or Physiological Reactions		24	41.4
Birth/miscarriage/hysterectomy	17		
Drug reaction	7		
Total	53	58	

Reprinted from Last CG, Barlow DH, O'Brien GT: Precipitants of agoraphobia: role of stressful life events. Psychological Reports 1984; 54:567-570. Copyright 1984 by Psychological Reports. Reprinted by permission.

for approximately 91 percent of the life events reported. Liebowitz and Klein (1979) also reported a large proportion of individuals developing panic attacks after experiencing endocrinological changes, and Klein, in an early survey (1964) noted "endocrine fluctuations" such as those associated with birth, menopause, gynecological surgery, and so forth, as events immediately preceding panic in a subgroup of patients.

Perhaps the best study in this group was also one of the earliest. Roth (1959) found that 96 percent of a sample of 135 agoraphobics reported some type of background stress preceding the development of their disorder. The stressors of 83 percent of these patients were categorized as follows: bereavement or a suddenly developing serious illness in a close relative or friend (37 percent); illness or acute danger to the patient (31 percent); and severance of family ties or acute domestic stress (15 percent). In an additional 13 percent of the women, panic began during pregnancy or after childbirth, and was characterized by an abrupt onset shortly after delivery. What makes this study strong is that Roth was the only one to employ a control group. He found that the incidence of identifiable stressors in his agoraphobic patients was significantly greater than that found in 50 control patients suffering from some other form of "neurosis." The incidence was also greater than that in 50 additional individuals who had recently recovered from a physical illness but had never suffered a psychiatric disorder. More recently, Roy-Byrne and colleagues (1986) partially replicated those findings comparing panic disorder patients with healthy controls.

These data, consistent as they are, have led many to assume that stress plays a major role in the etiology of panic (Margraf et al, 1986; Mathews et al, 1981; Tearnan et al, in press). But what can we conclude from these intriguing observations? While the consistency of these observations attests to the reliability of reports of this relationship, one cannot escape the fact that these reports are retrospective.

It is also becoming increasingly apparent that stress, defined as negative life events, seems to be associated with the onset or exacerbation of any number of physical and psychological disorders. For example, relationships have been demonstrated between stress and cardiovascular disease, complications associated with pregnancy and birth, tuberculosis, multiple sclerosis, diabetes, arthritis, chronic back pain, and depression to name only a few (Depue, 1979; Flor et al, 1985; Hammen et al, 1986; Lewinsohn et al, in press; Lloyd, 1980).

The most common explanation for the effects of stress is the well-known stress–diathesis model, wherein stress precipitates and facilitates a particular physical or emotional disorder to which the individual is already predisposed. In the case of psychophysiological stress responses such as hypertension, ulcers, and so on, the "weak organ" model best expresses this hypothesis. Essentially (and simplistically) the effects of stress overactivate one's (physiological) system until the weakest part of the system breaks down. This weakness might be constitutional or a result of earlier traumatic processes (Selye, 1976).

Within psychological disorders, such as panic disorder, this hypothetical process is a little less clear. Nevertheless, it is possible that a number of individuals are "prone" to panic attacks or false alarms during periods of stress, just as others are vulnerable to other types of disorders such as headaches or ulcers.

But a common finding across all disorders studied is that even acute stress, usually defined as a negative life event, correlates only modestly with psychopathology. That is, while there may be a clear association, as it certainly seems there is with panic, a large number of people even if "prone" to a disorder experience similar life events without developing panic or some alternatie disorder. Usually it is assumed that moderating variables such as certain cognitive and personality traits, as well as social support, diminish the effects of stress (Depue and Monroe, 1986; Sarason and Sarason, 1981).

Thus, a variety of evidence supporting a stress–diathesis model of panic suggests that certain individuals are susceptible to stress produced by negative life events. This vulnerability may be due to neurobiological factors, relatively low social support, and/or some combination of personality and cognitive dispositions. These individuals then react to negative life events in much the same way as they might react to physical threats from wild animals or snakes. That is, they evince a basic fear or panic response much as they would when confronted with any other threat to their well-being. Because the panic is not temporally associated within hours with the negative life event, the individual is unable to specify an antecedent to the fear, or a "cause." Indeed there is no antecedent which would require an immediate "alarm" reaction with all of its associated action tendencies of fight or flight. For that reason the alarm is false.

Although this is the stress–diathesis model, it is unlikely in the extreme that there is a direct link between a specific stressful event and panic. Rather, the initial panic is most likely mediated by biological and/or cognitive variables such as stress-related noradrenergic or serontonergic activity or information processing mechanisms. In this way, initial panic attacks may "spike off" a stress reaction in vulnerable individuals.

Separation Anxiety

Separation anxiety has occupied a prominent place in many theories of child development and psychopathology. Based on early clinical observations, some investigators (for example, Klein and Fink, 1962) suggested that panic attacks seen in agoraphobic patients may well be a "mature" expression of the type of distress and panic some children evince upon separation from their mothers. Rachel Gittelman has written most extensively on this topic and has pulled together a variety of evidence both affirming and denying the relationship of separation anxiety to the development of panic disorder and agoraphobia (Gittelman and Klein, 1985). Generally, there are three lines of evidence supporting this relationship: similarity of drug treatment effects for separation anxiety and adult agoraphobia; family concordance for separation anxiety and agoraphobia; and history of childhood separation anxiety in agoraphobic adults.

Gittelman and Klein (1973) treated 44 severely school-phobic children with imipramine and found that, when compared to placebo, most of the children reported feeling generally much better, had fewer complaints on schooldays, and experienced less distress at separation as reported by the mothers. Since studies indicate that imipramine is effective for panic disorder, the possibility exists that panic and separation anxiety may be similar.

Weissman and colleagues (1984) in a very strong study, examined the family concordance of separation anxiety and adult anxiety. They determined the prevalence of separation anxiety in the 6- to 18-year-old children of depressed and normal adults identified in community surveys. These adult patients, diagnosed by direct structured clinical interview, were classified into four groups: 1) depressed with no anxiety disorder; 2) depressed with agoraphobia; 3) depressed with panic disorder; and 4) depressed with generalized anxiety disorder at any time in their adult life. Separation anxiety was diagnosed in 24 percent of the children whose parents had a diagnosis of both depression and agoraphobia or panic. In contrast, none of the children of adults with pure depression, and only six percent of the children of parents with depression and generalized anxiety disorder, reported separation anxiety. This suggests a connection between separation anxiety and panic with or without agoraphobic avoidance.

Finally, in some recently analyzed data, Gittelman and Klein (1985) report on the incidence of separation anxiety in agoraphobic adults. These data were collected from clinical interviews with adult agoraphobics who were asked to recall separation anxiety in their childhood. This method, of course, suffers the weaknesses of any retrospective study. But it is one of the few studies of its type to employ a control group, in this case simple phobics. In both childhood and adolescence (the periods examined) agoraphobic patients recalled significantly more separation anxiety than the comparison group of patients with simple phobia who were also asked about these recollections. Intriguingly, this group difference was due entirely to a high prevalence of separation anxiety disorder in female agoraphobics. No differences were found between male agoraphobics and simple phobics.

Unfortunately for the theory, considerable evidence exists contradicting these positive results. For example, Thyer and colleagues (1986) administered carefully structured questionnaires to 23 panic disorder patients and 28 small-animal phobics and found essentially no differences in reports of childhood separation anxiety. This group, (Thyer et al, 1985) also found a lack of differences when examining agoraphobics compared to simple phobics. Other studies have also failed to find an increased incidence of reports of separation anxiety during the childhood of agoraphobics (Buglass et al, 1977; Parker, 1979). Examining it from another direction, no association has been found between forced childhood separations due to illnesses or other family circumstances and the later development of anxiety and depression (Tennant et al, 1982). Similarly, Gittelman-Klein (1975) failed to find any incidence of agoraphobia or panic disorder in the parents of 45 school-phobic children.

It is very difficult to establish strong evidence for this model without time-consuming and costly prospective studies. Nevertheless, the preliminary postive findings are intriguing. But even those favoring this model are suggesting only a correlation between separation anxiety and adult panic attacks. Both separation anxiety and panic attacks, if this relationship is established, might be due to more fundamental biological and/or psychological processes.

A Psychoanalytic Model

A consideration of separation anxiety turns our attention to the potential importance of early childhood experiences in the development of panic disorder. Psychoanalytic theory delves deeply into this overlooked but potentially important area. Indeed real or symbolic experiences of separation anxiety may be one trigger for adult panic attacks in the context of modern psychoanalytic theory.

It is also clear that Freud recognized and clearly described panic attacks, which he referred to as anxiety attacks. Freud also noted on several occasions that the maintenance of phobic behavior may well be due, in large part, to fear of having another anxiety attack, although he did not suppose that these attacks were crucial in every case. The emphasis in modern psychoanalytic thinking is on conscious or unconscious mental triggers to anxiety and anxiety attacks. The triggers are seen as symbolically related to infantile wishes and/or fears. Specifically, adult panic would be conceived as a response to cues that have been learned or associated with earlier fundamental innate psychological and biological threats to the organism. Thus, mental imagery involving symbolic representations of very frightening early themes such as castration, separation, or parental disapproval may be sufficient to trigger panic attacks.

For psychoanalytic theory, then, the cause of anxiety (and anxiety attacks) lies clearly in early developmental experiences. Specifically, an inability to control unconscious fantasies linked to infantile fears through adaptive defenses may be influential in the later appearance of adult panic (Freud, 1959). As we shall now see, themes of uncontrollability and helplessness are assuming increasing importance in theories of anxiety and panic from a number of different perspectives.

A VIEW FROM EMOTION THEORY

It is possible to integrate these models in a manner that recognizes the important contribution made by each. In this approach, developed at length elsewhere (Barlow, in press), one cannot understand panic without understanding the nature of anxiety and fear. In turn, one cannot understand anxiety and fear without referring to the accumulated wisdom of emotion theory. For panic and anxiety are primarily emotions. In their pathological expressions they become emotional disorders.

Anxiety

Emotion theorists generally agree that fear and anxiety refer to different phenomena. But these differences are not necessarily subsumed under the usual distinction of presence or absence of cue or stimuli. That is, anxiety is not simply fear without a cue. Almost all emotion theorists consider anxiety a loose association or blend of different emotional and cognitive processes. In the parlance this is sometimes called a cognitive-affective structure. Theorists as diverse as Izard (1977), Lang (1985), and Hallam (1985) consider anxiety (and depression) to be a pervasive, diffuse state that may represent either a blend of basic emotions (Izard, 1977) or a rather loose, widespread affective network stored in memory (Lang, 1985). The construct of anxiety may also have multiple referents. That is, the types of somatic, behavioral, or subjective experiences that are labeled "anxiety" may differ somewhat. In other words, what one individual construes as anxiety may refer to somewhat different sensations or experiences from what another individual construes as anxiety (Hallam, 1985).

In our view (Barlow, in press), this loose cognitive-affective structure is characterized by a variety of cognitive and behavioral operations not generally considered to be strictly within the purview of the study of emotion. These operations can be organized in a negative feedback cycle so that once initiated, it can become an intensifying process.

The primary ingredients of anxiety are high negative affect and an accompanying sense that both internal and external events are proceeding in an unpredictable, uncontrollable fashion. This sense of "uncontrollability" also seems to be accompanied by a shift in the focus of one's attention. Most usually attention shifts away from the task at hand to an internal, self-evaluative mode. This is partly responsible for difficulties in concentrating associated with anxiety. Specifically, attention is directed at the negative affect itself and its associated arousal and generally unpleasant characteristics. This results in self-preoccupation and worry and a further intensification of anxiety. Typically the process of anxiety begins after a disruption or interruption of ongoing behavior as might be occasioned by a stressful or negative life event.

Anxiety, then, may be best characterized as apprehension surrounding anticipation of uncontrollable, unpleasant, or dangerous events in the future: "That terrible event could happen again and I might not be able to deal with it." For this reason, the term anxious apprehension might refer more precisely to this diffuse future-oriented mood state. Anxiety also implies an effort to cope with difficult situations: "I've got to be ready to try and deal with it," and the physiology (arousal) is there to support active attempts at coping. The difficulty is that the sense of uncontrollability and unpredictability, which is a major part of anxiety, requires continued vigilance or preparation, resulting in chronic arousal.

Fear

If anxiety is a clinical manifestation of a diffuse cognitive-affective structure spanning a variety of emotional, cognitive, and behavioral operations, then what is fear? Most emotion theorists consider fear as a tightly organized focal, intense experience that may represent a very tightly organized, cohesive affective structure (Lang, 1985) or perhaps a distinct, primitive, basic emotion (Izard, 1977). Indeed, many emotion theorists consider fear to be a primary alarm in response to present danger characterized by high negative affect and arousal. There is general agreement that fear occurs when we are directly threatened with a dangerous, perhaps life threatening, event. An impending attack from wild animals is something few of us experience today, but our ancestors knew this threat well in centuries past. This may account for our somewhat greater susceptibility to becoming "alarmed" in the presence of snakes, mountain lions, and the like, than more modern-day threats as noted above (Cook et al, 1986; Seligman, 1971).

Relevant threats today include speeding vehicles, guns, drowning, seeing the safety of our children threatened, and so on. Under these conditions the emotion of fear mobilizes us physically and cognitively for quick action and sometimes "superhuman" efforts. Most typically, running or struggling are behavioral manifestations of fear. Occasionally, directed action to counter the threat is apparent, such as attacking a predator or single-handedly lifting an automobile so that a child trapped underneath can escape. We have already suggested that this response represents Cannon's emergency reaction characterized by the compelling action tendencies of "fight or flight." Sometimes these actions are counterproductive, as in the drowning victim vainly struggling when the rational response would be to lie still and attempt to float. This action tendency is experienced by most people as the undeniably overwhelming urge to "get out" of the situation as described above. There is no mistaking fear for other basic emotions such as sadness. Evidence exists suggesting that the basic emotion of fear is found invariantly across cultures, races, and species, and far down the phylogenetic scale (Izard, 1977).

Creative theorists such as Beck (Beck and Emery, 1985) have long insisted on considering the functional significance of the evolutionary purpose of behavior in general and emotions in particular. This has not been difficult to do with fear. To almost all observers, beginning with Darwin (1872), the alarm of fear has been responsible in large part for the survival of the species. Those individual organisms capable of becoming quickly alarmed, with the accompanying mobilization of the body for fight or flight, survived and won the day when those not so inclined perished. Based on this point of view, then, fear is an ancient, probably hard-wired alarm system enabling the organism to respond to emergencies (Cannon, 1929). But what is the clinical manifestation of fear? In our view, fear is panic and panic is the unadulterated, ancient, hard-wired alarm system we call fear.

When confronted with an immediate threat to our well-being, which, quite fortunately, is experienced very seldom these days, we share this reaction with our ancestors who lived in caves. It has been demonstrated again and again that our physical capacities to perform necessary actions are greatly enhanced during fear when our objective is clear. Our objective, of course, is fight or flight. But what if there is no objective? No cue? No threat? Under these circumstances, the same reaction can be considered a false alarm.

A THEORY OF PANIC

It is now possible to consider how some of these models might be integrated into a larger theory. But first there are several additional issues that seem important. One fascinating issue concerns who develops clinical disorders associated with panic attacks and who doesn't.

Now we have learned that panic attacks may be far more prevalent in the general population than we assumed. In fact, studies from around the world are converging to suggest that occasional panic attacks occur relatively frequently in the general population. The first study to suggest this was reported by Norton and colleagues (1985), who administered questionnaires to 186 presumably normal young adults. Of these subjects, 34.4 percent reported having had one or more panic attacks in the past year. The percentage reporting more frequent attacks during the past year decreased markedly. For example, of the original 34.4 percent, 17.2 percent reported two or more attacks in the past year; 11.3 percent reported 3 to 4 panic attacks; while 6 percent reported 5 or more attacks in the past year. In the past 3 weeks, 17.2 percent reported experiencing one panic attack, while 4.8 percent, or 9 subjects, reported 2 panic attacks; and only 4 subjects (2.1 percent) reported experiencing 3 or more panic attacks in the past past 3 weeks, a frequency that would meet *Diagnostic and Statistical Manual of Mental Disorders, Third Edition (DSM-III)* (American Psychiatric Association, 1980) criteria for panic disorder. In addition, 4 subjects, or 2.1 percent, reported avoiding some activities or situations because of panic attacks.

One interesting facet of these data is that the number reporting panic attacks that would meet clinical criteria is very close and even slightly less than what we might expect based on recent epidemiological investigations (Myers et al, 1984). This fact, as well as subsequent replication, lends credence to these data.

These infrequent panickers also reported significantly greater depression, anxiety, and phobic anxiety on the well-known and often-used Hopkins Symptom Checklist–90 (HSCL–90) (Deragotis et al, 1973) than those who had never panicked.

While assessment of the presence or absence of panic attacks by questionnaire can be justifiably criticized, more careful assessment by structured interview of 24 of these nonclinical subjects who reported panic revealed that 22 met DSM-III criteria for panic attacks. The remaining two subjects actually reported experiencing intense nonpanic anxiety (Harrison, 1985). This finding also supports the validity of these data.

In a cross-validation study reported by Norton and colleagues (1986), 256 subjects completed a variety of questionnaires, including a more sophisticated questionnaire than was utilized in the first study. This questionnaire assessed not only the presence or absence of panic attacks, but severity, temporal factors associated with the attacks, situations associated with the attacks, whether the attacks were predictable or unpredictable, and so on. Once again, panickers scored significantly higher than nonpanickers on general anxiety and depression as measured by a number of scales such as the State Trait Anxiety Inventory, the Beck Depression Inventory, as well as anxiety and depression subscales of the Profile of Mood States (POMS). Closely replicating the first study, 35.9 percent, or 92 subjects, reported experiencing one or more panic attacks in the past year, with 22.7 percent experiencing a panic attack within the past 3 weeks.

Another factor that builds confidence in the validity of these findings is data on the aggregation of panic and other psychopathology in the families of nonclinical infrequent panickers. For example, Norton and associates (1986) found that a significantly greater proportion of panickers than nonpanickers reported fathers, mothers, brothers, and sisters who had had panic attacks. These findings are particularly strong since the results were statistically significant for each class of relatives, rather than just in the aggregate. These data resemble results demonstrating a high familial aggregation of panic in the families of patients. For example, Crowe and colleagues (1983) found that 25 percent of first-order relatives of panic disorder patients also met DSM-III criteria for panic disorder. An additional 30 percent experienced infrequent panic attacks. In Norton and colleagues (1986), approximately 30 percent of first-order relatives were reported to experience panic. The data from Crowe and associates also attest to the seeming high prevalence of panic in the population at large.

Similar data on the prevalence of panic attacks in the normal population have recently been reported from Great Britain (G.L. Klerman, personal communication, 1985). Wittchen (1986) also reported a high rate of panic in the general population in Germany, albeit substantially lower than Norton and colleagues (1986) reported. Specifically, over nine percent of a random sample reported having experienced panic, a figure three times higher than the percentage of individuals eventually qualifying for a DSM-III diagnosis of panic disorder or agoraphobia with panic. There were many differences between these studies which could account for discrepancies. But Wittchen also concludes that the frequency of panic in the general population is much higher than one would expect.

It is possible, of course, particularly among those who were experiencing more frequent panics, that these would develop further in intensity and frequency to the point where a full-blown panic disorder would develop. However, another possibility is that they simply did not "fear" these alarms or, more accurately, they were not apprehensively anxious about them. What could account for this? Perhaps the alarms simply were not of sufficient intensity to elicit a negative affective response. But, another more likely possibility is that people who develop full-blown panic or phobic disorders are specifically susceptible to this type of learning due to individual biological vulnerabilities, or psychological factors, or a combination of the two. Among these factors could be baseline levels of arousal, perceptions of unpredictability and uncontrollability of the panic attack or other negative events, poor coping skills, lack of social support, and so on. In other words, if this panic or "false alarm" causes anxiety with its associated perceptions of unpredictability, uncontrollability, increased arousal surrounding the panic, and a shift of attention to internal self-evaluative modes, then it is possible that the conditions will be ripe for the development of an emotional disorder. If, on the other hand, one does not experience unpredictability or loss of control from this event, one might, as a consequence, attribute it to predictable events of the moment ("something I ate," "a fight with my boss"). In this case, one would not experience an internal self-evaluative shift in attention, and the false alarm would be just that. Life would then go on as before with perhaps an occasional rather mild false alarm reappearing from time to time under stressful conditions.

In other words, to develop panic disorder, one must be susceptible to developing anxiety or apprehension over the possibility of subsequent alarms or other negative events. Thus, the importance of anxiety mentioned above becomes apparent. The development of anxiety, in turn, depends upon specific vulnerabilities that are based on both neurobiological variables and specific early learning experiences (Barlow, in press; Mineka, 1985). Neurobiological variables would account for the familial aggregation of panic disorder. But early learning experiences are particularly crucial, based on recent evidence, just as psychoanalytic theory predicts (Insel et al, 1986; Mineka, Gunnar, Champoux, in press).

Specifically, if one develops a sense of control over one's world, including one's inner emotions, even if this sense is illusory, one will be less susceptible to developing anxiety over negative events such as panic attacks in later years. The vulnerability to perceive events as uncontrollable is based firmly in early behavioral experience. It is at this point, then, that separation experiences as well as other early experiences might contribute to the development of panic disorder. The loss of control inherent in early separation experiences may be one of the most significant contributions to anxiety proneness. Later cognitive distortions (catastrophic misinterpretations) are simply a reflection of these early experiences.

In panic disorder, then, the basic problem is anxiety or distress over the possibility of experiencing another hard-wired emotional response that is construed as being unpredictable or uncontrollable. A diagram of this model is presented in Figure 1.

REFERENCES

American Psychiatric Association: Diagnostic and Statistical Manual of Mental Disorders, Third Edition. Washington, DC, American Psychiatric Association, 1980

Aronson TA, Craig TJ: Cocaine precipitation of panic disorder. Am J Psychiatry 1986; 143:643-645

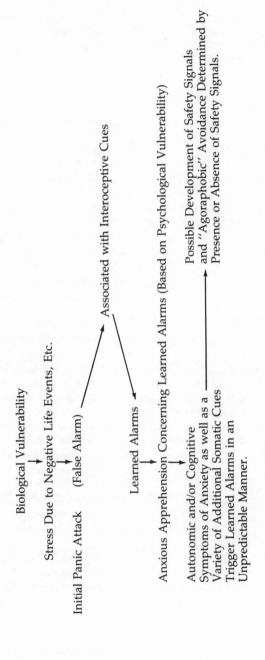

Figure 1. A model of panic disorder

Ballenger JC: Biological aspects of panic disorder. Am J Psychiatry 1986; 143:516-518

Barlow DH: The dimensions of anxiety disorders, in Anxiety and the Anxiety Disorders. Edited by Tuma GH, Maser JD. Hillsdale, NJ, Lawrence Erlbaum Associates, 1985

Barlow DH: In defense of panic disorder with extensive avoidance and the behavioral treatment of panic: a comment on Kleiner. Behavior Therapist 1986; 5:99-100

Barlow DH: Panic, Anxiety and the Anxiety Disorders. New York, Guilford Press (in press)

Barlow DH, Craske MG: The phenomenology of panic, in Panic: Psychological Perspectives. Edited by Rachman S, Maser JD. Hillsdale, NJ, Lawrence Erlbaum Associates (in press)

Beck AT, Emery G: Anxiety Disorders and Phobias: A Cognitive Perspective. New York, Basic Books, 1985

Buglass P, Clarke J, Henderson AS, et al: A study of agoraphobic housewives. Psychol Med 1977; 7:73-86

Cannon W: Bodily Changes in Pain, Hunger, Fear and Rage. New York, Appleton, 1929

Clark DM: A cognitive approach to panic. Behav Res Ther 1986; 24:461-470

Cook EW III, Hodges RL, Lang PJ: Preparedness and phobia: effects of stimulus content on human visceral conditioning. J Abnorm Psychol 1986; 95:195-207

Crowe RR, Noyes R, Pauls DL, et al: A family study of panic disorder. Arch Gen Psychiatry 1983; 40:1065-1069

Darwin CR: The expression of emotions in man and animals. London, Murray, 1872

Depue RA: The Psychobiology of the Depressive Disorders: Implications for the Effects of Stress. New York, Academic Press, 1979

Depue RA, Monroe SM: Conceptualizations and measurement of human disorder in life stress research: the problem of chronic disturbance. Psychol Bull 1986; 99:36-51

Deragotis LR, Lipman RS, Covi L: SCL-90: an outpatient psychiatric rating scale preliminary report. Psychopharmacol Bull 1973; 9:13-25

Doctor RM: Major results of large-scale pretreatment survey of agoraphobics, in Phobia: a Comprehensive Summary of Modern Treatments. Edited by DuPont RL. New York, Brunner/Mazel, 1982

Finlay-Jones R, Brown GW: Types of stressful life events and the onset of anxiety and depressive disorder. Psychol Med 1981; 11:801-815

Flor H, Turk DC, Birbaumer N: Assessment of stress-related psychophysiological reactions in chronic back pain patients. J Consult Clin Psychol 1985; 53:354-364

Freud S: Inhibition, symptoms, and anxiety (1926), in Complete Psychological Works, Standard Edition, vol 20. London, Hogarth Press, 1959

Fyer MR, UY J, Martiney J, et al: Carbon dioxide challenge of patients with panic disorder. Paper presented at the 139th Annual Meeting of the Amerian Psychiatric Association. Washington, DC, May 1986

Gelder MG: Panic attacks: new approaches to an old problem. Br J Psychiatry 1986; 149:346-352

Gittelman R, Klein DF: School phobia: diagnostic considerations in the light of imipramine effects. J Nerv Ment Dis 1973; 156:199-215

Gittelman R, Klein DF: Childhood separation anxiety and adult agoraphobia, in Anxiety and the Anxiety Disorders. Edited by Tuma AH, Maser JD. Hillsdale NJ, Lawrence Erlbaum Associates, 1985

Gittelman-Klein R: Psychiatric characteristics of the relatives of school phobic children, in Mental Health in Children, vol 1. Edited by Siva-Sankar PV. New York, PJD Publications, 1975

Hallam RS: Anxiety: psychological perspectives on panic and agoraphobia. New York, Academic Press, 1985

Hammen C, Mayol A, deMayo R, et al: Initial symptom levels and the life-event-depression relationship. J Abnorm Psychol 1986; 95:111-114

Harrison BJ: Anxiety provoked ideation in phobic and nonphobic panickers. Bachelor of Arts (honors) thesis. Winnipeg, University of Winnipeg, 1985

Insel TR, Champoux M, Scanlan JM, et al: Rearing condition and response to anxiogenic drug. Paper presented at the 139th Annual Meeting of the American Psychiatric Association. Washington, DC, May 1986

Izard CE (Ed): Human emotions. New York, Plenum Press, 1977

Klein DF: Delineation of two drug response anxiety syndromes. Psychopharmacologia 1964; 5:397-408

Klein DF, Fink M: Psychiatric reaction patterns to imipramine. Am J Psychiatry 1962; 119:438

Lang PJ: The cognitive psychophysiology of emotion: fear and anxiety, in Anxiety and the Anxiety Disorders. Edited by Tuma AH, Maser JD. Hillsdale, NJ, Lawrence Erlbaum Associates, 1985

Last CG, Barlow DH, O'Brien GT: Precipitants of agoraphobia: role of stressful life events. Psychol Rep 1984; 54:567-570

Lewinsohn PM, Hoberman HM, Rosenbaum M: A prospective study of risk factors for unipolar depression. J Abnorm Psychol (in press)

Liebowitz MR: Behavioral approaches to the treatment of agoraphobia and panic: the case for pharmacotherapy. Invited address presented at the 20th Annual Meeting of the Association for the Advancement of Behavior Therapy. Chicago, IL, 1986

Liebowitz MR: Klein DF: Clinical psychiatric conferences: assessment and treatment of phobic anxiety. J Clin Psychiatry 1979; 40:486-492

Lloyd C: Life events and depressive disorder review, II: events as precipitating factors. Arch Gen Psychiatry 1980; 37:542-548

Margraf J, Ehlers A, Roth W: Current biological models of panic disorder and agoraphobia: a look at evidence. Behav Res Ther 1986; 24:553-567

Mathews AM, Gelder MG, Johnston DW: Agoraphobia: Nature and Treatment. New York, Guilford Press, 1981

McNally RJ, Steketee GS: The etiology and maintenance of severe animal phobias. Behav Res Ther 1985; 23:431-435

Mineka S: Animal models of anxiety-based disorders: their usefulness and limitations, in Anxiety and the Anxiety Disorders. Edited by Tuma AH, Maser JD. Hillsdale, NJ, Lawrence Erlbaum Associates, 1985

Mineka A, Gunnar M, Champoux M: Control and early socioemotional development: infant rhesus monkey reared in controllable versus uncontrollable environments. Child Dev (in press)

Munjack DJ: The onset of driving phobias. J Behav Ther Exp Psychiatry 1984; 15:305-308

Murray EJ, Foote F: The origins of fear of snakes. Behav Res Ther 1979; 17:489-493

Myers JK, Weissman MM, Tischler CE, et al: Six-month prevalence of psychiatric disorders in three communities. Arch Gen Psychiatry 1984; 41:959-967

Norton GR, Harrison B, Hauch J, et al: Characteristics of people with infrequent panic attacks. J Abnorm Psychol 1985; 94:216-221

Norton GR, Dorward J, Cox BJ: Factors associated with panic attacks in non-clinical subjects. Behavior Therapy 1986; 17:239-252

Ohman A, Dimberg U, Ost LG: Animal and social phobias: a laboratory model, in Trends in Behavior Therapy. Edited by Sjoden PO, Bates S. New York, Academic Press, 1985

Parker G: Reported parental characteristics of agoraphobics and school phobics. Br J Psychiatry 1979; 135:555-560

Rapee RM: Differential response to hyperventilation in panic disorder and generalized anxiety disorders. J Abnorm Psychol 1986; 95:24-28

Rapee RM: The psychological treatment of panic attacks: theoretical conceptualization and review of evidence. Clinical Psychology Review (in press)

Razran G: The observable unconscious and the inferable conscious in current Soviet psychophysiology: interoceptive conditioning, semantic conditioning, and the orienting reflex. Psychol Rev 1961; 68:81-150

Reiman EM, Raichle ME, Robins E, et al: The application of positron emission tomography to the study of panic disorder. Am J Psychiatry 1986; 143:469-476

Rimm DC, Janda LH, Lancaster DW, et al: An exploratory investigation of the origin and maintenance of phobias. Behav Res Ther 1977; 15:231-238

Roth M: The phobic-anxiety-depersonalization syndrome. Proceedings of the Royal Society of Medicine 1959; 52:587-596

Roy-Byrne PP, Geraci M, Uhde TW: Life events and the onset of panic disorder. Am J Psychiatry 1986; 143:1424-1427

Salkovskis PM: Phenomenology assessment and the cognitive model of panic, in Panic: Psychological Perspectives. Edited by Rachman S, Maser JD. (in press)

Sarason JG, Sarason BR: Teaching cognitive and social skills to high school students. J Consult Clin Psychol 1981; 908-918

Seligman M: Phobias and preparedness. Behavior Therapy 1971; 2:307-320

Selye H: The Stress of Life, revised edition. New York, McGraw Hill, 1976

Shafar S: Aspects of phobic illness: a study of 90 personal cases. Br J Med Psychol 1976; 79:221-236

Sheehan DV, Sheehan KE, Minichiello WE: Age of onset of phobic disorders: a reevaluation. Compr Psychiatry 1981; 22:544-553

Snaith RP: A clinical investigation of phobia. Br J Psychiatry 1968; 117:673-697

Solyom L, Bech P, Solyom C, et al: Some etiological factors in phobic neurosis. Can J Psychiatry 1974; 19:69-78

Taylor CB, Sheikh J, Agras WS, et al: Self report of panic attacks: agreement with heart rate changes. Am J Psychiatry 1986; 143:478-482

Tearnan BH, Telch MJ, Keefe P: Etiology and onset of agoraphobia: a critical view. Compr Psychiatry (in press)

Tennant C, Hurry J, Bebbington P: The relation of childhood separation experiences to adult depressive and anxiety states. Br J Psychiatry 1982; 141:475-482

Thyer BA, Nesse RM, Cameron OG, et al: Agoraphobia: a test of the separation anxiety hypothesis. Behav Res Ther 1985; 23:75-78

Thyer BA, Nesse RM, Curtis GC, et al: Panic disorder—a test of the separation anxiety hypothesis. Behav Res Ther 1986; 24:209-211

Turner SM, Beidel DC, Jacob RG: Assessment of panic, in Panic: Psychological Perspectives. Edited by Rachman S, Maser JD. Hillsdale, NJ, Lawrence Erlbaum Associates (in press)

Uhde TW, Boulenger JP, Roy-Byrne PP, et al: Longitudinal course of panic disorder: clinical and biological considerations. Prog Neuropsychopharmacol Biol Psychiatry 1985; 9:39-51

van den Hout MA, van der Molen GM, Griez E, et al: Specificity of interoceptive fear to panic disorders. Journal of Behavior Assessment 1987; 9:99-106

Wambolt MZ, Insel TR: Pharmacologic models of anxiety, in Handbook of Anxiety Disorders. Edited by Last C, Hersen M. New York, Pergamon Press (in press)

Weissman MM, Leckman JF, Merikangas KR, et al: Depression and anxiety disorders in parents and children. Arch Gen Psychiatry 1984; 41:845-852

Wittchen HV: Epidemiology of panic attacks and panic disorders, in Panic and Phobias. Edited by Hand I, Wittchen HU. Berlin, Springer Verlag, 1986

Woods SW, Charney DS, Loke J, et al: Carbon dioxide sensitivity in panic anxiety. Arch Gen Psychiatry 1986; 43:900-909

Chapter 2

Biological and Psychopathologic Findings in Panic Disorder

by M. Katherine Shear, M.D., and Minna R. Fyer, M.D.

The way a clinician understands an illness will determine his or her approach to patients. Clinical models are enhanced by incorporating available data from systematic research. Experimental findings related to biological and psychopathological features of panic have implications for assessment, diagnosis, and treatment of panic patients. These data also form the basis for future research aimed at increasing treatment specificity, improving treatment techniques, providing primary prevention, and maximizing protection against relapse.

The last two decades have witnessed a major expansion of research efforts aimed at understanding pathogenic mechanisms in panic. Interest has been directed toward understanding both the mechanisms of panic and the special characteristics of the interpanic state (panic vulnerability). Biological studies have been done to elucidate neurotransmitter function, metabolic and respiratory activity, peripheral autonomic reactivity, and specific organ pathology (primarily cardiac and vestibular). Psychological studies have focused on identifying psychological triggers for panic, studying cognitive changes during the panic attack itself, and defining cognitive characteristics and personality traits of people who panic.

Researchers studying pathogenic mechanisms need to develop hypotheses and test them. Clinicians need to integrate available data into a clinically meaningful model, which can be used to identify patient subgroups, guide treatment planning, and optimize therapeutic efficacy. The purpose of this chapter is to provide the clinician with a detailed and practical review of current findings from biological and psychological studies of panic patients. We will do this by 1) providing an overview of research methodologies including their strengths and limitations; 2) reviewing the findings related to the leading hypotheses of panic pathogenesis; and 3) suggesting a model for integrating these findings into clinical practice.

OVERVIEW OF METHODOLOGIES

Methods for studying pathogenic mechanisms of panic include those which focus on eliciting panic and those which are directed toward identifying underlying abnormalities present in the absence of acute panic. The most widely used method for studying panic is laboratory provocation using pharmacologic agents. More recently, interest in nonpharmacologic provocation has developed. The latter include both laboratory and naturalistic studies. Efforts to elucidate biological aspects of underlying pathology have utilized measures of central neurotransmitter status, neurohormonal response patterns, and peripheral physiologic reactivity. Brain imagery techniques are also beginning to be used. Psychopathological studies of underlying mechanisms have based assessment on psychological response to a variety of stimuli, and on questionnaire measures of cognitive response patterns and personality traits.

Methodologies for Studying Panic Attacks

PHARMACOLOGICAL PROVOCATIVE TESTING. Pharmacologic provocation has afforded the opportunity to conduct detailed studies of the panic attack in a controlled experimental setting. The discovery of the specific vulnerability of panic patients to sodium lactate infusion marked the beginning of an important methodologic advance in understanding panic. The initial studies by Pitts and McClure (1967) led to a flurry of interest in the mechanism of this effect, but it was a decade later before researchers began to actively pursue studies using lactate provocation of panic. More recently a number of other agents have been identified which are capable of provoking panic in a high proportion of panic disorder patients. These include intravenous infusion of yohimbine, isoproterenol, caffeine, and possible benzodiazepine antagonists, and inhalation of 5–35 percent carbon dioxide.

Pharmacologic provocative testing is being used to study pathophysiologic mechanisms of panic and as a treatment outcome measure. It is important to note that these tests should not be used clinically for diagnostic purposes, since their sensitivity is relatively low (around 70 percent with sodium lactate and no higher with other agents) and their specificity has not been well studied. Similarly, it is not possible to use response to a pharmacologic provocative test to predict differential treatment response. Panic patients have a high response rate to the available treatment methods, regardless of their vulnerability to pharmacologic panic.

We will briefly describe each of the pharmacologic methods for provoking panic.

Sodium lactate. In 1967, Pitts and McClure conducted a landmark study showing that an infusion of 10mg/kg of 0.5 M racemic sodium lactate produced panic symptoms in 13 out of 14 anxiety neurotics and in only 2 out of 16 normal controls. Other investigators have replicated this finding, reporting, on average, 70 percent occurrence of panic in patients with panic disorder with and without agoraphobia compared to zero percent in normal controls. Patients described sodium lactate-provoked panic attacks as quite similar to naturally occurring episodes (Liebowitz et al, 1984). Patients with obsessive-compulsive disorder (Gorman et al, 1985) and social phobia (Liebowitz et al, 1985a) have panic rates slightly higher than normal controls, but significantly lower than panic patients.

Sodium lactate produces physiologic changes and altered bodily sensations in controls as well as in patients. Heart rate, systolic blood pressure, blood lactate, pyruvate, HCO_3, and prolactin increase with the infusion, while blood cortisol, $_pCO_2$, calcium, and phosphorus decrease (Liebowitz et al, 1985b; Bonn, 1973). Controls as well as patients experience palpitations, tingling, twitching, urinary urgency, and other bodily sensations (Kelly et al, 1971). Panic patients tend to experience more pronounced symptoms, even when they do not panic (Liebowitz et al, 1984). Lactate panic attacks are usually accompanied by an abrupt increase in heart rate and a further decrease in $_pCO_2$ and HCO_3. Patients who panic with sodium lactate show no difference in treatment outcome compared to those who do not panic. On the other hand, successful treatment with tricyclic antidepressant medication significantly decreases the frequency of lactate-provoked panic attacks (Kelly et al, 1971; Rifkin et al, 1981; Ortiz et al, 1985). Reemergence of lactate sensitivity occurs in some remitted patients who are off medication for several months or more (Fyer et al, 1985).

The mechanism of lactate panic is not known. The leading hypotheses (Levin et al, 1984) will be examined in this chapter. In addition, there are methodologic problems in studies to date. For example, reliability of assessor judgment has not been established either between or within individual laboratories. In most studies, panic attacks are rated as present or absent. Naturally occurring panic encompasses a range of severity. Lactate panic probably also varies along a dimensional severity scale. The specificity of lactate vulnerability also deserves further study. For example, vulnerability may be related to infusion concentration or rate. High doses of caffeine or yohimbine produce panic-like states in normal subjects. This may also be true of sodium lactate. Furthermore, we now know that panic attacks occur across diagnostic groups (see Chapter 4 in this volume). The question of whether lactate vulnerability is related to a history of panic attacks or to a special characteristic of panic disorder patients has not been answered.

In summary, sodium lactate has been clearly demonstrated to provoke panic attacks in most panic patients. The mechanism of vulnerability is not known and the sensitivity of the test is not high. Specificity issues also remain unanswered. In the absence of these data, lactate tests are probably most useful as a research tool and as an adjunct to clinical assessment in treatment outcome studies.

Caffeine. Caffeine can precipitate panic in panic disorder patients (Uhde et al, 1984a; Charney et al, 1985). Studies (for example, Boulenger, et al, 1984b) have documented an association between caffeine and anxiety in otherwise normal individuals, and panic-like states have also been reported as a consequence of caffeinism. Boulenger and Uhde (1982) provoked "unequivocal panic" in two normal subjects given a single dose of 720 mg caffeine (approximately the equivalent of 10 cups of percolated coffee). Several authors (Lee et al, 1985; Boulenger et al, 1984b) have noted caffeine sensitivity in panic patients and a tendency to reduce caffeine intake after the onset of panic disorder.

Biochemical actions of caffeine have been reviewed by Gould and colleagues (1984). Currently, investigators agree that the most likely mediator of the behavioral response to caffeine is the blockade of the adenosine receptor (see also Boulenger et al, 1984a).

Two useful conclusions have emerged from this work. First, people who consume extremely high doses of caffeine may develop symptoms of anxiety or even panic which remit when caffeine is discontinued. Second, patients with panic disorder are likely to be hypersensitive to caffeine. In these patients even small doses may trigger some panic attacks. Thus, panic patients should be advised to discontinue caffeine if they have not already done so.

The usefulness of caffeine in understanding panic mechanisms needs to be explored further. Interactive effects of small doses of caffeine and other pharmacologic or psychologic stimuli might be explored.

Yohimbine. A leading biological hypothesis of panic pathogenesis is brain noradrenergic activation. The locus coeruleus is the brain nucleus containing most of the noradrenergic neuron cell bodies. A complex system of excitatory and inhibitory inputs regulates locus coeruleus activity. One of these regulators is the alpha$_2$ autoreceptor. Activation of this autoreceptor leads to inhibition of locus coeruleus discharge. Yohimbine is an alpha$_2$ adrenergic antagonist which interferes with presynaptic receptor mediated inhibition of noradrenergic transmission. Yohimbine administration leads to increased anxiety in normal subjects as well as in panic patients. Yohimbine has also been used to provoke panic attacks in panic disorder patients and to demonstrate biological differences between panic patients and controls. Both alprazolam and imipramine block these effects, but do so in different ways (Charney et al, 1984b; Uhde et al, 1984b).

While yohimbine appears to be an effective panicogenic agent, it also clearly produces anxiety in normal subjects, even at low doses (Charney et al, 1982). Early studies of treatment effects suggest that yohimbine administration may be a useful research tool to help understand mechanisms of drug action. However, studies also suggest that the relationship between locus coeruleus activation by yohimbine and subsequent anxiety is not simple or direct. Yohimbine studies suffer from lack of sensitivity and specificity data. Similarity of yohimbine-induced anxiety to naturally occurring panic has not been demonstrated. Future studies might compare responses to yohimbine administration of panic patients who are vulnerable to sodium lactate with those who are not.

Isoproterenol.   Peripheral beta adrenergic receptor hypersensitivity is another possible etiologic mechanism for panic disorder. Patients with beta adrenergic hyperactivity have panic-like symptoms which are provoked by beta adrenergic agonists and respond well to treatment with beta blockers (Frohlich et al, 1969; Easton and Sherman, 1976). These patients have heightened cardiovascular and behavioral reactivity to infusion of isoproterenol, a beta adrenergic agonist. Isoproterenol crosses the blood–brain barrier poorly and is used to test peripheral responsiveness. Freedman and colleagues (1984) found that isoproterenol infusion produced panic in panic disorder patients. This finding has not been replicated and other work suggests that beta adrenergic hypersensitivity is not characteristic of panic patients (see below). Future studies might explore the psychological aspects of isoproterenol infusion.

Beta CCE.   Benzodiazepine receptor antagonists (such as betacarboline-3-carboxylicacidethylester (beta CCE) have been found to be potently "anxiogenic" in preclinical studies of primates (Ninan et al, 1984). A European report documented severe anxiety in normal human volunteers given a similar beta carboline ester (Dorow et al, 1983). Paul and Skolnick, in Volume 3 of the *American Psychiatric Association Annual Review* (Grinspoon, 1984) reviewed the subject of benzodiazepine antagonists as a model for anxiety. To our knowledge, no further human studies have been done, and the role of benzodiazepine receptors in panic has not been clarified.

CO$_2$ Inhalation.   Gorman and colleagues (1984a) reported provocation of panic by five percent CO$_2$ inhalation as a serendipitous finding from a study of room air hyperventilation. These researchers used five percent CO$_2$ as a control, which would cause increased respiratory rate without causing the blood alkalosis seen with room air hyperventilation. They were surprised to find that 7 out of 12 patients experienced panic attacks with CO$_2$, while only 3 out of 12 panicked with room air hyperventilation. This low rate of panic with hyperventilation occurred in spite of the development of clear metabolic alkalosis in all patients.

Control subjects did not report panic feelings. This study does not contain a description of specific reactions of normal subjects.

Gorman and colleagues (in press) challenged 31 panic disorder patients, 13 normals, and 12 patients with other anxiety disorders with five percent CO_2 and room air hyperventilation. The same subjects underwent sodium lactate infusion. Among the panic disorder patients, 58 percent panicked to lactate, 39 percent to 5 percent CO_2 and 23 percent to room air hyperventilation. Five percent CO_2 appears to be a potent panicogenic agent which is specific to panic disorder patients. The results with room air hyperventilation are inconclusive. Although 23 percent of the panic disorder patients experienced panic attacks, most did so before hypocapnia or alkalosis developed. Furthermore, the tendency to panic to five percent CO_2 and room air hyperventilation did not correlate. The authors suggest that room air hyperventilation panic attacks may represent the "effect of poor exercise tolerance and fatigue, rather than the effect of alkalosis," and that the CO_2 and room air hyperventilation panickers may represent different subgroups of panic disorder patients.

Patients in this study differed from controls in respiratory parameters. At baseline, panic disorder patients had a more chaotic breathing pattern (as reflected in greater standard deviation of tidal volume) and a trend toward lower $_pCO_2$. Panic disorder patients who panicked to five percent CO_2 had higher respiratory rates and norepinephrine levels during inhalation. Panickers showed increased sensitivity to CO_2 as a respiratory stimulant with a more rapid rise in minute ventilation during the first 2½ minutes of five percent CO_2. Finally, patients who panicked to five percent CO_2 or room air hyperventilation continued to hyperventilate during the recovery period. This abnormal response has been observed following hyperventilation-induced anxiety. The normal response is to decrease ventilation and allow $_pCO_2$ to rise to a normal level.

Woods and colleagues (1987) investigated CO_2 response in panic disorder patients using a rebreathing method in which subjects use a mouthpiece to breathe a mixture of 5 percent CO_2 and 95 percent O_2 in a spirometer bag. The nose is occluded with a clip. As the subject rebreathes, his or her expired CO_2 is returned to the mixture in the bag and the concentration of inspired CO_2 rises. Subjects continue rebreathing until: (1) they want to stop; (2) they reach an end tidal CO_2 of 70 mm Hg; or (3) they appear as if they might pass out.

These researchers found that panic disorder patients had a shorter duration of rebreathing and an exaggerated anxiety, but not an exaggerated ventilatory response to CO_2. Using stringent panic criteria, 8 out of 10 patients and 12 controls had panic attacks. There were no differences in baseline end tidal $_pCO_2$ between groups and both had values in the normal range. When rechallenged after successful treatment with alprazolam, only one out of seven panic disorder patients met stringent panic criteria. After alprazolam treatment there was a trend for panic disorder patients to have a lower ventilatory response to CO_2 than at pretreatment. There was no correlation between the ventilatory and anxiogenic response to CO_2 in either patients or controls.

Subsequently, Woods and colleagues (personal communication) administered 5 percent CO_2 to 14 panic disorder patients and 5 percent and 7.5 percent CO_2 to 8 normal controls. Panic disorder patients experienced more panic attacks and greater increases in anxiety and somatic symptoms in response to five percent CO_2 than healthy subjects. The controls' anxiety response to 7.5 percent

CO_2 was similar to the panic disorder patients' response to 5 percent CO_2. CO_2 inhalation did not affect plasma-free 3-methoxy, 4-hydroxyphenylglycol (MHPG) in either group. CO_2-induced panic was characterized by large increases in heart rate.

Margraf and colleagues (1986) have conducted respiratory challenge studies in patients with panic disorder. They examined the effects of room air hyperventilation in 25 panic disorder patients and 21 normal controls, and the effects of prolonged 5.5 percent CO_2 inhalation on 24 panic disorder patients and 18 normal controls. They report that room air hyperventilation is anxiogenic, but found no difference between patients and controls in behavioral or cardiovascular response. CO_2 inhalation was also anxiogenic, but again responses were similar in patients and controls. Patients had higher baseline levels of anxiety and arousal than controls.

Van den Hout and Griez (1984) have studied effects of single and double breath inhalation of a mixture of 35 percent CO_2 and 65 percent O_2. In normal controls, a single inhalation of 35 percent CO_2–65 percent O_2 reliably provoked the somatic sensations characteristic of panic attacks. Somatic anxiety symptoms occurred during the rapid drop in CO_2 subsequent to CO_2 expiration, not during the hypercapnia associated with inhalation, or during the ensuing rebound hypocapnia (van den Hout and Griez, 1985). A placebo controlled trial established that panic patients report higher levels of subjective anxiety after inhalation than normals (Griez and van den Hout, personal communication). The authors hypothesize that panic patients respond to somatic symptoms with a phobic reaction, which leads to a panic attack.

Fyer and colleagues (unpublished manuscript) report that 5 out of 8 panic disorder patients and 0 out of 5 controls panicked with double breath inhalation of 35 percent CO_2–65 percent O_2. Panic provoked by CO_2 closely resembled naturally occurring panic. These authors speculate that the rapidity with which panic occurs may reflect peripheral, in addition to central, CO_2 chemoreceptor hypersensitivity.

Possible panicogenic mechanisms for CO_2 are discussed below. Methodologic problems are similar to those of other pharmacologic challenge tests with regard to specificity and sensitivity. In addition, effects of method of administration of gas, such as use of nose clips or face masks, need to be compared.

NONPHARMACOLOGICAL INDUCTION OF PANIC. The development of nonpharmacologic techniques for provoking panic is an interesting new area of investigation. These studies promise to provide a useful counterpart to the pharmacologic provocation studies, which are inevitably complicated by the direct effects of the drugs. The initial reports of nonpharmacologic panic described patients who experienced spontaneous panic attacks while participating in experimental laboratory procedures unrelated to provocation of panic. More recently, experimental studies have been designed using in vivo exposure to panic-provoking situations. Ambulatory monitoring techniques have also been exploited to study panic attacks that occur during 24-hour monitoring. Finally, there are some beginning attempts to provoke panic using experimental nonpharmacologic techniques in a laboratory setting. We will briefly review each of these approaches.

Spontaneous Panic in a Laboratory Setting. Lader and Mathews (1970) reported panic attacks in three patients in a physiologic monitoring study. One patient experienced a sudden panic attack associated with a thought that she had been left alone. Another patient panicked suddenly after 50 minutes of study. A third patient described "coming to after a period of drowsiness" as her panic began. Another study (Cohen et al, 1985) described panic attacks in two patients during a physiologically monitored relaxation instruction. Panic measurements in both studies are simple, clear, and accurate. The reports of this small number of patients have contributed importantly to our understanding of panic. From a methodologic viewpoint, the major difficulty is the obvious one of unpredictability. Studies cannot be designed to expect unpredictable panic, and systematic assessment of panic triggers is not possible. Nevertheless, continued exploitation of those panic attacks that do occur in a well monitored laboratory setting undoubtedly will be of great value.

IN VIVO EXPOSURE. In vivo exposure to phobic stimuli is the primary method used in nonpharmacologic studies to date. Ko and colleagues (1983) reported the results of a study in which they measured biochemical changes after a panic attack provoked by exposure to a phobic situation. They found significant elevations in MHPG 30 minutes after the exposure experience. A second study from the same institution extended these findings (Woods et al, 1987). This study compared agoraphobic patients with panic attacks to matched controls during exposure to individually determined phobic stimuli. Significant increases in heart rate and anxiety ratings occurred in patients compared to controls. However, surprisingly little difference was found between patients and controls in blood pressure response or in any of a number of neurohormonal measures (for example, MHPG, cortisol, growth hormone, and prolactin).

Behavioral treatment and assessment procedures for agoraphobic patients include exposure to anxiety provoking situations. There are a number of studies by behavioral scientists that record heart rate changes during in vivo exposure (Mavissakalian and Michelson, 1982; Vermilyea et al, 1984).

AMBULATORY MONITORING OF AN ORDINARY DAY. Availability of ambulatory cardiovascular monitoring equipment makes it possible to study panic patients over extended periods of the day in their natural environment. Physiologic measures can be taken repeatedly during the patient's usual activities. Panic attacks occur in a substantial minority of patients studied in this way (7 out of 10 patients in Taylor et al, 1983; 5 out of 12 in Freedman et al, 1985; and 6 out of 25 in Shear et al, 1987). Physiologic changes measured during panic can be compared to recordings from anxious and nonanxious periods of the same day. These findings complement laboratory results. Interpretation of the more controlled laboratory findings can be confounded by effects of the experimental setting and the devices used to provoke panic.

Taylor and colleagues (1982) reported heart rate elevations in the absence of activity in 3 out of 8 panic attacks monitored in 10 patients. Freedman and colleagues (1985) monitored heart rate and skin temperature in panic patients and normal controls during a 24-hour period. They recorded a total of eight monitored panic episodes. No attack occurred during physical exercise, and all but one were associated with substantial heart rate increases (16–38 beats per minute). Shear and colleagues (1987) measured heart rate and rhythm during 12 panic episodes in 6 out of 24 patients. This group also studied changes that occurred during partial panic and anticipatory heart rate, and there was a statistically significant increase in arrhythmic beats during the symptomatic compared to nonanxious periods.

Taylor and associates (1986) studied heart rate changes in conjunction with activity levels using a Vitalog MC-2 ambulatory monitor that records both parameters simultaneously. Twelve patients and 12 matched controls wore monitors for at least 5 days each. Thirty-three panic attacks were measured in 12 patients monitored for at least 5 days. These authors created a physiologic criteria for panic, which they called "MC-2 panic." This criteria included a heart rate increase lasting at least 3 minutes, which was greater than 20 beats higher than the average heart rate of the surrounding 30 minutes, and was not accompanied by comparable degrees of activity. Nineteen of the 33 self-reported panics met the MC-2 criteria for definite or probable panic.

There are some methodologic difficulties in ambulatory monitoring studies. Data are based solely on patient self-report in both symptom identification and timing of symptom onset. There may be substantial variability between individuals in type and level of activity during a 24-hour period, since daily activities are not controlled. Bias may occur through selection of patients willing to wear a monitor, or through direct effect of the monitor on the psychological and/or physiological experience of the day. Future studies might include planned periods of different activities in the naturalistic environment (for example, physical exercise, relaxation, exposure to phobic stimulation). Findings could be compared with those from a parallel study of these activities in a laboratory (see below).

NONPHARMACOLOGIC PROVOCATION IN A LABORATORY SETTING.   Provocation of panic in a laboratory setting has the advantage of a greater number of measurements and greater accuracy of observation. Techniques to provoke panic include room air hyperventilation, imaginal fear, sudden loud noise, exercise, relaxation, and false feedback of heart rate. Of these, phobic imagery and hyperventilation have been most promising. Approximately 25 percent of patients panic with room air hyperventilation (for example, Gorman et al, 1984). A larger number may panic on imaginal exposure to feared situations (Sellew et al, 1987; Moreau et al, unpublished data). Studies by behavioral scientists (such as Lande, 1982; Robinson and Reading, 1985) have demonstrated physiologic changes during imaginal exposure, though the occurrence of panic was not described. In an ingenious study, Ehlers and associates (unpublished manuscript) obtained self-report anxiety measures following false heart rate feedback in panic patients and controls. At least one patient reported a panic attack during this procedure (Ehlers and Margraf, 1987).

Methodologically, the similarity of panic attacks provoked by exposure to one of these nonpharmacologic stimuli to naturally occurring panic still needs to be established. It is not yet clear how great a yield of panic can be obtained through these methods. Finally, the different maneuvers may cause physiologic changes in controls. Thus, comparison with normals will need to be explored.

Methodologic Approaches to Understanding Panic Vulnerability

Study of panic attacks provides important information about the pathophysiology and psychopathology of panic. The type, sequence, and intensity of changes during panic are clues to underlying pathogenic mechanisms. However, an equally important line of investigation addresses the problem of what panic patients are like between panic episodes. These data can help answer the intriguing question of what causes the enhanced vulnerability of these patients to experience panic. It is possible that different mechanisms are involved in panic pathogenesis and panic vulnerability. Studies to elucidate this question are being conducted from biological and psychological perspectives. We will review the different approaches.

BIOLOGICAL STUDIES OF PANIC PATIENTS. Panic attacks are associated with prominent physical symptoms which suggest an underlying autonomic instability. There are two main approaches to studying biologic aspects of autonomic regulation. One is to study central nervous system (CNS) function and the other is to measure peripheral reactivity. Each has been used with panic patients.

Assessment of Central Neurotransmitter Status and Neurohormonal Response Pattern. Brain neurotransmitter activity cannot be studied directly. Instead, peripheral measures must be used and inferences drawn. The strategy used to characterize neurotransmitter function is to measure some combination of 1) peripheral blood levels of circulating neurotransmitters and/or their metabolites; 2) in vitro activity of circulating blood cell receptors; and 3) in vivo activity of neurotransmitter-modulated physiologic and hormonal levels. Assays are performed with the patient in a resting state and following stimulation. Stimulation may be physiologic, pharmacologic, or psychologic. Pharmacologic stimulation may involve agents which have behavioral specificity (such as sodium lactate) or pharmacologic specificity (such as yohimbine). Some studies are designed to compare neurotransmitter function in patients to controls and others to compare patients' pretreatment to posttreatment measures.

Biochemical assay procedures now exist for a number of circulating neurotransmitters. The focus of studies in panic patients has been on the catecholamine system, although some studies of serotonin activity are also available. Catecholamine studies include resting and stimulated levels of norepinephrine, epinephrine, and MHPG. MHPG is a metabolic product of norepinephrine and is thought to reflect reliably central noradrenergic activity (Leckman and Maas, 1984), while circulating norepinephrine is derived primarily from peripheral sympathetic nervous activity. Catecholamine receptor activity has been characterized in panic patients using platelet alpha$_2$ adrenergic receptors (Cameron et al, 1984) and lymphocyte beta adrenergic receptors (Mann et al, manuscript in submission).

The recent techniques of brain imaging deserve some mention. A number of techniques are available and each has specific strengths and limitations. The imaging technique that has been used in panic patients is positron emission tomography (PET). Studies by Reiman and colleagues (1986) demonstrated abnormal asymmetry of parahippocampal blood flow in lactate-vulnerable panic patients, compared to patients who do not panic with lactate, and to controls.

The result of the neurotransmitter and neurohormonal studies to date do not clearly support any specific hypothesis of panic vulnerability. They do, however, suggest that underlying biological abnormalities are present in these patients.

Another aim of some of the neurobiologic studies is to compare results with findings for depressed patients. These studies are interesting in that they begin to address the issue of mechanism comorbidity, a problem which will undoubtedly be the focus of increasing research attention in the near future.

Measuring Peripheral Physiologic Reactivity. A series of studies has been done to characterize peripheral autonomic reactivity in panic patients. Early work by Lader and colleagues (for example, Lader and Wing, 1964) suggested there were differences in arousal and response to stimuli in agoraphobic patients compared to other anxious patients and normal controls. This work used baseline measures of heart rate and skin conductance and response to repeated auditory tones. A more recent study (Roth et al, 1986), investigated heart rate and electrodermal levels in agoraphobics with panic attacks. They measured tonic levels, spontaneous fluctuation, and reactivity to different stimuli. Reactivity was assessed in terms of level, recovery, and habituation to the different stimuli used.

Another method of studying peripheral reactivity is using physiologic levels at baseline and in reaction to simple physiologic maneuvers, such as standing and return to recumbency. Finally, cardiovascular measures are available from ambulatory monitoring studies, which reveal average heart rate level, heart rate and blood pressure range, and reactivity to ordinary daily events such as exercise, work, sleep, and various interpersonal activities. Findings from these studies will be reviewed as they relate to hypotheses discussed below.

PSYCHOPATHOLOGICAL STUDIES.   In recent years there has been growing interest in psychological aspects of panic. This interest has paralleled the development of effective psychological treatments for panic (see Chapter 6 in this volume). Several investigators have been troubled by the lack of control of psychological factors in pharmacologic provocative testing and by the lack of attention to psychological responses during testing. There are now available a series of studies which begin to address these problems. A second area of interest is in understanding psychological aspects of vulnerability to panic and the consequences of panic (such as phobic avoidance). There are only a few studies in this area to date, but the future promises expansion. We will review methodologic aspects to the studies here and outline the underlying hypotheses below.

Assessing Psychological Aspects of Provocative Testing.   A number of lines of evidence exist that there is a psychological component to sodium lactate vulnerability. Kelly et al (1971) noted that some patients reported only bodily sensations of panic, explaining that the presence of the physician reassured them and prevented the usually associated fear. Bonn and colleagues (1973) used repeated lactate infusions to conduct an effective desensitization treatment.

Guttmacher (1984) reported reversal of lactate vulnerability in a patient treated with behavioral treatment and placebo medication. We found reversal of lactate vulnerability in two patients successfully treated without medication (Fyer and Shear, unpublished data).

Margraf and associates (1986) provide a comprehensive review of the potential influence of psychological factors in lactate provocation of panic. They discuss the role of memory of past experiences, expectation and anticipation of the current situation, appraisal of external cues and bodily feelings, and perceptions of helplessness, uncertainty, threat, and lack of control. Several recent studies (Rappee et al, 1986; Ehlers et al, in press; van der Molen et al, 1986) test expectancy in pharmacologic provocation of panic by providing different instructions to patients and controls prior to infusion or CO_2 inhalation. They found that instruction and expectancy determined, in large part, the occurrence of panic.

Psychometric Methods.   A number of investigators have measured the degree of "fear of fear" in panic and agoraphobic patients using subjective report measures (Beck et al, 1974; Goldstein and Chambless 1978; Hibbert, 1984; Chambless et al, 1984a). In addition, structured interviews for making *The Diagnostic and Statistical Manual of Mental Disorders, Third Edition, Revised (DSM-III-R)* (American Psychiatric Association, 1987) diagnosis of personality disorders have been conducted in panic patients (Crowe and Noyes, 1987; Freedman et al, 1987). These studies suggest that there is a high prevalence of personality disorders in panic patients, and that dependent and compulsive features may contribute to exacerbation or protection, respectively, of phobic consequences of panic.

Information-Processing Studies. A third area of investigation of psychological aspects of panic is information-processing studies (Lang, 1985; Mathews and McLeod, 1985; Mathews and MacLeod, 1986). These studies look at cognitive functions of memory, attention, and accessing of fear constructs using experimental paradigms. The methods involve testing of automatic processes using rapid computerized presentation of stimuli and measuring reaction times. None of the studies to date has addressed these issues in patients with *DSM-III-R* panic disorder, but this group is included in larger populations of anxiety patients.

THE LEADING HYPOTHESES OF PANIC PATHOGENESIS

Central Noradrenergic Activation

A widely held biologic theory holds that panic results from abnormal central noradrenergic function. Support for this theory comes from a variety of sources. Clinical observations suggest that panic symptoms are related to surges in sympathetic nervous activity. Animal work supports a role for central noradrenergic activation in anxiety and fear states (Redmond, 1979). Pharmacologic studies show that agents which increase noradrenergic release are anxiogenic, and those which decrease firing of noradrenergic neurons are anxiolytic. These effects are reported in both normal and patient populations. Tricyclic antidepressant drugs, which have antipanic efficacy, have prominent effects on the central noradrenergic system.

Charney and colleagues have been interested in direct testing of the central noradrenergic hypothesis. They have done studies measuring biochemical, behavioral, and physiologic responses to yohimbine in panic patients compared to controls (Charney et al, 1984b) and in panic patients before and after effective treatment with alprazolam (Charney and Heninger, 1985b) or imipramine (Charney and Heninger 1985a). They have also compared panic patients to normals in response to clonidine administration. One study of response to yohimbine revealed a significant drug effect on plasma MHPG and a significant patient–control difference in MHPG response only for patients with frequent (more than 2.5 attacks per week) panics. However, all patients experienced a significantly greater number of yohimbine-induced anxiety and somatic symptoms than controls, and reported the anxiety to be similar to that experienced during naturally occurring panic. In low frequency panickers, MHPG elevations correlated with anxiety. A second study showed that, after treatment with alprazolam, there was a small, statistically significant fall in baseline MHPG and blunting of the yohimbine stimulated rise. Imipramine also induced a significant fall in baseline MHPG, but the decrement was substantial and there was no effect on the yohimbine provoked MHPG increase.

Clonidine stimulates alpha-2 receptor mediated inhibition of noradrenergic release. Clonidine infusion leads to growth hormone release and a fall in plasma free MHPG. Study of panic patients by Charney and Heninger (1986a) and Uhde (1984) resulted in blunted growth hormone release and greater decrements in MHPG levels compared to normals.

Additional evidence for central noradrenergic function in panic pathogenesis comes from studies of sodium lactate-induced panic. Liebowitz and colleagues (1985b) suggest that the pattern of changes occurring with acute lactate induced panic is most consistent with stimulation of central noradrenergic centers; that is, the locus coeruleus.

In studies by Uhde and associates (1984a), six of seven patients experienced profound anxiety following oral administration of low dose (20 mg) yohimbine. Five of these had panic attacks. Clonidine effectively blocked these yohimbine responses. However, the authors cite a previous study by Charney and colleagues (1982) demonstrating that yohimbine induced anxiety in normal subjects is blocked by 10 mg of diazepam, as well as by clonidine. Liebowitz and colleagues (personal communication) found that pretreatment with intravenous clonidine blocked sodium lactate induced panic in only 4 out of 10 subjects who had previously panicked with lactate. Furthermore, mianserin and buspirone, which, like yohimbine, are alpha$_2$ receptor antagonists (Sanghera et al, 1983; Hjoarth and Carlsson, 1982), do not appear to be anxiogenic. In fact, both are reported to possess anxiolytic properties (Klein, 1985). This suggests that the mechanism of yohimbine's anxiogenic effect has not been fully elucidated, and that the relationship between locus coeruleus activation by yohimbine and subsequent anxiety is not simple or direct.

Klein and associates (1985) suggest that neurotransmitter abnormalities in panic are best viewed from a systems theory perspective rather than from a rheostat model perspective. This means pathogenesis may relate to abnormal feedback circuits or changes in the character of responses, rather than to straightforward changes in transmitter release or receptor sensitivity. The findings related to noradrenergic function are, in fact, most consistent with a dynamic, interactive, systems theory model.

Peripheral Nervous Hypersensitivity

A second leading theory holds that peripheral autonomic hyperactivity is responsible for somatic symptoms of panic. This has been conceptualized as either beta adrenergic receptor hypersensitivity or more generalized autonomic nervous arousal. While this theory has not been disproved, evidence to date does not support its viability.

BETA ADRENERGIC ACTIVATION. Peripheral beta adrenergic hypersensitivity has been considered as a possible pathogenic mechanism for panic. Challenge studies with isoproterenol infusions have been used to investigate this hypothesis (see above).

Nesse and colleagues (1984) also used isoproterenol to compare the response of panic disorder patients and normals at low dose infusion. Patients had higher resting heart rates, but showed significantly less increase per unit dose of isoproterenol than controls. This response fails to support theories of beta adrenergic hypersensitivity in panic disorder. Instead, it suggests that there is receptor desensitization. In vitro studies of lymphocyte beta receptors by J. Mann and associates (manuscript in submission) have also shown decreased isoproterenol-stimulated production of cyclic AMP in panic disorder patients as compared with controls. Ambulatory monitoring studies (see above) fail to show cardiovascular hyperactivity in panic patients.

Oral propranolol has not been demonstrated as an effective pharmacologic treatment for panic (Noyes et al, 1984), and acute intravenous administration of propranolol does not block panic induced by sodium lactate (Gorman et al, 1983).

In summary, there is little evidence for beta adrenergic hypersensitivity in most panic patients. However, a subgroup with this characteristic may exist. Observed panicogenic effects of isoproterenol need to be explained. Direct central effects are unlikely, since isoproterenol crosses the blood-brain barrier so poorly. Panic may be related to cognitive factors.

AUTONOMIC AROUSAL. Although beta adrenergic hypersensitivity does not appear to be typical of panic patients, autonomic studies demonstrate physiological activation. It is not known whether the observed autonomic arousal is a cause or effect of anxiety and panic vulnerability. A series of studies has addressed the possibility that panic patients have an underlying autonomic imbalance (see above).

Baseline Measures. Baseline studies reveal heart rate, skin conductance, and blood pressure elevations in most laboratory settings. In general, these findings are correlated with increased anxiety or fearfulness. Roth and colleagues (1986) report a lower correlation between anxiety and arousal in panic patients than a normal control group. Interestingly, the lack of correlation is due to reported anxiety in the absence of physiologic arousal, not the reverse. Ambulatory monitoring studies fail to show heart rate, skin temperature, or blood pressure elevations in sleep or nonanxious periods of the day (Freedman et al, 1984; Shear et al, 1987; Shear et al, unpublished manuscript). Twenty-four-hour average values of these measures are not different from normals. Using the criteria for MC-2 panic described above, Taylor and colleagues (1986) found an equal number of sudden heart rate spikes in normals and panic patients. Together, these studies suggest that in most panic patients there is no underlying state of physiologic arousal in the absence of anxiety. When subjects experience anxiety, concomitant autonomic arousal will likely, but not inevitably, occur.

Response to Stimulation. Although baseline nonanxious autonomic activity is not high, it is still possible that panic vulnerability results from accentuated responses to minor everyday stimuli. However, Roy-Byrne and associates (1983) found normal pain sensitivity in panic patients and normal response to cold pressor. Taylor and colleagues (1986) found no difference between normals and panic patients on baseline or maximum heart rate during a treadmill test. Reports of cardiovascular reponses to orthostatic change have been normal (Charney et al, 1984b) or slightly elevated (Weissman et al, in press). Blood pressure during work, home, and sleep periods of the day are normal during ambulatory monitoring studies (Shear et al, unpublished manuscript).

However, a group of studies demonstrates physiologic changes during both in vivo exposure (Emmelkamp and Felton 1985; Mavissakalian and Michelson, 1982) and phobic imagery (Robinson and Reading, 1985; Marks et al, 1971). These will not be reviewed in detail here. Studies by Lande (1982) and Vermilyea et al (1984) provide examples of this work. Lande found increases in both heart rate and respiratory rate during imaginal exposure to phobic scenes in three agoraphobics. Anxiety ratings simultaneously increased more than 50 units on a 0–100 scale. Vermileyea and colleagues reported greater heart rate increases in agoraphobics during a pretreatment, compared to posttreatment, in vivo exposure. These findings, like the baseline findings, support the hypothesis that physiologic arousal occurs during anxiety rather than the reverse.

Other Neurotransmitter Abnormalities

It has been postulated that serotonin regulation is defective in panic patients. Evans and colleagues (1985) reported a preliminary study of six patients who met *DSM-III* criteria for agoraphobia with panic attacks. The patients had significantly lower blood serotonin levels than controls. Lingjaerde (1985) hypothesized a role for serotonergic mechanisms in sodium lactate-provoked panic. An unfinished study of the serotonergic agent, zimeldine, suggested antiphobic effects in a group of agoraphobic patients (Evans et al, 1986). Open studies of clomipramine (Gloge et al, 1981; Beaumont, 1981), fluoxitine (Gorman, personal communication), and 5-hydroxytryptophan (Kahn, 1985) provide further support for a possible role for serotonin in panic vulnerability. However, a recent report by Charney and Henniger (1986b) showed normal physiologic (prolactin) response to the serotonin precursor, tryptophan, in panic patients. Two studies showed normal platelet imipramine binding in panic patients (Uhde et al, 1987; Schneider et al, 1987). This preliminary biochemical evidence does not support a role for serotonin abnormalities in panic patients, but more studies are needed.

Identification of specific benzodiazepine receptors and related regulatory systems such as gamma aminobutyric acid (GABA) led to speculations about the possible role of these neurotransmitters in anxiety disorders. Benzodiazepines are well demonstrated to be effective antianxiety agents. However, their usefulness in panic is questionable. Most patients seen in panic disorder treatment centers have a history of receiving benzodiazepine treatment which was not fully effective. Klein (1981) has suggested that these agents ameliorate anxiety associated with panic but are not effective against panic attacks themselves. Betacarboline-3-carboxylicacidethylester (BCCE) is a recently developed high affinity benzodiazepine receptor antagonist which has been found to be potently "anxiogenic" in preclinical studies of primates. It seems likely that the BCCE model will best reflect the pathological syndrome of generalized anxiety correlated with animal models of arousal and conflict. Panic attacks may be more effectively studied using the agents described above, and may reflect animal models of alarm and fear.

Respiratory Dysfunction

Although it is commonly believed that hyperventilation causes anxiety or panic, there has been little rigorous investigation in this area. Renewed interest, due in part to the serendipitous finding that CO_2 inhalation provokes panic, has led to promising investigation of the role of respiratory dysfunction in the pathogenesis of panic. We will review the available findings and hypotheses.

There is now evidence that a subgroup of panic disorder patients are chronic hyperventilators. Two studies (Liebowitz et al, 1985b); and Gorman et al, 1986) reported blood gas findings prior to lactate infusion. Both found that panic patients, but not controls, had evidence of chronic hyperventilation: low mean venous carbon dioxide ($_pCO_2$) and bicarbonate (HCO_3) levels with normal pH. Rapee (1986) has reported that a group of panic disorder patients had lower resting end tidal CO_2 (ET CO_2) than controls with generalized anxiety disorders. Because HCO_3 and pH were not measured, this finding is difficult to interpret. It could indicate that generalized anxiety alone is not accompanied by significant chronic hyperventilation. Resting $_pCO_2$ for the generalized anxiety disorder group was low normal, but for the panic disorder group it was below the normal range (LaPuerta, 1976). Minute respiratory volume did not differ between groups, suggesting that acute hyperventilation alone did not account for the lower ET CO_2 in the panic disorder group. Chronic hyperventilation in the panic disorder group seems the most likely explanation. The fact that many patients do not appear to be overbreathing can be misleading, because once chronic hyperventilation is established, only a few sighs or deep breaths each hour are required to maintain this state.

Gorman and colleagues (1985) studied blood gas changes in 21 panic disorder patients receiving lactate infusion before and after successful pharmacologic blockade of panic. There were two subgroups of panic disorder patients: those blood chemistries indicating hyperventilation, and those which indicated hypoventilation. With pharmacologic treatment, blood gases of both groups normalized.

Examination of the respiratory concomitants of lactate-induced panic is another method used to examine the role of hyperventilation in the pathophysiology of panic. Gorman and colleagues (1986) studied 76 panic disorder patients and 22 normal controls, just prior to and during lactate infusion, and found that:

1) Immediately prior to the infusion, panic disorder patients had lower HCO_3 and $_pCO_2$ as well as higher pH, than controls. The increased pH suggests that patients are in transit from chronic hyperventilation (characterized by low HCO_3, low $_pCO_2$, and normal or near-normal pH to acute hyperventilation (characterized by low $_pCO_2$ and elevated pH). The acute hyperventilation was attributed to anticipatory anxiety and was greater in patients than controls.
2) During lactate infusion, all subjects developed metabolic alkalosis (reflected in increased bicarbonate levels) and hyperventilation (reflected in further decreased $_pCO_2$). Therefore, lactate caused mixed respiratory and metabolic alkalosis in everyone. However, panicking patients showed greater hyperventilation than controls, but not greater metabolic alkalosis.
3) At point of panic, only hyperventilation-induced hypocapnia differentiated panicking patients from nonpanicking patients and normal controls. Of interest, a low preinfusion plasma inorganic phosphate was characteristic of patients who panicked to lactate. Hypophosphatemia is a known correlate of hyperventilation.

Although there are many clinical reports of anxiety induced by voluntary hyperventilation, there have been only a few controlled studies in patients with panic disorder. Rapee (1986) found that in response to 90 seconds of voluntary hyperventilation, panic disorder patients experienced more "distress" and a greater number of somatic symptoms than generalized anxiety disorder patients. None of the subjects experienced panic attacks, although 80 percent of panic disorder patients reported that hyperventilation-induced sysmtoms resembled their usual panics. In contrast, only 20 percent of generalized anxiety disorder patients reported similarity to their usual anxiety symptoms. There were no significant differences between groups in hyperventilation-induced heart rate or ET CO_2 changes. Refinements of this research strategy are potentially useful in dissecting out the respiratory concomitants of particular forms of pathological anxiety.

The panicogenic mechanism of CO_2 is not understood. There are four main hypotheses. One is that CO_2 increases firing of locus coeruleus neurons. Second, panic patients may have a hypersensitive, CO_2-responsive "suffocation alarm mechanism" (Gorman et al, 1986). Patients become chronic hyperventilators in order to maintain low levels of $_pCO_2$ and avoid triggering their CO_2 receptors. A third possibility is a primary defect in the brain stem redox regulating system (Carr and Sheehan, 1984). CO_2 decreases brain stem intraneuronal pH. This stimulates central chemoreceptors, which may trigger panic in susceptible individuals. Finally, Griez and van den Hout (1983) suggest that patients panic with CO_2 inhalation because of a cognitive-behavioral response to the induced somatic sensations. With 35 percent CO_2 inhalation, almost everyone experiences somatic sensations that are commonly associated with anxiety; but susceptible patients have a phobic response to these interoceptive stimuli and thus experience a panic reaction.

Metabolic Imbalance

A number of investigators have pursued the search for a particular metabolic derangement in patients with panic disorder. Much, but not all, of this work has utilized sodium lactate provocative studies.

CALCIUM AND BICARBONATE. Over 30 years ago, Cohen and White (1951) found that patients with neurocirculatory asthenia, a disorder with resembles panic disorder, developed higher postexercise blood lactate levels than normal controls. They hypothesized that patients had a defect in the capacity for aerobic metabolism. Based on this, Pitts and McClure (1967) studied responses to sodium lactate and found panic reactions in anxiety neurotics but not in normal controls. Addition of 20mM of calcium chloride to sodium lactate infusion decreased the anxiety response. They theorized that lactate elevations lead to complexing of ionized calcium at the surface of neuronal membranes. They speculated that panic patients were sensitive to lactate because of overactivity of the CNS or because of a peripheral metabolic defect. Pitts and Allen (1979) infused EDTA, a powerful calcium chelator, and found that both anxiety neurotics and controls had hypocalcemic symptoms, but none of the subjects panicked. This suggested that lowering of ionized calcium might not be involved in the panicogenic mechanism of sodium lactate. Fyer and colleagues (1984), further investigating this hypothesis, took serial ionized calcium measurements during sodium lactate infusion of patients and normal controls. They did not find a significant decrease in ionized calcium in any of the subjects. Furthermore, no association between the occurrence of lactate-induced panic and the rate or amount of decrease in ionized calcium was found.

The study of bicarbonate infusion has not been conducted in panic patients; however, several lines of evidence suggest that alkalosis alone is not panicogenic. First, biochemical analyses by Liebowitz and associates (1985) have shown that there is no difference in blood pH between subjects who show lactate-induced panic and those who do not. Second, in the study of room air hyperventilation mentioned above, Gorman and colleagues (1984a) found a low incidence of panic episodes despite the development of profound alkalosis and associated peripheral symptoms. However, the possibility that abrupt changes in pH trigger panic, at least in some subjects (van den Hout and Griez, 1985), has not been ruled out.

HYPOGLYCEMIA. There has been a great deal of popular interest in the hypothesis that hypoglycemia causes panic attacks, but there is little data to support this idea. Uhde and associates (1984c) administered glucose tolerance tests to panic disorder patients. Although a number had blood glucose nadirs in the hypoglycemia range, none reported anxiety symptoms of panic attacks. Scweizer (1986) performed insulin tolerance tests on panic disorder patients. Again, although the majority experienced significant hypoglycemia, none had panic attacks. Gorman and colleagues (1984b) reported that lactate-induced panic is not accompanied by significant hypoglycemia. Overall, the evidence suggests that hypoglycemia is not routinely involved in the pathogenesis of panic. However, further investigation is warranted.

Specific Organ Pathology

Patients with panic attacks are often convinced that they have an underlying physical illness. Clinicians and researchers have also considered this a possibility. Neurogenic hypertension, idiopathic cardiac arrhythmias, mitral valve prolapse, hyperventilation, hypoglycemia, pheochromocytoma, and vestibular dysfunction have been cited as possibilities. Study results fail to show hypoglycemia as a cause of panic. Hyperventilation produces panic-like symptoms, but does not appear to be necessary or sufficient for panic pathogenesis. Prevalence of panic attacks was low in a recent study of pheochromocytoma (Starkman et al, 1985). Panic patients do not show blood pressure elevations typical of neurogenic hypertension (Harshfield et al, 1984). Cardiac arrhythmias are not common during or before panic episodes (Taylor et al, 1986). An interesting recent study of vestibular function in panic disorder patients revealed significant abnormalities (see Chapter 4 in this volume) but their significance is not yet clear.

Mitral valve prolapse (MVP) is the only specific medical condition that has been reported repeatedly to occur with a high prevalence in panic disorder patients. However, the meaning of this relationship remains unclear. Several studies are available that fail to support a strong relationship between the two disorders (Mavissakalian et al, 1983; Shear et al, 1984). It is possible that variations in diagnostic criteria lead to differences in the threshold of diagnosing MVP in some studies. This hypothesis was supported in a study that revealed striking differences in interpretation of echocardiograms at two institutions (Gorman et al, 1986b). Ascertainment bias may also explain prevalence differences. Hartman and associates (1982) reported a high prevalence of panic disorder in a group of probands (self-identified patients) with MVP. This relationship did not hold up in an unselected group of subjects with MVP who had a rate of panic disorder no higher than a control group of normals. Importantly, family studies (Crow et al, 1980) and treatment studies (Gorman et al, 1981) suggest that even when MVP and panic disorder are found in the same individual, there is no evidence that panic attacks are different from those that occur in patients without MVP. Together, these findings suggest that: 1) panic should not be conceptualized as a symptom of MVP; 2) treatment of panic attacks in patients with MVP should not be different from treatment in patients without prolapse; and 3) MVP may be overdiagnosed in patients with frequent panic symptoms.

In summary, studies to date indicate a high prevalence of nonspecific physiologic abnormalities in panic patients, but no evidence of a clearcut role for medical illness in explaining the pathophysiology of panic. It is still possible that an individual patient reporting panic symptoms may be suffering from a primary medical illness which must be diagnosed and treated appropriately (see Chapter 4 in this volume).

Psychological Disturbance

In 1974, Ackerman and Sachar suggested that psychological factors should be considered when thinking about possible mechanisms for lactate-provoked panic. They correctly observed that physiological abnormalities were neither necessary nor sufficient for the production of an anxiety state, and emphasized that even if a specific metabolic or physiologic disturbance were identified, its ability to provide a specific etiology for a change in mental state would still need to be explained. Their suggestion that peripheral physiologic changes may generate anxiety by way of a conditioned emotional response or a learned perceptual association remains central to psychological thinking about panic today.

The major current hypothesis of the psychological origin of panic is that panic patients respond to bodily changes with an alarm reaction. This response may be either conditioned or cognitively mediated (see Chapter 1 in this volume). There is some support for this hypothesis.

Cognitive features have been best characterized during and immediately preceding panic episodes. However, there is evidence that cognitive disturbances may also lead to panic vulnerability. Such disturbances may include chronic preoccupation with bodily sensations, excessive attention to environmental threat cues, overexpectation of the probability or harmfulness of threats, recurrent intrusive fear images or thoughts, or appraisal of loss of safety (enhanced vulnerability). The occurrence and origin of predisposing cognitive traits have not yet been clarified, but it is likely that cognitive patterns play a role in panic vulnerability in at least some patients.

Descriptive studies of cognitive aspects of panic have been done by Chambless and colleagues (1984b), Beck and colleagues (1974), and Rapee and colleagues (1986). These studies reveal a high prevalence of catastrophic thoughts and images at the inception of panic episodes. Panic patients tend to misinterpret specific types of bodily sensations. Clark's study (1986) showed increased likelihood of negative interpretations of bodily sensations but not of other ambiguous situations.

Cognitive mechanisms related to attention, evaluation, appraisal, valence, and cue sensitivity have been studied in anxious subjects and agoraphobics (Chambless, in press). Such studies provide a basis for hypotheses about panic mechanisms, but studies with panic patients have not yet been done. Work with anxiety patients predicts that panic patients may attend selectively to fear related cues either in or out of awareness. Attention to fear provoking cues may lead to heightened arousal and physiologic activation, which in turn, may predispose to panic through cognitive and/or physiologic mechanisms. Attention to fear relevant stimuli may also operate to distract the patient from task performance and lead to a sense of inadequacy or confusion. Such interference may generate anxiety or even trigger panic. Studies testing such hypotheses need to be done.

Another interesting experimental approach to panic is provided by Rachman and Lopatka (1986a, 1986b). They have conducted a series of studies of panic attacks in claustrophobic subjects, focusing on the role of predictions and consequences of panic in enhancing or diminishing the probability of panic. This work needs to be replicated in an agoraphobic or even nonphobic population of panickers.

Studies of nonpharmacologic provocation using phobic exposure or phobic imagery are of interest here because they provide further evidence that psychological changes alone can be associated with significant changes in physiologic activation. It is not known whether phobic imagery is prominent during pharmacologic provocative testing. Clearly this issue needs to be addressed.

In summary, it is likely that there are several cognitive-behavioral abnormalities that occur either alone or in combination to influence vulnerability to panic. Among these are altered quality and/or quantity of stimulus-response associations, excessive tendency to behavioral avoidance, and cognitive processing errors.

SUMMARY AND CLINICAL INTEGRATION

No hypothesis of panic pathogenesis has yet been confirmed as fully explanatory. It is clear that panic disorder patients demonstrate a variety of abnormal physiologic, biochemical, and cognitive-behavioral responses. It is likely that an integrated model is needed to explain these findings. It may also be the case that panic patients represent a heterogeneous population with different underlying pathophysiology.

Research findings in this area are of interest to the clinician, both because they shed some light on mind-body interactions, and because of specific information related to panic patients. This information can be used in initial phases of treatment, building a rapport, and initiating treatment planning.

Perhaps the most useful clinical application of this work is in the area of patient education. Panic patients are often very frightened by their symptoms and are convinced they are crazy to have them. If the treating physician is knowledgeable about current findings related to biological and psychological aspects of panic, he or she will be able to explain symptoms to the patient in a way that is both comprehensible and less frightening. This process of psycho-education is likely to be very helpful to patients treated in any modality.

Other clinical applications of research in pathogenesis are indirect. Mechanism studies have already guided development of new treatment strategies, and this process is likely to continue. Identification of psychological and biological subgroups of panickers should also lead to increased treatment specificity. Increased knowledge of psychobiologic underpinnings of panic should also lead to more efficient use of combined treatments and to identification of the active ingredients of currently available methods.

Our understanding of diagnosis, pathogenesis, and treatment of panic has dramatically increased in the last few decades. The future promises even more exciting developments as new techniques and collaborative investigative approaches are increasingly exploited.

REFERENCES

Ackerman SH, Sachar EJ: The lactate theory of anxiety: a review and reevaluation. Psychosom Med 1974; 36:69-79

American Psychiatric Association: Diagnostic and Statistical Manual of Mental Disorders, Third Edition, Revised (DSM-III-R). Washington, DC, American Psychiatric Association, 1987

Arbab AGB, Bonn JA, Hicks DC: Effect of propranolol on lactate induced phenomena in normal subjects. Br J Pharmacol 1971; 41:430-432

Barlow DH: Behavioral conception and treatment of panic. Psychopharmacol Bull 1986; 22:802-806

Basowitz H, Korchin SJ, Oken D, et al: anxiety and performance changes with minimal doses of epinephrine. Archives of Neurological Psychiatry 1956; 76:98-106

Beaumont G: A large open multicenter trial of clomimpramine (Anafranil) in the management of phobic disorders. J Int Med Res 1981; 5:116-123

Beck AT, Laude R, Bohnert M: Ideational components of anxiety neurosis. Arch Gen Psychiatry 1974; 31:319-325

Bonn JA: Progress in anxiety states. Proceedings of the Royal Society of Medicine 1973; 66:249-256

Bonn JA, Readhead CP: Enhanced adaptive behavioral response in agoraphobic patients pretreated with breathing retraining. Lancet 1984; 1:665-669

Bonn JA, Harrison J, Rees WL: Lactate induced anxiety: therapeutic application. Br J Psychiatry 1971; 119:468-470

Bonn JA, Harrison J, Rees L: Lactate infusion in the treatment of "free-floating" anxiety. Canadian Psychiatric Association Journal 1973; 18:41-46

Boulenger JP, Uhde TW: Caffeine consumption and anxiety: preliminary results of the survey comparing patients with anxiety neurosis and normal controls. Psychopharmacology 1982; 18:53-57

Boulenger J, Marangos PJ, Patel J, et al: Central adenosine receptors: possible involvement in the chronic effects of caffeine. Psychopharmacol Bull 1984a; 20:431-435

Boulenger JP, Uhde TW, Wolff EA III, et al: Increased sensitivity to caffeine in patients with panic disorder: preliminary evidence. Arch Gen Psychiatry 1984b; 41:1067-1071

Cameron OG, Smith CB, Hollingsworth PJ, et al: Platelet alpha adrenergic receptor binding and plasma catecholamines. Arch Gen Psychiatry 1984; 41:1144-1150

Carr DB, Sheehnan DV: Panic anxiety: a new biological model. J Clin Psychiatry 1984; 45:323-330

Chambless DL: Cognitive mechanisms in panic disorder, in Panic and Cognitions. Edited by Rachman J, Mazer J. Hillsdale, NJ, Laurence Erlbaum Associates (in press)

Chambless DL, Caputo GC, Bright P, et al: The assessment of fear in agoraphobics: the Body Sensations Questionnaire and the Agoraphobic Cognitions Questionnaire. J Consult Clin Psychol 1984b; 52:1090-1097

Charney DS, Heninger GR: Effect of long term imipramine treatment. Arch Gen Psychiatry 1985a; 42:473-481

Charney DS, Heninger GR: Noradrenergic function and the mechanism of action of antianxiety treatment, 1: the effect of long term alprazolam treatment. Arch Gen Psychiatry 1985b; 42:458

Charney DS, Heninger GR: Abnormal regulation of noradrenergic function in panic disorder; effects of clonidine in healthy subjects and patients with agoraphobia and panic disorder. Arch Gen Psychiatry 1986a; 43:1042

Charney DS, Heninger GR: Serotonin function in panic disorder. Arch Gen Psychiatry 1986b; 43:1059-1067

Charney DS, Heninger GR, Sternberg DE: Assessment of alpha 2 adrenergic autoreceptor function in humans: effects of oral yohimbine. Life Sci 1982; 30:2033-2041

Charney DS, Heninger GR, Redmond DE Jr: Yohimbine induced anxiety and increased noradrenergic function in humans: effects of diazepam and clonidine. Life Sci 1983; 33:19-29

Charney DS, Galloway MP, Heninger GR: The effects of caffeine on plasma MHPG, subjective anxiety, autonomic symptoms and blood pressure in healthy humans. Life Sci 1984a; 35:135-144

Charney DS, Heninger GR, Breier A: Noradrenergic function in panic anxiety. Arch Gen Psychiatry 1984b; 41:751

Charney DS, Heninger GR, Jatlow PL: Increased anxiogenic effects of caffeine in panic disorder. Arch Gen Psychiatry 1985; 42:233-243

Clark DM: A cognitive approach to panic. Behav Res Ther 1986; 4:461-470

Cohen AS, Barlow DH, Blanchard EB: Psychophysiology of relaxation-associated panic attacks. J Abnorm Psychol 1985; 95:96-101

Cohen ME, White PD: Life situations, emotions and neurocirculatory asthenia. Psychosom Med 1951; 13:335-357

Crowe RR, Pauls DL, Slymen DU, et al: A family study of anxiety neurosis: morbidity risk in families of patients with and without mitral valve prolapse. Arch Gen Psychiatry 1980; 37:77-79

Dorow R, Horowski R, Paschelk G, et al: Severe anxiety induced by FG 7142, a B-carboline ligand for benzodiazepine receptors. Lancet 1983; 1:98-100

Easton D, Sherman DG: Somatic anxiety attacks and propranolol. Arch Neurol 1976; 33:689-691

Ehlers A, Margraf J: Panic attack associated with perceived heart rate acceleration: a case report. Behavior Therapy 1987; 18:84-89

Ehlers A, Margraf J, Roth WP: CO2 as a trigger for panic in panic patients. Paper presented at the 138th Annual Meeting of the American Psychiatric Association, Dallas, May 1985

Ehlers A, Margraf J, Roth WT: Interaction of expectancy and physiologic stressors in a laboratory model of panic, in Neuronal Control and Bodily Function: Basic and Clinical Aspects, 11—Psychological and Biological Approaches to the Understanding of Human Disease. Edited by Helhammer D, Florin L. Boston, Martinus-Nijof (in press)

Emmelkamp PG, Felton M: The process of exposure in vivo: cognitive and physiologic changes during treatment of agoraphobia. Behav Res Ther 1985; 23:219-223

Evans L, Kernardy J, Schneider P, et al: Effect of a selective serotonin uptake inhibitor in agoraphobia with panic attacks. Acta Psychiatr Scand 1986; 73:49-53

Freedman RR, Ianni P, Ettedgui E, et al: Psychophysiologic factors in panic disorder. Psychopathology 1984; 17 (Suppl 1): 67-73

Freedman RR, Ianni P, Ettedgui E, et al: Ambulatory Monitoring of Panic Disorder. Arch Gen Psychiatry 1985; 42-244-248

Friedman K, Shear MK, Frances AJ: Prevalence of DSM-III personality disorder in panic disorder patients. Journal of Personality Disorders (in press)

Frolich ED, Tarazi RC, Dustan HP: Hyperdynamic B-adrenergic state. Arch Intern Med 1969; 123:1-7

Fyer AJ, Gorman JM, Liebowitz MR, et al: Sodium lactate infusion, panic attacks and ionized calcium. Biol Psychiatry 1984; 19:1437-1447

Fyer AJ, Liebowitz MR, Gorman JM, et al: Lactate vulnerability of remitted panic patients. Psychiatry Res 1985; 14:143-148

Garfield SL, Gershon S, Sletten I, et al: Chemically induced anxiety. Int J Neuropsychiatry 1967; 3:426-433

Garssen B, van Veedendaal W, Bloemink R: Agoraphobia and the hyperventilation syndrome. Behav Res Ther 1984; 21:643-649

Gloger S, Grunhaus L, Birmacher B, et al: Treatment of spontaneous panic attacks with clomipramine. Am J Psychiatry 1981; 138:1215-1221

Goldstein AJ, Chambless DL: A reanalysis of agoraphobia. Behavior Therapy 1978; 9:47-58

Gorman JM: The Biology of Anxiety, in Psychiatry Update: The American Psychiatric Association Annual Review, Vol. 3. Edited by Grinspoon L. Washington, DC, American Psychiatric Press, 1984

Gorman J, Fyer A, Glicklich J, et al: Effect of imipramine on prolapsed mitral valves of patients with panic disorder. Am J Psychiatry 1981; 138:997-998

Gorman JM, Levy GF, Liebowitz MR, et al: Effect of acute B-adrenergic blockade on lactate-induced panic. Arch Gen Psychiatry 1983; 40:1079-1082

Gorman JM, Askanazi J, Liebowitz MR, et al: Response to hyperventilation in a group of patients with panic disorder. Am J Psychiatry 1984a; 141:857-861

Gorman JM, Martinez JN, Liebowitz MR, et al: Hypoglycemia and panic attacks. Am J Psychiatry 1984b; 141:101-102

Gorman JM, Liebowitz MT, Fyer AJ: Lactate infusions in obsessive-compulsive disorder. Am J Psychiatry 1985; 142:864-866

Gorman JM, Liebowitz M, Fyer AJ, et al: Possible respiratory abnormalities in panic disorder. Psychopharmacol Bull 1986a; 2:797-801

Gorman J, Shear MK, Devereux RB, et al: Prevalence of MVP in panic disorder: effect of echocardiographic criteria. Psychosom Med 1986; 48:167-171

Gorman J, Fyer MR, Goetz R, et al: Ventilatory physiology of patients with panic disorder. Arch Gen Psychiatry (in press)

Gould RJ, Murphy KM, Katims JJ, et al: Caffeine actions and adenosine. Psychopharmacol Bull 1984; 20:436-440

Griez E, van den Hout MA: Treatment of phobophobia by exposure of CO_2 induced anxiety. J Nerv Ment Dis 1984; 171:506-508

Grinspoon L (Ed): Psychiatry Update: The American Psychiatric Association Annual Review, vol. 3. Washington, DC, American Psychiatric Press, 1984

Grossman P, DeSwart JGG: Diagnosis of hyperventilation syndrome on the basis of reported complaints. J Psychosom Res 1984; 28:97-104

Grosz JH, Farmer FB: Blood lactate in the development of anxiety symptoms. Arch Gen Psychiatry 1969; 21:611-619

Grosz HJ, Farmer BB: Pitts and McLure's lactate-anxiety study revisited. Br J Psychiatry 1972; 120:415-418

Guttmacher LB; In vivo desensitization alteration of lactate-induced panic: a case study. Behavior Therapy 1984 15:369-372

Guttmacher LB, Murphy DL, Insel TR: Pharmacologic models of anxiety. Compr Psychiatry 1983; 24:312-326

Hartman N, Kramer R, Brown WT, et al: Panic disorder in patients with mitral valve prolapse. Am J Psychiatry 1982; 139:669-670

Heide FJ, Borkovec TD: Relaxation induced anxiety: mechanisms and theoretical implications. Behav Res Ther 1984; 22:1-12

Hjorth S, Carlsson A: Buspirone: effects on central monoamine transmission—possible relevance to animal experiments and clinical findings. Eur J Pharmacol 1982; 83:299-303

Hibbert GA: Hyperventilation as a cause of panic attacks. Br Med J 1984; 288:263-264

Insel TR, Ninan PT, Aloi J, et al: A benzodiazepine receptor-mediated model of anxiety. Arch Gen Psychiatry 1984; 41:741-750

Jones M, Mellersh V: A comparison of the exercise response in anxiety states and normal controls. Psychosom Med 1946; 8:180-187

Kahn RS, Westenberg HGN: L-5 hydroxytryptophan in the treatment of anxiety disorders. J Affective Disord 1985; 8:197-200

Kelly D, Mitchell-Heggs SD: Anxiety and the effects of sodium lactate assessed clinically and physiologically. Br J Psychiatry 1971; 119:129-141

Klein DF: Anxiety reconceptualized, in Anxiety: New Research and Changing Concepts. Edited by Klein DF, Rabkin JG. New York, Raven Press, 1981

Klein DF, Rabkin J, Gorman J: Etiologic inferences from pharmacologic data, in Anxiety and the Anxiety Disorders. Edited by Tuma H, Mayer J. Hillsdale, NJ, Laurence Erlbaum Associates, 1985

Ko GN, Elsworth JD, Roth RH, et al: Panic induced elevation of plasma MHPG levels in phobic-anxious patients. Arch Gen Psychiatry 1983; 40:425-430

Lader M, Mathews A: Physiologic changes during spontaneous panic attacks. J Psychosom Res 1970; 14:377-382

Lader MH, Wing L: Habituation of the psychogalvanic reflex in patients with anxiety states and normal subjects. J Neurol Neurosurg Psychiatry 1964; 27:210-218

Lande S: Physiological and subjective measures of anxiety during flooding. Behav Res Ther 1982; 20:81-88

Lang P: The cognitive physiology of emotion: fear and anxiety, in Anxiety and the Anxiety Disorders. Edited by Tuma AH, Maser J. Hillsdale, NJ, Lawrence Erlbaum, 1985

LaPuerta L: Blood Gases in Clinical Practice. Springfield, IL, Charles C Thomas, 1976

Leckman JS, Maas JW: Plasma MHPG: relationship to brain noradrenergic systems and emerging clinical applications, in Neurobiology of Mood Disorders. Edited by Post RM, Ballenger J. Baltimore, Williams & Wilkins, 1984

Lee, MA, Cameron OG, Graeden JF: Anxiety and caffeine consumption in people with anxiety disorders. Psychiatry Res 1985; 15:211-217

Levin AP, Liebowitz MR, Fyer AJ, et al: Lactate induction of panic, hypothesized mechanisms and recent findings, in Biology of Agoraphobia. Edited by Ballenger JC. Washington, DC, American Psychiatric Press, 1984

Liebowitz MR, Fyer AJ, Gorman JM, et al: Lactate provocation of panic attacks, I: clinical and behavioral findings. Arch Gen Psychiatry 1984; 41:764-770

Liebowitz MR, Fyer AJ, Gorman JM: Specificity of lactate infusions in social phobia versus panic disorder. Am J Psychiatry 1985a; 142:947-950

Liebowitz MR, Gorman JM, Fyer AJ, et al: lactate provocation of panic attacks, II: biochemical and physiology findings. Arch Gen Psychiatry 1985b; 42:709-718

Lingjaerde O: Lactate induced panic attacks: possible involvement of serotonin reuptake stimulation. Acta Psychiatr Scand 1985; 72:206-208

Lum LC: Hyperventilation: the tip and the iceberg. J Psychosom Res 1975; 19:375-383

MacLeod C, Matthews A, Tata P: Attention bias in emotional disorders. J Abnorm Psychol 1986; 95:15-20

Margraf J, Roth, WT, Ehlers A: Respiratory challenges in anxiety research. Paper presented at the 139th Annual Meeting of the American Psychiatric Association. Washington, DC, May 1986

Margraf J, Ehlers A, Roth WT: Sodium lactate infusions and panic attacks: a review and critique. Psychosom Med 1986; 48:23-51

Marks IM, Marset P, Boulougouris J: Physiological accompaniments of neutral and phobic imagery. Psychol Med 1971; 1:299-307

Matthews A, McLeod C: Selective processing of threat cue in anxiety states. Behav Res Ther 1985; 23:563-569

Mavissakalian M, Michelson L: Patterns of psychophysiological change in the treatment of agoraphobia. Behav Res Ther 1982; 20:347-356

Mavissakalian M, Salerni R, Thompson M, et al: MVP and agoraphobia. Am J Psychiatry 1983; 140:112-114

McNally RJ, Lorenz M: Anxiety sensitivity in agoraphobics. J Behav Ther Exp Psychiatry 1987; 18:3-11

Michelson L: Treatment consonance and response profiles in agoraphobia: the role of individual differences in cognitive, behavioral and physiological treatments. Behav Res Ther 1986; 24:263-275

Missri JC, Alexander S: Hyperventilation syndrome: a brief review. JAMA 1978; 240:2093-2096

Nesse RM, Cameron OG, Curtis GC, et al: Adrenergic function in patients with panic anxiety. Arch Gen Psychiatry 1984; 41:771-776

Ninan PT, Insel TM, Cohen RM, et al: Benzodiazepine receptor mediated experimental "anxiety" in primates. Science 1984; 218:132-134

Noyes R, Anderson DG, Clancy J: Diazepam and propranolol in panic disorder and agoraphobia. Arch Gen Psychiatry 1984; 41:287-292

Ortiz A, Rainey JM, Frohman R, et al: Effects of imipramine on lactate induced panic anxiety. Abstract, World Congress of Biological Psychiatry, Philadelphia, Sept. 1985

Paul SM, Skolnick P: The biochemistry of anxiety: from pharmacotherapy to pathophysiology, in Psychiatry Update: The American Psychiatric Association Annual Review, Vol. 3. Edited by Grinspoon L. Washington, DC, American Psychiatric Press, 1984

Pitts FN, Allen RE: Biochemical induction of anxiety, in Phenomenology and Treatment of Anxiety. Edited by Fann WE, Karacan I, Pokorny AD, et al. New York, SP Medical and Scientific Books, 1979

Pitts FN, McClure JN: Lactate metabolism in anxiety neurosis. N Engl J Med 1967; 25:1329-1336

Rachman S, Lopatka C: Match and mismatch of fear in the prediction of fear, I. Behav Res Ther 1986a; 4:387-393

Rachman S, Lopatka C: Match and mismatch of fear in Gray's theory, II. Behav Res Ther 1986b; 4:395-401

Rainey JM, Nesse RM: Psychobiology of anxiety and anxiety disorders. Psychiatr Clin North Am 1985; 8:133-144

Rainey JM, Pohl RB, Williams M, et al: A comparison of lactate and isoproterenol anxiety states. Psychopathology 1984; 17 (Suppl):74-82

Rapee R: Differential response to hyperventilation in panic disorder and generalized anxiety disorder. J Abnormal Psychol 1986; 95:24-28

Rapee R, Mattick R, Murrell E: Cognitive medication in the affective component of a spontaneous panic attack. J Behav Ther Exp Psychiatry 1986; 4:245-253

Read DJC: A clinical method for assessing ventilatory response to CO2. Australian Annual of Medicine 1967; 16:20-32

Redmond DE: New and old evidence for the involvement of a brain norepinephrine system in anxiety, in Phenomenology and Treatment of Anxiety. Edited by Fann WE, Karacan I, Pokorny AD, et al. New York, SP Medical and Scientific Books, 1979

Reiman EM, Raichle ME, Butler FK, et al: A focal brain abnormality in panic disorder, a severe form of anxiety. Nature 1984; 310:683-685

Reiman EM, Raichle ME, Robins E, et al: The application of positron emission tomography to the study of panic disorder. Am J Psychiatry 1986; 143:469-475

Rifkin A, Klein DE, Dillon D, et al: Blockade by imipramine or desipramine of panic induced by sodium lactate. Am J Psychiatry 1981; 138:676-677

Robinson A, Reading C: Imagery in phobic subjects: a psychophysiological study. Behav Res Ther 1985; 23:247-253

Roth WT, Telch MJ, Taylor CB, et al: Autonomic characteristics of agoraphobia with panic attacks. Biol Psychiatry 1986; 21:1133-1154

Roy-Byrne, Uhde TW, Post RM, et al: The corticotropin releasing stimulation test in patients with panic disorder. Am J Psychiatry 1986a; 143:896-899

Roy-Byrne P, Uhde TW, Rubinow D, et al: Reduced TSH and prolactin response to TRH in patients with panic disorder. Am J Psychiatry 1986b; 143:503-507

Sanghera MK, McKillen BA, German DC: Buspirone: a nonbenzodiazepine anxiolytic increases locus coeruleus noradrenergic neuronal activity. Eur J Pharmacol 1983; 86:107-110

Schandry R: Heartbeat perception and emotional experience. Psychophysiology 1981; 18:483-488

Schneider IS, Munjack D, Severson J, et al: Platelet [^{3}H] imipramine binding in generalized anxiety disorder, panic disorder and agoraphobia with panic attacks. Biol Psychiatry 1987; 22:59-66

Schweider E, Winokur A, Rickels K: Insulin induced hypoglycemia and panic attacks. Am J Psychiatry 1986; 143:654-655

Sellew A, Low J, Shear MK, et al: Norepinephrine increase during panic attacks. Paper presented at the 140th annual meeting of the American Psychiatric Association, Chicago, May 1987

Shear MK, Devereux RB, Kramer FR, et al: Low prevalence of mitral valve prolapse in patients with panic disorder. Am J Psychiatry 1984; 302-303, 1984

Shear MK, Kligfield P, Harschfield G, et al: Cardiac rate and rhythm in panic patients. Am J Psychiatry 1987; 144:633-637

Starkman MN, Zelnik JC, Nesse RM, et al: Anxiety in patients with pheochromocytoma. Arch Int Med 1985; 154:248-252

Taylor CB, Telch MJ, Havvik D: Ambulatory heart rate changes during panic attacks. J Psychiatr Res 1983; 17:261-266

Taylor CB, Sheikh J, Agras WS, et al: Self report of panic attacks: agreement with heart rate changes. Am J Psychiatry 1986; 143:478-482

Uhde TW, Vittone BJ, Siever L, et al: Blunted growth hormone response to clonidine in panic disorder patients. Biol Psychiatry 1986; 1081-1085

Uhde TW, Boulenger JP, Jimerson DC, et al: Caffeine: relationship to human anxiety, plasma MHPG and cortisol. Psychopharmacol Bull 1984a; 20:426-430

Uhde TW, Boulenger JP, Vitton BJ, et al: Historical and modern concepts of anxiety: a focus on adrenergic function, in Biology of Agoraphobia. Edited by Ballenger JC. Washington, DC, American Psychiatric Press, 1984b

Uhde TW, Vittone BJ, Post RM: Glucose tolerance testing induces somatic symptoms but not panic attacks in panic disorder patients. Am J Psychiatry 1984c; 141:1461-1463

Uhde TW, Berrettini WH, Roy-Byrne PP, et al: Platelet [^{3}H] imipramine binding in patients with panic disorder. Biol Psychiatry 1987; 22:52-58

van den Hout MA, Griez E: Panic symptoms after inhalation of carbon dioxide. Br J Psychiatry 1984; 144:503-507

van den Hout MA, Griez E: Peripheral panic symptoms occur during changes in alveolar CO_2. Compr Psychiatry 1985: 26:381-387

van den Hout MA, Griez E, van der Molen GM, et al: Pulmonary carbon dioxide and panic-arousing sensations after 35% carbon dioxide inhalation: hypercapnia-hyperoxia versus hypercapnia-normoxia. J Behav Ther Exp Psychiatry 1987; 18:19-23

van der Molen GM, van den Hout MA, Vroemen J, et al: Cognitive determinants of lactate induced anxiety. Behav Res Ther 1986; 24:677-680

Vermilyea JA, Boice R, Barlow DH: Rachman and Hodgson (1974) a decade later; how do desynchronous response systems relate to the treatment of agoraphobia? Behavior Therapy 1984; 15:431-449

Watson JP, Marks IM: Physiological habituation to continuous phobic stimulation. Behav Res Ther 1972; 10:269-278

Weissman N, Shear MK, Devereux RB, et al: Contrasting patterns of autonomic function in patients with mitral valve prolapse and panic disorder. Am J Med (in press)

Wolkowitz OM, Paul SM: Neural and molecular mechanisms in anxiety. Psychiatr Clin North Am 1985; 8:145-158

Woods SW, Charney DS, Goodman WK, et al: Effects of alprazolam on CO2 induced anxiety. Abstract from the World Conference on Biological Psychiatry, Pittsburgh, Sept. 1985

Woods SW, Charney DS, McPherson CA, et al: Situational panic attacks. Arch Gen Psychiatry 1987: 44:365-375

Chapter 3

The Epidemiology of Panic Disorder and Agoraphobia

by Myrna M. Weissman, Ph.D.

. . . a group of phobias which is quite beyond our comprehension. When a strong grown-up man is unable owing to anxiety to walk along a street or cross a square in his own familiar home town.

The connection between anxiety and a threatening danger is completely lost to view . . . spontaneous attacks . . . represented by a single, intensely developed symptom . . . tremor, vertigo, palpitations of the heart . . .

Sigmund Freud, Lecture XXV, 1917*

RATIONALE AND DEFINITIONS

Epidemiologic data on panic disorder and agoraphobia are important for understanding the full clinical picture of these disorders, who is at risk for being ill, and who may need treatment. In panic disorder the presenting symptoms may be misconstrued by the patient as a cardiac problem or may be "self-treated" with alcohol and possibly never come to the attention of a psychiatrist. In agoraphobia the presenting symptoms include social withdrawal, which may inhibit the person from seeking treatment at all. Thus, inferences about these disorders based on limited samples of who comes to psychiatric treatment may lead to a distorted view of their nature, as well as to lost opportunities for treatment. This chapter will review our current understanding of the epidemiology of panic disorder and agoraphobia.

While epidemiology has many definitions and has recently been broadened to include some aspects of population genetics and of clinical research, traditionally it is considered the study of the distribution and determinants of disease prevalence in populations. Epidemiologic studies relate the distribution of disease (incidence and prevalence rates) to any conceivable factor (for example, time, place, person, families) existing in or affecting that population. By understanding the magnitude of a disorder and the patterns of risk for the occurrence of a disorder (risk factors), clues as to what alterations might lead to prevention of the disorder may be obtained. Ultimately, the purpose of epidemiology is to provide data that can be used to prevent the future occurrence of a disorder or to provide early treatment.

As noted before, the population samples in epidemiologic studies must go beyond the clinician's office and must include representative samples of both treated and untreated persons in order to obtain a true estimate of the disorder and a complete understanding of the clinical picture. For many disorders, only

---

* Reprinted from Anxiety: Introductory Lectures of Psychoanalysis. Complete Psychological Works, Standard Edition. Translated and edited by Strachey J. New York, W.W. Norton, 1977.

a small fraction of ill persons seek medical treatment (Boyd, 1986; Shapiro et al, 1984). Those persons who do seek treatment are usually not representative of the population with the disorder and may include the unusual or complicated cases.

Since the 1980s, when the first multisite, community-based survey of psychiatric disorders in the United States was initiated by the National Institute of Mental Health, epidemiologic topics have been of increasing interest in psychiatry (Regier et al, 1984). The data emerging from this survey have challenged the clinicians' view of the nature, frequency, risks, course, and comorbidity of many psychiatric disorders and especially panic and agoraphobia.

THE SOURCES OF EPIDEMIOLOGIC DATA

The division of the anxiety states into specific subtypes is quite recent. Therefore, the epidemiologic data based on older classification did not separate out panic disorder and agoraphobia and are of limited utility for this discussion.

There are four community surveys of treated and untreated persons which have incorporated the division of anxiety states into subtypes and use either Research Diagnostic Criteria (RDC) or *Diagnostic and Statistical Manual of Mental Disorders, Third Edition* (*DSM-III*) (American Psychiatric Association, 1980) criteria, as follows:

The New Haven survey was the first application of the new structured diagnostic interview techniques (Schedule for Affective Disorders and Schizophrenia-Lifetime [SADS-L] and RDC) in a community sample of persons. The study was conducted in the New Haven, Connecticut area in 1975, and included a sample of 511 persons (a follow-up of a probability study) who were interviewed by clinically trained persons using the SADS-L, which generated RDC (Weissman et al, 1978).

The National Survey of Psychotherapeutic Drug Use, conducted in 1979, was a survey of a probability sample of 3,161 adults living throughout the United States in which a symptom checklist, the SCL-90, was administered by survey interviewers. The primary interest was in drug use. However, based on an algorithm of symptoms, diagnostic counterparts of some *DSM-III* anxiety disorders, including panic and agoraphobia, were identified (Uhlenhuth et al, 1983).

The Zurich study, conducted by Angst and Dobler-Mikola (1985), was a population study of 3,902 19-year-old men and 2,391 20-year-old women. Approximately 50 percent of the total population in this age group completed the SCL-90. Ten percent of the total sample was selected to participate in a prospective interview study by having either high or low scores on the psychiatric self-rating instrument. Within one year of screening, about 500 persons were directly interviewed using a structured interview. *DSM-III* diagnoses were derived both from the checklist and the interview.

The NIMH Epidemiologic Catchment Area (ECA) Survey was a survey conducted between 1980 and 1984 of a probability sample of more than 18,000 adults, using the Diagnostic Interview Schedule (DIS), which generated *DSM-III* diagnoses. The study was independently conducted at five United States sites: New Haven, Connecticut (Yale University); Baltimore, Maryland (Johns Hopkins University); St. Louis, Missouri (Washington University); Piedmont area, North Carolina (Duke University); and Los Angeles, California (UCLA).

This study provides the most comprehensive epidemiologic data available on panic and agoraphobia in large samples of adults (Myers et al, 1984; Regier et al, 1984; Robins et al, 1984). This review will focus on the findings from the ECA data.

RATES AND RISKS

Panic Symptoms

There is good agreement that symptoms of panic are extremely common and that they occur in many psychiatric disorders. In an examination of panic attacks and panic disorder in three ECA sites, Von Korff and colleagues (1985) found an increase in the onset of panic attacks in the 15- to 19-year-old age group and rare onset in panic attacks after age 40. There was no clear demarcation between simple, severe, or recurrent panic attacks and DSM-III panic disorder in terms of autonomic symptoms, age of onset, and distribution of demographic factors. Panic attacks were quite common, with a six-month prevalence rate of 3/100. However, only 10 percent of the population reported any history of panic attacks.

In a separate examination of the ECA five-site data, it was found that about 10 percent of the sample (range 7.6 percent to 11.6 percent) answered positively to the question, "Have you ever had a spell when all of a sudden you felt frightened, anxious, very uneasy in situations, when most people wouldn't be afraid?"

The close association between current and lifetime rates of panic attacks noted by Von Korff and colleagues (1985) may be an artifact of reporting, or may suggest that only a small subgroup of persons have panic attacks but that these are recurrent. The investigators recommended a flexible approach to classifying panic attacks until there is evidence from longitudinal studies or other data that indicate a clear separation of disorder from attacks.

Boyd (1986), in a separate examination of ECA data, also found a high prevalence of panic attacks in persons with other psychiatric disorders.

Panic Disorder

There is a convergence of findings concerning the epidemiology of panic disorder. The range of prevalence rates (one month to one year) was 0.4–1.6/100 (see Table 1). The ECA study showed considerable consistency in six-month prevalence rates of panic disorder across the five sites.

In the ECA data, which was the only sample large enough to examine association of panic disorder with sociodemographic characteristics, the rates were higher in women, in persons aged 25–44, and in the separated and divorced. The increased risk in women as compared to men also has been found in family studies (Cloninger et al, 1981; Crowe et al, 1983; Noyes et al, 1978). The rates were lowest in persons over age 64. There was no consistent relationship to race or education. The mean age of onset was mid- to late thirties.

Agoraphobia

As shown in Table 1, the reported six-month prevalence rates of agoraphobia were more variable than for panic disorder and were also considerably higher. They ranged between 2.5/100 and 5.8/100, and were highest in the Baltimore

Table 1. Rates per 100 of Panic Disorder and Agoraphopia in Epidemiologic Studies Using RDC or *DSM-III* Criteria

	Rates per 100		
	Period (Months)	Panic Disorder	Agoraphobia
ECA (Myers et al, 1984; Regier et al, 1984; Robins et al, 1984):			
New Haven	6	0.6	2.8
Baltimore	6	1.0	5.8
St. Louis	6	0.9	2.7
Piedmont	6	0.7	5.4
Los Angeles	6	0.9	3.2
1975 Survey (Weissman et al, 1978)	1	0.4	2.5
Zurich (Angst and Dobler-Mikola, 1985)	12	1.6	—
National Survey (Uhlenhuth et al, 1983)	12	1.2	—

Table 2. Current *DSM-III* Agoraphobia and Panic Disorder by Place of Residence in the Piedmont ECA[1]

	Rates per 100	
	Rural	Urban
Agoraphobia	4.57	6.37*
Panic disorder	.24	1.02**

* = $p < .05$
** = $p < .001$
[1] Weighted data

and Piedmont sites of the ECA survey. In the ECA data, prevalence rates were two to four times higher in women, in less educated persons, and in nonwhites. The mean age of onset was approximately 25 years, earlier than for panic disorder. Rates were consistent across the age groups between 18 and 64 years, but declined after age 65.

A study by George and colleagues (1986) compared anxiety disorders in urban and rural communities of the Piedmont region of North Carolina and found that only agoraphobia and panic disorders were related to place of residence (see Table 2). There was a statistically significant higher prevalence of both these disorders among urban as compared to rural residents. Contrary to expectation, rural areas were more protective against anxiety disorders for whites, younger adults, and the better educated.

COMORBIDITY

Anxiety and Other Disorders

There is good evidence from epidemiologic and clinical studies that individuals who experience anxiety disorder tend to have other psychiatric disorders, including other anxiety disorders, over their lifetime. For example, in the 1975 survey, over 80 percent of persons with generalized anxiety disorder had at least one other anxiety disorder; 30 percent of persons with phobias had had panic disorder at some time. There was also an overlap between the anxiety disorders and major depression: Over seven percent of persons with generalized anxiety disorder, two percent with panic disorder, and four percent with phobia had experienced major depression.

Similarly, on the basis of data from three ECA sites, Boyd and colleagues (1984) found high comorbidity among disorders. There was an 18.8-fold increased risk of panic disorder and a 15.3-fold increased risk of agoraphobia, given a major depression (see Table 3). There was a 4.3-fold increased risk of alcohol abuse, given a panic disorder, and an 18-fold increased risk of panic disorder, given agoraphobia. The risk of major depression, given panic disorder, could not be calculated due to the exclusion criteria of *DSM-III*.

Panic Disorder and Agoraphobia

Of particular interest has been the relationship between panic disorder and agoraphobia. According to Klein's (1981) observations, agoraphobia is a conditioned reaction to the sudden onset of unexplained panic attacks—a view that has been adopted by many clinicians and researchers who state that agoraphobia does not occur without panic disorder. At least two epidemiologic surveys, however, have found a number of cases of agoraphobia in the absence of any known history of panic disorder, suggesting that agoraphobia may be heterogeneous (see Table 4). In a longitudinal study of young adults in Zurich, Angst and Dobler-Mikola (1985) found that the one-year prevalence rate of agoraphobia without panic disorder was 1.6 per 100, while the rate for agoraphobia with panic disorder was 0.7 per 100. In the data from the New Haven ECA site, the rate of agoraphobia with no history of panic disorder ever was 2.9 per 100, whereas the rate of agoraphobia plus panic was only 0.3 per 100.

A more intensive investigation of the New Haven ECA findings revealed that of the 144 subjects with agoraphobia and no history of panic disorder, 67 had experienced some panic symptoms (Weissman et al, 1985). These symptoms

Table 3. Odds Ratios for Coexistence of *DSM-III* Disorders, from Three ECA Sites

		Odds Ratio
Major depressive episode	Panic disorder	18.8
	Agoraphobia	15.3
Panic	Alcohol abuse	4.3
Agoraphobia	Panic disorder	18.0

Table 4. Prevalence Rates per 100 of Agoraphobia and Panic Disorder, Using *DSM-III* Criteria[1]

Diagnoses and Sites	Rates per 100
Agoraphobia only	
ECA, New Haven Site	2.9
Zurich	1.6
Agoraphobia plus panic	
ECA, New Haven site	0.3
Zurich	0.7

[1] The New Haven prevalence rate is annual and the Zurich prevalence rate is six-month.

were either of insufficient number or magnitude to meet the criteria for the *DSM-III*, or were of sufficient number but had not resulted in three panic attacks within three weeks.

Among the 77 subjects with agoraphobia and no symptoms of panic, 29 (38 percent) had at least one other psychiatric disorder; affective disorders were the most common diagnoses.

Thus, although many subjects in the New Haven ECA survey were identified by diagnostic criteria as having only agoraphobia and no panic disorder, in fact 47 percent did have some panic symptoms. Of the 53 percent with no symptoms of panic, more than one-third had another psychiatric disorder, usually major depression. Thus, only 33 percent of the overall group diagnosed as having agoraphobia without panic disorder had neither panic symptoms nor other psychiatric disorders. If we consider only these 48 subjects as the "true" cases of agoraphobia without panic, then the rate of 1.0 per 100 is close to the rate of 1.6 per 100 reported by Angst and Dobler-Mikola (1985).

Since the only epidemiologic data available in a large heterogeneous sample of adults are from the five ECA sites, we extended this exploration of the relationship between panic disorder and agoraphobia to the other ECA sites. The question explored was, "Is agoraphobia a variant of panic disorder, or does it occur in the absence of panic disorder, panic symptoms, or perhaps other psychiatric disorders? Is there a pure agoraphobia?" (Weissman et al, 1986).

The lifetime rates of agoraphobia with and without panic disorder or symptoms in the five-site ECA data were examined. The lifetime rates of agoraphobia with panic disorder or symptoms ranged from 1.7 to 2.6 per 100, and without panic disorder or symptoms ranged from 1.4 to 6.6 per 100 in the five sites. Thus, at all five sites, substantial portions of subjects with agoraphobia had no symptoms of panic disorder.

Figure 1 shows the percentage of subjects with agoraphobia plus panic disorder or symptoms, other psychiatric disorders, or no other disorder over a lifetime in the five ECA sites (see Figure 1). The excess risk of agoraphobia in Piedmont and Baltimore is largely accounted for by the subjects with pure agoraphobia. The pure agoraphobics comprise nearly 44 percent of the agoraphobics in Baltimore and 53 percent in Piedmont, but only 23 percent in New Haven, 34 percent in St. Louis, and 37 percent in Los Angeles. The subjects with agoraphobia and

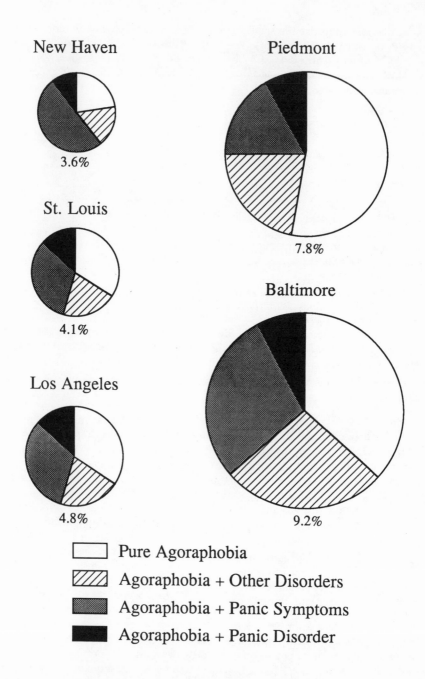

New Haven

3.6%

Piedmont

7.8%

St. Louis

4.1%

Baltimore

Los Angeles

4.8%   9.2%

☐ Pure Agoraphobia
▨ Agoraphobia + Other Disorders
▤ Agoraphobia + Panic Symptoms
■ Agoraphobia + Panic Disorder

Figure 1. Percentage of subjects with agoraphobia, with and without other disorders over a lifetime: ECA.

panic disorder comprise the smallest percentage of agoraphobics in all five sites (range, 6 percent to 13 percent). The range of persons with agoraphobia who also have other disorders is 16.5 percent to 28.1 percent across the five sites. There was more variability between sites of subjects with agoraphobia and panic symptoms (50.4 percent in New Haven, 22.5 percent in Baltimore, 32.4 percent in St. Louis, 16.8 percent in Piedmont, 28.0 percent in Los Angeles).

Not shown here, a range of other psychiatric disorders occurred in subjects with agoraphobia and no panic disorder or symptoms. The most common diagnoses were depression and alcohol and drug abuse.

FAMILIAL TRANSMISSION

There have been three reports of family data which include probands with panic disorder, and which used direct interviews and specified diagnostic criteria, either DSM-III or RDC (Cloninger et al, 1981; Crowe et al, 1983; Harris et al, 1983). These studies confirm the highly familial nature of panic disorder. The rates of illness obtained were higher than those reported in the earlier family history studies, but the patterns were the same (Carey and Gottesman, 1981; Pauls et al, 1980). The relatives of probands with panic disorder have markedly elevated rates of panic disorder in their first-degree relatives, and a greater number of females than males were affected. The lifetime risk for panic disorder in the relatives of probands with panic disorder was about 20.5 per 100, and were as high as 50 per 100 in a small sample of female relatives of panic probands (Cloninger et al, 1981). The study by Harris and colleagues (1983) included a sample of probands with agoraphobia and compared them to probands with panic only and no agoraphobia, as well as to medically ill controls without anxiety disorders, to determine the relationship between agoraphobia and panic disorder.

Specificity of transmission of agoraphobia was not found. However, specificity of transmission of panic disorder was, suggesting the association between agoraphobia and panic disorders within families, as has been clinically observed within patients.

Finally, the relationship between panic disorder and major depression was examined in the adult relatives (Leckman et al, 1983) as well as the children (Weissman et al, 1984) of probands with major depression and agoraphobia, major depression and panic disorder, major depression and no anxiety disorder, and normal, never psychiatrically ill controls. These studies suggested a strong relationship between major depression and anxiety disorders in relatives of all ages. Moreover, the relatives of probands with major depression plus panic disorder had higher rates of panic disorder and major depression when compared to the relatives of other probands groups. The findings on the high overlap between panic and depression have not been confirmed in all family studies, although this may be due to methodologic differences among studies (Crowe et al, 1984; Leckman et al, 1984).

There has been only one twin study of anxiety disorders using DSM-III criteria (Torgersen, 1983). In a study of 29 adult twins of the same sex, monozygotic twins had significantly higher rates of panic disorder or agoraphobia with panic attacks than did dizygotic twins. The monozygotic concordance rate was 31 percent compared to no concordance in dizygotic twins (see Table 5).

Table 5. Disorders in Co-Twins of Probands with Panic Disorder or Agoraphobia with Panic Attacks

| | Twin Diagnoses | | | |
Proband Diagnosis	With Panic Attacks	Without Panic Attacks	Other Psychiatric Disorder	Number Co-Twins
Panic disorder or agoraphobia with panic attack				
monozygotic twins	31%	15%	8%	13
dizygotic twins	0%	25%	6%	16

Results of these family and twin studies demonstrate the potential importance of genetic factors in familial transmission of the anxiety disorders, although methodologic factors limit the generalizability of findings. The only anxiety disorder for which specificity of transmission has been observed is panic disorder.

There have been attempts to explain the familial patterns of panic disorder using genetic models. However, no specific patterns of genetic transmission have been conclusively or consistently established (Pauls et al, 1979, 1980). Also, the twin studies suggest that environmental factors are also operating. The family data are also useful for suggesting the relationship among disorders, particularly the different anxiety disorders and panic disorder, and major depression.

CONCLUSIONS AND THEIR IMPLICATIONS FOR CLINICAL PRACTICE

From the epidemiologic data available now we can conclude that panic symptoms are common, experienced by about 10 percent of the adult population during their lifetime. They can occur frequently in association with a wide range of psychiatric disorders.

While panic symptoms are common, the full-blown panic disorder is considerably less so. The six-month and annual prevalence rate of panic disorder is approximately 1 per 100. The rates are fairly consistent across urban areas studied in the United States. The mean age of onset is in the mid-thirties.

The rates of agoraphobia are considerably higher than for panic disorder and there is greater variability in their prevalence, between 2 and 5 per 100 for six-month prevalence. The rates are also higher in women than in men. The mean age of onset for agoraphobia is younger than that for panic disorder, approximately the mid-twenties. Rural areas may be protective against agoraphobia and panic disorders.

The family and twin data, while limited, show that panic disorder is highly familial and that it most likely has a genetic component. The lower rate in rural areas and the concordance rate in monozygotic twins, considerably lower than 100 percent, suggest the importance of the environment and/or psychosocial factors.

The family and epidemiologic studies also suggest that agoraphobia is a heterogeneous disorder. While there is considerable overlap with panic disorder, a large number of persons report agoraphobia without ever having had a panic attack. However, clinicians who consider agoraphobia only as a variant of panic disorder, from their perspective, may be correct in that agoraphobia *usually* occurs with panic disorder or panic symptoms in clinical practice, especially in anxiety clinics.

From the clinician's perspective, agoraphobia is probably rarely seen without panic symptoms or disorder. The patient with agoraphobia and panic symptoms is more likely to be motivated to come for the treatment of the distressing symptoms of panic, whereas the patient with only agoraphobia is more apt to stay home (Boyd et al, in press). Moreover, those agoraphobics seen in tertiary care settings may represent the most severely ill cases, or may be individuals entering treatment due to the panic attacks.

The epidemiologic, family, and clinical data show high comorbidity between the panic disorders and other anxiety disorders, major depression, and alcoholism.

We conclude that there is:

1. an association between panic disorder and agoraphobia, but that both occur in pure forms
2. an association between panic disorder and major depression
3. an association between panic disorder and alcoholism; this may be due to use of alcohol as self-medication (Bibb and Chambless, 1986; Munjack and Moss, 1981)
4. an association between adult panic disorder and agoraphobia and childhood forms of anxiety.

The implications for these findings for treatment are still unclear (for discussion, see Klerman, 1985; Klerman, in press). If agoraphobia does occur in pure form and is not merely an avoidance of panic symptoms, there is controversy as to how agoraphobia should be treated. Pharmacologically? With behavior therapy? Should transient panic symptoms, if they are so prevalent, be treated at all?

The high comorbidity of these disorders and their familial nature probably have the most immediate clinical relevance. The findings suggest that systematic inquiry into the psychiatric status of the patient's family members should be made for both adults and children. An interview with an adult presenting with panic disorder or agoraphobia should lead to questions about similar problems in parents, children, and siblings.

For direct psychiatric examination of the patient, family, or both, several structured diagnostic interviews are available to make RDC or *DSM-III* diagnoses. These can also become a routine part of clinical practice. It is important to adopt a lifetime as well as a current perspective of psychopathology. For example, if there is a past history of alcohol abuse or depression in the patient presenting with panic disorder, this information has important implications for treatment planning.

The epidemiologic data show that most persons with these disorders do not receive treatment and that many of them can be found in the families of patients who come for treatment with the same disorders. Thus, systematic inquiry into the clinical status of close family members may offer the clinician opportunities for early detection and treatment and, it is hoped, for prevention of future episodes.

REFERENCES

American Psychiatric Association: Diagnostic and Statistical Manual of Mental Disorders, Third Edition (DSM-III). Washington, DC, American Psychiatric Association, 1980

Angst J, Dobler-Mikola A: The Zurich study: anxiety and phobia in young adults. Eur Arch Psychiatr Neurol Sci 1985; 235:171-178

Bibb JL, Chambless DL: Alcohol use and abuse among diagnosed agoraphobics. Behav Res Ther 1986; 24:49-58

Boyd JH: Use of mental health services for the treatment of panic disorder. Am J Psychiatry 1986; 143:1569-1574

Boyd JH, Burke JD, Gruenberg E, et al: Exclusion criteria of DSM-III: a study of co-occurrence of hierarchy-free syndromes. Arch Gen Psychiatry 1984; 41:983-989

Boyd JH, Regier DA, Burke JD: The contribution of epidemiology to the advancement of nosology, in International Classification in Psychiatry. Edited by Mezzich J, Von Cranach M. New York, Cambridge University Press (in press)

Breier A, Charney DS, Heninger GR: The diagnostic validity of anxiety disorders and their relationship to depressive illness. Am J Psychiatry 1985; 142:787-817

Carey G, Gottesman II: Twin and family studies of anxiety, panic and obsessive disorders, in Anxiety: New Research and Changing Concepts. Edited by Klein DF, Rabkin JG. New York, Raven Press, 1981

Cloninger CR, Martin RL, Clayton P, et al: A blind follow-up and family study of anxiety neurosis: preliminary analysis of the St. Louis 500, in Anxiety: New Research and Changing Concepts. Edited by Klein DF, Rabkin JG. New York, Raven Press, 1981

Crowe RR, Noyes R, Pauls DL, et al: A family study of panic disorder. Arch Gen Psychiatry 1983; 40:1065-1069

Crowe RR, Noyes R, Harris E, et al: Family study methodology. Arch Gen Psychiatry 1984; 41:919

George LK, Hughes DC, Blazer DG: Urban/rural differences in the prevalence of anxiety disorders. Am J Soc Psychiatry 1986; 6:249-258

Harris EL, Noyes R, Crowe RR, et al: Family study of agoraphobia: report of a pilot study. Arch Gen Psychiatry 1983; 40:1061-1064

Klein DF: Anxiety reconceptualized, in Anxiety: New Research and Challenging Concepts. Edited by Klein DF, Rabkin JG. New York, Raven Press, 1981

Klerman GL: Controversies in research on psychopathology of anxiety and anxiety disorders, in Anxiety and the Anxiety Disorders. Edited by Tuma AH, Maser JD. Hillsdale, NJ, Lawrence Erlbaum Associates, 1985

Klerman GL: Relationship between anxiety and depression, in Handbook of Anxiety, vol. 1: General Overview. Edited by Roth M, Noyes R, Burrows GD. Amsterdam, Elsevier Science Publishers (in press)

Leckman JF, Weissman MM, Merikangas KR, et al: Panic disorder and major depression: increased risk of depression, alcoholism, panic and phobic disorders in families of depressed probands with panic disorder. Arch Gen Psychiatry 1983; 40:1055-1060

Leckman JF, Weissman MM, Merikangas KR, et al: Methodologic differences in major depression and panic disorder studies. Arch Gen Psychiatry 1984; 41:722-723

Myers JK, Weissman MM, Tischler GL, et al: Six-month prevalence of psychiatric disorders in three communities: 1980-1982. Arch Gen Psychiatry 1984; 41:959-967

Munjack DJ, Moss HR: Affective disorder and alcoholism in families of agoraphobics. Arch Gen Psychiatry 1981; 38:869-871

Noyes R, Clancy J, Crowe R, et al: The familial prevalence of anxiety neurosis. Arch Gen Psychiatry 1978; 35:1057-1059

Pauls DL, Noyes R, Crowe RR: The familial prevalence in second-degree relatives of patients with anxiety neurosis (panic disorder). J Affective Disord 1979; 1:279-285

Pauls DL, Bucher KD, Crowe RR, et al: A genetic study of panic disorder pedigrees. Am J Hum Genet 1980; 32:639-644

Regier DA, Myers JK, Kramer M, et al: The NIMH Epidemiologic Catchment Area Program: historical context, major objectives, and study population characteristics. Arch Gen Psychiatry 1984; 41:934-941

Robins LN, Helzer JE, Weissman MM, et al: Lifetime prevalence of specific psychiatric disorders in three sites. Arch Gen Psychiatry 1984; 41:949-958

Shapiro S, Skinner EA, Kessler LG, et al: Utilization of health and mental health services: three epidemiologic catchment area sites. Arch Gen Psychiatry 1984; 41:971-978

Torgersen S: Genetic factors in anxiety disorders. Arch Gen Psychiatry 1983; 40:1085-1089

Uhlenhuth ED, Balter MB, Mellinger GD, et al: Symptom checklist syndromes in the general population: correlations with psychotherapeutic drug use. Arch Gen Psychiatry 1983; 40:1167-1173

Von Korff M, Eaton W, Keyl P: The epidemiology of panic attacks and disorder: results from three community surveys. Am J Epidemiol 1985; 122:970-981

Weissman MM, Merikangas KR: The epidemiology of anxiety and panic disorders: an update. J Clin Psychiatry 1986; 47 (6 Suppl):11-17

Weissman MM, Myers JK, Harding PS: Psychiatric disorders in a U.S. urban community. Am J Psychiatry 1978; 135:459-462

Weissman MM, Leckman JF, Merikangas KR, et al: Depression and anxiety disorders in parents and children: results from the Yale family study. Arch Gen Psychiatry 1984; 41:845-852

Weissman MM, Leaf PJ, Holzer CE, et al: The epidemiology of anxiety disorders: a highlight of recent evidence. Psychopharmacol Bull 1985; 21:538-541

Weissman MM, Leaf PJ, Blazer DG, et al: The relationship between panic disorder and agoraphobia: an epidemiologic perspective. Psychopharmacol Bull 1986; 22:787-791

This work was supported in part by the Yale Mental Health Clinical Research Center, National Institute of Mental Health Grant MH 30929; by the John D. and Catherine T. MacArthur Foundation Mental Health Research Network on Risk and Protective Factors in the Major Mental Disorders; and by the Epidemiologic Catchment Area Program at Yale University.

The Epidemiologic Catchment Area Program is a series of five epidemiologic research studies which were performed by independent research teams in collaboration with staff of the Division of Clinical Research, and the Division of Biometric and Applied Sciences, of the National Institute of Mental Health (NIMH). The NIMH principal collaborators were: Darrel A. Regier, M.D., M.P.H.; Ben Z. Locke, M.S.P.H.; and Jack D. Burke, Jr., M.D., M.P.H. The NIMH Project Officer was William J. Huber. The Principal Investigators and Co-Investigators from the five sites when the study was initiated were:

Yale University, New Haven, CT (U01 MH34224)—Jerome K. Myers, Ph.D.; Myrna M. Weissman, Ph.D.; and Gary L. Tischler, M.D.

Johns Hopkins University, Baltimore, MD (U01 MH33870)—Morton Kramer, Sc.D.; Sam Shapiro; and Shep Kellam, Ph.D.

Washington University, St. Louis, MO (U01 MH33883)—Lee N. Robins, Ph.D., and John Helzer, M.D.

Duke University, Durham, NC (U01 MH35386)—Linda George, Ph.D., and Dan Blazer, M.D., Ph.D.

University of California, Los Angeles (U01 MH35865)—Marvin Karno, M.D.; Richard Hough, Ph.D.; Javier Escobar, M.D.; Audrey Burnam, Ph.D.; and Dianne Timbers, Ph.D.

This work is currently supported at Yale by MH40603-01A1.

Chapter 4

Panic Disorder: Diagnosis and Assessment

by Rolf G. Jacob, M.D., and Samuel M. Turner, Ph.D.

Panic disorder has been under intense scientific investigation during the past few years. In 1986 alone, close to 200 publications appeared on the subject. Several factors have contributed to this productivity. First, panic disorder is a condition that causes a high degree of distress. Second, constituting the most common disorder for which patients received ambulatory mental health care (Boyd, 1986), panic disorder and agoraphobia with panic are highly prevalent conditions. Third, research on panic disorder has been rewarded by the emergence of treatments of increasing effectiveness (see Chapters 5 and 6 in this volume). Fourth, the establishment of specific diagnostic criteria for panic disorder and agoraphobia in the *Diagnostic and Statistical Manual of Mental Disorders, Third Edition (DSM-III)* (American Psychiatric Association, 1980) highlighted gaps in our knowledge, gaps which acted to stimulate further scientific inquiry. Finally, as other chapters in this volume will demonstrate, panic disorder is of interest for both biological and behavioral scientists. Research on panic disorder might therefore become a model for studying how the mind and body interface with respect to research and therapy.

DIAGNOSIS ACCORDING TO *DSM-III* AND *DSM-III-R* CRITERIA

One of the consequences of the research on panic disorder is that in the revised version of the *DSM-III* (*Diagnostic and Statistical Manual of Mental Disorders, Third Edition, Revised—DSM-III-R*) (American Psychiatric Association, 1987), substantial changes occurred in the diagnostic criteria for panic disorders. One of the main changes was the merging of the *DSM-III* categories of panic disorder and agoraphobia with panic into one major diagnostic category—panic disorder—with the subtypes of panic disorder without phobic avoidance, and panic disorder with agoraphobia (see Table 1).

The merging of agoraphobia with panic and panic disorder reflects the view that, in most cases, phobic avoidance can be conceptualized as a consequence of panic, thus making panic attacks the central disturbance in agoraphobia (Klein et al, 1978). This view was supported by retrospective life-charting studies which revealed that, in virtually all cases, phobic avoidance developed after the initial panic attack (Breier et al, 1986; Uhde et al, 1985). Furthermore, psychometric studies did not reveal major differences between panic disorder and agoraphobia; the differences found are consistent with the view that agoraphobia with panic is a more pervasive variant, or a later stage, of panic disorder (Buller et al, 1986; Turner et al, 1986a, 1986b; Thyer et al, 1985a). A recent family study showed that the relatives of patients with panic disorder, and agoraphobia with

Table 1. Comparison of Anxiety Disorder Categories in *DSM-III* and *DSM-III-R*

DSM-III	DSM-III-R
Panic disorder	Panic disorder without agoraphobia severity: mild moderate severe in partial remission in full remission
Agoraphobia with panic	Panic disorder with agoraphobia severity of panic, as above severity of phobic avoidance: mild moderate severe
Agoraphobia without panic	Agoraphobia without history of panic disorder: with limited symptom attacks without limited symptom attacks
Atypical anxiety disorder	Panic disorder, with current limited symptom attacks Anxiety disorder not otherwise specified
Major depression (with panic)	Major depression and panic disorder

panic, both had approximately a 20 percent risk for panic attacks (Noyes et al, 1986a); however, risk of agoraphobia was greater for relatives of agoraphobics (12 percent) than for relatives of patients with panic disorder (1.6 percent). This pattern could again be consistent with the notion that agoraphobia is a more pervasive variant of panic disorder.

In the *DSM-III-R*, diagnostic criteria for panic disorder (without agoraphobia) were also changed. Table 2 juxtaposes the old and new criteria. The new criteria reflect the notion that panic attacks occur suddenly (criterion D) and, at least some of the time, unexpectedly (criterion A). One major change is the recognition of limited symptom attacks, in which less than "4 of 12" *(DSM-III)* or "4 of 13" *(DSM-III-R)* autonomic or cognitive symptoms are present. Thus, panic disorder can now be diagnosed even if the four symptoms were not present in more than a few attacks (criteria C, D).

Finally, *DSM-III's* frequency criterion of "at least three panic attacks during a three-week period" was made less stringent. The frequency criterion can now be fulfilled if "one or more attacks were followed by a period of at least one month of persistent fear of having another attack." This change appears to be in recognition of findings that panic attacks occurring in clusters or at frequencies of less than three per three-week period are common. Furthermore, individuals with infrequent attacks are more anxious than normals; the topography of panic symptoms of individuals with infrequent attacks does not appear to differ from the panic attacks of *DSM-III* panic disorder patients (Katon et al, 1987; Norton et al, 1986; von Korff et al, 1985).

Like panic disorder, the diagnostic criteria for agoraphobia with panic *(DSM-III)*/panic disorder with agoraphobia *(DSM-III-R)* have been modified (Table 3). In particular, while *DSM-III* was noncommittal as to the cause of the phobic avoidance, criterion B of *DSM-III-R* clearly relates phobic avoidance to the fear of panic. The criterion of "constriction of normal activities" in *DSM-III* agoraphobia has been replaced by three gradations of phobic avoidance: mild, moderate, and severe.

Agoraphobia without panic was kept as a separate category, "Agoraphobia without History of Panic Disorder." *DSM-III-R* requires specification of presence or absence of a history of limited symptom attacks to accompany the diagnosis. Agoraphobia without panic is believed to be rare. However, Weissman and colleagues (1985) reported a prevalence of 2.9 percent in the general population, higher than the rate for panic disorder with agoraphobia (0.3 per 100). Upon closer examination, 47 percent of these actually had a history of some panic, but of insufficient frequency or number of symptoms to meet *DSM-III* criteria for panic disorder. Of the 53 percent without history of any panic symptoms, 40 percent had at least one other psychiatric disorder, most often depression. Thus, the prevalence of agoraphobia without panic and without other psychiatric diagnosis was approximately one percent, much lower but still more than is commonly assumed.

DIFFERENTIAL DIAGNOSIS

The differential diagnosis of panic disorder includes organic mental disorders (organic anxiety syndrome, *DSM-III-R*), depression, hypochondriasis, and other anxiety disorders. The differential diagnosis between panic disorder and other nonorganic mental disorders was markedly changed in *DSM-III-R* because of the elimination of hierarchical rules in which other mental disorders, such as depression and hypochondriasis, would be diagnosed preferentially if the panic symptoms were considered "due to" the other disorder. For a further discussion of hierarchical rules, see Boyd and colleagues (1984) and Spitzer and Williams (1985). Hierarchical rules were maintained with respect to organic factors that might cause anxiety, such as cardiac arrythmias, hyperthyroidism, or substance intoxication; however, mitral valve prolapse (MVP) may coexist with panic disorder.

Other Anxiety Disorders

Panic attacks occur in virtually all anxiety disorders (Barlow et al, 1985). The differential diagnosis between panic disorder and other anxiety disorders is based on a judgment as to whether the occurrence of or preoccupation with panic attacks constitutes the principal feature of the patient's disorder.

SOCIAL PHOBIA. Social phobia involves "a persistent fear of one or more situations in which the individual is exposed to possible scrutiny by others and

Table 2. Panic Disorder Criteria in *DSM-III* and *DSM-III-R*

DSM-III	*DSM-III-R*
A. At least three panic attacks within a three-week period in circumstances other than during marked physical exertion or in a life-threatening situation. The attacks are not precipitated only by exposure to a circumscribed phobic stimulus.	A. At some time during the disturbance, one or more panic attacks (discrete periods of intense discomfort or fear that were (1) unexpected, i.e., did not occur immediately before or on exposure to a situation that almost always caused anxiety, and (2) not triggered by situations in which the individual was the focus of others' attention) occurred within a four-week period, or one or more attacks were followed by a period of at least a month of persistent fear of having another attack.
B. Panic attacks are manifested by discrete periods of apprehension or fear and at least four of the following symptoms appear during each attack: (1) dyspnea (5) dizziness, vertigo, or unsteady feelings (2) palpitations (11) trembling or shaking (9) sweating (4) choking or smothering sensations . . . (10) faintness (6) feelings of unreality (7) paresthesias (tingling in hands or feet) (8) hot and cold flashes (3) chest pain or discomfort (12) fear of dying, going crazy, or doing something uncontrolled during an attack	C. At least four of the following symptoms developed during at least one of the attacks: (1) shortness of breath (dyspnea) or smothering sensations (2) dizziness, unsteady feelings, or faintness (3) palpitations or accelerated heart rate (tachycardia) (4) trembling or shaking (5) sweating (6) choking (7) nausea or abdominal distress . . . (8) depersonalization or derealization (9) numbness or tingling sensations (paresthesias) (10) flushes (hot flashes) or chills (11) chest pain or discomfort (12) fear of dying (13) fear of going crazy or doing something uncontrolled

Table 2. Panic Disorder Criteria in *DSM-III* and *DSM-III-R (continued)*

DSM-III	*DSM-III-R*
C. Not due to a physical disorder or another mental disorder, such as Major Depression, Somatization Disorder, or Schizophrenia	D. During at least some of the attacks, at least four of the C symptoms developed suddenly and increased in intensity within ten minutes of the beginning of the first C symptom in the attack.
D. The disorder is not associated with Agoraphobia	E. It cannot be established that an organic factor initiated and maintained the disturbance, e.g., Amphetamine or Caffeine intoxication, hyperthyroidism. Note: Mitral valve prolapse may be an associated condition but does not rule out a diagnosis of Panic Disorder.

Table 3. *DSM-III* Criteria for Agoraphobia with Panic and *DSM-III-R* Criteria for Panic Disorder with Agoraphobia

DSM-III: Agoraphobia	*DSM-III-R*: Panic Disorder with Agoraphobia
A. The individual has marked fear of and thus avoids being alone or in public places from which escape might be difficult or help not available in case of sudden incapacitation, e.g., crowds, tunnels, bridges, public transportation.	A. Meets criteria for Panic Disorder. B. Agoraphobia: Fear of being in places or situations from which escape might be difficult (or embarrassing) or in which help might not be available, in the event of a panic attack. . . . As a result of this fear, there are either travel restrictions or need for a companion when away from home, or there is endurance of agoraphobic situations despite intense anxiety. Common agoraphobic situations include being outside of the home alone, being in a crowd or standing in a line, being on a bridge, traveling in a bus, train, or car.
B. There is increasing constriction of normal activities until the fears or avoidance behavior dominate the individual's life.	Mild agoraphobic avoidance: some avoidance (or endurance with distress), but relatively normal lifestyle, e.g., travels unaccompanied when necessary, such as to work or to shop; otherwise avoids traveling alone. Moderate: Avoidance results in constricted lifestyle, e.g., the person is able to leave house alone, but not go more than a few miles unaccompanied. Severe: Avoidance results in being nearly or completely housebound or unable to leave house unaccompanied.
C. Not due to a major depressive episode, Obsessive Compulsive Disorder, Paranoid Personality Disorder, or Schizophrenia.	

fears that he or she may do something or act in a way that will be humiliating and embarrassing" *(DSM-III-R)*. Social phobics may avoid parties, eating in public, or speaking in public, situations in which they feel that their performance is scrutinized by others. Social fears and social avoidance also occur in panic disorder; patients with panic disorder might avoid social situations from which they cannot leave quickly without embarrassment should they have a panic attack. The *DSM-III-R* makes a distinction between the fear of panic and the fear of negative evaluation of performance. Social phobia is diagnosed only if the social fears are "unrelated to" the fear of having a panic attack *(DSM-III-R)*.

SIMPLE PHOBIA. Panic attacks or extreme anxiety can occur in simple phobia, such as claustrophobia (Rachman et al, 1985). The main difference between panic disorder and simple phobia, according to *DSM-III-R*, is that in simple phobia the fear is always related to a circumscribed stimulus other than the fear of panic. The panic attacks of panic disorder, on the other hand, are characterized by their unexpected occurrence, at least during a phase of the disorder. If panic occurs in simple phobia, it will occur immediately upon or immediately before exposure to the phobic stimulus. Panic in agoraphobia, on the other hand, may occur at any time during exposure to the phobic situation, or not at all. The differential diagnosis between panic disorder and simple phobia may be difficult in cases where the panic attacks currently are situation-specific and there are no "spontaneous" panic attacks. Usually, however, there is a history of unexpected attacks in the past in these cases, thus justifying a diagnosis of panic disorder with agoraphobia. Conceptually, agoraphobia without panic may be closer to simple phobia than to agoraphobia with panic. If the prevalance data for agoraphobia without panic described earlier are confirmed, the relationship between this condition and simple phobia would need to be studied.

GENERALIZED ANXIETY DISORDER. The elimination of the concept of anxiety neurosis by differentiating between panic disorder and generalized anxiety disorder (GAD) remains controversial (Tyrer, 1984; Editorial, 1986). The distinction between panic and anxiety was intially based on hypotheses of differential responsivity of panic and anxiety to treatment with antidepressants and minor tranquilizers (Freedman et al, 1981); however, recent drug trials demonstrating the reduction of panic with benzodiazepines do not always confirm this distinction (Noyes et al, 1984; Rickels and Schweizer, 1986; Speir et al, 1986). Rather, the case can be made that panic represents an extreme form of anxiety (Turner et al, in press).

If panic disorder and GAD are separate conditions, one should be able to find differences between the disorders not only with respect to the defining characteristics, but also with respect to other variables. One such difference, independently found by several investigators, appears to be the distribution of age of onset. While panic disorder and agoraphobia typically have onsets peaking in the mid-twenties, the age of onset of GAD was more evenly distributed over the entire age range below 40 (Rapee, 1985; Thyer et al, 1985b). The differences in age distribution were due to the fact that GAD often had a childhood onset. It is therefore not surprising that in a study by Barlow and colleagues (1986) one of the major differences between panic disorder and GAD was that the duration of generalized anxiety in GAD (243 months, or 56 percent of the patient's life) was significantly longer than in panic disorder (62.4 months, or 15 percent of the patient's life) or agoraphobia (136 months, or 32 percent of the patient's life). An earlier onset for GAD was also found by Anderson and associates (1984).

This research on GAD was based on the criteria in *DSM-III*. Because the criteria for GAD were substantially revised, the results of these studies are not necessarily generalizable to GAD as defined in the *DSM-III-R*. According to *DSM-III-R*, GAD is defined as "a period of six months or longer during which the individual has been bothered more days than not by unrealistic or excessive worry . . . about two or more life circumstances . . ."; furthermore, that "if another Axis I disorder is present, the focus of the worry is unrelated to it." Thus, according to *DSM-III-R*, panic disorder and GAD can be diagnosed simultaneously if the patients worry about things other than panic. If preoccupation with panic is their only concern, a separate diagnosis is not made.

Depression

Panic attacks can occur in patients diagnosed as having major depression in the *DSM-III*. If *DSM-III's* hierarchical rule of not diagnosing panic disorder when the panic attacks are considered "due to" depression were valid, one would expect depression without panic to be similar to depression with panic in all essential respects (Boyd et al, 1984). However, several investigations have shown that depression with panic and depression without panic differ. In particular, depression with panic appears to have a different prognosis and family history pattern than depression without panic.

For example, Leckman and colleagues (1983) found that relatives of individuals with anxious depressions had a higher prevalance of depression (as well as anxiety associated with depression) than did relatives of individuals having depression without anxiety. Furthermore, children of patients with depression and panic showed a higher prevalence of depression and anxiety, particularly separation anxiety, than did children of pure depressives. Van Valkenburg and associates (1984) found that patients with depression and panic had significantly more enduring chronic depression (exceeding two years), more family history of alcoholism, and significantly poorer response to treatment and psychosocial outcome, than patients with "pure" depression. Finally, Grunhaus and colleagues (1986) studied the sleep architecture of depressives and patients with simultaneous depressions and panic. The sleep data suggested that while depression with panic was a heterogeneous group, on the average, sleep latencies were (nonsignificantly) longer in this group.

The weight of the evidence suggests that it is useful to make a distinction between unipolar depression and depression with panic. Therefore, the differential diagnosis between panic disorder and depression was greatly simplified in the *DSM-III-R*. There is no longer a need to establish whether the panic disorder can be considered "due to" depression. Instead, both diagnoses are given in cases with a coexisting depression and panic disorder.

Hypochondriasis

Somatic symptoms and hypochondriacal concerns are common in panic disorder (Noyes et al, 1980; Sheehan et al, 1980). Before the revision of *DSM-III*, the practice was not to diagnose panic disorder when the panic attacks were "due to" a somatization disorder, a hierarchical rule that was eliminated in the *DSM-III-R*. Furthermore, the diagnostic criteria for hypochondriasis in the

DSM-III-R were modified to rule out a diagnosis of hypochondriasis if the hypochondriacal concerns "are not only symptoms of panic attacks." Thus, hypochondriacal concerns in panic disorder do not warrant a diagnosis of hypochondriasis unless they occur independently of the panic disorder. In a recent study, Noyes and associates (1986b) found that panic disorder patients scored similarly to hypochondriacal patients on the Pilowsky Illness Behavior Questionnaire, an instrument developed to measure abnormal illness behavior (see Jacob and Turner, 1984, for a review of this instrument). Those patients who responded to treatment with alprazolam also showed significant reductions in their abnormal illness behaviors.

Organic Anxiety Syndrome

Organic anxiety syndrome is a new category in *DSM-III-R*. Coined by Dietch (1981) and Mackenzie and Popkin (1983), this diagnosis is given if panic is due to a physical disorder. In patients with panic disorder, the differential diagnosis of organic anxiety syndrome confronts the physician with two contradicting tasks. The first and overriding task is not to overlook treatable medical conditions, as required by prudent medical practice. This goal is particularly important, because preliminary research findings suggest an increased prevalance of physical disorders, particularly cardiovascular disease, in panic disorder (Coryell et al, 1986). Vittone and Uhde (1985) reported that 58 percent of panic patients seen in their program had previously unrecognized physical illnesses. The illnesses, which usually appeared to be unrelated to the panic attacks, included mild conditions such as iron deficiency anemia as well as major disorders, such as multiple endocrine adenomas or strokes.

The second task is to address the hypochondriacal attributions that panic patients make with respect to their symptoms. These attributions make many panic patients seek out medical clinics as their primary source of care. For example, Beitman (in press) found that a large percentage of cardiology patients with functional chest complaints fulfilled diagnostic criteria for panic disorder. As mentioned earlier, the hypochondriacal concerns of panic patients often improve with treatment (Noyes et al, 1986b).

The possibility that medical disorders may cause panic has intrigued not only the panic patients themselves (they often are surprisingly well-informed even of the latest research), but also the investigators in the field. A number of conditions have been implicated, the best-known being mitral valve prolapse, but none has as yet been proven to cause panic disorder (see Jacob and Rapport, 1984, and Chapter 2 in this volume, for reviews). Most of the conditions implicated also occur in normals, in which they may cause transient anxiety, but not panic disorder. It may be that a certain predisposition, anxiety- or panic-proneness is necessary for a medical condition to cause panic. In panic-prone individuals, medical conditions could serve as a nonspecific stressor triggering the onset of panic (Jacob et al, 1985; Jacob and Rapport, 1984; Turner et al, in press). In considering the causal direction of a hypothesized relationship between panic and a medical condition, one also needs to explore the possibility of reverse causality (that is, panic causing physiological abnormalities) and of a third factor causing both panic and the medical condition (for example, medication use). For example, hyperventilation can cause vasoconstriction, which significantly reduces cerebral and coronary blood flow.

Mitral valve prolapse (MVP) has a special status with respect to the diagnosis of panic disorder. It has been found to be associated with panic disorder in some studies but not in others (see Chapter 2 in this volume). The significance of MVP for panic is unknown; *DSM-III-R* permits the diagnosis of panic disorder in the presence of MVP (see note to criterion E, Table 2). Mitral valve prolapse is not the only cardiac condition that has been implicated in panic. Other cardiac conditions that can present with panic-like symptoms include cardiac arrythmias and angina pectoris. Because these conditions can be treated medically, and furthermore because if left untreated they may pose significant risk to the patient, clinicians should continue to be concerned about cardiac arrythmias and angina, although, according to a recent study involving ambulatory electrocardiographic monitoring, clinically significant arrythmias are found infrequently (Shear et al, 1987).

We recently demonstrated that *vestibular abnormalities* appeared to be common in a selected group of 21 patients with panic disorder whose panic attacks included sensations of vertigo or movement, or who experienced episodes of dizziness between full-blown panic attacks. The abnormalities included cases of peripheral vestibular dysfunction (for example, labyrinthitis) and others in which the source of the dysfunction could not be established (Jacob et al, 1985). Vestibular involvement has long been suspected in agoraphobia (Gordon, 1986), but the significance of vestibular dysfunction is as yet unclear. In no case did we identify underlying neurological disorders.

Anxiety is a common symptom of *hyperthyroidism*. For example, Kathol and colleagues (1986) reported that 80 percent of hyperthyroid patients showed symptoms of generalized anxiety disorder; these symptoms responded to treatment for hyperthyroidism. *Hypothyroidism* likewise may be associated with anxiety. Lindemann and associates (1984) found 14 cases of hyperthyroidism and 13 cases of hypothyroidism among 295 patients treated for phobic disorders; in a similar study, however, Fishman and colleagues (1985) found no thyroid abnormalities in 82 panic patients.

Hypoglycemia can present with symptoms similar to panic. Uhde and associates (1985) found hypoglycemia (glucose nadir < 60) during a five-hour glucose tolerance test in seven out of nine nondiabetic women with panic disorder; during the test, the patients reported symptoms but did not develop panic. Schweizer and colleagues (1986) induced hypoglycemia in 10 patients with panic disorder by administering intravenous insulin. In none of these cases did panic symptoms develop. Thus, in a laboratory setting, panic patients do not develop panic attacks in response to hypoglycemia. It remains an open question whether unexpected hypoglycemia in the "free-living" panic patient may trigger panic. In any case, caution should be exerted in attributing panic symptoms to hypoglycemia, as this condition was, at one time, quite overdiagnosed (Yager and Young, 1974).

Partial complex seizures (temporal lobe seizures) may present with symptoms similar to panic (Volkow et al, 1986). This diagnosis has recently become particularly interesting because of the demonstration of an abnormal asymmetry of parahippocampal blood flow in lactate-sensitive panic patients (Reiman et al., 1986). Vittone and Uhde (1985) recommended that panic patients whose panic attacks are accompanied by psychomotor or psychosensory signs of temporal lobe epilepsy be subjected to appropriate electroencephalographic (EEG) examinations. However, we are not aware of a study estimating the actual prevalence of temporal lobe epilepsy in panic patients.

Possible sources of organic anxiety syndrome other than those mentioned above include pheochromocytoma, hypoparathyroidism, hyperparathyroidism, Cushing's syndrome, and substance abuse/dependence. Given the multitude of rare conditions that can cause anxiety or panic, how aggressive should one be in the routine medical workup in panic patients? To re-emphasize, panic patients are at increased risk for having medical disorders, disorders which are not necessarily related to panic. The presence of panic should not preclude appropriate medical evaluation; positive clinical findings should not be "written off" as being due to panic disorder. In our opinion, therefore, a thorough medical history, review of systems and physical examination, as well as laboratory tests including complete blood count (CBC) and differential thyroid function tests, liver function tests, serum calcium and phosphate urine analysis, urine drug screen, and an electrocardiogram (EKG) with rhythm strip would be a useful minimum screening assessment. Further tests, such as EEG, computerized tomography (CT) scan, ambulatory EKG, vestibular and audiological examinations, as well as referrals to appropriate medical specialists, could then be ordered based on the clinical findings.

Substance Abuse and Dependence

A frequent problem in panic disorder patients is alcohol abuse. Thyer and associates (1986) found that 27 percent of agoraphobics and 8 percent of panic disorder patients scored in the problem drinking range of the Michigan Alcoholism Screening Test. Similarly, Bibb and Chambless (1986) reported that alcohol dependence occurred in 12 percent of agoraphobic patients. The onset of problem drinking preceded agoraphobia by an average of one year. Alcohol was often used as self-medication.

Conversely, panic attacks are frequently found in alcoholics. Cox and colleagues (in press) found that 31 percent of inpatient alcoholics fulfilled diagnostic criteria for panic disorder and 13 percent reported being treated previously for panic attacks. In 40 percent, the panic attacks began before the onset of problem drinking. Most panickers reported using alcohol to relieve panic, a self-treatment believed by them to be quite effective.

Thus, clinicians should have a high index of suspicion for alcohol abuse or dependence when assessing patients with panic disorder. Other forms of drug abuse are also thought to contribute to panic, including marijuana abuse (Moran, 1986), caffeine abuse (Boulenger et al, 1984), and cocaine abuse (Aronson and Craig, 1986).

ASSESSMENT

The role of assessment in panic disorder, of course, depends on the purpose of one's inquiry. New questions often necessitate new assessment techniques before the questions can be answered. The clinician, however, usually is primarily concerned with three questions: those of diagnosis, severity, and effect of treatment.

Diagnosis involves the establishment of qualitative differences between patients and typically involves the classification of a large number of categorical data.

An alternative to diagnosis is a dimensional approach in which individuals are classified along a number of dimensions, such as anxiety, depression, and psychotism. While diagnoses are useful as shorthand behavioral descriptions and as hypothesis generators for further inquiry, dimensional approaches often do greater justice to atypical or mixed cases, such as anxious depressions (Strauss, 1973; Strauss et al, 1979). The dimensional approach, however, quickly becomes impractical when more than a few dimensions are considered.

Determining severity involves a quantitative assessment of a relatively limited number of dimensions relevant to the disorder being studied. Measurement of treatment effects involves comparing severity before and after treatment. In this section we will discuss assessment techniques necessary to determine diagnosis as well as severity; assessments pertaining to other types of questions (such as neuroendocrinology of panic, anxiety proneness) will not be covered here.

Diagnostic Interview Schedules

The delineation of specific criteria for psychiatric disorders, as exemplified by the early work on the Feighner criteria and research diagnostic criteria (RDC), culminating in the publication of the *DSM-III* and *DSM-III-R*, represents a trend toward increased precision in descriptive psychopathology and psychiatric diagnosis. Another expression of this trend is the recent development of structured and semi-structured interviews. Use of these instruments should serve to increase the reliability of psychiatric diagnosis, to increase the confidence in the diagnostic process, and to make comparisons across various research studies more meaningful.

The Anxiety Disorders Interview Schedule (ADIS; DiNardo et al, 1983) is a structured interview schedule designed specifically to differentiate among different anxiety disorders. The ADIS also has sections designed for the diagnosis of major depression and psychosis. In addition, the schedule incorporates the Hamilton Anxiety and Depression Scales, making it possible to obtain a quantitative assessment of the anxiety and depression dimensions. Barlow (1985) reported that the reliabilities for individual anxiety disorders was kappa = 0.91 for social phobia, 0.85 for agoraphobia with panic, 0.83 for obsessive compulsive disorder, 0.65 for panic disorder, 0.57 for generalized anxiety disorder, and 0.56 for simple phobia.

The ADIS has been updated to include *DSM-III-R* criteria (DiNardo et al, unpublished manuscript). Barlow (personal communication) reported that in the revised version of the ADIS, the reliabilities for generalized anxiety disorder and panic disorder were considerably improved, although the exact kappa coefficients are not available at this time. A potential drawback to the ADIS is that information necessary for the Axis I diagnoses other than anxiety disorders may be less than adequate, and Axis II personality disorders cannot be diagnosed.

The Structured Clinical Interview for *DSM-III-R* (SCID; Spitzer et al, in press) is a structured clinical interview recently revised to secure the information necessary to establish a broad spectrum of *DSM-III-R* diagnoses. The interview schedule lists all of the criteria necessary for accurate *DSM-III-R* diagnoses. Thus, by following the line of questioning, the interviewer is assured of conducting a thorough clinical interview. There are several different versions of this interview schedule, suitable for different purposes. There is the SCID-P (for inpatients when there is a need for differential diagnosis of a psychotic disorder); the

SCID-OP (for use in outpatient settings when psychotic disorders are presumed to be rare); and the SCID-NP (for use with subjects not identified as psychiatric patients). The major difference among these various versions pertains to the emphasis placed on questions regarding psychosis. An additional version, the SCID-II, can be used for evaluating 12 of the *DSM-III-R* personality disorders and can be used in conjunction with any of the other SCIDs.

One positive feature of the SCID is that there is a version that can be administered to a nonpatient group. Similarly, the ability to arrive at personality disorder diagnoses is an asset. However, at this time, there are no published data on reliability or on how well the different versions work with the populations for which they are designed.

A third structured interview, the *Diagnostic Interview Schedule* (DIS; Robins et al, 1981) was developed for use in the Epidemiologic Catchment Area (ECA) project. The DIS is highly structured and is suitable for use by clinicians or lay interviewers. It differs from the ADIS and SCID in that it is possible to derive diagnoses not only according to *DSM-III*, but also according to the Feighner criteria and RDC. There are now several versions of the DIS. The test-retest reliability and concordance between lay interviewers and psychiatrists for the anxiety disorders has not been very good. This is particularly true with respect to panic disorder, a problem which might be due to the fact that the interview schedule includes only one screening question for panic (see Robins, 1985, for a review of issues related to the use of structured interviews.

The use of structured interviews for the purpose of diagnosing panic disorder has certain positive as well as negative features. Issues of reliability, validity, sensitivity, and specificity must be addressed before the full utility of a given diagnostic schedule can be determined. The interview schedules discussed here differ with respect to how well the criteria for panic disorder are covered and how well the criteria for other diagnoses are addressed. At our clinic, we have found it helpful to use a semistructured interview, the Initial Evaluation Form, (Mezzich and colleagues, 1981) to obtain information pertinent for general psychiatric diagnosis; we then conduct a second interview, using the ADIS, for the final anxiety disorders diagnosis. We decided on the ADIS because of its published reliability data, because it comprehensively covers *DSM-III* criteria for anxiety disorders, because it provides quantitative estimates of anxiety and depression levels, and because it is relatively time-efficient.

Dimensional Approaches to Panic Assessment

Structured interviews are most useful for establishing a particular diagnosis but are not well suited for assessing various quantitative parameters of a disorder, or for assessing how these parameters change over time as a function of treatment. Anxiety, including panic anxiety, is multidimensional in nature, having behavioral, somatic/physiological, and cognitive dimensions. The somatic and cognitive features have repeatedly been found to account for most of the variance of anxiety (Barrett, 1972; Buss, 1962; Hamilton, 1959); for phobic conditions, however, behavioral avoidance is an equally important dimension.

It is not our purpose here to examine all of the instruments and methods used to assess anxiety and phobic states. Rather, we will focus on those instruments and strategies that have been developed recently and used in the study of the psychopathology of panic disorder, as well as in treatment outcome studies. We will begin by discussing various methods involving self-report.

INSTRUMENTS BASED ON SELF-REPORT. The difficulties inherent in using self-report inventories in psychiatric research are well documented. The requirements to properly construct and validate such an instrument are considerable. Yet, Agras and Jacob (1981) found such inventories to be among the most sensitive to changes over the course of treatment. Self-report inventories should be an integral part of efforts to assess panic disorder patients. We will not discuss several recently developed self-report inventories particularly relevant to panic disorder and/or agoraphobia.

Chambless and colleagues have developed three inventories highly relevant for the assessment of panic and agoraphobia. Two of these inventories, the Body Sensations Questionnaire (BSQ) and the Agoraphobic Cognitions Questionnaire (ACQ), were developed by Chambless and associates (1984). Together, the individual items of the scales also provide a comprehensive and clinically useful description of the phenomenology of panic/agoraphobia. The BSQ consists of 17 items measuring fear of bodily sensations, such as dizziness, nausea, and heart palpitations. The test-retest reliability of the BSQ was 0.67; the internal consistency as determined by Chrohnbach's alpha was .87. The ACQ is a 14-item questionnaire designed to measure agoraphobic cognitions, such as fear of passing out or of having a heart attack. Test-retest reliability was reported to be .79, with an internal consistency of .80.

The two inventories described above are focused on panic phenomenology. Inventories have also been developed to assess avoidance behavior. One such inventory is the Mobility Inventory for Agoraphobia (MI; Chambless et al, 1985). The MI consists of 27 items and provides measures of Avoidance Alone (AAL), Avoidance Accompanied (AAC) and Panic Frequency (PF). Test-retest reliability for AAL and AAC were consistently good over three to five days of retesting (ranging from .83 to .84). Panic frequency test-retest reliability was variable due to the highly variable nature of panic attacks (ranging from 0.65 to 0.87). There is also evidence of concurrent as well as construct validity. The MI has been found to be highly sensitive to changes occurring as a function of exposure treatment over a six-month period (Chambless et al, 1985) and a 12-month period (Goldstein, 1982).

Two other often used inventories for phobic avoidance are the Fear Questionnaire (FQ; Marks and Matthews, 1979) and the Fear Survey Schedule (FSS; Wolpe and Lang, 1964). The FSS is a general measure of fearfulness that can be used both as a quantitative index and as a clinical device to determine the presence or absence of certain fears. The FQ generates a total fear score as well as several subscores. Both instruments are widely used and considerable data are available on their usage (Mavissakalian, 1986).

ASSESSMENT OF COGNITIONS. Although cognitions have received less attention than somatic symptoms in the study of panic, it is clear that the cognitions of panic patients are extremely important in understanding the phenomenology of the disorder and in conducting treatment (Beck and Emery, 1985; Borkovec, 1985; Chambless et al, 1984). Cognitive events can be examined with structured self-report inventories such as the ACQ developed by Chambless and her colleagues. In addition, a number of methods may be employed to assess the occurrence of specific cognitions of panic patients and others. Several retrospective methods are available including self-statement inventories, thought-listing procedures, and a relatively new strategy known as post-performance videotape reconstruction (Schwartz and Garamoni, 1986). The post-performance videotape procedure is designed to assist the patients in recalling their thoughts during an episode of fear by replaying a videotape of the fear event.

Each of the measures of cognitive events has some limitation. Self-statement inventories, by virtue of providing the subject with a list of possible thoughts, may prompt overrecording. In contrast, thought-listing relies solely on the patient's memory and thus may lead to underreporting. The postperformance videotape procedures might be difficult to employ in treatment studies but would be ideal for the assessment of cognitions resulting from laboratory-induced panic.

ASSESSMENT OF THE BEHAVIORAL DIMENSION OF FEAR. The instruments described thus far have been based on patient self-report. In this section, we will consider the measurement of fear related behavior. Fear related behavior includes verbal or nonverbal expression of fear as well as avoidance behaviors.

Observational Measures of Panic Expression. Observer checklists constitute the main avenue for the measurement of behavioral fear expression. They have the advantage of producing data relatively unaffected by the patient's judgement or recollections. However, checklists have their own sources of bias. A discussion of such biases can be found in Harris and Lahey (1982a, 1982b). Ideally, checklists should be employed under double blind conditions.

One checklist that has been widely used in lactate infusion studies of panic is the Acute Panic Inventory (Liebowitz et al, 1984). This checklist consists of 17 items designed to assess the presence of panic symptoms. Such checklists can be valuable in the study of laboratory panic as well as naturally occurring panic. However, we are unaware of any reliability and validity data for this checklist. Thus, it should be employed with caution until such data are forthcoming.

Assessment of Avoidance Behavior. Observer checklists may also be used to assess avoidance behavior. Such measures are commonly employed in behavioral studies of phobic and anxiety states. They require the listing of appropriate behaviors and a trained observer. The use of such measures is particularly appropriate in measuring the effects of treatment.

Another method for assessment of avoidance behavior is the Behavioral Avoidance Test (BAT; Lang and Lasovick, 1963). The Behavioral Avoidance Test may be arranged in any number of ways. The basic strategy is to arrange for the patient to confront the feared stimuli in the laboratory or in the natural setting. The patient's behavior is then rated on a number of dimensions, including whether or not he or she avoided a particular step in the test. Self-report of fear as well as various behavioral and physiological indicants of anxiety (for example, sweating, tremors) may also be monitored.

PHYSIOLOGICAL ASSESSMENT. Psychophysiological correlates of anxiety include heart rate increases and changes in skin conductance (Agras and Jacob, 1981; Roth et al, 1986). Of these, heart rate has been used extensively, although the reliability of heart rate as a fear measure (Holden and Barlow, 1986) is not as high as for most self-report measures. Heart rate can increase dramatically during a panic attack. Lader and Matthews (1970) found sudden heart rate increases of 35–40 beats per minute during panic attacks recorded incidentally during a physiological experiment. Cohen and colleagues (1985) reported similar changes during panic attacks occurring during the course of relaxation training (relaxation-induced panic).

Interest in heart rate has recently been stimulated by the availability of monitors that can measure heart rate in the ambulatory patient. For example, Taylor and associates (1986) reported increases in heart rate by approximately 30 beats per minute during self-reported panic attacks in patients wearing an ambulatory heart rate monitor. However, the sensitivity and specificity of heart rate as a measure of panic was low. Only 58 percent of the panic attacks were accompanied by characteristic heart rate changes; conversely, only four of 14 heart rate episodes identified in the heart rate record as signifying panic actually were accompanied by subjective reports of panic. Thus, using verbally reported panic as a yardstick, the sensitivity of ambulatory heart rate was approximately 60 percent, and the specificity, 30 percent.

While heart rate is not a sufficient measure of anxiety or panic in isolation, it is of interest as the physiological component of the "triple response" measurement of fear (see Himadi et al, 1985, for a comprehensive review). The behavioral avoidance test constitutes a forum for studying the relationship between heart rate and the other two channels of anxiety, behavior and the subjective experience of fear. The relationship between heart rate and other measures of anxiety is not a simple one. It is often found that some patients improve behaviorally and also report less anxiety after treatment, while heart rate *increases*, indicating greater anxiety (Mavissakalian and Michelson, 1982). Such a pattern is called *desynchrony*. Desynchrony may prove to be a negative predictor of maintenance of treatment gains during follow-up (Mavissakalian, in press; Michelson and Mavissakalian, 1985).

Another research use of the tripartite assessment of fear in agoraphobia may be in the prediction of treatment response to different types of treatment. If such predictions were possible, then one could match patients with the appropriate treatment based on a pretreatment assessment. For example, Michelson (1986) classified agoraphobic patients into behavioral, cognitive, and physiological "reactors," depending upon which of the three dimensions was the most deviant before treatment, and assessed the effect of three different behavioral treatments within these three types. He found that individuals who had been assigned to the "consonant" treatment (that is, the one that was thought to more specifically address the most deviant dimension, such as relaxation therapy for the physiological reactors, or graduated exposure for the behavioral reactors) improved the most. A similar study was performed by Öst and colleagues (1984), however, with less clear-cut results.

SUMMARY AND CONCLUSIONS

The accumulation of data on panic disorder is reflected in the recent changes in the *DSM-III-R*. One major change was that of combining panic disorder and agoraphobia with panic into one major category. Furthermore, the differential diagnosis between panic disorder and other anxiety disorders also was sharpened; there continues to be debate, however, as to whether the distinction between panic disorder and other anxiety disorders is as clear-cut as implied in the *DSM-III-R*. The boundary between panic attacks in normals and panic disorder also remains somewhat arbitrary.

The new category of organic anxiety syndrome reflects the fact that anxiety can be a presenting complaint in a number of medical disorders. Furthermore, patients with panic disorder are at high risk for medical diseases unrelated to panic. Therefore, the presence of panic disorder should prompt appropriate medical evaluation. In addition, the possibility of drug and alcohol abuse or dependence, including caffeine abuse, should be considered. The causal nature of the relationship between panic disorder and medical disorders is still unknown.

The assessment of panic involves psychiatric diagnosis as well as quantitative evaluations of anxiety related variables. The quantitative assessment spans over the subjective (self-report), behavioral, and physiological dimensions. In the near future, we will most likely see refinements in the assessment of cognitive factors in panic, in biological correlates of panic, and in the assessment of anxiety proneness or factors predisposing an individual to develop panic.

REFERENCES

American Psychiatric Association: Diagnostic and Statistical Manual of Mental Disorders, Third Edition (DSM-III). Washington, DC, American Psychiatric Association, 1980

American Psychiatric Association: Diagnostic and Statistical Manual of Mental Disorders, Third Edition, Revised (DSM-III-R). Washington, DC, American Psychiatric Association, 1987

Agras WS, Jacob RG: Phobia: nature and measurement, in Phobia, Psychological and Pharmacological Treatment. Edited by Mavissakalian M, Barlow DH. New York, Guilford Press, 1981

Anderson DJ, Noyes R, Crowe RR: A comparison of panic disorder and generalized anxiety disorder. Am J Psychiatry 1984; 141:572-575

Aronson TA, Craig TJ: Cocaine precipitation of panic disorder. Am J Psychiatry 1986; 143:643-645

Barlow DH: The dimensions of anxiety disorders, in Anxiety and the Anxiety Disorders. Edited by Tuma HC, Maser J. Hillsdale NJ, Lawrence Erlbaum Associates, 1985

Barlow DH, Vermilyea J, Blanchard EB, et al: The phenomenon of panic. J Abnorm Psychol 1985; 94:320-329

Barlow DH, Blanchard EB, Vermilyea JA, et al: Generalized anxiety and generalized anxiety disorder: description and reconceptualization. Am J Psychiatry 1986; 143:40-44

Barrett ES: Anxiety and impulsiveness: toward a neuropsychological model, in Anxiety: Current Trends in Theory and Research, vol. 1. Edited by Spielberger CD. New York, Academic Press, 1972

Beck AT, Emery G: Anxiety Disorders and Phobias: A Cognitive Perspective. New York, Basic Books, 1985

Beitman BD, DeRosar L, Basha I, et al: Panic disorder in cardiology patients with atypical or non-anginal chest pain: a pilot study. Journal of Anxiety Disorders (in press)

Bibb JL, Chambless DL: Alcohol use and abuse among diagnosed agoraphobics. Behav Res Ther 1986; 24:49-58

Borkovec TD: Worry: a potentially valuable concept. Behav Res Ther 1985; 23:481-482

Boulenger JP, Uhde TW, Wolff EA, et al: Increased sensitivity to caffeine in patients with panic disorders. Arch Gen Psychiatry 1984; 41:1067-1071

Boyd JH: Use of mental health services for the treatment of panic disorder. Am J Psychiatry 1986; 143:1569-1574

Boyd JH, Burke JD, Gruenberg E, et al: Exclusion criteria of DSM-III: a study of co-occurrence of hierarchy-free syndromes. Arch Gen Psychiatry 1984; 41:983-989

Breier A, Charney DS, Heninger GR: Agoraphobia with panic attacks. Arch Gen Psychiatry 1986; 43:1029-1037

Buller R, Maier W, Benkert O: Clinical subtypes of panic disorder: their descriptive and prospective validity. J Affective Disord 1986; 11:105-114

Buss AM: Two anxiety factors in psychiatric patients. Journal of Abnormal and Social Psychology 1962; 65:426-427

Chambless DL, Caputo C, Bright P, et al: Assessment of fear in agoraphobics: The Body Sensations Questionnaire and Agoraphobics Cognitions Questionnaire. J Consult Clin Psychol 1984; 62:1090-1097

Chambless D, Caputo GC, Jasin SE, et al: The mobility inventory for agoraphobia. Behav Res Ther 1985; 23:35-44

Cohen AS, Barlow GH, Blanchard EB: Psychophysiology of relaxation-associated panic attacks. J Abnorm Psychol 1985; 94:96-101

Coryell W, Noyes R, House JD: Mortality among outpatients with panic disorder. Am J Psychiatry 1986; 143:508-510

Cox BJ, Norton GR, Dorward J, et al: The relationship between panic attacks and chemical dependencies. Addict Behav (in press)

Crowe RR: The genetics of panic disorder and agoraphobia. Psychological Development 1985; 2:171-186

Dietch JT: Diagnosis of organic anxiety disorders. Psychosomatics 1981; 22:661-669

DiNardo PA, O'Brien GT, Barlow DH, et al: Reliability of DSM-III anxiety disorder categories using a new structured interview. Arch Gen Psychiatry 1983; 40:1070-1074

Editorial: Panic Disorders: A separate entity? Lancet 1986; 1:1014-1015

Freedman AM, Dornbush RL, Shapiro B: Anxiety: here today and gone tomorrow. Compr Psychiatry 1981; 22:44-53

Fishman SM, Sheehan DV, Carr DB: Thyroid Indices in Panic Disorder. J Clin Psychiatry 1985; 46:432-433

Grunhaus L, Rabin D, Harel Y, et al: Simultaneous panic and depressive disorders: clinical and sleep EEG correlates. Psychiatry Res 1986; 17:251-259

Goldstein AJ: Agoraphobia: treatment success, treatment failures and theoretical implications, in Agoraphobia: Multiple Perspectives on Theory and Treatment. Edited by Chambless DL, Goldstein AJ. New York, Wiley 1982

Gordon AG: Otoneurological abnormalities in agoraphobia. Am J Psychiatry 1986; 143:807

Hamilton M: The assessment of anxiety states by rating. Br J Psychiatry 1959; 32:50-55

Harris FC, Lahey BB: Recording systems bias in direct observational methodology: A review and critical analysis of factors causing inaccurate coding behavior. Clinical Psychology Review 1982a; 2:539-556

Harris FC, Lahey BB: Subject reactivity in direct observational assessment: a review and critical analysis. Clinical Psychology Review 1982b; 2:523-538

Himadi WG, Boice R, Barlow DH: Assessment of agoraphobia: triple response measurement. Behav Res Ther 1985; 23:311-323

Holden A, Barlow DH: Heart rate variability recorded in vivo in agorophobics and nonphobics. Behav Ther 1986; 17:26-42

Jacob RG, Rapport M: Panic disorder, in Behavioral Treatment of Anxiety Disorders. Edited by Turner, SM. New York, Plenum, 1984

Jacob RG, Turner SM: Somatoform disorders, in Handbook of Psychopathology. Edited by Suther P, Adams HE. New York, Plenum, 1984

Jacob RG, Moller MB, Turner SM, et al: Otoneurological examination of panic disorder and agoraphobia with panic attacks: a pilot study. Am J Psychiatry 1985; 142:715-720

Kagan J, Reznick JS, Clarke C, et al: Behavioral inhibition to the unfamiliar. Child Dev 1984; 55:2212-2225

Katon W, Vitaliano PP, Russo J, et al: Panic disorder: spectrum of severity and somatization. J Nerv Ment Dis 1987; 175:12-19

Kathol RG, Turner R, Delahunt J: Depression and anxiety associated with hyperthyroidism: response to antithyroid therapy. Psychosomatics 1986; 27:501-505

Klein DF, Zitrin CM, Woerner M: Antidepressants, anxiety, panic and phobia, in Psychopharmacology: A generation of Progress. Edited by Lipton MA, DiMascio A, Killam KF. New York, Raven Press, 1978

Lader M, Mathews A: Physiological changes during spontaneous panic attacks. J Psychosom Res 1970; 14:377-382

Lang PJ, Lazovik AD: Experimental desensitization of a phobia. Journal of Abnormal and Social Psychology 1963; 66:519-525

Leckman JF, Merikangas KP, Pauls DL, et al: Anxiety disorders and depression: contradictions between family study and DSM-III convention. Am J Psychiatry 1983; 140:880-882

Liebowitz MR, Fyer AJ, Gorman JM, et al: Lactate provocation of panic attacks, I: clinical and behavioral findings. Arch Gen Psychiatry 1984; 41:764-770

Lindemann CG, Zitrin CM, Klein DF: Thyroid dysfunction in phobic patients. Psychosomatics 1984; 25:603-606

Mackenzie TB, Popkin MK: Organic anxiety syndrome. Am J Psychiatry 1983; 140:342-343

Marks IM, Mathews AN: Brief standard self-rating for phobic patients. Behav Res Ther 1979; 17:263-267

Mavissakalian M: The fear questionnaire: a validity study. Behav Res Ther 1986; 24:83-85

Mavissakalian M: Trimodal assessment in agoraphobia research: further observations on heart rate and synchrony/desynchrony. Journal of Psychopathology and Behavioral Assessment 1987; 9:89-98

Mavissakalian M, Michelson R: Patterns of psychophysiological change in the treatment of agoraphobia. Behav Res Ther 1982; 20:347-356

Mezzich JE, Dow JT, Rich CL: Developing an effective clinical information system for a comprehensive psychiatric institute, II: Initial Evaluation Form. Behavior Research Methods and Instrumentation 1981; 13:464-478

Michelson L: Treatment consonance and response profiles in agoraphobia: the role of individual differences in cognitive, behavioral and physiological treatments. Behav Res Ther 1986; 24:263-275

Michelson R, Mavissakalian M: Psychophysiological outcome of behavioral and pharmacological treatments of agoraphobia. J Consult Clin Psychol 1985; 53:229-236

Moran C: Depersonalization and agoraphobia associated with marijuana use. Br J Med Psychol 1986; 589:187-196

Norton GR, Dorward J, Cox BJ: Factors associated with panic attacks in nonclinical subjects. Behavior Therapy 1986; 17:239-252

Noyes R, Clancy J, Hoek P, et al: The prognosis of anxiety neurosis. Arch Gen Psychiatry 1980; 37:173-178

Noyes R, Anderson DJ, Clancy M, et al: Diazepam and propranolol in panic disorder and agoraphobia. Arch Gen Psychiatry 1984; 41:287-292

Noyes R, Crowe RR, Harris EL, et al: Relationship between panic disorder and agoraphobia. Arch Gen Psychiatry 1986a; 43:227-231

Noyes R, Reich J, Clancy J, et al: Reduction in hypochondriasis with treatment of panic disorder. Br J Psychiatry 1986b; 149:631-635

Ost LG, Jerremalm A, Jansson L: Individual response patterns and the effects of different behavioral methods in the treatment of agoraphobia. Behav Res Ther 1984; 22:697-707

Rachman S, Levitt K: Panics and their consequences. Behav Res Ther 1985; 23:585-600

Rapee RM: Distinctions between panic disorder and generalized anxiety disorder: clinical presentation. Aust NZ J Psychiatry 1985; 19:227-232

Reiman EM, Raichle ME, Robins E, et al: The application of positron emission tomography to the study of panic disorder. Am J Psychiatry 1986; 143:469-477

Rickels K, Schweizer EE: Benzodiazepines for treatment of panic attacks: a new look. Psychopharm Bull 1986; 22:93-99

Robins LN: Epidemiology: reflections on testing the validity of psychiatric interviews. Arch Gen Psychiatry 1985; 42:918-924

Robins LN, Helzer JE, Croughan J, et al: National Institute of Mental Health Diagnostic Interview Schedule. Arch Gen Psychiatry 1981; 38:381-389

Roth WT, Telch CB, Taylor CB: Autonomic characteristics of agoraphobia with panic attacks. Biol Psychiatry 1986; 21:1133-1154

Schwartz RM, Garamoni GL: Multitrain-multimethod issues in cognitive assessment: the case of assertiveness. Journal of Psychopathology and Behavioral Assessment (in press)

Schweizer E, Winokur A, Rickels K: Insulin-induced hypoglycemia and panic attacks. Am J Psychiatry 1986; 143:654-655

Shear MK, Kligfield P, Harshfield G, et al: Cardiac rate and rhythm in panic disorder patients. Am J Psychiatry (in press)

Sheehan DV, Ballenger J, Jacobsen G: Treatment of endogenous anxiety with phobic, hysterical and hypochondriacal symptoms. Arch Gen Psychiatry 1980; 37:51-59

Speir SE, Tesar GE, Rosenbaum JF, et al: Treatment of panic disorder with clonazepam. J Clin Psychiatry 1986; 47:238-242

Spitzer RL, Williams JBW: Proposed revisions in the DSM-III classification of anxiety disorders based on research and clinical experience, in Anxiety and the Anxiety Disorders. Edited by Tuma AH, Maser J. Hillsdale, NJ, Lawrence Erlbaum Associates, 1985.

Spitzer RL, Williams JBW: The Structured Clinical Interview for DSM-III-R. New York, Biometric Research Institute, New York State Psychiatric Institute (in press)

Strauss JS: Diagnostic models and the nature of psychiatric disorder. Arch Gen Psychiatry 1973; 29:445-449

Strauss JS, Gabriel R, Kokes RF, et al: Do psychiatric patients fit their diagnoses? J Nerv Ment Dis 1979; 167:105-113

Taylor CB, Sheikh J, Agras WS, et al: Ambulatory heart rate changes in patients with panic attacks. Am J Psychiatry 1986; 143:478-482

Thyer BA, Himle J, Curtis GC, et al: A comparison of panic disorder and agoraphobia with panic attacks. Compr Psychiatry 1985a, 26:208-214

Thyer B, Parrish R, Curtis G, et al: Ages of onset of DMS-III anxiety disorders. Compr Psychiatry 1985b; 26:113-122

Thyer BA, Parrish RT, Himle J, et al: Alcohol abuse among clinically anxious patients. Behav Res Ther 1986; 24:357-359

Turner SM, McCann BS, Beidel DC, et al: DSM-III classification of anxiety disorders: a psychometric study. J Abnorm Psychol 1986a; 95:168-172

Turner SM, Williams SL, Beidel DC, et al: Panic disorder and agoraphobia with panic attacks: covariation along dimensions of panic and agoraphobic fear. J Abnorm Psychol 1986b, 95:384-388

Turner SM, Beidel DC, Jacob RG: Assessment of panic, in Panic: Psychological Perspectives. Edited by Rachman S, Maser J. Hillsdale, NJ, Lawrence Erlbaum Associates (in press)

Tyrer P: Classification of anxiety. Br J Psychiatry 1984; 144:78-83

Uhde TW, Vittone BJ, Post RM: Glucose tolerance testing in panic disorder. Am J Psychiatry 1984; 141:1461-1463

Uhde TW, Boulenger JT, Roy-Byrne PP, et al: Longitudinal course of panic disorder: clinical and biological considerations. Prog Neuropsychopharmacol Biol Psychiatry 1985; 9:39-51

van Valkenburg C, Akiskal HS, Puzantian V, et al: Anxious depressions: clinical, family history and naturalistic outcome—comparisons with panic and major depressive disorders. J Affective Disord 1984; 67-82

Vittone BJ, Uhde T: Differential diagnosis and treatment of panic disorder: a medical model perspective. Aust NZ J Psychiatry 1985; 19:330-341

Volkow ND, Harper A, Swann AC: Temporal lobe abnormalities and panic attacks. Am J Psychiatry 1986; 143:1484-1485

von Korff MR, Eaton WW, Keyl PM: The epidemiology of panic attacks and panic disorder: results of three community surveys. Am J Epidemiol 1985; 122:970-981

Weissman MM, Leckman JF, Merikangas KR, et al: Depression and anxiety disorders in parents and children. Arch Gen Psychiatry 1984; 41:845-853

Weissman MM, Leaf PJ, Holzer CE, et al: Panic disorder and major depression: epidemiology, family studies, biologic, and treatment response similarities. Psychopharmacol Bull 1985; 21:539-541

Wolpe J, Lang P: A Fear Survey Schedule for use in behavior therapy. Behav Res Ther 1964; 2:27-30

Yager J, Young RJ: Nonhypoglycemia is an epidemic condition. N Engl J Med 1974; 291:907-908

Chapter 5

Pharmacologic Treatment of Panic Disorder

by Abby J. Fyer, M.D., and Diana Sandberg, M.D.

The discovery of effective drug treatments for panic disorder is one of the major recent advances in psychopharmacology.

Panic disorder is a common and disabling illness. Therefore, availability of successful treatment has had considerable impact on the lives of many individuals. In addition, the observation that drugs such as imipramine and phenelzine eliminate panic while having little or no effect on generalized anxiety has contributed significantly to the development of a qualitative as opposed to quantitative approach to the nosology and etiology of anxiety disorders.

A number of medications are now known to effectively block panic attacks. This chapter reviews the available efficacy data on these agents, clinical guidelines for their use, and management of common difficulties.

TREATMENT STRATEGY

The theoretical context of pharmacologic treatment of panic disorder is the three-phase structure of the illness delineated by Klein (1981). The core symptom is recurrent, unpredictable panic attacks. Repeated experience of unexpected panic attacks leads to worry or anticipatory anxiety about where and when the next one will occur. Often, to alleviate their distress, patients begin to avoid situations in which help might be unavailable or escape difficult should a panic attack occur. Events and places frequently associated with previous panic attacks are also avoided.

Treatment is a reversal of this process. The initial goal is to block the panic attacks with medication. Patients are then encouraged to reenter phobic situations in order to demonstrate to themselves that they will no longer panic. The persistent absence of panic in spite of a return to normal activity extinguishes anticipatory anxiety.

Most patients arrive at the psychiatrist's office frightened, confused, and with no idea of what is happening to them. Typically they have already had several medical evaluations—electrocardiogram (EKG), neurological workup, ENT exam, and so on, and been told that "there is nothing wrong." Since there is no tangible evidence of illness, family and friends can't understand what is going on and are often skeptical and impatient with the patient's fears.

The first steps in pharmacologic treatment of panic disorder are:

1. to undo this process by acknowledging the patient's experience (this often

The authors wish to thank Donald F. Klein, M.D., for his review of the manuscript, and Peggy Ray for editorial assistance.

includes educating the family and correcting their misrepresentation of the patient's behavior as lazy, exploitative, or childish)
2. to explain the three-stage development of the illness and how the treatment will reverse it
3. to develop a descriptive terminology for the patient's symptoms that is understood by both the doctor and the patient.

Developing an accurate terminology for the patient's symptoms is crucial for successful treatment. The drug is expected to block panic attacks but not anticipatory anxiety. If the patient doesn't know the difference or the doctor misunderstands, the result will be incorrect assessments of progress and mistaken dosage adjustments. The best way to establish a common terminology is to start from the patient's descriptions of specific episodes. The patient should be encouraged to give a detailed sequential account of thoughts, feelings, and physical symptoms that occur during the anxiety episodes (for example, Can you tell me about your last attack? The last time you avoided going out? Where were you? What happened first? and so on). The doctor can then translate the phenomenological descriptions into psychiatric terminology and explain to the patient *in terms of the patient's own symptoms* what psychiatrists mean by panic attack, anticipatory anxiety, and phobia. (For example, "What happened to you at the bus stop yesterday is what we call a panic attack because. . . .") These examples can be referred back to as treatment progresses in order to clarify interpretation of changes in the patient's condition.

It is particularly important to be very explicit in describing what is meant by panic attack. Some patients feel that to panic indicates weakness or loss of control and are therefore reluctant to use the label. They may call only their most severe episodes panic attacks. Milder attacks may be termed "anxiety" or "nervousness." In other cases, the term panic is used to describe a variety of intense emotional experiences ranging from temper tantrums to realistic fear.

Confusion about the distinction between panic and anticipatory anxiety is also common. One approach is to have the patient recall a recent situation in which he or she expected to panic but didn't, and compare it to one where panic did occur. Contrasting characteristics of anticipatory anxiety versus panic attack can be highlighted and used as an example to refer back to if necessary.

Another useful strategy that contributes to all aspects of history taking is to have a family member or friend who lives with the patient present for at least part of the interview and to involve them in the treatment. Patients are often embarrassed or ashamed of their actions and may tend to minimize or "forget" them. This is particularly true for avoidance behavior.

The next task is to ensure compliance in regular use of the prescribed antipanic medication. Most patients are intensely relieved when they find out that theirs is a common disorder which the doctor has frequently treated with great success. A number are further pleased to find out that the relatively simple procedure of daily medication will alleviate the cause of their distress. However, some panic patients have a variety of fears about medication that evolve from the symptoms of their illness. Awareness of these fears is helpful in getting the patient through the beginning phase of treatment, during which both symptoms and side effects are often evident despite medication.

A common fear is that medication will in some way affect the ability to control oneself and one's environment. Fear of loss of control is often a central panic attack symptom. By association, any threat to the patient's ability for self-control is seen as likely to either precipitate a panic or increase the possibility of loss of control during it. It is not uncommon for patients to report avoidance of alcohol and/or nonprescription drugs on these grounds. Psychiatric medications are also often feared since among many people they have acquired a reputation for being sedating and/or changing one's personality. Empathy, reassurance, and clarification from the physician will enable most patients to take medication regularly and without undue anxiety. However, severe cases may require added intervention. Strategies include: 1) arranging for the patient to talk with another panic patient who has previously taken the medication, and 2) arranging for participation in a short-term educational support group with other patients who are also currently starting medication.

Finally, the physician should be as available as possible during the initial phases of medication treatment. We routinely provide 24-hour telephone coverage. In our experience patients rarely call outside of normal working hours. However, the knowledge of the constant availability of help is important. It counteracts the panic-induced atmosphere of constant fearfulness and unpredictability in which most of these patients live.

Once the medication is started, somatic side effects can cause further difficulties. New and apparently inexplicable physical sensations are a prominent feature of panic attacks. For many panic patients, any strange sensation becomes associated with the imminent possibility of panic. The significance of all physical symptoms may become overrated so that minor complaints are seen as harbingers of medical disaster. The intensity of these responses can be contagious. If the physician does not have a clear assessment at the start of treatment of the patient's actual medical problems and the real medical difficulties that may arise from the medication, a vicious cycle of new symptoms, fruitless medical evaluations, and ultimately unnecessary premature termination of treatment may ensue. This problem and strategies for its management are further discussed below in the section on imipramine course of treatment.

ASSESSMENT OF DRUG EFFECT

Since antipanic medications block panic attacks but usually have little direct effect on anticipatory anxiety or avoidance, patients frequently report little or no improvement during the initial phase of pharmacologic treatment. It is therefore important in assessing drug effect to inquire specifically at each contact about each component of the illness: panic attacks, anticipatory anxiety, and avoidance.

Worry about the possibility of an attack and the limitations imposed by phobic behavior are often so overwhelming that the absence of panic attacks themselves can be overlooked during a particular week. Further, since the course of panic attacks is erratic, most patients derive no relief from a cessation of only a week or two. They remain on guard against the next episode that they are certain is just around the corner.

An extremely helpful strategy is to have patients keep a daily diary of their anxiety symptoms throughout the course of treatment. Panic attacks, avoidance due to fear of panic, and level of anticipatory anxiety are recorded on a daily basis. Review of the diary can guide medication dose changes by indicating the extent to which panics are blocked. A diary is also helpful in demonstrating to patients that in spite of persistent anticipatory fears, they are no longer having panic attacks and can therefore safely reenter phobic situations.

MEDICAL WORKUP

As in all of medicine, the medical evaluation of patients with probable panic disorder must be individualized. Panic patients, due to the multiplicity of their physical symptoms, are often convinced that they have a serious physical illness. Such convictions can be contagious, and physicians must use their best clinical judgment in deciding how far to pursue a medical workup. Many patients come to their psychiatric evaluation with an extensive medical workup in hand (one recent case of ours had even undergone nuclear magnetic resonance [NMR] scanning).

There are three major reasons to pursue medical testing: 1) to rule out other medical diagnoses masquerading as panic attacks; 2) to ensure that medication can be safely administered; and 3) to make sure concomitant illnesses are well cared for as part of routine good health care.

The major medical diagnosis to rule out is hyperthyroidism, which can present with episodic anxiety or agitation. Hypothyroidism should also be considered since panic attacks may have their onset during waning thyroid function. Every patient should have a T_3, T_4, and thyroid-stimulating hormone (TSH) test. If the patient does not respond to medication as expected, a thyrotropin-releasing hormone (TRH) test and basal metabolic rate should be considered.

Another common cause of anxiety to be ruled out is caffeinism or the use of diet pills or other sympathomimetics. Rarer causes to be considered are paroxysmal atrial tachycardia and pheochromocytoma. For patients with prominent depersonalization, derealization, and faintness, temporal lobe epilepsy is a rare possibility. For these patients as well as for those with unilateral symptoms, neurological consultation may be warranted.

Before beginning medication, we recommend that a physical examination, complete blood count (CBC), and routine blood chemistries be done unless the patient has had a normal result within the past year. Many advise patients beginning tricyclic drugs to have an EKG, since use of tricyclic antidepressants is contraindicated in individuals with preexisting bundle branch disease (Glassman and Bigger, 1981).

Persons with known medical illness or persons over the age of 40 usually warrant a discussion between the psychiatrist and the patient's internist.

Narrow angle glaucoma is also a contraindication to tricyclics; therefore, many clinicians believe that persons with a positive family history for narrow angle glaucoma should see an ophthalmologist prior to treatment.

Patients with a history of asthma should receive monoamine oxidase (MAO) inhibitors with caution, since sympathomimetics are incompatible and may be emergently necessary. Similar awareness applies to individuals with incompletely diagnosed severe allergic reactions who may also unexpectedly require epinephrine treatment. Nevertheless, if the MAO inhibitor is the best therapy for the patient's condition, and both the patient and his or her internist understand the pharmacology (including use of phentolamine if necessary), we believe the benefit is worth the minimal risk.

TRICYCLIC ANTIDEPRESSANTS

Imipramine

There are now six double blind placebo controlled trials that establish the antipanic efficacy of imipramine.

Klein (Klein and Fink, 1962; Klein, 1964) first noted the antipanic efficacy of imipramine during a study of its behavioral effects on hospitalized phobic anxiety patients. Imipramine blocked panic attacks but had little effect on anticipatory anxiety and phobic avoidance. A subsequent double blind study comparing imipramine, chlorpromazine, and placebo confirmed these results (Klein, 1967).

Klein and colleagues (Zitrin et al, 1978; Zitrin et al, 1980; Zitrin et al, 1983; Klein et al, 1983) replicated and extended these findings in two large studies that compared imipramine and placebo in the context of various forms of psychotherapy.

The first study (Zitrin et al, 1978; Zitrin et al, 1983) compared three treatments: imipramine plus behavior therapy, placebo plus behavior therapy, and imipramine plus supportive psychotherapy in patients classified as agoraphobics with panic ($N = 77$), simple phobics ($N = 81$), or mixed phobics ($N = 70$). The latter group had spontaneous panic attacks and circumscribed phobias. Dose of imipramine was on a fixed flexible schedule, with a maximum of 300 mg/day (mean, 204 mg/day).

The great majority of patients in all groups showed moderate to marked global improvement (50 to 90 percent depending upon the rater). In agoraphobics and mixed phobics (both groups experiencing spontaneous panic attacks), imipramine was significantly superior to placebo. There was no difference between behavior therapy plus imipramine and supportive psychotherapy plus imipramine, both resulting in high improvement rates (70 to 96 percent depending upon the rater). For specific phobics there were no significant differences between imipramine and placebo or behavior therapy and supportive therapy.

In the second study by this group, 76 agoraphobic women were treated with combined group exposure in vivo, and imipramine or placebo in a randomized double blind design (Zitrin et al, 1980). Groups of patients accompanied by a therapist would enter phobic situations; the course of therapy was 10 weekly sessions lasting three to four hours each.

The majority of patients in both groups showed marked to moderate improvement. However, imipramine was significantly superior to placebo on improvement measures for spontaneous panic, primary phobia, and global improvement. In addition, a much greater proportion of imipramine than placebo treated patients were markedly improved. For example, at 26 weeks, the percentage of patients with marked global improvement was 62 percent for the imipramine group and 29 percent for placebo. The figures for marked improvement in spontaneous panic and primary phobia were 63 percent versus 27 percent, and 78 percent versus 23 percent, respectively.

Three additional centers have now reported positive studies of efficacy of imipramine in panic patients.

The earliest (Ballenger, 1977; Sheehan et al, 1980) compared imipramine to both placebo and the MAO inhibitor phenelzine in treatment of patients with panic attacks and multiple phobias. All subjects also participated in supportive group psychotherapy. Length of treatment was 12 weeks. Both active drugs were significantly superior to placebo. Phenelzine was significantly superior to imipramine on scales for global improvement, social and work disability. The proportion of patients markedly as compared to moderately improved was also greater on phenelzine.

The two more recently completed investigations were conducted by groups whose previous work had focused mainly on behavioral treatment with agoraphobics (Marks et al, 1983; Mavissakalian and Michelson, 1986). Both are 2 × 2 designs contrasting imipramine versus placebo and therapist-aided exposure, plus systematic self-directed exposure versus systematic self-directed exposure alone.

In the first study, Marks and colleagues (1983) treated 45 agoraphobic patients for 28 weeks. Initial analyses of these data showed no imipramine effect and a slight advantage for the therapist-aided exposure condition. However, subsequent reanalyses found a significant positive effect of imipramine over placebo (Raskin, 1983).

Mavissakalian and Michelson (1986) studied 62 agoraphobics in a second trial of similar design but shorter duration (12 weeks). Imipramine was used in doses up to 200 mg/day (mean daily doses 80 in month 1, 125 in month 2, 123 in month 3). All treatment groups showed significant improvements in all outcome measures over time. Imipramine was significantly superior to placebo with respect to global outcome, reduction of subjective distress during excursions, and two phobic measures. As discussed in detail below (see Dosage), dosage of imipramine was an important variable. Seventy-five percent of patients on ≥150 mg/day imipramine had no or minimal symptomatology during the last month of treatment, as compared to 25 percent of patients on ≤125 mg/day imipramine and 29 percent of those on placebo.

UNRESOLVED ISSUES. While the studies discussed above confirm the clinical efficacy of imipramine in treatment of patients with panic attacks and multiple phobias, there are several questions that are unanswered or remain a subject of controversy in the literature.

One question is whether similar positive results will be seen in patients who suffer recurrent panic attacks without secondary phobias. The only controlled trial that addresses this issue is the 1983 study by Zitrin and colleagues, which included a group of mixed phobics (panic attacks plus circumscribed phobias). This group did as well or better than the agoraphobic patients on most outcome measures.

Two open trials also indicate a high degree of imipramine efficacy in this group. Gerakani and associates (1984) openly treated 10 *Diagnostic and Statistical Manual of Mental Disorders, Third Edition* (*DSM-III*; American Psychiatric Association, 1980) panic disorder patients with 50–300 mg/day of imipramine for 5–12 months. The eight patients who took imipramine for at least three weeks all had a complete remission of panic attacks. This study is unique in that a medical management model was used (that is, patients saw the doctor for approximately 15 minutes at each visit. There was no additional psychotherapy). Liebowitz and colleagues (1984) reported on open treatment of 43 patients (17 panic disorder and 26 agoraphobia with panic) with imipramine or desipramine as part of a study of pre- and posttreatment vulnerability to sodium lactate. Thirty-nine (91 percent) became panic free. There was no significant difference between clinical outcome or rate of panic on sodium lactate reinfusion for the two diagnostic groups.

A large body of clinical experience corroborates these findings. However, controlled trials now in progress will provide a definitive answer to the question.

A second issue is determination of the specific action by which imipramine produces improvement. One group of investigators (Klein, 1981; Zitrin, 1981) believes that imipramine has a direct panic blocking effect. However, most published controlled studies of imipramine have been in the context of some form of psychotherapy. Other researchers have therefore suggested that the concomitant treatment (usually behavioral or supportive psychotherapy) is responsible for the decrease in panic, anxiety, and phobia while imipramine either 1) exerts a nonspecific facilitatory effect (Telch et al, 1983) or 2) improves functioning by improving mood (Marks et al, 1983).

Several studies have attempted to address the effects of imipramine and psychotherapeutic interventions on panic and avoidance (Klein et al, 1987; Telch et al, 1985; Mavissakalian et al, 1983; Garakani et al, 1984). However, methodologic issues and/or small sample size limit interpretation of the data. Large controlled trials that document panic frequency and report outcome in terms of numbers of patients recovered are greatly needed.

In terms of clinical practice, the studies by Garakani and colleagues (1984) and Mavissakalian and colleagues (1983) suggest that imipramine plus medical management is an effective treatment for many panic disorder patients. Heuristically, the problem is more complicated and remains an unresolved area for future research.

Marks (1981) has been the main proponent of the theory that the differences between imipramine and placebo groups in various combined treatment studies were a result of imipramine's antidepressant action. Many agoraphobic patients, demoralized because of their limitations, exhibit some depressive symptomatology. Concurrent affective depressive disorder also occurs in some. Marks hypothesized that imipramine relieved depressive symptoms, enabling patients to make better use of psychotherapy. It was the psychotherapy (in particular, exposure) which eliminated anxiety, panic attacks, and phobias. However, a subsequent reanalysis of Marks' data found no relationship between imipramine-induced improvement and depression (Raskin, 1983).

Studies by other investigators have also shown that improvement of agoraphobia while taking imipramine is independent of the presence or severity of preexisting depressive symptomatology (Mavissakalian and Michelson, 1986; Zitrin et al, 1983).

DOSE.   In most patients, effective treatment of panic attacks requires 150–250 mg/day of imipramine. However, the range of effective doses is very wide (10–400 mg/day). In addition, panic patients tend to be both more sensitive to and more upset about the common side effects of tricyclic antidepressants. It is therefore best to start imipramine at a low dose and build slowly to a therapeutic range. We generally use a starting dose of 10 mg at bedtime and increase at a rate of 10 mg every 1–2 days so that the patient reaches 50 mg/day by the end of the first week. Usually patients will have no or few difficulties on this slow regimen and can be switched over at this point to a more rapid rate of increase (25 mg every 2–4 days, up to 150–200 mg/day). Patients who continue to panic at 200 mg/day are raised 25 mg every 2–4 days (or 50 mg every 4–7 days) to 300 mg/day. The exact rate of increase depends upon the patient's level of residual symptoms and side effects. Patients who continue to panic after two weeks on 300 mg/day and six weeks on imipramine should have an imipramine blood level and EKG. If EKG is normal, dose may be increased in 25 mg or 50 mg increments to 350 and then 400 mg/day if necessary. The EKG should be repeated after 1–2 weeks on 350 mg/day if further increase is anticipated. Guidelines for evaluation of imipramine effects on EKG are discussed below under section entitled Side Effects.

There is some disagreement about the dose of imipramine usually necessary for treatment of panic attacks. Klein (1984) and Zitrin (1981) have stressed the importance of trying up to 300 mg/day. Mean daily doses in their clinical trials are 200–225 mg/day. In contrast, other investigators (Mavissakalian and Michelson, 1986; Marks et al, 1983; Sheehan et al, 1980) used maximum daily doses of 150–200 mg, with means in the range of 125–160 mg/day.

The consistently better outcome reported by Klein and Zitrin (Zitrin et al, 1983; Klein et al, 1983) may reflect this willingness to use higher doses in some patients. Supporting this is a report by Mavissakalian and Perel (1985). In a comparative study of imipramine and placebo in conjunction with behavioral treatments (Mavissakalian and Michelson, 1986), 76 percent of subjects whose mean dose of imipramine in the last month of the study was 150 mg or more had no or minimal symptoms at termination. Only 23 percent of subjects on 125 mg/day or less of imipramine had a similarly good outcome.

The few studies correlating plasma imipramine levels and clinical outcome have had inconsistent results. Mavissakalian and colleagues (1984) found a positive relationship between imipramine, but not desipramine, levels and clinical outcome in 15 agoraphobics treated with imipramine and behavior therapy. In contrast, Ballenger (1986) found no significant differences in clinical outcome between two groups of panic disorder patients maintained at two different serum levels (100–150 ng/ml and 200–250 ng/ml) of imipramine plus its principal metabolite, desipramine. Several case reports have also suggested that effective antipanic treatment can be seen in conjunction with very low imipramine plasma levels. Further studies are indicated. However, at present there is no indication that routine plasma levels are useful in the treatment of panic.

COURSE OF TREATMENT. There are several types of difficulties sometimes encountered in starting panic patients on imipramine. If correctly assessed these difficulties are almost always transitory and do not interfere with positive outcome. However, frequently a mistaken interpretation of the patient's condition leads to premature unnecessary termination of treatment. These distinctions are important, since *inadequate dosage and premature termination of medication trials are probably the major causes of failure in tricyclic antidepressant (TCA) treatment of panic patients.* Therefore, before describing the usual course of response, we discuss these situations here in some detail.

A small percentage of panic patients (about 15 percent) (Zitrin et al, 1981) have what is known as a "hypersensitivity" response to imipramine. This is characterized by insomnia, a sense of inner agitation, and the feeling of "jumping out of my skin." A number of patients also report flushing and sweating.

This response usually occurs within 24 hours of the critical dose being reached. Its cause is not known, though there is some speculation that it may be related to the serotonergic system (Gorman et al, in press). If a hypersensitivity response occurs, the dose of imipramine should be decreased until the syndrome resolves. In some individuals, the lowered dose will also be effective in blocking panics. However, others will continue to panic. In these cases, a small increase in dose should be tried after an interval of several days to a week. Often a habituation-like effect occurs and patients are able to tolerate a dose they were previously hypersensitive to. Further increases can be made at a similar slow rate until panics are blocked.

A second group of patients will metabolize the drug very slowly and have a disproportionately high level of side effects to a given dose. This is relatively uncommon and is not specific to panic patients. Usually the side effects complained about are anticholinergic (dry mouth, sweating, constipation, urinary retention, difficulty with visual accommodation). If this is suspected the dose is reduced and confirming evidence obtained through imipramine plasma level. If the patient cannot tolerate an effective antipanic dose of imipramine, then one approach is to use adjunctive urecholine. Alternatively, the patient can be switched to either a less anticholinergic TCA (for example, desipramine) or an MAOI or alprazolam.

The third and most common difficulty is an anxious overreaction to the usual mildly uncomfortable side effects of imipramine. Patients who experience recurrent panic attacks often develop both hypochondriacal fears and an overawareness of somatic symptoms. In this setting, a slight imipramine-induced tachycardia, which might be overlooked by another patient, becomes a symptom of impending heart failure. Any unusual sensation becomes intolerable since it is associated with a panic attack and therefore with the fear of dying, losing control, or going crazy. This situation is, of course, exacerbated by the fact that with imipramine (and MAO inhibitors) patients experience side effects but little clinical improvement during the first two weeks of treatment.

Often the doctor's response to this type of patient unintentionally escalates the situation. This usually happens in one of two ways. A common approach used by physicians is a scientifically appropriate dismissal of the clinical significance of the symptoms and a blanket assurance of eventual recovery. However, with many panic disorder patients this is unproductive, since it only serves to reevoke their previous experience of having panic attacks disregarded at numerous doctor visits, which ended in the mistaken diagnosis of "nothing wrong." On the other hand, these patients can be so persistent and agitated that their hypochondriasis and fear become contagious. The doctor may find himself ordering a variety of tests to rule out conditions that were often *already* eliminated *before* the patient started treatment. This insecurity can be communicated to the patient, setting up a vicious cycle of increased anxiety and frustration. Unnecessary discontinuation of medication often occurs at this point.

Effective management depends on the particular patient. However, several frequently applicable strategies are described here.

A simple and extremely helpful procedure is to arrange for the patient to speak with others who have undergone the same treatment and had a positive outcome. Most individuals find this enormously reassuring. Unlike the doctor, the fellow patient does not have any apparent vested interest in promoting pill taking. Further, a fellow patient understands what it's *really* like to be in this position. Some clinics and self-help groups routinely assign new patients to 1) a "partner" who is slightly further along in the program, or 2) an educational support group whose members are all at varying stages of treatment. In one program we know of, partners talk on the phone while taking nightly medication, then check with each other later to ensure there have been no subsequent ill effects.

Another technique is to use very low doses of alprazolam (.25–.5 four times daily) or clonazepam (.25–.5 twice daily) in conjunction with imipramine during the first 3–4 weeks of treatment. High potency benzodiazepines appear to have a very rapid (four to seven days) onset of antipanic action. Relatively low doses of these drugs will often "take the edge off" of a patient's symptoms. This in turn may make both the side effects and fears related to taking medication more tolerable. Once the imipramine takes effect the benzodiazepine can usually be tapered without difficulty.

It is also possible for some patients, through experience and discussion with the physician, to develop a self-critical capacity which gradually enables them to modify this aspect of their behavior. In most cases this is achieved only during a second or third episode. However, since panic disorder is usually a recurrent episodic illness, and since an overanxious hyperalert response style often pervades other areas of the patient's life, this capacity can be extremely helpful to both the patient and his doctor and is worth the effort to cultivate.

The antipanic effect of imipramine usually starts about the third week on medication. Often the first sign is the patient's report of a partially aborted panic attack: "It seemed about to start but suddenly it just went away." Following this there usually will be a gradual reduction in frequency and intensity of episodes as the dose is increased. Panic attacks tend to have an irregular pattern of occurrence (Uhde et al, 1985). Therefore, during the later phases of treatment it is sometimes hard to tell whether a panic-free interval between visits is due to blockage by the drug or to the irregular rhythm of the illness. One approach is to have the patient test the drug effect by entering situations which, in their past experience, were almost always associated with a panic attack. However, patients are at times extremely demoralized by recurrent attacks. For some, even a single panic attack may lead to persistent renewed anxiety and/or avoidance. In these cases it is probably better (provided side effects are not problematic) to use an alternative strategy of raising the medication slightly (10–15 percent) above the level at which a patient became panic free (for example, for a patient who became panic free at 150, raise to 175; for one who did so at 250, raise to 275 or 300).

SIDE EFFECTS. The usual side effects of imipramine are dry mouth and constipation. Other less common effects are increased sweating, orthostatic hypotension, slowness of visual accommodation (blurred vision), moderate weight gain, and cardiac conduction delays.

Management of dry mouth, constipation, and blurred vision is generally symptomatic. However, substitution of a less anticholinergic TCA (for example, desipramine) may also reduce these side effects. Increased sweating can be an embarrassing, uncomfortable, and difficult to control symptom. There is no specific antidote. In severe cases, a change to another TCA, an MAO inhibitor, or alprazolam may be necessary. Nortriptyline may be less likely to cause orthostatic hypotension than imipramine. Therefore, a trial of this drug may be merited in patients for whom this side effect is severe. Otherwise the management of orthostatic hypotension on imipramine is similar to that discussed in detail in the section on MAO inhibitors below. A small number of individuals develop prolongation of PR and QRS intervals on their EKG. Clinically significant increases are rarely seen in patients who do not have preexisting conduction delays or other cardiac disease. Increases are usually dose dependent. Discontinuation of imipramine (or other TCA) is usually recommended if PR or QRS prolongation is equal to or greater than 30 percent of baseline value (Glassman and Bigger, 1981).

DISCONTINUATION AND FOLLOW-UP. Systematic studies of optimal length of imipramine treatment for panic patients have not been carried out. However, several reports (Zitrin et al, 1981; Zitrin et al, 1980; Garakani et al, 1984) indicate that most patients may continue to improve for at least six months and in many cases up to a year.

We recommend a minimum of six months of continuous treatment. Usually we begin gradual discontinuation of imipramine at the earliest point between 6 and 12 months on drugs, when the patient has returned to, and shown assurance in, his or her normal level of activity for 6 months. If relapse occurs the patient should be restarted on medication and taper reattempted in another six months.

Discontinuation of imipramine is usually at a rate of 25–50 mg/day unless a more rapid taper is required for medical reasons. In some cases a more gradual reduction is used because it is psychologically acceptable to the patient. Withdrawal symptoms are not usually seen during imipramine taper; however, in a small number of patients, a transitory flu-like syndrome (Kramer et al, 1961; Dilsaver and Greden, 1984) accompanies abrupt discontinuation of tricyclic antidepressants. If this occurs, the dose should be reraised and a more gradual taper undertaken.

Only three follow-up studies are available. Results are contradictory and inconclusive.

Zitrin and Klein (1983) reported a relapse rate of 19 to 30 percent in patients who had been at least moderately improved after 6 months of treatment on imipramine and behavioral or supportive psychotherapy and who were followed for two years after discontinuation of medication. Relapse was defined as the return of avoidance behavior. In contrast, Sheehan and colleagues (personal communication) found that over 70 percent of subjects treated for six months with imipramine or phenelzine relapsed after being taken off the drug. However, in this study, the definition of relapse was any return of unexpected anxiety or avoidance which led the patient to request restarting of medication on at least two separate occasions.

Cohen and colleagues (1984) reported a two-year follow-up of 40 of the 45 agoraphobics who had participated in a treatment study comparing imipramine versus placebo, and therapist-aided exposure versus relaxation (Marks et al, 1983). A comprehensive criterion for relapse is not given. The authors state that at follow-up all groups remained significantly improved from pretreatment. There were no significant between-group differences with respect to clinical condition or degree of improvement. Significant placebo versus imipramine and relaxation versus exposure differences were not found. Mean scores on severity of spontaneous panics were 1.1 for imipramine and 1.8 for placebo (8 = several a·day and 0 = none) as compared to 3.1 and 3.3 at pretreatment. The number of patients panic-free or relapsed is not stated. History of further treatment was assessed from both subjects and their family doctors. No between-group differences were found. However, the authors do not state how many subjects reentered treatment.

Clomipramine

Clomipramine is a tricyclic antidepressant not currently marketed in the United States but widely used in Europe, Canada, and South America for treatment of depression and anxiety disorders. Two small controlled studies (Karabanow, 1977; Escobar and Landbloom, 1976) and a number of open trials (Colgan, 1975; Waxman, 1975; Carey et al, 1975; Beaumont, 1977) conducted during the 1970s suggested that clomipramine was an effective treatment for agoraphobia. However, interpretation of these results is limited by small sample size, comorbidity for other psychiatric disorders, and absence of both operationalized diagnostic criteria and specific panic attack assessments.

Recent open trials with patients who meet *DSM-III* criteria for panic disorder or agoraphobia with panic attacks support these earlier findings and indicate that low dose clomipramine may be an effective and well tolerated antipanic agent.

Gloger and colleagues (1981) treated 20 patients who met *DSM-III* criteria for panic disorder (PD) (N = 8) or agoraphobia with panic attacks (PDA) (N = 12) with clomipramine up to 100 mg/day for 8 weeks. Seventy-five percent of the subjects in both diagnostic groups were asymptomatic at week eight. Another 15 percent had only mild symptoms.

Grunhaus and associates (1984) administered clomipramine 25–150 mg/day to 20 subjects with either PD or PDA. At eight weeks, 17 (85 percent) of the 20 had "none or minimal symptoms."

Caetano (1985) also reported positive results in the majority of 22 panic patients openly treated with clomipramine 10–50 mg/day. However, subjects in this trial were allowed to continue previously taken benzodiazepines whose amount and frequency of dose were not specified.

Results of these trials are very promising; however, larger placebo controlled trials as well as comparative trials with imipramine and phenelzine are needed.

DOSAGE, COURSE OF TREATMENT, AND SIDE EFFECTS. Panic patients appear to have a particular sensitivity to clomipramine that is not seen in patients with depressive or obsessive compulsive disorders. Successful treatment of panic attacks may not require doses of clomipramine as high as those usually used in other groups. Gloger and colleagues (1981) and Grunhaus and colleagues (1984) reported that 45 percent and 65 percent of their respective samples required 50 mg/day or less. Mean daily dose in Caetano's trial was 26.4 mg.

In addition, both Gloger and Caetano noted that a number of patients had exacerbations of panic symptoms during the first two weeks of treatment on doses of 25 mg/day or greater. Caetano recommends a starting dose of 5 mg/day followed by slow, carefully monitored increases (increments of ≤ 10 mg are best). The beginning of antipanic efficacy was noted to be in the second week of treatment.

Higher doses of clomipramine are often associated with multiple uncomfortable side effects (Rapoport and Ismond, 1982; Insel et al, 1983). However, the lower dosage requirement observed for panic patients may circumvent this difficulty. None of the three recent trials reported dropouts due to side effects. However, specific side effect frequencies were not reported.

Other Tricyclic Antidepressants

Clinical experience and numerous case reports suggest that other tricyclic antidepressants may have antipanic effects similar to those of imipramine and clomipramine. However, controlled studies have not been reported.

Two investigators have described systematic use of desipramine. Lydiard (1985) found desipramine to be an effective antipanic agent in a small open trial. Liebowitz and colleagues (1984), in a study of the effects of medication treatment on vulnerability to sodium lactate-induced panic, used desipramine as a second choice drug in those patients who could not tolerate imipramine. Desipramine was as effective as imipramine both clinically and in blocking lactate-induced panic. However, the mean dose of desipramine was somewhat higher (271 mg/day versus imipramine 178 mg/day).

MONOAMINE OXIDASE INHIBITORS

Another class of drugs effective in blocking panic attacks is the monoamine oxidase inhibitors (MAOIs). The most commonly used MAOI is the hydrazine derivative, phenelzine (Nardil). Other available MAOIs are the hydrazine derivative, isocarboxazid (Marplan), and the nonhydrazine, tranylcypromine (Parnate). Eutonyl is another MAOI that is used only to treat hypertension.

These drugs were first developed as antidepressants. Early investigators, including West and Dally (1959) and Sargant and Dally (1962), noted that iproniazid especially helped "anxious" depressives. Later, Robinson and colleagues (1973) and Ravaris and colleagues (1976) observed that their nonendogenous depressives with prominent anxiety symptoms had significantly greater improvement in anxiety symptoms on phenelzine 60 mg/day than on placebo. These depressed patients as described in 1959 by West and Dally were characterized by prominent anxiety and phobic features, emotional overreactivity, self-reproach, fatigue, initial insomnia, reverse diurnal variation, poor electroconvulsive therapy (ECT) response, and adequate premorbid personality.

This led several researchers to investigate the efficacy of MAOIs in anxiety disorders, including Tyrer and associates (1973), Lipsedge and co-workers (1973), Mountjoy and Roth (1974), and Solyom and colleagues (1973). These studies are well summarized by Klein and associates (1980). They all showed either no difference between the MAOI and placebo, or a suggestion of MAOI effectiveness for panic but not for avoidance. The studies suffered from low dosages, short treatment periods, and mixed diagnostic groups (that is, social phobics and simple phobics included in sample). Nor did they include adequate measures to differentiate the treatment response of the various components of the agoraphobic syndrome, including phobic avoidance, anticipatory anxiety, and panic attacks.

The first placebo controlled, double blind comparison of imipramine versus phenelzine was undertaken in the mid-1970s (Ballenger et al, 1977; Sheehan et al, 1980). The study was a 12-week trial of 150 mg imipramine versus 45 mg phenelzine, versus placebo in a sample of 57 agoraphobic patients. It showed marked benefits over placebo for both drugs. Phenelzine was somewhat more efficacious than imipramine on disability and avoidance scales, and phenelzine had fewer side effects.

There is continued interest regarding the interface between panic disorder and depression. In 1982, Paykel and colleagues compared amitriptyline and phenelzine in depressives and found phenelzine superior for patients who also had an anxiety disorder.

Liebowitz and associates (1985) conducted a study of 120 patients meeting criteria for atypical depression. They found that a lifetime history of panic attacks predicts high MAOI response, moderate TCA response, and poor placebo response. Patients without a history of panic responded moderately well to all three drugs. The criteria for atypical depression include: 1) meets criteria for Research Diagnostic Criteria (RDC) major, minor, or intermittent depressive disorder; 2) maintains mood reactivity while depressed; 3) two of the following: increased appetite or weight gain while depressed; oversleeping or spending more time in bed while depressed; severe fatigue to the point of a sensation of leaden paralysis, or extreme heaviness of arms or legs while depressed; and hypersensitivity to rejection as a trait throughout adulthood.

Patients were randomized separately according to whether or not they had a lifetime history of panic attacks. Each group was randomized to imipramine up to 300 mg/day versus phenelzine up to 90 mg/day versus placebo. The outcome strongly suggests that atypical depressives with a history of panic attacks respond preferentially to MAOIs.

Treatment

Phenelzine is begun at 15 mg daily in the morning for three days, followed by 30 mg in the morning for four days, followed by 45 mg each morning for one week. The target symptom is the panic attack. If at the end of a week on 45 mg the patient continues to have panic attacks, the dose should be raised to 60 mg and held there for two weeks. Again, if the patient is not panic free, one can progress to 75 mg each morning, and one week later, if necessary, to 90 mg per day. Our experience is that once a patient is panic free, support and encouragement are enough to get the patient to enter phobic situations, redevelop a sense of mastery, and rapidly become mobile and free of anticipatory anxiety. However, the addition of a benzodiazepine may be useful in helping patients with high levels of residual anticipatory anxiety to overcome their reluctance.

Parnate is begun at 10 mg in the morning, and may be raised if necessary by 10 mg per week to 60 mg/day. If the drug is tolerated well and the patient does not respond, it may be raised to 80 mg/day.

Side Effects

Common autonomic side effects include dry mouth, constipation, blurred vision, sweating, tremor, and palpitations. Urinary hesitancy occurs at higher doses, and may progress to retention, especially if the patient has prostatic hypertrophy. A variety of sexual side effects may develop, including difficulty with erection and ejaculation, anorgasmia, and loss of desire. Cyproheptadine (Periactin) is often helpful in restoring sexual functioning.

A stimulant effect is often seen. This includes insomnia (for this reason the drug is given in the morning), but may progress to overtalkativeness, increased aggression, impaired judgment, hyperactivity, euphoria, irritability, and frank hypomania. Unlike the tricyclic induced hypomania, phenelzine induced hypomania rarely progresses to mania and may be treated by careful observation and dose reduction or, if necessary, discontinuation of the drug. Small doses of neuroleptic are rarely necessary. If insomnia is the only problem, we have found trazodone 50 mg just before sleep to be quite effective. One may alternately add a benzodiazepine. Occasionally a patient is sedated rather than activated by phenelzine. This patient requires evening dosing.

Another more troublesome side effect is orthostatic hypotension. A good practice is to ask patients whether they salt-restrict themselves. In its milder forms it is easily controlled by adding salt to food or taking salt tablets. In patients without cardiac contraindication, Florinef, a mineralocortoid, may be quite effective. Usual doses are 0.1 mg one to three times daily. In refractory cases of orthostatic hypotension, small doses of Ritalin or dextroamphetamine (2.5 mg/day to start) can be safely added and can be highly effective (Feighner et al, 1985).

Phenelzine can also induce pyridoxine (vitamin B_6) deficiency (Stewart et al, 1984). Some clinicians routinely add 150–300 mg/day of this vitamin to the regimen; others wait for the symptoms of pyridoxine deficiency to develop. Usual symptoms include electric shock sensations in the limbs and numbness. Carpal tunnel syndrome is a rare complication. Doses of pyridoxine higher than 300 mg per day are not recommended, as they have been associated with neurotoxicity.

Peripheral edema is another rare but problematic side effect of phenelzine. Support hose and diuretics may be helpful, but it is our experience that this development usually necessitates discontinuation of the drug.

A more serious and, again, rare, side effect of the hydrazine derivative MAOIs, including phenelzine, is hepatic toxicity. Iproniazid, the first MAOI investigated, was withdrawn from the market due to several cases of fatal hepatic necrosis. Occasionally patients on phenelzine develop elevated liver function tests. Discontinuation of the drug usually leads to fairly rapid normalization. However, if a hydrazine compound is given again, elevations will recur. Therefore, MAOI treatment in these cases is not recommended.

Of course, the side effect of most concern with MAOIs is the hypertensive crisis. This sudden rise in blood pressure is due to inhibition of gut monoamine oxidase which usually inactivates dietary tyramine. In order to avoid tyramine's pressor effect, foods containing tyramine must be strictly avoided, along with many medications (see Table 1). Cheese and red wine are the foods with the highest tyramine content, but any preserved, fermented, or aged protein can cause a reaction. Demerol is strictly contraindicated. Sympathomimetics are also traditionally forbidden although, as discussed, Feighner has reported their safe use. Patients should be given a wallet card stating they are on the drug and cautioned to inform all doctors *including* their dentists, since epinephrine (or noreprinephine) may be injected with a local anesthetic.

The hypertensive reaction is heralded by a severe throbbing headache which may be associated with nausea, vomiting, stiff neck, and high blood pressure. The incidence of such paroxysmal headaches is about 2.1 percent. More rarely (0.3 to 0.5 percent), this will progress to severe hypertension, chest pain, palpi-

Table 1. Instructions to Patients on MAO Inhibitors (Nardil, Parnate, Eutonyl)

1. *Foods and beverages to avoid*
   — Matured or aged cheeses such as blue, Swiss, cheddar, American, as well as processed cheeses and spreads, are particularly to be avoided. However, cottage, cream, or farmer cheese is permissible.
   — Red wines (Chianti in particular) and rose wines
   — Sherry, vermouth
   — Beer
   — Marmite, Bovril and similar yeast or meat extracts (beware of drinks, soups, or stews made with these products)
   — Yogurt not made by a reliable manufacturer
   — Broad bean, fava bean, or Chinese pea pods
   — Banana skins and overripe bananas
   — Any meat, fish, poultry or other protein food that is not fresh, freshly canned, or freshly frozen. (This includes game meats, offal, lox, salami, sausage, corned beef, and liver, including pate.)
   — Meat prepared with tenderizers
   — Pickled herring and pickled lox
   — Any food that previously produced unpleasant symptoms

2. *The following foods and beverages should be used with moderation, as they are occasionally associated with adverse reaction*
   — Caffeinated beverages, such as coffee, tea, cola
   — Chocolate
   — Alcoholic beverages of any kind*
   — Avocados
   — Soy Sauce
   *Distilled liquors (vodka, gin, rye, Scotch) will not produce a hypertensive reaction but will interact with Nardil to produce more rapid intoxication.

3. *Medications to avoid*
   — Cold tablets or drops
   — Nasal decongestants (tablets or drops)
   — Hay fever medication
   — Sinus tablets
   — Weight reducing preparations—pep pills
   — Anti-appetite medicine
   — Asthma inhalants
   — Demerol
   — Other antidepressants
   — Epinephrine in local anesthesia (includes dental)

4. Do not take any medicine, drugs, proprietary preparations (including cough and cold cures), or any other medication whatever without consulting your doctor.

5. Follow these instructions (and carry this with you) all the time while taking MAO inhibitors and continue to do so for two weeks after stopping medication.

tations, and loss of consciousness. The incidence of progression to intracranial bleeding is very rare, with the fatality rate less than one in 100,000 (Klein et al, 1980).

Many clinicians routinely give patients who are taking MAO inhibitors 100 mg of oral chlorpromazine to carry with them and use before proceeding to the emergency room in case of a severe headache or known dietary error. The alpha blocking properties of chlorpromazine will counteract the hypertension while the patient is in transit. The treatment of choice for hypertensive reactions is intravenous phentolamine, a pure alpha antagonist.

Discontinuation and Follow-up Studies

In responders, discontinuation should be at a psychologically acceptable pace for the particular patient. Nonresponders or patients discontinuing due to side effects may be tapered at 15–30 mg/day phenelzine (or another, equivalent, MAOI). There is risk of hypertensive crisis for two weeks after discontinuation of the drug, so the diet *must be continued* during this time.

It should also be kept in mind that the *different MAOIs are incompatible*. Therefore, to avoid a hypertensive crisis, a 10–14 day washout period is required before switching from one to the other.

Two discontinuation studies have been reported. The study by Sheehan (personal communication) is discussed above in the section on Discontinuation and Follow-up studies of imipramine. A second study by Kelly (1970) retrospectively assessed outcome in a large series of phobic anxiety patients treated with phenelzine. Thirty percent of patients who had been well for at least one year on medication were able to taper without recurrence. However, the length of follow-up is not stated. A second 30 percent relapsed during taper. The remaining subjects were advised not to attempt taper.

BENZODIAZEPINES

Alprazolam

Currently available data indicate the triazolobenzodiazepine alprazolam has an antipanic efficacy comparable to that of imipramine and phenelzine. Its rapid onset of action and low side effect profile make it a potential therapeutic advance. However, as discussed below, the frequent occurrence of relapse and withdrawal symptoms during discontinuation constitute problems in the use of this drug.

Three controlled trials have reported that alprazolam is superior to placebo in the treatment of panic patients. Chouinard and colleagues (1982) studied 20 patients with *DSM-III* panic disorder in an 8-week trial. Eight of the 14 patients on active drug as compared to one of six on placebo had a moderate to excellent response in four weeks. This study was limited by its small sample size and the lack of specific ratings on occurrence of panic. However, its findings are confirmed and extended by preliminary results from a multicenter study initiated by the Upjohn Company (Ballenger, 1986). Five hundred sixty patients with *DSM-III* panic disorder or agoraphobia with panic attacks were randomized under double blind conditions to alprazolam or placebo and treated for eight weeks. Eighty-eight percent of alprazolam-treated, but only 38 percent of those on placebo, were at least moderately improved at week 8. Alprazolam had a significantly greater effect than placebo in reducing panic attacks, phobic avoidance, and social and work disability.

Sheehan and associates (1984a) conducted a 10-week 4-cell trial of 108 patients with agoraphobia and panic attacks. Results indicated that alprazolam, imipramine, and phenelzine were comparable and significantly more effective than placebo in producing improvement. These data were presented but are not yet published in full, so that a more detailed review of the findings is not possible at this time.

Four reported open trials have also had positive results. Alexander and Alexander (1986) reported on 27 retrospectively rated panic patients treated with alprazolam in a private practice setting for 4–14 weeks. Eighty-five percent became panic free within the first week of treatment. Liebowitz and colleagues (1986) reported a 73 percent response rate in an open 12-week trial of alprazolam in 30 panic patients. Fifteen of the 22 were panic free for the last three weeks of the study. The remaining seven had occasional panics which were less frequent and/or intense than prior to treatment. Sheehan and co-workers (1984b) conducted a single blind 8-week comparison of alprazolam and ibuprofen in 37 patients with agoraphobia and panic attacks. The alprazolam group showed a significantly greater global improvement and reduction of anticipatory anxiety, as well as a trend toward greater panic reduction, which did not reach significance.

The studies by Liebowitz and colleagues (1986) and Sheehan and colleagues (1984b) also indicated that clinically effective treatment with alprazolam was able to block the panicogenic effects of sodium lactate.

Though a number of trials are currently underway, there are only three published reports that compare alprazolam to another established antipanic agent. The trial by Sheehan and associates (1984a) just mentioned found alprazolam to be as effective as either phenelzine or imipramine. More detailed comparisons of imipramine and alprazolam are available from two recent studies (Rizley et al, 1986; Charney et al, 1986). Rizley and co-workers (1986) conducted a small double blind trial in a mixed group of patients: 13 panic disorder (with and without phobias), 11 agoraphobia with panic, and 2 agoraphobia without panic. Mean daily doses of alprazolam and imipramine were 2.8 and 132.5 mg respectively. At the end of the 12-week trial, effects of the two drugs were equivalent on phobia measures and on two out of three panic measures. However, doctors' ratings during the first five weeks showed a superiority for alprazolam, suggesting an earlier onset of action. In addition, alprazolam-treated subjects reported significantly fewer side effects and a greater sense of global improvement. Results of this study must be considered with some reservation since the sample size is small and imipramine doses are modest. Further, the 26 completers represent only 60 percent of the patients who entered the study. The data reported are on completers only. The authors state that they undertook an endpoint analysis ($N = 35$) but do not report its results in detail. They state that both types of analyses (completer and endpoint) yielded similar results with the exception that there were fewer significant findings favoring alprazolam in the former.

Charney and colleagues (1986) compared efficacy of imipramine, alprazolam, and trazodone in 74 *DSM-III* panic disorder patients. All subjects received an initial three weeks of placebo treatment, following which those still ill were assigned to eight weeks on one of the three active drugs. Drug assignment was not random but was based on neurobiological rather than clinical characteristics of subjects. Patients, clinicians, and raters were aware of drug assignments but not of the sequence of placebo and active treatment. Mean daily doses of imipramine, alprazolam, and trazodone at week 8 of active treatment were 141 mg., 3.1 mg, and 250 mg respectively. Seventy percent (17 out of 24) of the imipramine and 56 percent (13 out of 23) of the alprazolam-treated subjects were judged as good or complete responders. Only 4 out of 27 trazadone-treated patients completed treatment and only 2 out of 27 were responders. Therapeutic effects of alprazolam were seen in the first week of active treatment. Efficacy of imipramine was not apparent until week four.

Klein (1981) has hypothesized that the anticipatory anxiety and phobic avoidance experienced by patients with panic disorder and agoraphobia are secondary complications of recurrent spontaneous panic. Benzodiazepines are helpful for generalized anxiety. The introduction of alprazolam, therefore, evoked great interest since it was hoped that one medication would be effecive against both the panic and anticipatory anxiety components of the illness. In contrast to this expectation, Liebowitz and colleagues (1986) reported that the major therapeutic effect of alprazolam for patients with agoraphobia was panic blockade. At the end of the trial, many responders still had at least a moderate level of phobic avoidance and anticipatory anxiety, even though they were panic free. However, Alexander and Alexander (1986) argue that alprazolam can treat both components but that higher doses are required to alleviate anticipatory anxiety than those needed to block panic attacks. The mean effective antipanic dose for their 27 patients was 2.2. mg/day. However, the mean optimal dose (that which treated anticipatory anxiety as well) was 3.9 mg/day. Within this dose range, 21 of the 23 subjects who had clinically significant phobic avoidance became asymptomatic on alprazolam without psychotherapeutic intervention.

DOSAGE AND COURSE OF TREATMENT.   Alprazolam is usually started at a dose of .25 or .5 mg three times a day and raised .5 mg every 2–3 days. For patients who are new to the drug, one strategy is to start with a .5 mg bedtime dose and begin the three-times daily schedule the next day. Patients who have a marked sedation effect from the first nighttime dose can be started on .25 three times a day. Those who do not can begin directly with .5 mg three times a day.

As is the case for most psychiatric medications, individuals appear to vary considerably in the dose of alprazolam required to block their panic attacks. Mean effective antipanic doses of alprazolam in reported clinical trials range from 2.2 mg/day (range .25–6.9) (Alexander and Alexander, 1986) to 6.3 (range 3–9 mg) (Sheehan et al, 1984a).

In our experience, the majority of patients seem to need 3–6 mg/day to block their panic attacks. However, some patients do recover at lower doses (1–2 mg) (Alexander and Alexander, 1986; Chouinard et al, 1982) while others require over 6 mg/day (Ballenger, 1986; Sheehan et al, 1984a).

Since its half-life is relatively short (12–20 hours), alprazolam is generally taken on a three-times daily schedule. However, even on this regimen, some patients report a "wearing off" of therapeutic effect and/or a withdrawal-like syndrome in the hour or two before their next dose (Tesar and Rosenbaum, 1986). Changing to a four-times daily schedule usually alleviates these symptoms. However, for a few individuals, more frequent dosing may be necessary.

Several reports corroborate the finding by Rizley and associates (1976) that alprazolam has a more rapid onset of antipanic efficacy than is usually seen with antidepressant antipanic agents. Alexander and Alexander (1986) found that 24 out of 28 (85 percent) patients became panic free after two weeks on this drug. In the study by Liebowitz and colleagues (1986), 10 out of 22 responders had reached response level in the second week of treatment. Sheehan and co-workers (1984a) and Chouinard and associates (1982) reported significant improvement during week one on the physicians' global clinical and Hamilton anxiety scales respectively.

Though there is little systematic data as yet, tolerance to the antipanic effects of alprazolam does not appear to be a common problem. Clinical experience and reports from trials indicate that most responders appear to be controlled at the same or even lower doses over a six-month to one-year period (Liebowitz et al, 1986; Alexander and Alexander, 1986).

The optimum length of alprazolam treatment for panic patients is not known. Based on experience with other antipanic agents, we recommend an initial trial of six months. However, systematic studies are required to provide data-based guidelines in this area.

SIDE EFFECTS. Sedation is the most common side effect and is managed by decreasing the dose and/or slowing the rate of increase. In some patients, however, sedation and drowsiness have been reported to interfere to the extent that increase of dose to a therapeutically effective level is prevented. For example, Liebowitz and colleagues (1986) reported that 4 out of 8 nonresponders were unable to have their dose raised due to daytime sedation. Less frequent side effects include depressed mood and loss of sexual desire.

In a small number of patients, alprazolam appears to have a paradoxically stimulant effect. Pecknold and Fleury (1986) reported two cases of alprazolam-induced mania in patients with panic disorder. They suggest that alprazolam-induced mania is related to a history of affective disorder since two of the three cases fell into this category. A case of alprazolam-induced hypomania was also noted by Alexander and Alexander (1986). Another type of stimulant effect, paroxysmal excitement, has been observed in three cases by Strahan and associates (1985).

DISCONTINUATION AND FOLLOW-UP. Three systematic studies (Pecknold and Swinson, 1986; Mellman and Uhde, 1986; Fyer et al, 1987) and a number of case reports indicate that in many patients discontinuation of alprazolam is accompanied by a withdrawal syndrome and/or recurrence of panic attacks.

Pecknold and Swinson (1986) compared discontinuation results in 197 panic disorder patients who participated in a comparative treatment trial of alprazolam and placebo. Fifty-eight patients had been treated for 8 weeks with alprazolam; 33 of these completed the discontinuation. For placebo these figures were 49 and 21, respectively. Taper was at a rate of 1 mg every 3 days and generally lasted 4 weeks. During discontinuation, panic attacks returned to at least baseline level of severity in the majority of patients in both groups. About one-quarter of the alprazolam but only 1 of the placebo group had a rebound effect (increase of at least 50 percent over baseline and a change of at least 3 panic attacks).

Withdrawal symptoms were defined as those that appeared during discontinuation but that had not occurred prior to, or during, treatment. Typical benzo-diazepine withdrawal symptoms were seen at mild to moderate severity in a small number of alprazolam-treated patients.

Mellman and Uhde (1986) reported on the double blind gradual discontinuation of alprazolam in 10 hospitalized patients (8 panic disorder, 2 bipolar disorder). Assessments were made during tapering (withdrawal period) and at postwithdrawal. During the postwithdrawal period, patients had returned to their usual pretreatment clinical condition. All subjects had greatly increased anxiety symptoms and plasma cortisol levels during withdrawal as compared to postwithdrawal.

Fyer and colleagues (1987) tapered 17 panic patients from alprazolam at a rate of decrease of 10 percent of starting dose every three days. Only 4 out of 17 patients were able to complete discontinuation at this rate (4–5 weeks). Another 4 patients were able to complete taper at a slightly slower rate (7–13 weeks). The remaining 9 subjects were either unwilling to discontinue or did so only with use of adjunctive medication (tricyclic antidepressant).

Nine of the 17 patients reported clinically significant newly occurring withdrawal symptoms during discontinuation. Panic attacks recurred or increased in 15 out of 17 subjects. None of the subjects had seizures, delirium or hallucinations. Clinically significant neurological or electroencephalogram (EEG) changes were also not seen.

Case reports of abrupt alprazolam discontinuation (Breier et al, 1984; Levy, 1984) indicate that seizures and delirium can occur after only eight weeks of treatment. A severe withdrawal syndrome similar to that observed with conventional benzodiazepines has also been reported (Noyes et al, 1985).

These findings indicate that patients using alprazolam must be strongly cautioned not to stop medication abruptly.

The occurrence of a withdrawl syndrome during alprazolam discontinuation is consistent with its benzodiazepine structure. Observed withdrawal symptoms and onset are similar to those seen with other short to intermediate elimination half-life benzodiazepines. The significance of panic recurrence during tapering is less clear, and may be an interaction with the underlying illness. Anecdotal reports indicate that alprazolam withdrawal in depressives has been much easier.

Clonazepam

The antipanic efficacy of alprazolam has renewed interest in possible usefulness of other benzodiazepines in this patient group. Clonazepam is a high potency 1,4 benzodiazepine widely used in the treatment of minor motor epilepsy (Browne, 1978). It is of interest as a potential antipanic drug because, unlike other marked high potency drugs in this family, clonazepam is an intermediate-long acting compound with an elimination half-life of 20–40 hours in humans (twice that of alprazolam). The lengthier half-life may enable less frequent dosing than alprazolam. In addition, discontinuation from longer half-life benzodiazepines is associated with less frequent and less severe withdrawal, relapse, and rebound than is tapering of shorter half-life drugs.

The first report of antipanic efficacy of clonazepam was from an open clinical trial by Fontaine and Chouinard (1984). Twelve panic disorder patients were treated with daily doses of 6–9 mg of clonazepam. Ten of the 12 improved markedly while 2 continued to panic and required further treatment. Subsequently, Spier and associates (1986) have reported a retrospective uncontrolled trial of clonazepam in 50 patients with panic disorder or agoraphobia with panic. Forty-one of the 50 had failed or done poorly in previous pharamcologic treatment (MAO inhibitor, TCA, or alprazolam). Of the 50 patients, 39 (78 percent) responded, 5 (10 percent) did not respond, and 7 (12 percent) dropped out. Response was defined as having at least a two-week drug trial and a two-level improvement on the clinician's global response scale. Thirty-three of the 39 responders were rated "normal" or "borderline ill."

DOSAGE, COURSE OF TREATMENT, AND SIDE EFFECTS. Clonazepam has only recently been used to treat panic disorder. Therefore, dosage regimens are not well established. In most cases at present, clonazepam is started in doses of .25 or .5 mg twice a day and raised one pill every 2–3 days. There is a considerable discrepancy in the range of effective antipanic dose reported by the two groups cited above. Fontaine and Chouinard (1984) used 6–9 mg/day. Spier and colleagues (1986) had an average daily dose of 1.9 mg/day. Many patients appear to recover on doses in the range of 1.5–3 mg/day. Since clonazepam is a benzodiazepine and discontinuation may be problematic, it is probably best to increase the dose at a very slow rate above the range of 3–4 mg/day in order to maximize the patient's chance of being treated with the lowest effective dose.

The most common side effects of clonazepam appear to be drowsiness, nausea, and depression. Of these, depression is the most troublesome.

Spier and co-workers (1986) reported that 4 out of 50 patients became depressed during clonazepam treatment. Three of these had a history of depressive or dysthymic disorder. Anecdotal clinical reports corroborate this experience. Close monitoring for depressive symptomatology is recommended. Tesar and Rosenbaum (1986) have reported that drowsiness occurs in most patients transiently during the first two to three days of treatment, but it resolves and does not recur on further dose increases.

DISCONTINUATION. There are no reported systematic studies of clonazepam discontinuation in panic patients. Clonazepam is a high potency benzodiazepine. Therefore, it is expected that abrupt discontinuation would be accompanied by a withdrawal syndrome and possibly relapse or rebound similar to that seen with alprazolam. For this reason, discontinuation should be gradual (.5 mg every 4–7 days). It is hoped that the longer elimination half-life of clonazepam may reduce the occurrence and severity of withdrawal and relapse during discontinuation, as is seen in the case of conventional benzodiazepines. However, controlled studies are required to test these expectations.

Other Benzodiazepines

Clinical experience suggests that conventional benzodiazepines given in low and middle range doses do not effectively block panic attacks in most patients (Klein and Davis, 1969; Beaudry et al, 1985). However, the recent discovery of the antipanic efficacy of high potency benzodiazepines has led to a renewed interest in this question (Rickels and Schwetzer, 1986).

Whether conventional benzodiazepines can block panic is of interest for both therapeutic and heuristic reasons. From the standpoint of treatment, the low side effect profile and more rapid onset of benzodiazepines make them easier to administer to panic patients than TCA or MAO inhibitors. Long half-life, lower potency compounds may also be more easily tapered. Heuristically, Klein has hypothesized that panic and generalized anxiety are qualitatively distinct. Considerable data from family/genetic and biological studies support this distinction. If high enough doses of any benzodiazepine are able to treat both types of anxiety, then some rethinking of current classifications may be necessary. However, currently unknown qualitative distinctions between benzodiazepines may account for differences in antipanic efficacy.

Relatively few studies using conventional benzodiazepines in panic patients have been reported in the literature. Only one placebo controlled study has been done; the comparative trials are somewhat contradictory and as yet inconclusive.

McNair and Kahn (1981) reported an 8-week comparison of moderate doses of chlordiazepoxide (mean 55 mg/day) and imipramine (mean 132 mg/day) in 26 patients with agoraphobia and panic attacks. Imipramine was significantly superior to chlordiazepoxide in reducing panic symptoms. There were no significant between-drug differences on measures of agoraphobia or self-report of global improvement.

In contrast, Noyes and colleagues (1984) recently demonstrated that moderate doses of diazepam reduce frequency and severity of panic attacks but did not stop them over a two-week period. Twenty subjects meeting *DSM-III* criteria for panic disorder or agoraphobia with panic were given diazepam and propranolol in a double blind crossover design. Each subject took each drug for two weeks. Median daily doses were 30 mg diazepam (range 5–40 mg) and 240 mg propranolol (range 80–320 mg).

Diazepam reduced the average number of weekly panic attacks from 8.5 ($\pm$ 2.79) at baseline to 2.9 ($\pm$ 0.84) at week 2. At week 2 of propranolol, the number of weekly panics was not significantly different from baseline. Whether, and if so, how many subjects became panic free on either medication is not stated.

Somewhat equivocal results were reported by Dunner and colleagues (1986) who conducted a six-week double blind randomized trial comparing slightly higher doses of diazepam to alprazolam and placebo. Forty-eight patients with diagnosis of either *DSM-III* panic disorder ($N = 16$), agoraphobia with panic attacks ($N = 16$), or generalized anxiety disorder (GAD) ($N = 16$) were studied. All subjects were experiencing "panic or anxiety attacks" at the start of the study. However, the frequency of these for the GAD group is not stated. Mean daily doses of diazepam and alprazolam during the last treatment week were 44 mg (range 20–70) and 4 mg (range 1–10), respectively. Endpoint analysis did not show a significant between-treatment group difference for frequency of panic attacks. However, significant differences between baseline and endpoint panic frequency were found for diazepam (3 to .6 per week) and alprazolam (4.5 to .8 per week) but not placebo (5.9 to 4.3 per week). Neither the number of panic free subjects nor outcome by diagnostic group are presented.

Taken together, these data suggest that moderate daily doses of benzodiazepines may alleviate panic to some extent in some patients. Additional controlled trials of longer duration are needed. In particular, it would be of interest to know whether conventional benzodiazepines block the panic attack itself, or merely reduce the propensity to panic by way of a reduction of generalized anxiety.

BETA-BLOCKERS

Current data indicate that while beta-blockers may have some limited antianxiety effects, they are not effective antipanic agents. However, since placebo controlled trials with adequate sample size have not been reported, final conclusions cannot be drawn.

Studies carried out in mixed groups of anxiety patients prior to the *DSM-III* suggested that beta-blockers had some positive effect, particularly in patients with prominent somatic symptoms. Of seven placebo controlled propranolol trials, five showed a superior drug over placebo effect and two did not (Noyes et al, 1981).

In 1976 Heiser and DeFrancisco reported mixed results in the first propranolol trial in which the specific effect of propranolol on panic attacks was an outcome measure. Ten patients (3 panic disorder, 3 agoraphobia, 1 anxiety without panic, and 3 panic with depression) were openly treated. The 3 panic disorder patients became panic free on 20–60 mg/day propranolol. The remaining patients either did not benefit or refused an adequate medication trial.

Recently two small controlled trials have been reported. Results were contradictory. In the first, Noyes and colleagues (1984) found that two weeks of treatment with propranolol had little effect on panic attacks or global clinical condition of 20 panic patients. Propranolol was significantly inferior to 30 mg/day of diazepam.

In contrast, Munjack and associates (1985) found that propranolol and imipramine were equally effective in a double blind crossover comparing 6-week trials of each drug in 23 panic patients. Maximum daily doses of imipramine and propranolol were 300 and 160 mg per day, respectively. However, only 57 percent (13 out of 23) of patients became panic free on imipramine, and 43 percent (10 out of 23) on propranolol (χ^2 = .78 NS). The recovery rates on both agents are considerably lower than the 70–80 percent figures reported by other investigators using imipramine (Sheehan, 1980; Klein et al, 1983; Zitrin et al, 1983). As Munjack and colleagues (1985) point out, their study suffered from several methodologic limitations, which probably account for the low imipramine effect. Six weeks is probably too short a time to observe full imipramine effects (Zitrin et al, 1983). In addition, doses of imipramine used were somewhat low (mean 126 mg/day). Sixty-seven percent of subjects taking over 50 mg/day of imipramine became panic free, compared to only 20 percent of those taking less than this amount. The mean propranolol dose is not stated. However, 12 out of 23 subjects reached the maximum dose of 160 mg per day. The small sample size and lack of placebo control are further shortcomings.

An additional negative piece of evidence is the finding by Gorman and associates (1983) that acute beta-adrenergic blockade with propranolol does not prevent previously sodium lactate-vulnerable panic patients from panicking under the influence of sodium lactate.

CHOOSING AMONG MEDICATIONS

Imipramine, phenelzine, and alprazolam are effective antipanic agents. Although in most cases controlled studies are not available, clinical experience suggests that other compounds in these families (for example, desipramine, parnate, clonazepam) also block panic. Each drug (tricyclic antidepressant, MAO inhibitor, and high potency benzodiazepine) has advantages and disadvantages compared to the others (see Table 2). In choosing a medication, these advantages and disadvantages are considered with respect to the particular patient's 1) medical history; 2) concomitant psychiatric disorder (current and/or past); 3) current severity of illness; and 4) attitude toward medication and medication side effects.

In most cases, a tricyclic antidepressant is our first choice. Tricyclic antidepressants (TCAs) have been marketed and widely used for depression, panic, and other disorders for a number of years. Their side effects and safety profiles are well known. The once-daily dosage schedule is easy to follow, and use of TCAs rarely interferes with daily functioning. Relapse and withdrawal syndrome during discontinuation are unusual. Imipramine is the best studied antipanic agent. However, we feel that in most patients desipramine is equally effective, and its lower sedative and anticholinergic effects may make it more acceptable.

Patients in whom a TCA would not be a first choice are those with medical contraindications (see Table 2), a history of nonresponse, or well-documented adverse side effects.

Another possible exception is the patient suffering from panic disorder and atypical depression. This combination appears to have a considerably higher rate of response to phenelzine than imipramine (Liebowitz et al, 1985). A small number of patients do well on imipramine but prediction of response is not possible. The final decision is left to the clinician who must weigh the risk of delaying effective treatment against the greater difficulties of using an MAO inhibitor.

Because of its rapid onset of action, some physicians use alprazolam instead of imipramine or phenelzine for very anxious patients whom they feel will not tolerate the delay in onset of action. We do not feel this is necessary. Most patients can tolerate the delay with supportive reassurance alone. In those who cannot, we recommend adjunctive use of low doses of alprazolam (.25–.5 four times a day) during the first 2–4 weeks of antidepressant treatment. Once the TCA or MAO inhibitor takes effect, the alprazolam is gradually discontinued.

The choice between an MAO inhibitor and alprazolam depends to a large extent on the clinician's evaluation of the specific situation and the relative acceptability of each medication to the patient (see Table 2).

Most patients recover during their first medication trial. However, an important, often neglected point is that panic patients who don't get better or who can't tolerate the first medication will almost always recover on the second.

TREATMENT OF ANTICIPATORY ANXIETY AND AVOIDANCE

More than 70 percent of panic patients seen in clinical settings develop secondary phobias. Why some patients with recurrent panic attacks become avoidant while others do not remains one of the more intriguing questions in anxiety disorders research. Similarly, it is not known why successful pharmacological blockade of panic in some individuals is accompanied by rapid return to normal activity, while in others there is little apparent change in the level of anticipatory anxiety or phobic avoidance (Muskin and Fyer, 1981).

Table 2. Advantages and Disadvantages of Antipanic Medications

Medication	Advantages	Disadvantages	Side Effects	Contraindications
Imipramine	Well-studied antipanic agent. Once daily dosage. Older, widely used drug with well-known side effect and safety profile.	2–3 week delay in onset of action.	Dry mouth, constipation, orthostatic hypotension, urinary hesitancy, blurred vision, mania, or hypomania in bipolar patients	Acute M.I., narrow angle glaucoma, cardiac conduction delays (bundle branch disease), prostatic hypertrophy
Phenelzine	Established drug with known side effects and safety profile. Effective in atypical depression. May have more marked effect on phobic avoidance than other antipanic agents.	Dietary restrictions. 2–3 week delay in onset of action.	Insomnia, orthostatic hypotension, anorgasmia, hypomania, hypertensive reaction to food containing tyramine.	Asthma, history of undiagnosed allergic anaphylactic reaction
Alprazolam	Rapid onset of action. Low side effect profile. May also help anticipatory anxiety.	Possible withdrawal syndrome and recurrence of panic during discontinuation; multiple daily doses required.	Sedation, loss of sexual desire, paradoxical excitation.	History of benzodiazepine abuse

The theoretical premise of a pharmacologic approach to panic disorders is that patients develop anticipatory fear and avoidance not because they fear the avoided situation itself, but because they are afraid of what will happen if they panic while there. From this it follows that the goal in treating secondary avoidance behavior is to get the patients to go back "into the street" as Freud (1955) put it, and prove to themselves that panic will not recur. The clincian's task is to find the quickest way to get each particular patient to accomplish this.

For many patients an explanation of the relationship between the panic attacks and phobias, assurance that the medication has blocked the panic, and encouragement to reenter avoided situations is sufficient to extinguish anticipatory anxiety and reestablish normal activity. Since it is not possible to predict the course of any particular patient, we routinely begin treatment with this strategy. If after being panic free for 8–12 weeks the patient has made no progress, then a reevaluation is done and, if indicated, an additional treatment directed specifically at phobias and anticipatory anxiety is instituted. Reevaluation should also consider the possibility of 1) persistent unrecognized panic attacks; 2) undiagnosed atypical depression; and 3) existence of interpersonal or psychodynamic reasons for maintaining avoidant behavior.

There are two main types of treatment for avoidance in panic patients: psychotherapy and adjunctive medication.

Behavior therapy techniques developed for independent use (without medication) in treatment of phobias are often used to treat avoidance in panic patients. These techniques can be divided according to two parameters, depending upon whether the exposure is imaginal or in vivo (that is, the real situation) and whether it is graduated or sudden (that is, flooding). In vivo techniques are further divided into those in which the therapist works with the patient in the situation (therapist-aided), and those in which the patient is given exposure assignments to carry out either on his own or with a friend or family member between sessions (self-practice). Common to all of these treatments is a structured approach and repeated scheduled entry (real or imagined) into the phobic situation. The therapist sets the pace. The patient is required to learn to tolerate anxiety and stay in the situation in spite of it.

In contrast, supportive psychotherapy provides the patient with a realistic but nonjudgmental arena to discuss problems related to phobias as well as those in other areas of his or her life. The therapist is encouraging but does not set specific goals or deadlines. For example, if a patient who avoids trains were discussing a possibility of undertaking a business trip requiring a train ride, the therapist might say, "You haven't had a panic in a very long time. In fact, last time you went on a train you were fine. I understand that it's still frightening you. I think you will be OK, but if you don't feel you can do it this time, don't worry, another opportunity will arise."

There has been some controversy as to whether behavioral treatments have a specific efficacy over supportive psychotherapy for the treatment of phobias in panic patients. A number of studies have reported no difference between supportive or psychodynamic psychotherapy and imaginal desensitization. Klein (1983) has argued that the specific ingredient in the psychotherapy of phobic panic patients is getting them into the situation. In vivo techniques force the patient to reenter situations more quickly. Therefore, in vivo exposure may look more effective than supportive or imaginal techniques in the short term, but gains may equalize over time. Comparison of results from two studies of agoraphobic patients by Klein and colleagues (Zitrin et al, 1983; Klein et al, 1983) described above indicated that, at 13 weeks, group in vivo exposure was superior to supportive psychotherapy or imaginal desensitization with regard to reducing avoidance. However, at 26 weeks (after a 13-week hiatus in group exposure), there were no significant differences among the three, and the group exposure patients had suffered significant relapse.

A particularly interesting recent development is the use of programmed self-practice exposure (Mathews et al, 1981). In this approach, the patient is given a programmed manual explaining the theory and practice of exposure. The therapist spends only a few initial sessions with the patient reviewing the material and helping him or her develop exposure hierarchies. Thereafter, the patient practices alone or with the help of a family member or friend.

Programmed self-practice has been found in some cases to be surprisingly effective as an adjunct to medication treatment or office based supportive psychotherapy (Mathews et al, 1981). It is highly cost-effective since it provides an individualized exposure program for each patient without the cost of continuous therapist visits.

Benzodiazepines are sometimes used to decrease anticipatory anxiety. Their efficacy has not been studied. However, clinical experience suggests that benzodiazepines are an adjunct to, rather than a substitute for, encouragement to exposure.

The choice of benzodiazepines depends upon patient and physician preference.

COMMON CAUSES OF TREATMENT FAILURES

Panic blocking drugs are usually well tolerated and extremely effective. In our experience over 85 percent of patients can become panic free on medication. The remaining few will have significant improvement. Treatment failures are not commonly due to the refractory nature of the illness but to the way the drug is administered or the basis upon which outcome is assessed. Specifically, the most common causes of treatment failure are: 1) insufficient dosage; 2) insufficient length of drug treatment; 3) misassessment of residual symptoms (that is, confusion of panic and anticipatory anxiety); and 4) misdiagnosis of concomitant psychiatric disorders (for example, atypical depression, social phobia).

It is natural for a patient to expect that a successful treatment will make him or her feel well again. However, medication treatments block panic but usually do not have a direct effect on worry about the panic or avoidant behaviors. Patients who have persistent anticipatory anxiety and phobias will often complain that the treatment doesn't work. An unsophisticated clinician often mistakenly concurs and stops the drug. Conversely, patients who tend to minimize their symptoms may mislead the physician into believing that partially blocked panics are anticipatory anxiety.

One useful approach to these distinctions is to have the patient keep a diary of anxiety symptoms and situations surrounding them over a period of one to two weeks. Careful review usually provides both a diagnosis and a persuasive context in which to explain the treatment plan to the patient.

Concomitant atypical depression that is unresponsive to TCA or benzodiazepine is another cause of apparent treatment failure. The usual presentation of this is inability to resume normal activity even though panics have been in remission for a long time. These patients may appear euthymic while with family, friends, or doctor. However, when alone, the depressed mood reasserts itself and the patient has no motivation. The treatment for this is to change the patient to an MAO inhibitor. If this is not possible, then a combination of a more activating heterocyclic antidepressant and a high potency benzodiazepine may be a viable alternative.

A number of individuals also suffer simultaneously from both panic disorder and social phobia. Clinical experience suggests that imipramine and benzodiazepines have only minimal effects in this disorder. However, pilot data (Liebowitz et al, 1985) suggest that phenelzine is often significantly helpful. Panic patients who continue to complain of severe situational anxiety after adequate treatment on imipramine or alprazolam should be reassessed for possible coexisting social phobia. In certain cases a change to phenelzine may be merited.

CONCLUSION

Pharmacologic treatment of panic disorder is straightforward and extremely effective. Several types of drugs have been shown to block panic attacks in 75–90 percent of patients. These include the tricyclic antidepressant imipramine, the MAO inhibitor phenelzine, and the triazolobenzodiazepine alprazolam. Other agents with similar chemical structures, though not well studied, may also be useful. For many patients, the combination of medication, education about the illness, and supportive encouragement to reenter phobic situations are sufficient. For others, adjunctive treatment (for example, systematic exposure exercises) may be required. Treatment failures are most commonly due to inadequate dosage, insufficient medication trial, or misdiagnosis of concomitant psychiatric disorder, rather than the refractory nature of the illness.

REFERENCES

Alexander PE, Alexander DD: Alprazolam treatment for panic disorder. J Clin Psychiatry 1986; 47:301-304

Ballenger J: Pharmacotherapy of the panic disorders. J Clin Psychiatry 1986; 47(6 Suppl): 27-31

Ballenger JC, Sheehan DV, Jacobson G: Antidepressant treatment of severe phobic anxiety, in Abstracts of Scientific Proceedings of the 130th Annual Meeting of the American Psychiatric Association, Toronto, 1977

Beaudry P, Fontaine R, Chouinard G, et al: Clonazepam in the treatment of patients with recurrent panic attacks. Prog Neuropsychopharmacol Biol Psychiatry 1985; 9:589-592

Beaumont G: A large open multicentre trial of clomipramine (Anafranil) in the management of phobic disorders. J Int Med Res 1977; 5:116-123

Breier A, Charney DS, Nelson JC: Seizures induced by abrupt discontinuation of alprazolam. Am J Psychiatry 1984; 141:1606-1607

Browne TR: Drug therapy: clonazepam. N Engl J Med 1978; 299:812-816

Caetano D: Treatment for panic disorders with clomipramine (Anafranil): an open study of 22 cases. Ciba-Geigy reprint. J Brasileiro de Psiquiatria 1985; 34:125-132

Carey MS, Hawkinson R, Kornhaber A, et al: The use of clomipramine in phobic patients. Preliminary Research Report. Current Therapeutic Research 1975; 17:107-110

Charney DS, Woods SW, Goodman WK, et al: Drug treatment of panic disorder: the comparative efficacy of imipramine, alprazolam, and trazodone. J Clin Psychiatry 1986; 47:12

Chouinard G, Annable L, Fontaine R, et al: Alprazolam in the treatment of generalized anxiety and panic disorders: a double blind, placebo controlled study. Psychopharmacology 1982; 77:229-233

Cohen SD, Monteiro W, Marks IM: Two-year follow-up of agoraphobics after exposure and imipramine. Br J Psychiatry 1984; 144:276-281

Colgan A: A pilot study of Anafranil in the treatment of phobic states. Scott Med J 1975; 20 (Suppl 1):55-60

Dilsaver SC, Greden JF: Antidepressant withdrawal phenomena. Biol Psychiatry 1984; 19:237-255

Dunner DL, Ishiki D, Avery DH, et al: Effect of alprazolam and diazepam on anxiety and panic attacks in panic disorder: a controlled study. J Clin Psychiatry 1986; 47:458-460

Escobar JI, Landbloom RP: Treatment of phobic neurosis with clomipramine: a controlled clinical trial. Current Therapeutic Research 1976; 20:680-685

Feighner J, Herbstein J. Damlouji N: Combined MAOI, TCA and direct stimulant therapy of treatment resistant depression. J Clin Psychiatry 1985; 46:206-209

Fontaine R, Chouinard G: Antipanic effect of clonazepam (letter). Am J Psychiatry 1984; 141:149

Freud S: On infantile neurosis and other works in Complete Psychological Works, Standard Edition, vol 17. London, Hogarth Press, 1955

Fyer AJ, Liebowitz MR, Gorman JM, et al: Discontinuation of alprazolam treatment in panic patients. Am J Psychiatry 1987; 144:303-308

Garakani H. Zitrin CM, Klein DF: Treatment of panic disorder with imipramine alone. Am J Psychiatry 1984; 141:446-448

Glassman AH, Bigger JT: Cardiovascular effects of therapeutic doses of tricyclic antidepressants: a review. Arch Gen Psychiatry 1981; 38:815-820

Gloger S, Grunhaus L, Birmacher B, et al: Treatment of spontaneous panic attacks with clomipramine. Am J Psychiatry 1981; 138:1213-1217

Gorman JM, Levy GF, Liebowitz MR, et al: Effect of acute beta-adrenergic blockade on lactate-induced panic. Arch Gen Psychiatry 1983; 40:1079-1082

Gorman JM, Liebowitz MR, Fyer AJ, et al: An open trial of fluoxetine in the treatment of panic attacks. J Clin Psychopharmacol (in press)

Grunhaus L, Gloger S, Birmacher B: Clomipramine treatment for panic attacks in patients with mitral valve prolapse. J Clin Psychiatry 1984; 45:25-27

Heiser JF, DeFrancisco D: The treatment of pathological panic states with propranolol. Am J Psychiatry 1976; 133:1389-1394

Insel TR, Murphy DL, Cohen RM, et al: Obsessive-compulsive disorder: a double blind trial of clomipramine and clorgyline. Arch Gen Psychiatry 1983; 40:605-612

Karabanow O: Double-blind controlled study in phobias and obsessions. J Int Med Res 1977; 5(Suppl 5):42-48

Kelly D, Guirguis W, Frommer E, et al: Treatment of phobic states with antidepressants. Br J Psychiatry 1970; 116:387-398

Klein DF: Delineation of two drug-responsive anxiety syndromes. Psychopharmacologia 1964; 5:397-408

Klein DF: Importance of psychiatric diagnosis in prediction of clinical drug effects. Arch Gen Psychiatry 1967; 16:118-126

Klein DF: Anxiety reconceptualized, in Anxiety: New Research and Changing Concepts. Edited by Klein DF, and Rabkin J. New York, Raven Press, 1981

Klein DF: Psychopharmacologic treatment of panic disorder. Psychosomatics 1984; 25 (Suppl 10):32-35

Klein DF, Davis JM: Diagnosis and Drug Treatment of Psychiatric Disorders. Baltimore, Williams & Wilkins, 1969

Klein DF, Fink M: Psychiatric reaction patterns to imipramine. Am J Psychiatry 1962; 119:432-438

Klein DF, Gittelman R, Quitkin F, et al: Diagnosis and Drug Treatment of Psychiatric Disorders: Adults and Children. Second edition. Baltimore, Williams & Wilkins, 1980

Klein DF, Zitrin CM, Woerner MG, et al: Treatment of phobias, II: behavior therapy and supportive therapy—are there specific ingredients? Arch Gen Psychiatry 1983; 40: 139-145

Klein DF, Ross DC, Cohen P: Panic and avoidance in agoraphobia. Arch Gen Psychiatry 1987; 44:377-385

Kramer JC, Klein DF, Fink M: Withdrawal symptoms following discontinuation of imipramine therapy. Am J Psychiatry 1961; 118:549-550

Levy B: Delirium and seizures due to abrupt alprazolam withdrawal: case report. J Clin Psychiatry 1984; 45:38-39

Liebowitz MR, Fyer AJ, Gorman JM, et al: Lactate provocation of panic attacks, I: clinical and behavioral findings. Arch Gen Psychiatry 1984; 41:764-770

Liebowitz MR, Quitkin F, Stewart J, et al: Effect of panic attacks on the treatment of atypical depression. Psychopharmacol Bull 1985; 21:558-561

Liebowitz MR, Fyer AJ, Gorman JM, et al: Alprazolam in the treatment of panic disorders. J Clin Psychopharmacol 1986; 6:13-20

Lipsedge JS, Hajjoff J, Huggins P, et al: The management of agoraphobia: a comparison of iproniazid and systematic desensitization. Psychopharmacologia 1973; 32:67-80

Lydiard RB: Desipramine in panic disorder: an open fixed-dose study. Presented at the Annual Meeting of the American Academy of Clinical Psychiatry, San Francisco, October 1985

Marks IM: Behavioral treatment plus drugs in anxiety syndromes, in Anxiety: New Research and Changing Concepts. Edited by Klein DF, Rabkin J. New York, Raven Press, 1981

Marks IM, Gray S, Cohen D, et al: Imipramine and brief therapist-aided exposure in agoraphobics having self-exposure homework. Arch Gen Psychiatry 1983; 40:153-162

Mathews AW, Gelder MG, Johnston DW: Agoraphobia: Nature and Treatment. New York, Guilford Press, 1981

Mavissakalian M, Michelson L: Agoraphobia: relative and combined effectiveness of therapist-assisted in vivo exposure and imipramine. J Clin Psychiatry 1986; 47:117-122

Mavissakalian M, Perel J: Imipramine in the treatment of agoraphobia: dose-response relationships. Am J Psychiatry 1985; 142:1032-1036

Mavissakalian M, Michelson L, Dealy RS: Pharmacological treatment of agoraphobia: imipramine versus imipramine with programmed practice. Br J Psychiatry 1983; 143: 348-355

Mavissakalian M, Perel JM, Michelson L: The relationship of plasma imipramine and N-desmethylimipramine to improvement in agoraphobia. J Clin Psychopharmacol 1984; 4:36-40

McNair DM, Kahn RJ: Imipramine compared with a benzodiazepine for agoraphobia, in Anxiety: New Research and Changing Concepts. Edited by Klein DF, Rabkin J. New York, Raven Press, 1981

Mellman TA, Uhde TW: Withdrawal syndrome with gradual tapering of alprazolam. Am J Psychiatry 1986; 143:1464-1466

Mountjoy CQ, Roth MA: A controlled trial of phenelzine in anxiety, depression, and phobic neuroses, in Proceedings of the IX Congress of the Collegium International Neuropsychopharmacologium. Amsterdam, Excerpta Medica, 1974

Munjack DJ, Rebal R, Shaner R, et al: Imipramine versus propranolol for the treatment of panic attacks: a pilot study. Compr Psychiatry 1985; 26:80-89

Muskin PR, Fyer AJ: Treatment of panic disorder. J Clin Psychopharmacol 1981; 1:81-90

Noyes R Jr, Kathol R, Clancy J, et al: Antianxiety effects of propranolol: a review of clinical studies, in Anxiety: New Research and Changing Concepts. Edited by Klein DF, Rabkin J. New York, Raven Press, 1981

Noyes R Jr, Anderson DJ, Clancy J, et al: Diazepam and propranolol in panic disorder and agoraphobia. Arch Gen Psychiatry 1984; 41:287-292

Noyes R Jr, Clancy J, Coryell WH, et al: A withdrawal syndrome after abrupt discontinuation of alprazolam. Am J Psychiatry 1985; 142:114-116

Paykel ES, Rowan PR, Parker RR, et al: Response to phenelzine and amitriptyline in subtypes of outpatient depression. Arch Gen Psychiatry 1982; 39:1041-1049

Pecknold JC, Fleury D: Alprazolam-induced manic episode in two patients with panic disorder. Am J Psychiatry 1986; 143:652-653

Pecknold JC, Swinson RP: Taper withdrawal studies with panic disorder and agoraphobia. Psychopharmacol Bull 1986; 22:173-176

Rapoport J, Ismond DR: Biological research in child psychiatry. J Am Acad Child Psychiatry 1982; 21:543-548

Raskin A: The influence of depression on antipanic effects of antidepressant drugs. Presented at Conference on Biological Considerations in the Etiology and Treatment of Panic Related Anxiety Disorders, Boston, Nov. 4-6, 1983

Ravaris CL, Nies A, Robinson DS, et al: A multiple dose controlled study of phenelzine in depression-anxiety states. Arch Gen Psychiatry 1976; 33:347-350

Rickels K, Schweizer EE: Benzodiazepines for treatment of panic attacks: a new look. Psychopharmacol Bull 1986; 22:93-99

Rizley R, Kahn RJ, McNair DM, et al: A comparison of alprazolam and imipramine in the treatment of agoraphobia and panic disorder. Psychopharmacol Bull 1986; 22:167-172

Robinson DS, Nies A, Ravaris L, et al: The monoamine oxidase inhibitor phenelzine in the treatment of depressive anxiety states. Arch Gen Psychiatry 1973; 29:407-413

Sargant W, Dally PJ: Treatment of anxiety states by antidepressant drugs. Br Med J 1962; 1:6-9

Sheehan DV, Ballenger J, Jacobsen, G: Treatment of endogenous anxiety with phobic, hysterical, and hypochondriacal symptoms. Arch Gen Psychiatry 1980; 37:51-59

Sheehan DV, Claycomb JB, Surman OS, et al: The relative efficacy of alprazolam, phenelzine, and imipramine in treating panic attacks and phobias, in Abstracts of the Scientific Proceedings of the 137th Annual Meeting of the American Psychiatric Association, Los Angeles, May 1984a

Sheehan DV, Coleman JH, Greenblatt DJ, et al: Some biochemical correlates of panic attacks with agoraphobia and their response to a new treatment. J Clin Psychopharmacol 1984b; 4:66-75

Solyom L, Heseltine GFD, McClure DJ, et al: Behavior therapy vs drug therapy in the treatment of phobic neurosis. Canadian Psychiatric Association Journal 1973; 18:25-31

Spier SA, Tesar GE, Rosenbaum JF, et al: Treatment of panic disorder and agoraphobia with clonazepam. J Clin Psychiatry 1986; 47:238-242

Strahan A, Rosenthal J, Kaswan M, et al: Three case reports of acute paroxysmal excitement associated with alprazolam treatment. Am J Psychiatry 1985; 142:859-861

Stewart J, Harrison W, Quitkin F, et al: Phenelzine induced pyridoxine deficiency. J Clin Psychopharmacol 1984; 4:225-226

Telch MJ, Tearnan BH, Taylor CB: Antidepressant medication in the treatment of agoraphobia: a critical review. Behav Res Ther 1983; 21:505-517

Telch MJ, Agras WS, Taylor CB, et al: Combined pharmacological and behavioral treatment for agoraphobia. Behav Res Ther 1985; 23:325-335

Tesar GE, Rosenbaum JF: Successful use of clonazepam in patients with treatment-resistant panic disorder. J Nerv Ment Dis 1986; 174:477-482

Tyrer P. Candy J, Kelly DA: A study of the clinical effects of phenelzine and placebo in the treatment of phobic anxiety. Psychopharmacologia 1973; 32:237-254

Uhde TW, Boulenger JP, Roye-Byrne PP, et al: Longitudinal course of panic disorder. Prog Neuropsychopharmacol Biol Psychiatry 1985; 9:39-51

Waxman D: An investigation into the use of Anafranil in phobic and obsessional disorders. Scott Med J 1975; 20 (Suppl 1):61-66

West ED, Dally PJ: Effects of iproniazid in depressive syndromes. Br Med J 1959; 1:1491-1494

Zitrin CM: Combined pharmacological and psychological treatment of phobias, in Phobia: Psychological and Pharmacological Treatments. Edited by Mavissakalian M, Barlow DH. New York, Guilford Press, 1981

Zitrin CM, Klein DF, Woerner MG, et al: Behavior therapy, supportive psychotherapy, imipramine, and phobias. Arch Gen Psychiatry 1978; 35:307-316

Zitrin CM, Klein DF, Woerner MG: Treatment of agoraphobia with group exposure in vivo and imipramine. Arch Gen Psychiatry 1980; 37:63-72

Zitrin CM, Klein DF, Woerner MG, et al: Treatment of phobias, I: comparison of imipramine hydrochloride and placebo. Arch Gen Psychiatry 1983; 40:125-138

Chapter 6

Cognitive-Behavioral Treatment of Panic

by Michelle G. Craske, Ph.D.

It has been shown repeatedly that the most effective form of psychological treatment for agoraphobic avoidance is in vivo exposure therapy (Barlow and Waddel, 1985). Currently, the focus of agoraphobic research is upon treatment enhancement and relapse prevention, both of which involve consideration of treatment of panic attacks as well as other factors. Current definitions and theoretical models view panic as central to the phenomenon of agoraphobia, in contrast to the earlier emphasis upon behavioral avoidance of situations. Indeed, psychological procedures for the treatment of panic attacks have been developed only recently.

In this chapter, the results from research concerning the cognitive-behavioral treatment of agoraphobia, and the treatment of panic and anxiety within agoraphobia, are updated. The various cognitive-behavioral methods for the treatment of "spontaneous" panic not necessarily associated with agoraphobic avoidance are described. Suggestions for combining these methods with the exposure-based procedures for agoraphobic avoidance are made.

EFFICACY OF IN VIVO EXPOSURE FOR AGORAPHOBIA

The basic procedure for the psychological treatment of agoraphobia entails repeated approach to situations that are feared and/or avoided in the event of a panic attack or sudden incapacitation, or from which it is difficult to escape or receive help. This therapy is termed in vivo exposure. Various mechanisms have been hypothesized to account for the efficacy of in vivo exposure, including weakening of physiological arousal, extinction of conditioned responses, development of self-confidence, and restructuring of cognitions. While the mechanisms remain unclear, in vivo exposure is considered to be substantially more effective than any number of other alternative psychotherapeutic techniques (Emmelkamp, 1982; Emmelkamp et al, 1983; Marks, 1985; Mathews et al, 1981; Mavissakalian and Barlow, 1981. For example, controlled research regarding the efficacy of psychoanalytical approaches for the treatment of agoraphobia and panic is unavailable. The analytical approach is based on the development of insight by association. By recalling events and thoughts that precede anxiety, associations are made with repressed impulses that allow catharsis to occur (Dittrich et al, 1983). This follows from the analytical view that anxiety signals the potential eruption of threatening impulses into conscious awareness and, in effect, helps to keep the impulses repressed by directing attention toward the symptomology of anxiety (Nemiah, 1981). Chambless and colleagues (in press) conclude that traditional psychoanalytical or supportive therapy result in stable recovery for approximately 24 percent of the patients. Freud believed firmly in the value of in vivo exposure: "One can hardly ever master a phobia if one waits until a patient lets the analysis influence him to give it up" (Freud, 1919, pp. 399-400).

The results from outcome investigations of exposure-based treatments indicate that, when drop-outs are excluded, from 60 to 70 percent of agoraphobics completing treatment show some clinical benefit which is maintained on average for periods of four years or more (Burns et al, 1983; Cohen et al, 1984; Hafner, 1976; Jansson et al, 1986; Jansson and Ost, 1982; Marks, 1971; Munby and Johnston, 1980). For example, Jansson and colleagues (1986) found that, using a conservative composite criterion of outcome based on extensive assessment procedures, 50 percent of their 33 agoraphobics benefited clinically from treatment by postassessment, as did 66 percent by the 15-month follow-up assessment. Cerny and associates (in press) reported that 65 percent of their 28 agoraphobics were substantially improved one year after treatment and 68 percent two years after treatment.

However, various factors argue for continued attempts to enhance treatment effectiveness. The median drop-out rate from exposure-based treatments, for example, is 12 percent, with a rate from 25 to 40 percent recorded when exposure is conducted in an intensive fashion (Jansson and Ost, 1982; Zitrin et al, 1980). Also, the data reflect that 30 to 40 percent of all agoraphobics who complete treatment fail to benefit, and of the remaining 60 to 70 percent, a substantial proportion may not attain clinically meaningful levels of functioning. Marks (1971), for example, reported that only 3 of 65 patients were symptom-free at follow-up. McPherson and colleagues (1980) reported that only 18 percent of improvers were symptom-free at posttreatment. Finally, relapse may occur in as many as 50 percent of patients who have benefited clinically, although in most cases, these patients are able to return to the level of clinical improvement reached previously in treatment (Munby and Johnston, 1980).

Research issues pertinent to the enhancement of traditional in vivo exposure therapy include 1) the manner in which exposure is conducted; 2) inclusion of significant others in treatment; and 3) management of panic attacks.

ENHANCEMENT OF IN VIVO EXPOSURE THERAPY

Gradual versus Intense Exposure

In vivo exposure therapy can be conducted in an intensive fashion by massing practices over short periods of time, enforcing immediate approach to highly feared situations, or by using therapist-assisted exposure. At its most intensive, exposure therapy may be conducted three to four hours a day, for five consecutive days, with the therapist urging the patient to enter and remain in the most feared situation for prolonged periods. Alternatively, therapy sessions may be conducted weekly for 15 weeks, where the patient is instructed to practice between therapy sessions, graduating from the least to the most distressing feared situations, perhaps initially with the therapist present, but primarily in a self-directed manner.

Early research indicated that intensive forms of treatment produced more rapid reductions in avoidance behavior (Stern and Marks, 1973; Foa et al, 1980). However, graduated self-directed exposure seems to represent the treatment of choice for agoraphobic avoidance, as it results in continuing improvement beyond treatment completion, and less attrition and relapse than intensive exposure (Barlow and Waddell, 1985). Indeed, it appears that self-directed treatment that is conducted in the patient's home environment and involves little contact with the therapist can be as successful as therapist-aided clinic-based treatments (Mathews et al, 1981). This is particularly true if agoraphobic severity is no greater than moderate (Holden et al, 1983) and detailed instructions regarding exposure practices are provided (Ghosh and Marks, in press). Ghosh and Marks (in press) concluded that "clinicians . . . may help many agoraphobics by a few brief but appropriate instructions plus a self-help manual."

Involving the Family

The importance of the interpersonal context for the maintenance and treatment of agoraphobia is evident from the behavioral pervasiveness of agoraphobia and its profound influence upon home management, family activities, and interactions. Nonphobic partners, usually spouses, have been included in treatment in order to aid generalization from clinic-based treatment to the home setting, to improve interpersonal conflict surrounding the agoraphobic problem, and to encourage exposure practice. Spouses or other partners are taught to serve as coaches to help patients design and carry out exposure practices, to prompt use of anxiety control strategies, and to give appropriate reinforcement and support. This seems to enhance agoraphobic outcome at posttreatment (Barlow et al, 1984b) and up to two years following treatment (Cerny et al, in press). The one study in which inclusion of the spouse was not found to be more effective than a comparison nonspouse treatment (Cobb et al, 1984) may have been confounded by greater involvement on the part of the spouse than was intended in the nonspouse group.

Poor marital satisfaction seems to be a negative predictor of treatment outcome in cases in which the spouse is not included, but is unrelated to outcome when the spouse is included. Generally, marital satisfaction tends to improve with agoraphobic improvement. Hence, it has been hypothesized that improvement in couple interaction during the course of spouse treatment in turn contributes to phobic improvement (Himadi et al, 1986). Arnow and colleagues (1985) examined the effectiveness of the addition of communication training to in vivo exposure for agoraphobia. After receiving four weeks of therapist- and self-directed in vivo exposure, one-half of their 25 agoraphobics received communication skills training, while the remainder received relaxation training for a further 8 weeks. In accordance with the hypothesis stated above, the communication group responded more favorably than the relaxation group in terms of various self-report and behavioral measures of agoraphobic dysfunction.

Together, the data suggest that while completely home-based treatment may not be effective for severe agoraphobics, treatment effects are wider reaching and longer lasting when exposure is graduated. These effects are enhanced further for some by inclusion of a significant other in treatment.

Managing Anxiety

In vivo exposure therapy is conducted typically with the addition of various methods of anxiety control. Until recently, the anxiety was construed as fear of particular situations. The related anxiety control techniques usually include cognitive methods such as distraction to "take one's mind off" the anxiety (by counting, conversation, and so on), coping self-statements (instructions to oneself to remain in the situation, to accept feelings of anxiety, to discount unrealistic fears of being trapped, and so forth), or paradoxical intention (instructions to confront rather than avoid or fight the experience of fear, and to exaggerate fearful imagery and thereby render it less fearful). Somatic methods of anxiety reduction include relaxation and meditation.

Research has shown that while the combination of in vivo exposure and these methods of anxiety control is very effective (Vermilyea et al, 1984), the methods do not reliably reduce levels of anxiety during in vivo exposure in comparison to exposure conducted without such methods. Furthermore, the inclusion of such methods does not produce a more favorable outcome overall (Michelson et al, 1985; Jansson et al, 1986). Finally, these methods of anxiety control are of very limited usefulness when conducted without structured exposure practice (Emmelkamp et al, 1978).

The ineffectiveness of these techniques may lie in their lack of specificity for the kind of fear that predominates during in vivo exposure. Recent conceptualizations of agoraphobia construe the fear as fear of panic in particular situations as opposed to fear of a situation per se. Techniques that have been designed specifically for the management of panic may, therefore, indeed enhance in vivo exposure for agoraphobia.

The major benefit derived from the methods of anxiety control described previously appears to be to improve compliance with an exposure regimen. Michelson and associates (1985) reported that drop-out rates were twice as high in exposure-only treatments than in exposure treatments combined with anxiety control strategies. In addition, Michelson and co-workers (1986) found that clients trained in progressive muscle relaxation practiced exposure more frequently than clients trained in methods of exposure only, both during treatment and at follow-up assessment. The knowledge that techniques for controlling intensive subjective distress are available (despite their apparent ineffectiveness to date) may provide the motivation necessary to comply with or endure exposure to a situation that has been feared and avoided for a long period of time, especially in those individuals very unwilling to experience any form of discomfort.

The importance of having at one's disposal methods for control of fear is demonstrated further by studies which have shown that exposure proceeds equally well when conducted in two different ways: first, exposure may be continued until anxiety subsides (Marks, 1985; Foa and Kozak, 1986); second, exposure may be terminated when anxiety heightens followed by re-exposure after anxiety has subsided during a rest period (Agras et al, 1968; Emmelkamp, 1982; De Silva and Rachman, 1984; Rachman et al, 1986). The latter form of exposure incorporates a behavioral method of anxiety control, and indeed seems to enhance estimates of control beyond those associated with continuous exposure (Rachman et al, 1986). These results are consistent with suggestions made by Barlow in Chapter 1 that the development of a sense of control is crucial to fear reduction.

Treatment outcome may be optimized, therefore, by including techniques that not only lower attrition rates from exposure therapy, but also effectively reduce levels of anxiety during in vivo exposure. Anxiety levels have been shown to account for 30 to 50 percent of variance in the outcome from such treatment

(Michelson et al, 1986). This suggests the need for effective panic management strategies.

PANIC IN AGORAPHOBIA

The significance of panic attacks in the treatment of agoraphobia has been given little attention. However, the absence of procedures that target panic directly in the treatment for agoraphobia may account to some extent for drop-outs, treatment failures, and relapse. Panic can occur in association with particular situations, or can occur with seeming unpredictability. Agoraphobics experience both forms of panic, to which they have developed an avoidant strategy. Individuals who have panic disorder without agoraphobia experience panic attacks but have not developed a pattern of extensive avoidance of particular situations.

There is some evidence to suggest that in vivo exposure alleviates panic attacks. Linder (1981), for example, reported on four agoraphobics who monitored their excursions away from home and panic attacks during the course of a 12-week treatment program. Following imaginal exposure to feared situations and instructions for self-directed exposure, panic frequency reduced from a range of 2 to 29 per week at pretreatment to near zero at posttreatment. Maintenance of treatment gains up to six months posttreatment were established during telephone contact with the therapist. Unfortunately, the reliability and validity of the follow-up assessment is poor, especially as information regarding the frequency of panic is absent. Ghosh and Marks (in press) reported that ratings of panic–tension decreased from 6.3 (marked) to 1.5 (slight) six months after a program of exposure to feared situations.

Reports based on individual analyses rather than group averages suggest that panic is not alleviated in all patients who undergo in vivo exposure. As early as 1973, Stern and Marks found that some patients continued to experience panic despite reductions in avoidance behavior. Also, Arnow and colleagues (1985) reported that panic frequency did not change as a result of four weeks of in vivo exposure despite improvements in all other measures of agoraphobic avoidance (although the ratio of panics to number of excursions decreased markedly). In one of the first reports involving the systematic measurement of panic in the treatment of agoraphobia, Barlow and associates (1984b) found that treatment responders improved significantly on an overall rating of the frequency, intensity, and duration of panic in comparison to nonresponders. Chambless and co-workers (in press) reported that 29 percent of 35 agoraphobics continued to experience panic six months after treatment despite significant improvement in agoraphobic avoidance. Finally, Michelson and colleagues (1985) found that 45 percent continued to experience "spontaneous" panic attacks three months after in vivo exposure therapy.

Klosko and Barlow (1987, unpublished manuscript) examined in detail the occurrence of panic in 16 agoraphobics and 16 panic disorder patients. Agoraphobics received 12 sessions of training in self-directed in vivo exposure and coping self-statements. Panic disorder patients received 15 to 20 sessions of techniques designed specifically for the reduction of panic attacks. Eighty-five percent of the panic disorder patients who panicked in the two weeks pretreatment did not panic after treatment, in comparison to 44 percent of the agoraphobics. Together, the data lead to the conclusion that in vivo exposure is of some benefit but is not sufficient to treat panic in agoraphobia. Not surprisingly, procedures designed specifically for panic are more effective. In addition, there is evidence to suggest that the occurrence of panic may impede treatment progress and result in relapse in agoraphobics. Rachman and associates (1986) noted that the occurrence of panic between treatment sessions resulted in decreased estimates of safety and control regarding the performance of specific exposure tasks at subsequent treatment sessions in comparison to estimates made following a week without panic. Arnow and co-workers (1985) noted that in each instance of relapse, "those subjects whose gains were erased attributed their renewed avoidance to one or more significant episodes of panic" (p. 465). The results emphasize the importance of long-term follow-up assessment and the inclusion of procedures for measuring and treating panic attacks.

DIRECT TREATMENT OF PANIC

Several case studies report the successful use of hypnotherapy and psychoanalytical dream analysis for the treatment of panic attacks (Woods, 1972; Van Pelt, 1975; Fewtrell, 1984). However, their methods and outcome are specified poorly, and experimental control is lacking.

Multicomponent Treatment

The first systematic attempts to research the effectiveness of psychological treatment for panic attacks utilized multicomponent packages, with almost all containing cognitive, relaxation, and specialized exposure techniques. Newer treatments highlight specific components that have become more finely focused as our understanding of the nature of panic attacks and panic disorder progresses.

Gitlin and colleagues (1985) treated 11 patients with panic disorder who kept daily diaries of anxiety and panic attacks. They received from 6 to 32 individual group sessions in which they were provided with education about panic attacks, relaxation training, diaphragmatic breathing training, in vivo exposure, and assertiveness training. Patients were required to practice daily their relaxation, breathing exercises, and in vivo exposure. The pretreatment panic average of 4.6 per week reduced markedly—10 patients were free of panic after treatment. The panic outcome was reportedly maintained at an assessment five months after treatment, which, however, was conducted during telephone contact. These results are very impressive, but the study was uncontrolled. In an equally impressive set of results, Shear and associates (in press) treated 17 patients with panic disorder for an average of 17 sessions. Eighty-seven percent of the patients were free of spontaneous full panic attacks at posttreatment where panic was defined clearly as four or more symptoms from the *Diagnostic and Statistical Manual of Mental Disorders, Third Edition (DSM-III)* (American Psychiatric Association, 1980) checklist. All reported reductions in limited symptom attacks and situational panic attacks. Unfortunately, follow-up data are not yet available.

In two controlled studies, the effects of multicomponent treatment have been shown to be superior to the passage of time alone. After demonstrating the success with which episodes of intense anxiety were reduced in three patients by a combination of relaxation training, coping self-statement training, and challenging irrational belief sets (Waddell et al, 1984), Barlow and colleagues (1984a) conducted a study in which they assigned five patients with panic disorder to treatment and six to a wait-list control group. Treatment consisted of 18 weekly sessions in which patients were taught progressive muscle relaxation, muscle tension biofeedback, and cognitive restructuring as means of coping with anxiety induced imaginally within treatment sessions, and with anxiety that occurred naturally between treatment sessions. It was found that a composite measure of panic that included intensity, duration, and frequency estimates from self-monitoring data decreased significantly in the treated patients and did not change in the wait-list over the same period of time. This was accompanied by a general, broad-based improvement in the treated group, involving decreased muscle tension and heart rate during a standard physiological assessment, and reduced severity based on independent clinician's ratings. The improvements were maintained three months after treatment completion. It is noteworthy, however, that the decreases in muscle tension were not correlated with any outcome measure, suggesting that progressive muscle relaxation and biofeedback were not effective through their intended mechanisms, and highlighting the need for nonspecific treatment comparisons.

Several other studies have been conducted but lacked specific measures of panic. Jannoun and associates (1982) reported that a multicomponent treatment was more effective than the passage of time alone for 27 patients who experienced generalized anxiety and panic. Tarrier and Main (1986) reported some effectiveness from one session of training in breathing regulation, progressive muscle relaxation, and positive mental imagery (to control physical symptoms and to distract attention from anxiety-associated thoughts) followed by directions for five weeks of daily home practice in comparison to a wait-list control group.

In conclusion, the multicomponent treatment for panic seems to be more effective than time alone, with success rates (that is, free of panic) of up to 91 percent at posttreatment. Follow-up status is crucial to the evaluation of these procedures—in the one study where long term effects were measured, the results were very promising. However, more substantial follow-up data are required, and it is not known whether these procedures are any more effective than other forms of treatment. The specificity of treatment effects requires investigation, particularly as muscle reduction techniques form a large part of the multicomponent approach, and yet do not appear to yield positive outcome through functional reduction in muscle tension (Barlow et al, 1984a; Tarrier and Main, 1986). The current direction of research is toward the evaluation of the specific treatment components, as based on more advanced conceptualizations of panic disorder.

Specific Panic Treatments

The development of greater specificity in the treatment of panic emerged from the recognition of several aspects of panic disorder that seem particularly important to target in treatment, and which are consistent with the conceptualization of panic disorder as a phobic-like reaction to somatic sensations associated with panic and/or their perceived consequences.

INTEROCEPTIVE EXPOSURE. Extreme sensitivity to and fear of interoceptive cues in panic may well result from interoceptive conditioning, as suggested in Chapter 1. This development in the understanding of the nature of panic disorder is followed by a treatment that entails repeated exposure to the physical sensations. The purpose of this approach, as in the case of exposure to external phobic stimuli, is to disrupt associations between specific cues and panic reactions. The treatment procedures incorporate methods that induce panic-related symptoms reliably, such as physical exercise, inhalations of carbon dioxide, and hyperventilation, and is known as interoceptive exposure. It is interesting to note that some earlier reports used this type of procedure. For example, Orwin (1973a) introduced the notion of running therapy and CO_2 inhalations, believing that breathlessness would inhibit the anxiety response.

In two early studies, interoceptive exposure was used systematically as a form of treatment, but specific measures of improvement in panic were not included. Bonn and associates (1973) "successfully" treated 33 patients by repeated exposure to symptoms induced through infusions of sodium lactate. Haslam (1974) reported that 9 out of 10 people who experienced panic in response to sodium lactate infusions responded favorably to six weeks of repeated inhalations of carbon dioxide.

Griez and van de Hout (1983) described the successful treatment of an agoraphobic using CO_2 and hyperventilation induction. In 1986, they reported the first controlled study of interoceptive exposure. In their crossover design, 14 panickers and agoraphobics received 1) six sessions of repeated, graded CO_2 inhalation over two weeks, and 2) a two-week regimen of propranolol (a beta blocker), chosen because it suppresses symptoms that are induced during inhalations. The inhalation treatment proceeded from therapist modeling, to gradual approximation, to placing the mask over the face and taking a deep breath, to various elaborations of vital capacity breaths. The entire treatment package resulted in a mean reduction from 12 to 4 panic attacks over a very short two-week period. A mean reduction of 50 percent was achieved from the inhalation condition as compared to 38 percent from the medication condition. In addition, the inhalation treatment was superior in terms of ratings of fear of sensations. Data obtained six months after treatment suggested that the effects were generally maintained, although no information regarding panic frequency was provided. The authors noted that the rapid effects from CO_2 treatment may have operated through mechanisms of habituation or reduced chemoreceptor sensitivity, but a comparison control is required to test those hypotheses and alternative possibilities.

This treatment technique seems to parallel in vivo exposure that is conducted without anxiety control strategies. The strategies that have been developed for management of panic (or fear of its recurrence) include corrective information/ cognitive reinterpretation and breathing training.

COGNITIVE REATTRIBUTION.   Beck (1986) extended his cognitive model of depression to anxiety and panic, in which he focuses on the role of catastrophic interpretations of panic-related internal cues, especially related to death or loss of control. Cognitive treatment involves the establishment of more realistic interpretations of sensations through the provision of corrective information and more extensive analysis of cognitive factors that produce the misinterpretations (Rapee, 1987). Again, this has been part of almost all treatments reviewed above, but the procedure has become more focused upon specific misinterpretations that prevail in panic disorder (for example, "I am dying," "I am going crazy," and "I will lose control").

Several uncontrolled reports exist that employ mostly cognitive techniques

(Hollon, 1981). In the work reported by Beck and his colleagues, the cognitive therapy is conducted in conjunction with behavioral techniques, but the effective mechanism of change is assumed to lie in the cognitive realm. Sokol and Beck (1986), cited in Beck (in press) reported the results from 25 panic disorder patients who were treated with cognitive techniques combined with interoceptive exposure and in vivo exposure for an average of 17 sessions. Panic response was extremely good in the 17 patients who did not have additional diagnoses of personality disorder, reducing from 5.4 to 0 per week. These results were maintained 12 months after treatment. The study was uncontrolled but the results were uniform. However, the use of exposure precludes discussion of the effectiveness of cognitive techniques alone, and the absence of controlled comparisons prevents the conclusion that the treatment effect was greater than that achieved from time alone, or from any alternative procedure.

BREATHING TRAINING. Several researchers have examined the effectiveness of breathing training in light of the similarity of hyperventilatory symptoms to those that characterize panic attacks. It is believed that hyperventilation may produce the various somatic sensations that occur during panic attacks for a certain proportion of patients (Rapee, 1985). In the conception of panic that emphasizes hyperventilation, panic attacks are viewed as stress-induced respiratory changes that provoke fear because they are perceived as frightening, or augment fear already elicited by other stimuli. The increased apprehension produces further hyperventilation and a vicious cycle results (Salkovskis et al, 1986a).

Breathing training has been applied singly and in combination with cognitive strategies, and involves the development of slow and diaphragmatic breathing. As early as 1971, Suinn and Richardson advocated the use of relaxation and slowed breathing upon recognition of internal arousal cues in order to prevent the development of a full-blown panic attack (in Fewtrell, 1984). Kraft and Hoogduin (1984) found that 6 biweekly sessions of a combination of breathing retraining and progressive muscle relaxation reduced the frequency of self-monitored panic attacks from 10 to 4 per week. This treatment was no more effective than either repeated hyperventilation and control of symptoms by breathing into a bag, or identification of life stressors and problem-solving to eliminate precipitants to anxiety and tension, in terms of severity and number of hyperventilatory symptoms. However, important initial group differences, plus the fact that all three groups were given corrective information regarding the relationship between hyperventilatory patterns and panic sensations, make these results difficult to interpret.

At least two case reports have described the successful application of breathing training in the context of a cognitively oriented treatment in which patients are taught to reinterpret the sensations as nondangerous and nonthreatening. Rapee (1985) reported that three sessions of information about hyperventilation, cognitive reattribution, and breathing training resulted in a reduction of self-monitored panic attacks from 22 to 2 per week. The patient then received six additional sessions of lifestyle changes including smoking cessation and an exercise regimen, so that the maintenance of treatment effects at follow-up cannot be attributed solely to breathing training and cognitive reattribution. Salkovskis and colleagues (1986b) treated an individual who began to panic during dialysis due to the fear of dying associated with marked hyperventilation. Forced hyperventilation, with corrective information and breathing training, produced immediate response in controlling panic.

Two larger scale investigations provide impressive evidence for the effectiveness of the combination of breathing training and cognitive reattribution. Clark and associates (1985) reported on 18 panickers who received two weekly sessions of respiratory control training, including the application of corrective breathing and reinterpretation after brief hyperventilation. From a stable baseline period, panic attacks were found to reduce on average from 10 to 5 per week in those whose panic was associated with specific situations (that is, agoraphobics) and from 5 to 2 per week in "nonsituational" panickers. Patients received an average number of 10 additional sessions involving cognitive-behavioral treatment and in vivo exposure, during which the frequency of panic continued to diminish and stabilized at zero. A two-year follow-up assessment indicated that panic and generalized anxiety ratings had maintained. However, the study does not allow examination of the long-term effects of respiratory control alone, given the nature of the additional treatment sessions.

In an attempt to establish the specificity of the effects from respiratory control training, Salkovskis and co-workers (1986a) measured pCO_2 levels during the treatment of 9 panicking patients. Measures of pCO_2 reflect levels of expired CO_2, which is a good indicator of breathing regularity. Patients received four weekly sessions of forced hyperventilation, corrective information, and breathing training, after which they received in vivo exposure if necessary. Panic frequency on average reduced from 7 to 3 per week after respiratory control and maintained at that level during in vivo exposure. Levels of pCO_2 normalized during the course of respiratory control training. While this result is more encouraging than the weak relationship between muscle tension and outcome from progressive muscle relaxation or EMG biofeedback training, the normalization of pCO_2 cannot be used as an indicator of specificity of treatment effects yet. Normalization of pCO_2 must be shown to differentiate among groups that receive different forms of treatment, as pCO_2 may be an indicator of general arousal.

Conclusions

All of the specific components reviewed have shown to be effective in controlling panic attacks. These recent developments defy the claim by Marks (1985) that "behavioral psychotherapy is probably the treatment of choice for most phobic and obsessive-compulsive disorders and plays a lesser role in the management of panic disorder without agoraphobia . . ." (p. 25).

Of the various strategies, breathing training has received the most empirical support. Two issues, however, tend to mitigate the findings. In both the case studies and the larger scale investigations, patients were included only if they reported symptoms during panic attacks that were similar to hyperventilatory symptoms. Moreover, Salkovskis and colleagues (1986a) reported that the similarity between naturally occurring panic and hyperventilatory symptoms was a good predictor of response to respiratory control treatment. Not all patients experience hyperventilatory symptoms (Gelder, 1986). This form of treatment will be highly credible in a group of people who experience hyperventilatory symptoms. The efficacy of breathing training requires examination in a group who do not experience hyperventilatory symptoms, or comparison to an equally credible alternative treatment, if it is to be proclaimed a successful and specific treatment method for panic disorder. Second, these treatments have all included some form of exposure to internal sensations, through forced hyperventilation or exercise programs. It will be necessary to separate these procedures before concluding which techniques are most effective in the treatment of panic and the mechanisms through which they operate.

Interoceptive exposure is designed to allow individuals to experience repeatedly the feared stimuli (physical sensations) and to replace fearful responding with nonfearful responding. Breathing control and cognitive strategies, on the other hand, are methods by which fearful responding can be reduced. Hence, these approaches to the treatment of panic parallel in vivo exposure and the various anxiety-control strategies applied in the treatment of agoraphobia. As mentioned previously, the anxiety-control strategies alone do not seem to be sufficient for the treatment of agoraphobia (either because they are not the best available methods or agoraphobia requires more comprehensive treatment) but it is uncertain whether this will be the case for panic disorder. Corrective information, for example, may be all that is required to eliminate panic in some patients. Kraft and Hoogduin demonstrated the effectiveness of breathing training and relaxation techniques, but the extent to which exposure was involved in this treatment is unclear. Positive self-instruction training alone was found to be ineffective in the treatment of six panicking patients (Ramm et al, 1982). This form of cognitive therapy, however, was not designed specifically for panic attacks.

Therefore, it remains to be shown whether breathing training and corrective information are sufficient treatment procedures, and, if so, for whom; whether interoceptive exposure is a necessary treatment condition; whether specific panic management strategies enhance the effectiveness of interoceptive exposure; and whether these recent specializations in the treatment of panic are more effective than the multicomponent approach or nonspecific alternatives. The recently developed techniques do seem capable of producing marked reductions in panic frequency in a relatively short period of time. The multicomponent approach averages 17 sessions, whereas interoceptive exposure and breathing training with corrective information average 4 sessions (with an additional 4 to 10 sessions for situational fear and avoidance). It is also possible that the relevance of each specific component will differ across individuals, and that the choice of treatment will be dependent upon a thorough initial assessment. For example, the absence of hyperventilatory patterns might argue against the use of breathing retraining, whereas the inability to identify fears of going crazy or death would suggest that cognitive reattribution is inappropriate. Alternatively, an individual with all three elements may require all three treatment components.

The Albany Study

At the Center for Stress and Anxiety Disorders, we have begun addressing some of these empirical questions by examining the differential effects of four treatment conditions for panic disorder patients: 1) training in progressive muscle relaxation that is used as an active coping skill during in vivo exposure to feared situations; 2) cognitive restructuring and breathing training which are applied during interoceptive and in vivo exposure; 3) a combination of the first two conditions; and 4) a wait-list control. When complete, this study will enable the comparison of a treatment, including components specialized for the treatment of panic (cognitive reattribution, breathing training, and interoceptive exposure) to the more general and perhaps more basic component of the multi-component approach (relaxation). It will also allow an examination of enhancement deriving from the addition of relaxation to the specific skills, and a comparison with a wait-list control. This study is not sufficiently complete to analyze separate treatment effects, but the results from the combined treatment condition ($n = 18$) can be compared with those from the wait-list ($n = 14$) in a preliminary fashion, as a first controlled examination of the effectiveness of panic management techniques over and above the effects derived from an equivalent period of time in which patients merely monitored their anxiety and panic.

In treatment, specific feared internal cues are assessed by having patients engage in a variety of exercises designed to produce different patterns of physiological symptoms. Motor activity is used to activate cardiovascular symptoms (for example, running in place); voluntary hyperventilation is practiced for respiratory symptoms; and dizziness is induced for audiovestibular symptoms (for example, spinning in a chair). When feared patterns are identified, they become a part of treatment. Exposure is administered both imaginally and in vivo. During imaginal exposure patients visualize an anxiety provoking event or situation. Symptom induction using the above mentioned exercises within the controlled setting of the clinic and, subsequently, during assigned exposure tasks, comprises in vivo exposure. For example, patients might be instructed to run up a flight of stairs, enter a sauna, or engage in vigorous exercise. Following provocation of symptoms and subjective fear, patients are instructed to apply relaxation and slow diaphragmatic breathing and to reinterpret the symptoms as nonthreatening or nondangerous.

In general, the results indicate that this treatment is very effective in reducing both overall severity of the disorder and panic symptomology in comparison to the wait-list control condition. The average severity rated by an independent assessor was reduced from 5.0 to 2.5 (0–8 point scale) in the treatment group, taking them well below the level of clinical severity, in contrast to the stability of the wait-list averages. Seventy-five percent of the treated patients were free of panic attacks at posttreatment assessment in comparison to 31 percent of the wait-list group. The treatment group also reported greater improvement than the wait-list group in terms of clinician's ratings of anxiety and depression, questionnaire scores of social adjustment, and self-ratings. Follow-up data will be of crucial importance to the study. Of the few patients who have completed follow-up assessment, all have reported maintenance of treatment effects.

SUMMARY OF COGNITIVE-BEHAVIORAL TREATMENT FOR PANIC WITH AND WITHOUT AGORAPHOBIA

In vivo exposure has been shown to be very successful in the treatment of agoraphobic avoidance behavior, especially when conducted in a graduated and self-directed manner, but is not reliably effective in the treatment of panic attacks. It follows that techniques which target panic directly would enhance the effectiveness of current procedures for the treatment of agoraphobia. Bonn and colleagues (1984) randomly allocated 12 agoraphobics to either in vivo exposure, or respiratory control training plus in vivo exposure. While a trend was apparent, those who received respiratory control did not experience significantly fewer panic attacks at posttreatment. However, at follow-up, the exposure-alone group had deteriorated and the difference between the groups was significant. Breathing control training may have helped prevent relapse that occurs from the recurrence of panic.

The treatment of panic attacks alone is unlikely to be effective for agoraphobia, as the evidence suggests that only mild reductions in avoidance result from the various panic management techniques (Clark et al, 1985; Salkovskis et al, 1986; Griez and van den Hout, 1986), possibly through a reduction in the fear of panic. Avoidance continues to reduce when in vivo exposure is added to those treatments (Clark et al, 1985; Salkovskis et al, 1986a). In addition, the panic management techniques are not as effective with panic attacks that are elicited by specific situations as they are with panic attacks that seem to occur unpredictably (Clark et al, 1985; Shear et al, in press).

The techniques of interoceptive exposure, cognitive reattribution, and breathing retraining could be included prior to and simultaneously with in vivo exposure (again, the choice may depend upon individual assessment), in order to increase compliance with in vivo exposure instructions (by the availability of a means of coping with intense fear), to enhance the development of emotional control, and to reduce the occurrence of panic attacks. The success with which these techniques reduce anxiety during in vivo exposure (in comparison to the standard procedures of relaxation or coping self-statements) awaits empirical investigation. Also, the interpersonal context of the agoraphobic problem may warrant the inclusion of additional treatment techniques, such as communication skills training.

Panic management techniques in the treatment of panic without agoraphobic avoidance have been shown to be very successful and easy to apply. The generalizability of their effectiveness remains to be assessed. Alternative psychotherapeutic procedures may also be important for aspects of panic disorder in combination with cognitive-behavioral procedures. For example, it is possible that analytical procedures may be important in the treatment of panic disorder that is accompanied by Axis II disorders. Sokol and Beck (1986, cited in Beck, in press) found that the implementation of specific panic management techniques was considerably less effective for panic disorder patients who presented with various personality disorders.

The avoidance component of panic disorder has been given little attention. Currently, panic disorder and agoraphobia are differentiated in terms of the degree of behavioral avoidance of external situations. However, panickers often engage in subtle forms of avoidance: of activities that elicit sensations similar to those that occur during panic (for example, physical exercise, sexual arousal), of events that provoke strong emotionality, or even remembering what it feels like to panic. Interoceptive exposure suppresses such avoidance by forcing confrontation with feared sensations through structured exercises. However, this behavioral quality may warrant further investigation. Salkovskis (in press) suggests that not only agoraphobics but also panic disorder patients "sit down, hold on to walls, seek medical attention, take deep breaths, and generally engage in behaviors which they believe may abort imminent disaster . . . panic-related and catastrophy-avoiding behavior may also have the effect of maintaining preoccupation. For as long as efforts are directed at the avoidance of feared disasters, then cognitive activity is likely to remain centered on the possible disasters." Hence, an important part of exposure treatment for both agoraphobics and panic disorder patients may be the modification of fearful behavioral action tendencies (Barlow, in press). These parallels between agoraphobia and panic disorder have implications for future research. For example, as with in vivo exposure, interoceptive exposure may yield more enduring effects if conducted in a graduated self-directed manner than when it is intensive and therapist-directed.

In any case, pending further evidence, it seems that we have an effective nondrug treatment for panic that can be administered in a relatively brief period of time (15 sessions) in the therapist's office. Treatment manuals are now appearing describing these procedures in sufficient detail to allow most clinicians to immediately incorporate these procedures into their treatment programs (Cerny and Barlow, in press). This should prove an important addition to the armamentarium of therapists seeking effective methods for treating debilitating panic.

REFERENCES

Agras WS, Leitenberg H, Barlow DH: Social reinforcement in the modification of agoraphobia. Arch Gen Psychiatry 1968; 19:423-427

American Psychiatric Association: Diagnostic and Statistical Manual of Mental Disorder, Third Edition (DSM-III). Washington, DC, American Psychiatric Association, 1980

Arnow BA, Taylor CB, Agras WS, et al: Enhancing agoraphobia treatment outcome by changing couple communication patterns. Behavior Therapy 1985; 16:452-467

Barlow DH: Panic, Anxiety and the Anxiety Disorders. New York, Guilford Press (in press)

Barlow DH, Cerny JA: Psychological Treatment of Panic. New York, Guilford Press (in press)

Barlow DH, Waddell MT: Agoraphobia, in Clinical Handbook of Psychological Disorders. Edited by Barlow DH. New York, Guilford Press, 1985

Barlow DH, Cohen AS, Waddell MT, et al: Panic and generalized anxiety disorders: nature and treatment. Behavior Therapy 1984a; 15:431-449

Barlow DH, O'Brien GT, Last CG: Couples treatment of agoraphobia. Behavior Therapy 1984b; 15:41-58

Beck A: Cognitive approaches to panic disorder: theory and therapy, in Panic: Cognitive Views. Edited by Rachman SJ, Maser JD. Hillsdale, NJ, Lawrence Erlbaum Associates (in press)

Bonn JA, Harrison J, Rees L: Lactate infusion in the treatment of 'free-floating' anxiety. Canadian Psychiatric Association Journal 1973; 18:41-45

Bonn JA, Readhead CPA, Timmons BH: Enhanced adaptive behavioural response in agoraphobic patients pretreated with breathing retraining. Lancet 1984; 2:665-669

Burns LE, Thorpe GL, Cavallaro A: Agoraphobia eight years after behavioral treatment: a follow-up study with interview, questionnaire, and behavioral data. Paper presented at The World Congress of Behavior Therapy, Washington DC, 1983

Cerny JA, Barlow DH, Craske MG, et al: Couples treatment of agoraphobia: a two-year follow-up. Behavior Therapy (in press)

Chambless DL, Goldstein AJ, Gallagher R, et al: Integrating behavior therapy and psychotherapy in the treatment of agoraphobia. Psychotherapy (in press)

Clark MD, Salkovskis PM: A cognitive-behavioural treatment for panic attacks. Based on a paper presented at SPR 2nd European Conference on Psychotherapy Research, Louvain-la-Neurve, Belgium, Sept. 3-7, 1985

Clark DM, Salkovskis PM, Chalkley AJ: Respiratory control as a treatment for panic attacks. J Behav Ther Exp Psychiatry 1985; 16:23-30

Cobb JP, Mathews AM, Childs-Clarke A, et al: The spouse as co-therapist in the treatment of agoraphobia. Br J Psychiatry 1984; 144:282-287

Cohen SD, Monteiro W, Marks IM: Two-year follow-up of agorphobics after exposure and imipramine. Br J Psychiatry 1984; 144:276-281

De Silva P, Rachman S: Does escape behaviour strengthen agoraphobic avoidance? a preliminary study. Behav Res Ther 1984; 22:87-91

Dittrich J, Houts AC, Lichstein KL: Panic disorder: assessment and treatment. Clinical Psychology Review 1983; 3:215-225

Emmelkamp PMG: Phobic and Obsessive-Compulsive Disorders. New York, Plenum Press, 1982

Emmelkamp PMG, Kuipers ACM: Agoraphobia: follow-up study four years after treatment. Br J Psychiatry 1979; 134:352-355

Emmelkamp PMG, Kuipers ACM, Eggeraat JB: Cognitive modification versus prolonged exposure in vivo: a comparison with agoraphobics as subjects. Behav Res Ther 1978; 16:33-41

Emmelkamp PMG, van den Hout A, De Vries K: Assertive training for agoraphobics. Behav Res Ther 1983; 21:63-68

Fewtrell WD: Psychological approaches to panic attack—some recent developments. British Journal of Experimental and Clinical Hypnosis 1984; 1:21-24

Foa EB, Kozak MJ: Emotional processing of fear: exposure to corrective information. Psychol Bull 1986; 99:20-35

Foa EB, Jameson JS, Turner RM, et al: Massed vs. spaced exposure sessions in the treatment of agoraphobia. Behav Res Ther 1980; 18:333-338

Freud S: Turnings in the ways of psychoanalytic therapy, in Collected Papers, vol. 2. New York, Basic Books, 1919

Gelder MG: Panic attacks: new approaches to an old problem. Br J Psychiatry 1986; 149: 346-352

Gitlin B, Martin M, Shear K, et al: Behavior therapy for panic disorder. J Nerv Ment Dis 1985; 173:742-743

Ghosh A, Marks IM: Self-treatment of agoraphobia by exposure. Behavior Therapy (in press)

Griez E, van den Hout MA: Treatment of phobophobia by exposure to CO_2-induced anxiety symptoms. J Behav Ther Exp Psychiatry 1983; 14:297-304

Griez E, van den Hout MA: CO_2 inhalation in the treatment of panic attacks. Behav Res Ther 1986; 24:145-150

Hafner RJ: Fresh symptom emergence after intensive behaviour therapy. Br J Psychiatry 1976; 129:378-383

Hand I, Lamontagne Y: The exacerbation of interpersonal problems after rapid phobia-removal. Psychother Theory Res Prac 1976; 13:405-411

Haslam MT: The relationship between the effect of lactate infusion on anxiety states and their amelioration by carbon dioxide inhalation. Br J Psychiatry 1974; 125:88-90

Himadi WG, Cerny JA, Barlow DH, et al: The relationship of marital adjustment to agoraphobia treatment outcome. Behav Res Ther 1986; 24:107-115

Holden AE, O'Brien GT, Barlow DH, et al: Self-help manual for agoraphobia: a preliminary report of effectiveness. Behavior Therapy 1983; 14:545-556

Hollon SD: Cognitive-behavioral treatment of drug-induced pansituational anxiety states, in New Directions in Cognitive Therapy. Edited by Emery G, Hollon SD, Bedrosian RC. New York, Guilford Press, 1981

Jannoun L, Oppenheimer C, Gelder M: A self-help treatment program for anxiety state patients. Behavior Therapy 1982; 13:103-111

Jansson L, Ost L: Behavioural treatments for agoraphobia: an evaluative review. Clinical Psychology Review 1982; 2:311-337

Jansson L. Jerremalm A, Ost LG: Follow-up of agoraphobic patients treated with exposure in vivo or applied relaxation. Br J Psychiatry 1986; 149:486-490

Kraft AR, Hoogduin CAL: The hyperventilation syndrome: a pilot study on the effectiveness of treatment. Br J Psychiatry 1984; 145:538-542

Linder LH: Group behavioral treatment of agoraphobia: a preliminary report. Compr Psychiatry 1981; 22:226-233

Marks I: Phobic disorders four years after treatment: a prospective follow-up. Br J Psychiatry 1971; 118:683-688

Marks I: Behavioral psychotherapy for anxiety disorders. Psychiatr Clin North Am 1985; 8:25-35

Mathews AM, Gelder MG, Johnston DW: Agoraphobia: Nature and Treatment. New York, Guilford Press, 1981

Mavissakalian M, Barlow DH: Phobia: Psychological and Pharmacological Treatment. Edited by Mavissakalian M, Barlow DH. New York, Guilford Press, 1981

McPherson FM, Brougham L, McLaren S: Maintenance of improvement in agoraphobic patients treated by behavioral methods—a four-year follow-up. Behav Res Ther 1980; 18:150-152

Michelson L, Mavissakalian M, Marchione K: Cognitive and behavioral treatments of agoraphobia: clinical, behavioral, and psychophysiological outcomes. J Consult Clin Psychol 1985; 53:913-925

Michelson L, Mavissakalian M, Marchione K, et al: The role of self-directed in vivo exposure in cognitive, behavioral, and psychophysiological treatments of agoraphobia. Behavior Therapy 1986: 17:91-108

Milton F, Hafner J: The outcome of behavior therapy for agoraphobia in relation to marital adjustment. Arch Gen Psychiatry 1979; 36:807-811

Munby J, Johnston DW: Agoraphobia: the long-term follow-up of behavioural treatment. Br J Psychiatry 1980; 137:417-418

Nemiah JC: The psychoanalytic view of anxiety, in Anxiety: New Research and Changing Concepts. Edited by Klein DF, Rabkin J. New York, Raven Press, 1981

Orwin A: Augmented respiratory relief: A new use for CO$_2$ therapy in the treatment of phobic conditions: a preliminary report on two cases. Br J Psychiatry 1973a; 122:171-173

Orwin A: 'The running treatment': a preliminary communication on a new use for an old therapy (physical activity) in the agoraphobic syndrome. Br J Psychiatry 1973b; 122: 175-179

Rachman SJ, Craske MG, Tallman K, et al: Does escape behavior strengthen agoraphobic avoidance? a replication. Behavior Therapy 1986; 17:366-384

Ramm E, Marks IM, Yuksel S, et al: Anxiety management training for anxiety states: positive compared with negative self-statements. Br J Psychiatry 1982; 140:367-373

Rapee RM: A case of panic disorder treated with breathing retraining. J Behav Ther Exp Psychiatry 1985; 16:63-65

Rapee RM: The psychological treatment of panic attacks: theoretical conceptualization and review of evidence. Clinical Psychology Review 1987; 7:427-438

Salkovskis PM: Phenomenology, assessment and the cognitive model of panic, in Panic: Cognitive Views. Edited by Rachman S. Maser JD. Hillsdale, NJ, Lawrence Erlbaum Associates (in press)

Salkovskis PM, Jones DRO, Clark DM: Respiratory control in the treatment of panic attacks: replication and extension with concurrent measurement of behaviour and pCO$_2$. Br J Psychiatry 1986a; 148:526-532

Salkovskis PM, Warwick HMC, Clark DM, et al: A demonstration of acute hyperventilation during naturally occurring panic attacks. Behav Res Ther 1986b; 24:91-94

Shear KM, Ball G, Josephson S: Cognitive-behavioral treatment of panic: an empirical approach. International Journal of Eclectic Psychotherapy (in press)

Stern R, Marks I: Brief and prolonged flooding: a comparison in agoraphobic patients. Arch Gen Psychiatry 1973; 28:270-276

Suinn RN, Richardson F: Anxiety management training: a nonspecific behavior therapy program for anxiety control. Behavior Therapy 1971; 2:498-510

Tarrier N, Main CJ: Applied relaxation training for generalised anxiety and panic attacks: the efficacy of a learnt coping strategy on subjective reports. Br J Psychiatry 1986; 149:330-336

Van Pelt SJ: Hypnosis and panic. Journal of the American Institute of Hypnosis 1975; 16:39-46

Vermilyea JA, Boice R, Barlow DH: Rachman and Hodgson (1974) a decade later: how do desynchronous response sytems relate to the treatment of agoraphobia? Behav Res Ther 1984; 22:615-621

Waddell MT, Barlow DH, O'Brien GT: A preliminary investigation of cognitive and relaxation treatment of panic disorder: effects on intense anxiety vs 'background' anxiety. Behav Res Ther 1984; 22:393-402

Woods MM: Violence: psychotherapy of pseudohomosexual panic. Arch Gen Psychiatry 1972; 27:255-258

Zitrin CM, Klein DF, Woerner MG: Treatment of agoraphobia with group exposure in vivo and imipramine. Arch Gen Psychiatry 1980: 37:63-72

AFTERWORD

by M. Katherine Shear, M.D. and David Barlow, Ph.D.

Recognition of panic attacks as a discrete symptom, and of panic disorder as a diagnostic category, represents an important development in psychiatric thinking. Delineation of panic from other anxiety disorders was one of the major changes in diagnostic thinking reflected in the *Diagnostic and Statistical Manual of Mental Disorders, Third Edition (DSM-III)* (American Psychiatric Association, 1980). This distinction emerged initially from pharmacologic treatment studies of agoraphobics. These studies showed that antidepressant medication blocked panic attacks and enabled many severely phobic patients to resume normal activities. An argument was made that agoraphobia is a complication of panic disorder. Clinical experience supports this view (see Chapter 3 for a discussion of contrary epidemiologic findings), and the *Diagnostic and Statistical Manual of Mental Disorders, Third Edition, Revised (DSM-III-R)* (American Psychiatric Association, 1987) highlights the presumed pathogenic sequence by subsuming agoraphobia under the panic disorder designation.

The central pathogenic role of the initial panic attack in the panic-agoraphobia syndrome should not obscure the fact that much of the morbidity of the syndrome results from panic complications. Panic attacks usually last about 20 minutes. Some are much shorter. Even individuals with multiple episodes a week would not be very symptomatic if they had only panic symptoms. In fact, it is interpanic symptoms of anticipatory anxiety and phobic avoidance which are most debilitating to these patients. Again, *DSM-III-R* acknowledges this observation by removing the panic frequency criterion and replacing it with a criterion of persistent anticipatory anxiety (see Chapter 4).

One of the things we have learned recently is that panic attacks are not synonymous with panic disorder. Panic attacks are frequent in nonclinical populations and in other psychiatric disorders (see Chapters 1 and 3). Studies comparing panic disorder patients to infrequent panickers may help elucidate biological and psychological underpinnings of panic mechanisms. The initial observation of antipanic efficacy of antidepressant class drugs has held up nicely. Moreover, the pharmacologic armamentarium for panic has now been expanded, with newer and better drugs continually being developed (see Chapter 5). A more recent and particularly interesting development is the emergence of data showing that cognitive-behavioral treatment is also effective in ameliorating panic (see Chapter 6).

Much has been written about biological aspects of panic disorder in recent years, and most readers are likely to be aware of at least some of the exciting developments in this area (see Chapter 2). However, amidst the initial flurry of interest in biological treatment and mechanisms of panic, some of the psychological features were ignored. Most researchers in the field now acknowledge the need to better understand psychological as well as physiological aspects of panic. Our aim as editors of this section was to integrate a review of psychologically oriented assessment techniques, treatment strategies, research findings, and theoretical models into the now more familiar biomedical approach to panic. We hope to encourage readers to focus on psychological factors in designing and interpreting research studies and in working with panic disorder patients. This focus is meant to augment, not to displace, interest in biological aspects of panic.

In Chapter 1, Dr. Barlow examined different models of panic. In addition to the usual neurobiologic models, he reviewed several psychological models based on cognitive, conditioning, and psychodynamic theories. He pointed out that an integrated model is needed to explain all of the observed features, such as the tendency of panics to recur in consistent settings, the observation of a high familial prevalence of panic, the phenomenon of nocturnal panics, and the occurrence of panic with and without physiologic accompaniments. He noted that a large number of people have infrequent panic, and many fewer develop panic disorder. This point is echoed later in Dr. Weissman's chapter. Any model of panic needs to explain the basis of vulnerability to recurrent panic attacks.

Barlow also discussed the role of life stresses in precipitating a panic disorder. He listed types of life events which are typical, sources of personal vulnerability to negative life events, and a possible mechanism for the relationship of stress to panic onset. He noted that while stress commonly leads to exacerbation of medical and psychiatric disorders, life stress is even more common prior to onset of panic. Moreover, the stressor rarely precipitates an immediate panic attack, but rather sets the stage for an initial panic some months later. Barlow proposed an interesting new version of an integrated model, based on the principles of emotion theory. According to this model, panic is conceptualized as an inborn, hard-wired fear reaction, which is designed to function as an alarm. Panic attacks are conceived as false alarms (see also Klein, 1981). Panic disorder develops because of fear of uncontrollability of the false alarm. Some kinds of childhood experiences may predispose to fear of uncontrollability, which may be what differentiates the infrequent panicker from a panic disorder patient.

Chapter 2, by Drs. Shear and Fyer, reviewed the data relating to pathogenic mechanisms of panic. This chapter focused heavily on biological studies, especially in the area of respiratory function. Studies using carbon dioxide provocation of panic, along with exploration of respiratory parameters of panic, represent one of the exciting new developments in the field. The authors reviewed the latest findings in neurotransmitter, neurohormonal, and autonomic function testing. There is also a review of findings from psychological studies. These studies focus on psychological aspects of pharmacologic provocative testing, psychophysiologic studies, and psychometric approaches. The authors suggested that collaborative efforts between biologically and psychologically oriented investigators have an important role in panic research. Practitioners need to integrate findings from both areas into a working model which informs clinical treatment programs.

In Chapter 3, Dr. Weissman reviewed findings from epidemiologic and family studies. These data should be particularly useful in developing preventive approaches to treatment. Epidemiologic findings also provide insight into symptoms prevalence and patterns, which can be obscured in clinical populations by factors that determine patienthood. An example of this situation is the differing findings regarding the relationship between agoraphobia and panic. Epidemiologic studies reveal a substantial population of individuals who suffer from agoraphobia without panic. Drs. Jacob and Turner also commented on this observation. Weissman suggested that agoraphobia occurs in connection with other psychiatric disorders, particularly depression. It is likely that clinicians treating depression or other psychiatric or medical conditions may fail to focus on phobic symptoms. Patients are often reluctant to discuss phobias (see Chapter 5) and need to be asked about avoidance directly. Studies of prevalence of phobias in patients presenting with nonphobic disorders should be done. It is also possible that anxiety and panic prone individuals are likely to seek treatment, while phobia prone individuals are avoidant of treatment settings.

Epidemiologic studies reported by Weissman provide support for several clinical observations discussed by other chapter authors. These include a high prevalence of comorbidity with other anxiety disorders, depression, and substance abuse, as well as a high prevalence of infrequent panic episodes in the general population. Family and twin studies show a high familial prevalence of panic disorder and an identical twin concordance of about 30 percent. The latter finding suggests that there is both a constitutional predisposition to panic and a substantial environmental contribution.

Chapter 4, by Drs. Jacob and Turner, introduced issues of diagnosis and assessment. They review changes in diagnostic criteria reflected in the *DSM-III-R*. These include the important decision to place agoraphobia with panic attacks under the heading of panic disorder, the elimination of a frequency criterion for panic, a stronger emphasis on the sudden, unexpected quality of at least some symptoms, and the addition of limited symptom attacks as a diagnostic consideration. A major change in *DSM-III-R* is the elimination of the hierarchy rules allowing comorbidity to be identified. This is important because we now know that there is high comorbidity of panic with other anxiety disorders, depression, and substance abuse. The authors addressed the important issue of organic anxiety disorders. Several conclusions are warranted from this discussion: 1) physical illness which is unrelated to panic symptoms is common, and should be treated; 2) panic patients frequently have hypochondriacal concerns which must be addressed (see also Chapter 5); and 3) no medical illness has been found to account for panic symptoms in the majority of patients.

In the second section of this chapter, Jacob and Turner reviewed structured diagnostic interviews and dimensional symptom rating scales. They advocated a multidimensional approach to patient assessment that includes cognitive, behavioral, and physiologic measures, as well as careful diagnosis.

Chapters 5 and 6 outlined treatment strategies for panic patients. In Chapter 5, Drs. Fyer and Sandberg presented a thorough and highly useful compendium of pharmacologic agents that are effective in panic disorder. They outlined the medical evaluation needed in preparation for a pharmacologic trial and reviewed the pros and cons of the different agents. In addition, these authors provided a particularly important discussion of psychological factors involved in treating panic patients with medication. A psychological approach is particularly important in the initial phases of treatment. The authors stressed the need for an empathic approach in this patient group, as these patients tend to be highly fearful. Behavioral assessment, including direct questioning about phobias and inquiry into other behavioral patterns such as caffeine, nicotine, or alcohol use, is needed. There is a need to carefully define symptoms with patients in order to evaluate drug efficacy accurately. Perhaps most important, the authors believe that the most common side effect and reason for medication failure is *anxious overreaction*. The authors described ways to identify this problem and some innovative ways to manage it.

Chapter 6, by Dr. Craske, outlined the history and current findings in non-pharmacologic treatment of panic. This approach grew out of early cognitive-behavioral treatment of agoraphobia, which has been modified to address panic attacks directly. Studies are now being reported from sites around the world showing excellent results with nonpharmacologic treatment. Each approach differs slightly, but all have in common some form of panic management along with exposure to interoceptive cues.

The clinician evaluating a panic disorder patient now has a good deal of information available to provide the patient with a comprehensive assessment and a thorough psychoeducational introduction to treatment. In addition, there are a number of promising treatment approaches, which means that there is good reason for optimistic expectations. Several issues should be kept in mind when treating and evaluating these patients. First, a good medical evaluation is an essential part of the psychiatric assessment, although, in fact, most panic patients have already seen many internists before arriving in the psychiatrist's office. Second, a high index of suspicion of possible substance abuse is warranted. If it is present and significant, treatment of the substance abuse takes priority. Next, the clinician should question carefully for phobic avoidance. This must often be done by asking directly about avoidance and fear of specific situations. Phobic patients can underestimate (or avoid discussing) the extent of avoidance and mislead even the most experienced clinician. Treatment planning should target symptoms of panic, anticipatory anxiety, and phobic avoidance. If depression is present, it may play an important role in deciding on the treatment strategy.

Following the initial contact with the patient, the therapist must decide on a treatment approach. There are currently three possibilities. The clinician can choose to use pharmacotherapy alone, cognitive-behavioral treatment alone, or a combination of the two. Since there are currently no available studies to guide this choice, we will describe our own preferences. As a first principle, we feel that combination treatments are not generally warranted as an initial approach. For the most part, they should be reserved for patients who fail to respond to a simple medication or cognitive behavioral approach (see Muskin and Fyer, 1983, for a discussion of this principle). Second, patient preference plays an important role in the treatment decision. For example, some patients have considerable knowledge about medication efficacy and want a drug treatment. Others are highly fearful of medication and strongly prefer a nonpharmacologic approach. Other considerations include the following: Medication treatment requires less participation by the patient, and may work more quickly. Thus, medication may be warranted for patients who are severely ill and unlikely to be able to do the homework required by the cognitive-behavioral treatment. Patients with multiple severe daily panics and extremely high levels of anticipatory anxiety, hypochondriasis, and demoralization fall into this category. Similarly, patients who have very busy lives and are unlikely to practice panic management and homework assignments should be given medication as a first choice. On the other hand, cognitive-behavioral treatment lacks the problematic side effects of medication. Nonpharmacologic treatment is indicated for patients who have mild to moderate symptom intensity and good motivation to participate actively in the treatment. Special instances, such as a desire for pregnancy in a woman or the presence of relative medical contraindications to medications, also indicate a cognitive-behavioral approach.

We find that when panic disorder patients are free of panic symptoms, they often are able to resume normal activities and phobic avoidance disappears. Gentle encouragement and support may be all that is needed to accomplish this. As the panic and phobic symptoms subside, anticipatory anxiety and demoralization also resolve. We explain to patients that these symptoms tend to lag in responding to the treatment, but will diminish with time. However, some patients do not have such a favorable course. Phobic avoidance may persist even with good evidence for panic-blocking medication effects. In this case a behavioral treatment for the phobias should be added. Similarly, in some patients, the cognitive-behavioral treatment has good antiphobic effects, but panic is not blocked. These patients may experience further improvement if medication is added. When efficacy of single medication, cognitive-behavioral, and combined treatments is considered, a very high proportion of panic patients will be effectively treated. Studies comparing the three approaches are underway in several centers and promise to further enhance our ability to plan effective treatments and to increase our understanding of panic mechanisms.

REFERENCES

American Psychiatric Association: Diagnostic and Statistical Manual of Mental Disorders, Third Edition (DSM-III). Washington, DC, American Psychiatric Association, 1980

American Psychiatric Association: Diagnostic and Statistical Manual of Mental Disorders, Third Edition, Revised (DSM-III-R). Washington, DC, American Psychiatric Association, 1987

Klein DF: Anxiety reconceptualized, in Anxiety: New Research and Changing Concepts. Edited by Klein DF, Rabkin JG. New York, Raven Press, 1981

Muskin PR, Fyer AJ: Treatment of panic disorder. J Clin Psychopharmacol 1981; 1:81-93

II

Unipolar Depression

L

II

nipolar
epression

Section II

Unipolar Depression

Foreword

by Martin B. Keller, M.D., Section Editor

In biblical days, Nebuchadnezzar and Saul suffered from the despair and hopelessness of severe depression, as have world renowned leaders such as Abraham Lincoln and Winston Churchill. Moreover, in the past few years, many well known public figures in the arts, entertainment, sports, and politics have had their depressive or manic turmoil exposed to the public eye. Clinical and literary descriptions of depression and mania date to antiquity. The earliest hypothesis about the etiology of these states was the black bile theory of Hippocrates. More rigorous scientific inquiry into depression and mania began over 100 years ago and has had a tremendous upsurge in the past three decades following the discovery of antidepressant medication in the late 1950s. Prior to that, people with depression usually had to choose between two treatments: electroconvulsive therapy (ECT) and psychoanalysis. As will be discussed in this section, there is now a wide diversity of theories about the etiology and mechanisms of causality that lead to these conditions, and a broad array of somatic and psychotherapeutic treatments.

The terms "mood disorder" or "affective disorder" are usually used synonymously to group together a variety of syndromes in which there are disturbances in a person's emotional state ranging from dysphoria or severe irritability to elation, euphoria, or expansiveness. Such feelings are often accompanied by difficulties in cognition, psychomotor activity, physiological functioning and interpersonal activities. There is a tremendous range in the severity, duration, and treatment response of these disturbances. On one extreme, depression that meets *Diagnostic and Statistical Manual of Mental Disorders, Third Edition, Revised (DSM-III-R)* (American Psychiatric Association, 1987) criteria for an episode of "major depression" may be relatively mild with five symptoms, a duration limited to two weeks, remission without treatment, or a rapid response to psychotherapy or somatic treatment. On the other extreme, depression may be of marked severity with psychosis or impaired functioning, require hospitalization, have a duration of many years, be resistant to intensive treatment with medication or ECT, have a lifetime course of multiple recurrences with residual symptoms and psychosocial dysfunction in the intervals between episodes, and have a lifetime suicide rate as high as 15 percent.

Since the late 19th century, when Kraepelin (1921) included unipolar and bipolar affective disorder in his definition of manic-depressive illness, the terms "affective disorder" and "mood disorder" have most commonly referred to patients who had depression with or without a history of mania or hypomania as part of the present illness or past history. In 1962, Leonhard separated manic-depressive psychosis into two groups of patients—a unipolar group, who only had episodes of depression, and a bipolar group, who had episodes of depression and mania. The chapters in this section will concentrate almost exclusively on unipolar depression, also known as nonbipolar depression, although there will also be some discussion of mania and hypomania. The rationale for this is that although definitive etiological evidence separating bipolar disorder and unipolar disorder into distinct disease entities is lacking, there are substantial differences in epidemiology, familial and genetic transmission, neurophysiology, biochemistry, phenomenology, clinical course, and treatment response to warrant distinguishing these groups for clinical and research purposes. Moreover, Volume 6 of the *Psychiatry Update: The American Psychiatric Association Annual Review* (1987) has a superb section on bipolar disorders.

This section will also be restricted to states of sadness or depression that are of sufficient severity and duration to be considered "clinically meaningful." It is often extremely difficult to distinguish between the "blahs" and "blues" of everyday life or the passing periods of sadness, brooding, frustration, or even despair that most people experience and a state of depression that is of sufficient severity to be considered a clinical syndrome. This is a distinction that we are frequently asked to make by patients and their families, nonmental health professionals and third parties such as the media or health insurance companies. We need to acknowledge that this boundary is at times arbitrary and difficult to discern. *DSM-III-R* will be used in this section to make such distinctions, since in the absence of a "blood" depression level we need an explicitly defined system of criteria to refer to so that we may speak a common language. Although the criteria in *DSM-III-R* will probably be modified over time, it is likely that the current definitions of the various unipolar depressive disorders will not undergo substantial change.

Unipolar depression is probably the most widespread, most extensively studied and best understood major psychiatric disorder. In particular, there have been substantial advances in the last decade in our knowledge about the epidemiology, transmission, clinical course, psychobiology and treatment of this condition. The chapters in this section will systematically review current information that is known in each of these domains and will elucidate the unanswered questions that require further research.

REFERENCES

American Psychiatric Association: Diagnostic and Statistical Manual of Mental Disorders, Third Edition, Revised (DSM-III-R). Washington, DC, American Psychiatric Association, 1987

Hales RE, Frances AJ (Eds): Psychiatry Update: The American Psychiatric Association Annual Review, Volume 6. Washington, DC, American Psychiatric Press, Inc., 1987

Kraepelin E: Manic-Depressive Illness. Edinburgh, E&S Livingstone, 1921

Leonhard K, Korff I, Schultz H: Die temperamente in den familien der monopolaren und bipolaren phasischen psychosen. Psychiatry and Neurology 1962; 143:416

Chapter 7

The Genetic Epidemiology of Major Depressive Illness

by Lynn R. Goldin, Ph.D., and Elliot S. Gershon, M.D.

Major depressive illness, or unipolar depression, is a common psychiatric disorder in most populations. The disorder is more common in relatives of patients who have had an episode of major depression than it is in the general population. Monozygotic (MZ) twins are more often concordant for depressive illness than are dizygotic (DZ) twins. These observations are consistent with a genetic etiology. However, there are several factors that complicate genetic interpretations. The risk of depression is not only affected by the diagnostic criteria used, but also by factors such as age, sex, birth cohort, and possibly other cultural variables such as urban residence and socioeconomic status. There have been a substantial number of genetic studies of depression, but many issues are still unresolved. The most important of these are: 1) the genetic relationship between unipolar and bipolar illness; 2) evidence for heterogeneity of depression based on clinical characteristics of patients or pattern of illness in their families; 3) mode of inheritance; that is, single gene or polygenic trait; 4) association or linkage with known genetic marker traits; and 5) underlying biological risk factors.

In this chapter we will review epidemiological, family, twin, and adoption studies that have addressed these various issues. In addition, we will review studies that have examined the mode of transmission of depression and the relationship of depression to genetic marker traits and biological traits. Finally, we will consider which genetic strategies currently hold the most promise for our ability to answer these basic questions.

DEFINITIONS OF MAJOR DEPRESSIVE ILLNESS

Throughout this chapter, we will refer to major depression and unipolar depression synonymously. The diagnosis of depression is based on an individual's experiencing a depressed mood for at least two weeks, which is characterized by the following symptoms: appetite/weight disturbance, insomnia or hypersomnia, psychomotor agitation or retardation, loss of interest in usual activities, loss of energy, feelings of worthlessness and guilt, diminished ability to think or concentrate, and thoughts of death or suicide. During the last 15 years, several classification systems and standardized interviews have been developed to apply to family and population studies. These systems overlap but differ in stringency. We will briefly summarize the differences among the systems most commonly used in research.

Some systems allow for uncertainty of diagnosis by having categories for "definite" and "probable." In addition, criteria for past episodes may differ from that of current episodes. The first standardized criteria to be used in the

United States were those developed in St. Louis by Feighner and colleagues (1972). A diagnosis of depression required the presence of five symptoms for a period of four weeks. The Research Diagnostic Criteria (RDC) (Spitzer et al, 1978) were derived from the Feighner system. The diagnosis of depression requires five symptoms for two weeks and noticeable impairment in work, school, or social functioning. The most commonly used classification of mental disorders in the United States is the *Diagnostic and Statistical Manual of Mental Disorders, Third Edition (DSM-III)* (American Psychiatric Association, 1980), the current version being the *Diagnostic and Statistical Manual of Mental Disorders, Third Edition, Revised (DSM-III-R)* (American Psychiatric Association, 1987). The DSM-III was derived from the RDC and provides the category Major Depressive Episode, which requires four depressive symptoms that persist for at least two weeks. Clearly, rates of depression in the population and in relatives of patients will depend, in part, on which criteria are used. Absolute rates also depend on many other epidemiological and methodological factors; these will be discussed later in this chapter. A more detailed examination of *DSM-III-R* depressive disorders can be found in Chapter 9.

In genetic studies it is critical for diagnoses to be replicable over time, since the familial transmission of lifetime diagnoses are analyzed. Mazure and Gershon (1979) interviewed a small sample of patients, relatives, and controls six months apart and found very good reliability for major depression using modified RDC criteria. These criteria require either: 1) four weeks of symptoms and significant impairment in the individual's major social role, or 2) incapacitation if the episode is of shorter duration than four weeks. However, there was poor reliability for minor depression, suggesting that inferences should not be made based on the latter diagnosis. A study by Rice and colleagues (in press) examined the reliability of RDC for major depression based on interviews repeated several years apart, in relatives of patients. They found that those individuals meeting "minimal" criteria (that is, two weeks' duration, three symptoms, and no medication) for past episodes of depression were least likely to be stable over time. As the number of symptoms, number of episodes, and the extent of treatment increased, the case definition became more stable. Both the Mazure and Gershon (1979) and the Rice and colleagues (in press) studies suggest that past episodes of "mild" depression cannot be reliably diagnosed, which should be taken into account in population and family studies.

Another aspect of the consistency of major depression over time is the proportion of patients who are diagnosed initially as unipolar (or major depression) and who will at some time experience an episode of mania, thereby being rediagnosed as bipolar. In a 40-year follow-up of patients from the Iowa 500 study, it was found that 10 percent of patients diagnosed with unipolar depression were rediagnosed as having bipolar disorder (Winokur et al, 1982). This must also be kept in mind in family studies, since it suggests that any population of unipolar patients is always contaminated with a small proportion that will eventually become bipolar. With increasing age and a greater number of depressive episodes, the probability of a person developing mania or hypomania decreases.

One important methodological issue in diagnosing depression in family studies is whether the clinical data on relatives are collected by direct interview (family study method) or by family history from one or more informants (family history method). This issue is reviewed in detail by Weissman and associates (1986b). Structured family history interview methods to arrive at RDC and *DSM-III-R* diagnoses have been developed. Even if relatives are being directly interviewed, family history methods will have to be used for those individuals who are not available for interview. In addition, family history information is a good supplement to direct interviews because individuals may deny certain symptoms. Comparative studies have shown the family history method has high specificity but low sensitivity. However, underestimation of the prevalence of major depression in relatives can be improved by the use of multiple informants (Gershon and Guroff, 1984). Nonetheless, the sources of data must be taken into account when analyzing the results of family studies.

EPIDEMIOLOGY

Prevalence Estimates

The prevalence of depression has been studied in many community based epidemiological studies. As stated previously, the prevalence partially depends on the criteria used. In addition, different measures of prevalence are often reported, depending on how individuals were surveyed. Studies tend to report three-month, six-month, and one-year prevalence. In addition, a quantity of importance is the lifetime prevalence, which is the proportion of individuals in whom a disorder would develop if they all reached a specified age. This prevalence can be estimated by counting all individuals who have ever been ill and then weighting the denominator according to the amount of risk that the sample population has passed, which is a function of their ages. This calculation requires making assumptions about the distribution of the age of onset in the population. Alternative life table approaches can also be used to avoid making distributional assumptions (Thompson and Weissman, 1981). Whatever the method used, the lifetime prevalence is most important in genetic studies because we categorize individuals as ill or well based on whether or not they have ever been ill with the disorder of interest.

Sex Differences

While the prevalence of bipolar illness is the same in males and females, most studies find the prevalence of depression to be approximately twofold higher in women than in men. In a recent, multicenter study sponsored by the National Institute of Mental Health Epidemiological Catchment Area Study (ECA), the lifetime risk for *DSM-III* major depressive episode varied from 4.9–8.7 percent in women and from 2.3–4.4 percent in men (Robins et al, 1984). Surveys from the United States and other countries find rates from 4.7–25.8 percent in women and from 2.1–12.3 percent in men (Boyd and Weissman, 1981). One exception is a survey in the Amish population of Pennsylvania, which found equal frequency of depression in men and women (Egeland and Hostetter, 1983). Angst and Dobler-Mikola (1984) have suggested that case definition should be different for males and females. They found that in individuals experiencing two weeks of depression and social impairment, women reported a median of five symptoms and men reported a median of three symptoms. They conclude that if different thresholds were used for men versus women, then a 1:1 sex ratio would be found. However, in this study, male and female patients meeting Feighner, RDC, or *DSM-III* criteria did not differ in the median number of symptoms, which would not support separate thresholds. Angst and Dobler-Mikola also found that the female:male sex ratio was higher for depressions occurring over the last year than in those occurring over the last three months, suggesting that males preferentially forget depressive symptoms. However, Weissman and colleagues (1984b) found similar sex ratios no matter which prevalence estimates were used. In summary, the vast majority of studies, in a wide range of cultural settings, find approximately twofold higher frequency of depression in women than in men, suggesting that sex differences are not an artifact of differential treatment seeking behavior, but are due to underlying biological causes.

Birth Cohort Differences

Recently, birth cohort has been shown to play a large role in explaining variable rates of depression within populations. Several population and family studies have found that successive cohorts defined by decade of birth starting at about 1940 have significantly higher rates of depression, and in some studies an earlier age of onset, than earlier born cohorts (Robins et al, 1984; Weissman et al, 1984b; Hagnell et al, 1982). This is true for both males and females. Figure 1 shows the rates of depression by age in males and females from four different cohorts from the study of Weissman and colleagues (1984b). This may represent a true finding in the sense that for some "environmental" reason, more recently born individuals are more susceptible to depression. (Similar trends have also been found for suicide [Murphy and Wetzel, 1980], alcoholism, and mania [Robins et al, 1984.]) This effect could also be explained by overreporting in younger individ-

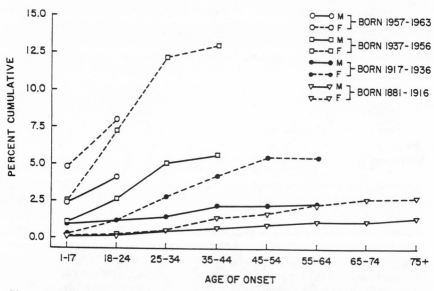

Figure 1. Age of onset of major depression by birth cohort and sex. Reprinted from Weissman MM, Leaf PJ, Holzer CE III, et al: The epidemiology of depression: an update on sex differences in rates. J Affective Disord 7:179-188, 1984. Reprinted by permission of Elsevier Science Publishers and the authors.

uals or underreporting in older ones. There may also be a tendency of older individuals with a history of depression to have earlier mortality or otherwise be lost to population studies. Whatever the explanation, the cohort effect will bias genetic studies, since relatives from several cohorts will be pooled for risk estimates. We will return to this issue later in this chapter.

Other Risk Factors

Race and social class do not seem to affect the risk for depression (Robins et al, 1984). In the St. Louis site of the ECA study, an urban population did not differ from a rural population (Robins et al, 1984), but a site in North Carolina found an increased six-month prevalence of major depression in urban residents in individuals younger than age 45 (Crowell et al, 1986).

FAMILIAL FINDINGS

Twin Studies

Bertelsen and colleagues (1977) studied both unipolar and bipolar twins for concordance of affective disorder. The concordance rates for unipolar twin probands were 54 percent in MZ twins and 24 percent in DZ twins. This greater than twofold difference suggests that genetic factors play a significant role in the etiology of unipolar illness. Torgersen (1986) recently studied the co-twins of 151 twin probands with affective illness. The twins were diagnosed according to *DSM-III* criteria. He found that the concordance rates for major depression in a sample of 92 twin pairs were 45 percent in MZ twins and 22 percent in DZ twins. The heritability (that is, the proportion of liability factors due to genetic factors) of major depression was calculated to be 54 percent. However, there was evidence of heterogeneity in the concordances for major depression, suggesting that the diagnostic category is too broad. For example, heritability for major depression with hysterical personality features could not be demonstrated. In addition, heritability for dysthymia (milder depression of at least two years' duration, equivalent to RDC chronic and intermittent depression or minor depression of two years' duration) could also not be demonstrated in this study.

It is clear that there is significant heritability to unipolar illness, although not to the same extent as bipolar illness (Bertelsen et al, 1977). Milder disorders such as dysthymia do not appear to be heritable, although depressive symptoms in the normal population have a heritable component.

Adoption Studies

A recent adoption study in Sweden examined the heritability of depression and substance abuse disorders (von Knorring et al, 1983). It was based on registrations for disability leave with the National Health Insurance Board. Adoptees were ascertained who had had disability leave for a psychiatric disorder lasting for at least two weeks. The individuals had to have been treated as outpatients or inpatients in a psychiatric department or mental hospital. Hospital and treatment records were obtained in order to classify the probands into subgroups using explicit criteria. The psychiatric adoptees were matched with control adoptees. The records of the biological parents of the adoptees were searched to determine whether they had had any psychiatric disability leave. It was found that there was no increase in psychiatric disorders in biological parents of adoptees with depression, except in the mothers of female adoptees. This study suggests that genetic factors do not play a role in depression. However, most of the adoptees with affective disorders had nonpsychotic, neurotic depression (defined in this study as a depression clearly associated with environmental precipitants or acute episodes in persons with maladaptive personality traits), suggesting that it is specifically milder depressions that are not heritable.

Wender and colleagues (1986) carried out an adoption study in Denmark similar to their earlier study of schizophrenia. They ascertained adoptees who had been hospitalized for an affective disorder and then searched for hospitalization records for biological relatives of these adoptees and those of a matched control group. They found an increase of affective disorders in the biological relatives of the affectively ill patients if they considered only relatives whose affective disorders were severe (bipolar, unipolar, and suicide) to be affected. Both this study and the Swedish study indicate low heritability of "mild" depression. The Danish adoption study was able to detect heritability of more severe diagnoses, whereas the Swedish study did not have a large enough sample of severely ill probands or biological relatives to be able to demonstrate heritability of severe affective disorder. In general, the results of the adoption studies of unipolar disorder are not as clear-cut as were the adoption studies of schizophrenia (Kety et al, 1975). What is needed is an interview study for affective disorders because of the large variation in severity of the disorder and the large number of patients who are never hospitalized.

Family Studies

RATES OF ILLNESS IN RELATIVES.   Table 1 shows the rates of bipolar and unipolar illness in first-degree relatives of unipolar probands from four studies that were based on direct interviews of all available first-degree relatives and that also included control groups. The rates are fairly consistent across studies despite the fact that different populations were sampled. The prevalence of bipolar illness (in some studies this includes bipolar II) in relatives of patients is two to three percent, which is clearly higher than in relatives of controls. The prevalence of unipolar ranges from 11–18 percent in relatives of patients, which is approximately threefold higher than in controls (five to six percent). The one exception is in the Israeli study by Gershon and colleagues (1975), where there is a very low rate (less than one percent) of unipolar illness in relatives of controls. One important observation is the very high correspondence of rates between the Bethesda and New Haven studies. These two studies were done collaboratively using identical instruments and criteria. This demonstrates that very similar results can be obtained when the same methodologies are used. The fact that the risk for bipolar illness is increased in relatives of unipolars is not surprising, because the rate of unipolar illness in relatives of bipolars is very high, and it would be expected that some unipolar probands ascertained in family studies come from bipolar families. The increased prevalence of major affective disorder in relatives of patients indicates that the disorder is familial and is consistent with the presence of genetic components. However, family study data do not rule out environmental and cultural liability factors.

As in population studies, factors such as age, sex, and birth cohort affect rates

Table 1. Summary of Controlled Family Studies of Unipolar Illness

Study	Diagnostic Criteria	Proband Diagnosis	Risk to First-Degree Relatives	
			Bipolar	Unipolar
Gershon et al, 1975 (Jerusalem)	Feighner	Unipolar	2.1	14.2
		Control	0.2	0.7
Tsuang et al, 1980 (Iowa)	Feighner	Unipolar	2.2	11.0
		Control	0.2	4.8
Gershon et al, 1982 (Bethesda)	Modified RDC*	Unipolar	3.0	16.6
		Control	0.5	5.8
Weissman et al, 1984a** (New Haven)	Modified RDC	Unipolar (severe)	2.0	18.4
		Unipolar (mild)	3.3	17.2
		Control	1.3	5.9

*Modified RDC criteria described in text

**This study was a collaboration with Gershon and colleagues (1982). The same methods and diagnostic criteria were used. "Severe" probands were hospitalized; "mild" probands were treated as outpatients.

in relatives. The studies presented here show age corrected rates of illness in relatives. Many studies find the rates of unipolar illness in female relatives to be higher than those in male relatives as compared to what is seen in the population (for example, Weissman et al, 1982). Most recent family studies have found that the rate of unipolar illness in relatives also depends to a large extent on birth cohort (Gershon et al, 1987; Klerman et al, 1985), with individuals born after 1940 reporting significantly higher rates than those born earlier. In addition, younger cohorts appear to have an earlier age of onset of unipolar illness than did older cohorts.

AFFECTIVE SPECTRUM. Family study data are also used to infer which other disorders are associated with the main disorder of interest. In studies of affective disorder, inferences can be made as to which other diagnoses should be included in the "affective spectrum," according to which ones aggregate in relatives of patients. RDC minor depression and depressive personality aggregate in families of unipolar probands in the Yale–NIMH study (Weissman et al, 1984a), but minor depression could not be reliably diagnosed in the NIMH study. Patients with anorexia have high rates of affective disorder in their relatives (Gershon et al, 1983, 1984) but some argue that increased rates are only found in families in which the anorexic proband is also depressed (Strober and Katz, in press) although this was not the case in the study by Gershon and colleagues (1983). There is no positive evidence that anorexia is found more frequently in relatives of affective disorder patients (Strober and Katz, in press) but the rate of anorexia in the population is very low and no study has been performed with a large enough sample size to detect even a two- or threefold increase in relatives. The study of Gershon and colleagues (1983), with less than 200 relatives, found a nonsignificant increase in the rate of bulimia in relatives of affective patients compared to controls. Thus, whether or not anorexia/bulimia should be considered as part of the affective spectrum must await additional family and biological studies.

Most studies do not find increased alcoholism in relatives of affective disorder (either unipolar or bipolar) patients (Gershon et al, 1982; Weissman et al, 1984a). However, alcoholism in a proband with major depression is associated with higher rates of both depression and alcoholism in the relatives in one study (Weissman et al, 1986b).

There have been many studies of psychopathology in children of parents with affective disorders which demonstrated that these children were at significant risk for developing psychopathology (reviewed by Beardslee et al, 1983). Many of these early studies were carried out before structured assessments for children were available. In addition, children were not always directly interviewed, control groups were not always included, and sample sizes were often small.

Using direct child interviews and additional information from parents, Decina and colleagues (1983) found an increased frequency of major and minor affective disorders in children of bipolar patients compared to controls. Gershon and associates (1985), based on direct interviews of children, found an increase in nonspecific diagnoses in children of bipolars compared with children of controls, but no difference in the frequency of major depression. Weissman and collaborators are currently carrying out a longitudinal study of 220 children aged 6–23, including children having a parent with a history of treated major depression and a group of controls having psychiatrically normal parents (Weissman, in press). DSM-III diagnoses were made based on direct interviews with the children. The results to date indicate that the children of affectively ill parents had a significantly increased prevalence of major depression and anxiety disorders, and a higher mean number of diagnoses than did the control children. Results of this and other longitudinal studies should clarify to what extent and for which disorders the children of affectively ill parents are at increased risk. In addition, such studies should be able to clarify the clinical and etiological relationship between childhood major depression and adult major depression.

POSSIBLE SUBTYPES. It has been proposed that unipolar depression is a genetically heterogeneous disorder, but it has been very difficult for investigators to demonstrate this by consistently distinguishing among different types of unipolar patients. Winokur and colleagues (1978) first proposed a classification of patients based on family history of depression and other disorders in first degree relatives. He divided unipolar patients into those with a family history of depression only (familial pure depressive disease, those with a family history of alcoholism or sociopathy (depression spectrum disease, and those with no ill family members (sporadic depressive disease). Patients having relatives with mania were excluded from this classification. Winokur and colleagues originally proposed that there were clinical differences among these patients. For example, the sporadic group tended to have a later age of onset and the familial pure depressive disease group were more severe than the depression spectrum disease group (Behar et al, 1981). However, these differences were not very large and were based on retrospective review of records. Perris and associates (1983) could not find any substantial differences in symptoms upon admission among patients classified in this manner. Zimmerman and co-workers (1986) recently studied a prospective series of patients and concluded that depression spectrum disease patients had more "neurotic" symptoms (such as more life events and nonserious suicide attempts) and that familial pure depressive disease patients had more endogenous symptoms. They found that sporadic depressive disease was not different from familial pure depressive disease. Patients with depression spectrum disease are also much less likely to be dexamethasone nonsuppressors in some studies (Zimmerman et al, 1985) but not others. This is examined in greater detail later in this chapter. In summary, these subtypes of unipolar patients clearly overlap a great deal. Until some unique biological or genetic etiology can be attributed to one subgroup or part of a subgroup, this method of classifying patients has limited clinical utility. Additional discussion of depression spectrum disease is provided in Chapter 9.

Weissman and colleagues (1984c) found that depressed probands with early age of onset (younger than age 20) had the greatest proportion of ill first degree relatives; probands with age of onset over 40 had the lowest proportion of ill first degree relatives, and those in between had an intermediate risk. The relatives of early onset patients also tended to have early onset themselves. The effect of age of onset of the proband was found to be independent of the birth cohort effect. In this same data base, Leckman and associates (1983) reported that probands with concomitant panic disorder had a greater number of relatives with depression, anxiety, and alcoholism. Weissman and associates (1986b) considered the overlap among groups of probands defined in different ways. They found that the only classifications that independently increased the risk to relatives was age of onset younger than 30, concomitant anxiety disorder, and secondary alcoholism. Endogenous depression, suicidal ideation, and recurrent depression did not contribute increased risk to relatives after the probands' early age of onset, co-morbidity with anxiety, or alcoholism were taken into account. A Canadian study (Bland et al, 1986) also found an increased risk to relatives of early-onset, recurrent probands. The predictability of these characteristics needs to be further examined.

Other characteristics of unipolar patients have been examined in relation to familial morbidity. Winokur and co-workers (1985) found that unipolar probands with psychosis were no more likely to have relatives with psychosis than were nonpsychotic probands. Some studies have examined the effect of the endogenous/nonendogenous classification on familial morbidity, but no consistent evidence for increased familial risks when the proband has endogenous depression have emerged (Andreasen et al, 1986).

One study found that the severity of the depressive syndrome was related to "familial" depression. Gershon and colleagues (1986) reanalyzed data from the NIMH–Yale collaborative study (Gershon et al, 1982; Weissman et al, 1982) and found that affectively ill relatives of both unipolar and bipolar probands were more likely to be impaired or incapacitated and to have multiple episodes than were affectively ill relatives of normal controls. That is, control relatives tended to meet *DSM-III* criteria but not more stringent criteria, including the modified RDC criteria used in the original studies. These findings are shown in Table 2 and the differences can be seen to be very significant. That is, 32 percent of depressed relatives of controls, compared to 64 and 72 percent of depressed relatives of unipolars and bipolars, respectively, met stringent criteria. While

Table 2. Association of Severity of Depression in Relatives with Type of Proband*

Proband Type	Number of Depressed Relatives	Number Meeting *DSM-III* But Not Modified RDC Criteria	Number Meeting Modified RDC Criteria
Bipolar/ Schizoaffective	111	31	80
Unipolar	100	36	64
Normal control	47	32	15

*Data of Gershon and colleagues (1986)

Note: Combining bipolar/schizoaffective and unipolar, $\chi^2 = 21.45$ (1 d.f.), $p < .0001$.

these findings need to be replicated, they suggest that stringent criteria should be used for diagnosis in biological and genetic studies.

GENETIC ANALYSES OF FAMILIAL DATA

Many studies have utilized family data to test hypotheses about the mode of inheritance of depressive illness. There are several approaches to this problem; but whatever the approach used, it is necessary to test for the effects of epidemiological factors that are known to affect the risk for developing the disorder in the population, in order to determine whether these effects are also operating in families. The importance of these factors will define the approach of further testing of genetic hypotheses.

Preliminary Approaches

The first step in most studies is to test whether or not the probability of a relative being ill is related to factors such as the sex, age, and cohort of the relative, and characteristics of the proband such as sex and age of onset. Some studies have used logistic regression models to test these hypotheses. Smeraldi and colleagues (1981) considered all affective illness in relatives and found that there was no effect of diagnosis of proband (that is, risk to relatives of unipolar probands was not different from risk to relatives of bipolar probands) or sex of proband. There was a borderline effect of sex of relative and an effect due to type of relative. In this case, the risk to siblings was greater than to parents. Weissman and associates (1982, 1984a) found no sex of proband effect, but found effects due to age and sex of relative and source of information (interview versus family history). Merikangas and co-workers (1985) reanalyzed these data and concluded that sex of relative and cohort were significant after correcting for age as a covariate. The results of these studies are not surprising since we know that age and sex affect the risk for depression. However, the fact that sex of proband is not significant is important because it allows us to rule out a class of models that assume different genetic liabilities for males and females.

Multifactorial and Major Locus Threshold Models

One way to approach genetic hypothesis testing is to assume that inheritance can be multifactorial or polygenic, which means that a large number of genes, each with small effect, along with random environmental factors act additively to produce liability to illness. These models have been applied to affective disorders by proposing that severity of illness is related to genetic liability and that unipolar and bipolar illness are two disorders on the same continuum of liability (Reich et al, 1972). Each illness represents a threshold on the liability scale so that bipolar illness, being the more severe disorder, would require a greater number of liability factors than unipolar illness. Thus, the relatives of bipolar probands would have a greater number of liability factors than the relatives of unipolar probands and would be expected to have higher rates of illness. Alternatively, the liability scale can be hypothesized to be due to the effects of one single locus with genotypic distributions that overlap. These models can be tested by first computing the expected rates of unipolar and bipolar illness in relatives based on the parameters of the model and then comparing them to the rates actually observed. Gershon and colleagues (1982) found that a three-threshold multifactorial model fit the rates of illness in relatives of affective disorder patients, with the severity of disorders being in the order of unipolar < bipolar < schizoaffective. Similarly, Tsuang and associates (1985b) found that unipolar and bipolar also fit a multifactorial model, with unipolar having less liability than bipolar. Price and co-workers (1985) combined the data of Gershon and colleagues (1982) with that of Weissman and colleagues (1984a), which had been collected collaboratively, and attempted to fit major locus and multifactorial threshold models to unipolar and bipolar illness. The schizoaffective threshold was eliminated by reclassifying such individuals as either unipolar or bipolar. They found that neither model fit the data. In both data sets, the prevalence of illness in offspring was much higher than the prevalence in parents, which is not predicted by the model. The difference from the analysis of Gershon and colleagues (1982) may have been a result of the cohort effect since the offspring are from a younger cohort than the parents. Recently Reich (1986) found that similar multifactorial models of liability did not fit their data on unipolar and bipolar illness. That is, unipolar and bipolar do not share multifactorial liability factors. However, if only early onset probands were considered, then a common liability model did fit, suggesting that an early age of onset defines a more homogeneous illness. It should be noted that all of these studies consist of different populations and different criteria. It is possible that some forms of unipolar illness share common liability factors with bipolar, but that unipolar illness is heterogeneous and more complicated by cohort effects. Results of analyses will also depend on how broad or stringent a definition of unipolar illness was used.

Tests of Single Locus Models by Segregation Analysis

Segregation analysis has long been used in the study of genetic diseases to determine whether the distribution of an illness in families corresponded to some simple Mendelian mode of transmission. In this way, diseases could be shown to be either dominant, recessive, and autosomal or sex-linked. Many common diseases (defined as a prevalence greater than one percent)—a class to which psychiatric disorders belong—are known to be familial but do not appear to conform to simple Mendelian models. However, methods have been developed to test Mendelian hypotheses for such disorders allowing for reduced penetrance (that is, not all persons having a susceptible genotype will develop the illness) and the probability of being ill depending on age or sex. Elston and Stewart (1971) developed a maximum likelihood method for testing genetic hypotheses in multigenerational families without having to break them down into nuclear families. The parameters for each model are estimated by maximum likelihood methods. That is, they are iterated until the likelihood of the observed family data is the greatest. Genetic hypotheses are tested by comparing likelihoods of models in which transmission in pedigrees must follow Mendelian rules to likelihoods of transmission following no rules at all.

A few studies have applied these methods to data on families of unipolar probands. Crowe and associates (1981) analyzed a single, large unipolar pedigree consisting of approximately 100 individuals using this method. First, they tested which diagnostic classification gave the best fit to a dominant model allowing for age of onset dependent risk. They found that including unipolar, alcoholism, and drug dependence gave the best fit to the model, indicating that this pedigree fit Winokur's definition of depression spectrum disease. However, they could not reject either a Mendelian hypothesis or an environmental (nongenetic) hypothesis. Since both a single gene and purely nongenetic hypothesis fit the data, it was not possible to conclude that a major locus accounted for affective disorder in this family. Tsuang and colleagues (1985a) applied similar models to the transmission of affective disorders (including unipolar and bipolar) in the families of unipolar probands. Both dominant and recessive hypotheses could be rejected, but a nongenetic hypothesis was not rejected. Goldin and co-workers (1983) applied similar analyses to data on the families of unipolar probands reported by Gershon and colleagues (1982). They also were able to reject all single locus genetic hypotheses, even when the diagnostic classification scheme was varied. It is clear that this method of segregation analysis has allowed us to reject single locus hypotheses for affective disorder in unipolar families. Similar results have been obtained for bipolar families (Bucher et al, 1981; Goldin et al, 1983).

The fact that multifactorial models are consistent with some studies and that single locus models are usually rejected does not necessarily rule out single locus inheritance. The power of these methods to detect major loci in complex diseases may be low. Goldin and associates (1984) found by simulation that a single locus for a disease could not be identified for certain modes of inheritance, especially "quasi-recessive" inheritance in which the heterozygote individuals have low, but not zero, penetrance. In addition, if affective disorders are genetically heterogeneous, the detection of single genetic mechanisms will be difficult with current methods.

GENETIC ANALYSES USING ASSOCIATION AND LINKAGE MARKERS

An alternative way to detect single locus components of diseases is to find association or genetic linkage of the disease to a genetic marker locus.

Genetic Markers

Genetic marker loci are normal variants of genes or proteins that are due to a single locus, some of which are mapped to human chromosomes. Some of the most commonly studied markers are ABO blood types, which are detected on red cells, and HLA antigens, which are detected on leukocytes. In addition, there are several other blood groups and many electrophoretic variants of red cell and serum enzymes and proteins that have been commonly used.

DNA Probes as Genetic Markers

The development of a set of powerful methods of molecular genetics has revolutionized the study of human genetic diseases. These breakthroughs are a result of the discovery of restriction endonucleases, development of methods for cloning genes, and the detection of fragments of DNA separated by gel electrophoresis and by Southern blotting, followed by hybridization with cloned DNA sequences. Variations in DNA sequences (called restriction fragment length polymorphisms, or RFLPs) can thus be identified. This technique has produced hundreds of new marker loci and it is expected that before long there will be markers covering the entire human genome (Kidd, in press). Thus, if a susceptibility gene for a disease exists, it will be detectable by linkage if enough markers are tested. Of special interest to psychiatry are cloned genes of neuroactive peptides such as pro-opiomelanocortin (POMC), neuropeptide Y, and somatostatin.

Association Studies

Association of genetic markers to diseases are detected by comparing the frequency of a given marker in samples of unrelated patients and unrelated controls. If the frequency is significantly different, then there may be some etiologic association between the marker and the disease. For example, specific HLA antigens are associated with diseases such as juvenile diabetes and multiple sclerosis (Thomson, 1981). These associations have been consistently found in different populations and suggest some etiologic determinants in the HLA region. However, it is possible to find spurious associations due to unknown differences between the control and patient populations. In addition, significant results can be found by chance, especially in small samples. It is therefore very important to be able to replicate a potential association in a new study. Several studies have looked for ABO and HLA associations to affective disorders but no consistent results have been found (Goldin and Gershon, 1983). Often, these studies have had small samples of patients, especially after they are divided into unipolar and bipolar subtypes.

Linkage Studies

If a disease gene is chromosomally linked to a marker locus, then in families, the marker type will be transmitted along with the disease in a predictable manner that can be analyzed statistically. Linkage will lead to association of phenotypes in families but not in the population. The nonrandom association in families can also be analyzed in sibships, and different methods are available for testing for linkage in affected sibling pairs (Goldin and Gershon, 1983). There have been many linkage studies in affective disorders but, for the most part, studies have been done in bipolar families or in samples containing both unipolar and bipolar families. A few studies have focused on linkage in unipolar families. Tanna and colleagues (1979) reported possible linkage of the haptoglobin locus to depression spectrum disease in 14 families. They also reported possible linkage of familial pure depressive disease to the secretor locus (Tanna et al, 1977). However, neither of these results were very strong and have not been replicated. Crowe and co-workers (1981) found no evidence of linkage in a large pedigree with depression spectrum disease to any of 30 markers. Weitkamp and associates (1980) studied a large pedigree with 19 individuals affected with primary depression but found no evidence of linkage to any of 29 markers, including haptoglobin and secretor.

In general, association and linkage studies have not demonstrated evidence of single gene susceptibility for unipolar illness. However, the disorder is likely to be heterogeneous and different investigators have used different diagnostic criteria. With the large number of available RFLP markers, it may be useful to do linkage studies in families with a well defined depressive illness. This strategy has begun to be followed in bipolar illness. For example, Detera-Wadleigh and colleagues (in press) found no association of variants of somatostatin and neuropeptide Y with bipolar affective disorder in a sample of unrelated patients and controls, and no linkage of these variants to affective disorder in two families.

BIOLOGICAL STUDIES

Many biological traits have been studied in depressed patients but generally they have been examined only as state markers and not as trait markers. These are discussed in detail in Chapter 8. Here we will discuss those traits that have been examined in relation to genetic susceptibility.

Dexamethasone Suppression Test

Abnormality of the dexamethasone suppression test (DST) is commonly found in depressed patients. Some studies have found that a much larger proportion of patients are abnormal on the DST if they fall into Winokur's category of familial pure depressive disease than if they are classified as depression spectrum disease. However, other studies have found no difference. This has been reviewed by Zimmerman and colleagues (1985), who argue that the difference among studies may be the result of different stringencies for diagnosing depression, alcoholism, and antisocial personality in the family members. Studies using stricter criteria for these disorders tended to find a significant difference between familial pure depressive disease and depression spectrum disease patients. In their own study, they found that the difference in nonsuppression rates was only borderline if family history RDC criteria were used to diagnose relatives, but highly significant if they required relatives to have hospitalization for depression, treatment for alcoholism, and legal consequences for antisocial personality in order to get a positive diagnosis. These results are provocative, but subtyping patients based on various diagnoses in relatives remains problematic for several reasons. In most populations, alcoholism is very common in males (Robins et al, 1984) and thus could easily be found by chance in a first-degree relative of a depressed patient. In addition, the prevalence of both depression and alcoholism is also increased in younger cohorts (Robins et al, 1984). Also, families cannot always be classified in such a straightforward manner. A unipolar proband could have only unipolar first-degree relatives but a bipolar second-degree relative (that is, a grandparent, aunt, or uncle). Unipolar patients may have relatives with other major diagnoses such as schizophrenia, and it is not clear whether such patients should be eliminated from the sample. Whether or not these subtypes can be validated will depend on finding a genetic or biological trait that reliably distinguishes these patient subgroups.

Platelet Monoamine Oxidase

There have been many studies of platelet monoamine oxidase (MAO) activity in psychiatric patients in hopes that this would be a trait marker of an illness. However, MAO is affected by many environmental variables and has not turned out to be a reliable marker for either affective disorders or schizophrenia (Goldin and Gershon, 1983). The MAO studies in affective disorders have found inconsistent results in both unipolar and bipolar patients (von Knorring et al, 1985). In a study in Sweden, a sample of affective disorders patients (mostly unipolar) was divided into the lowest versus the highest quartile of platelet MAO activity (von Knorring et al, 1985). The morbid risk of various disorders in relatives was determined on the basis of family history information supplemented by medical records. Relatives of "low" MAO patients had a higher morbid risk of neurotic depression and alcoholism than did relatives of "high" MAO patients. However, they did not differ with respect to the frequency of unipolar disorder. The authors suggest that "low" MAO is related to Winokur's depression spectrum disease. These results are interesting but the study was small and needs further replication.

Cerebrospinal Fluid Monoamine Metabolites

There have also been several studies relating cerebrospinal fluid (CSF) monoamine metabolites, such as 5-hydroxyindoleacetic acid (5-HIAA) and homovanillic acid (HVA) to subtypes of depression. CSF 5-HIAA levels have often been found to be bimodally distributed in depressed patients. Those patients in the low subgroup have a higher frequency of suicidal behavior (Asbert et al, 1984). Van Praag and de Haan (1979) classified affective disorder patients (including both unipolar and bipolar) into groups with "low" versus "high" CSF 5-HIAA. From family history information and examination of medical records, they found that the relatives of patients in the "low" group had a significantly greater number of hospitalizations for depression than did the relatives of patients in the "high" group. Unfortunately, the total number of hospitalizations in relatives is not a meaningful statistic. The quantity of interest is the risk of illness to relatives in the two subgroups. In addition, the "low" group contained twice as many bipolar individuals as did the "high" group, and the risk for affective disorders in relatives of bipolar patients is often found to be higher than the risk for relatives of unipolar patients.

Sedvall and colleagues (1980) studied CSF monoamine metabolites in 60 control individuals. They also gathered family history information on the relatives of the controls and determined which controls had had a relative hospitalized for a psychiatric disorder. They did not find any overall differences between those controls with and those without a family history, although the controls with depressed relatives tended to be at the low end of the 5-HIAA and HVA distributions, while the controls with schizophrenic relatives tended to be at the high end of the distributions. However, these subgroups contained only a very small number of controls (four to five) so it is difficult to make a strong conclusion about the relationship of these metabolites to susceptibility to depression. Recently, this same group of investigators (Oxenstierna et al, 1986) found no evidence for heritability of CSF 5-HIAA or HVA in a large twin study. Thus, it is not likely that these traits can be useful as genetic markers of depression.

Cholinergic Rapid Eye Movement Induction

Defects in the cholinergic system have been proposed to be related to bipolar illness (Janowski et al, 1972). For example, the cholinergic agonist, arecoline, decreases the time between the first and second rapid eye movement (REM) cycles in bipolar patients compared to normal controls (Sitaram et al, 1982). This trait is concordant in MZ twins, suggesting that it is under genetic control (Nurnberger et al, 1983). Recently, the association of this trait with affective illness has been tested in families. Sitaram and colleagues (in press) studied 66 first-degree relatives of affectively ill probands (unipolar and bipolar), who themselves had "early" REM induction. A significantly greater number of the affected relatives (both unipolar and bipolar) were "early" as compared to the unaffected relatives (Table 3). This study suggests that "early" REM induction is a potential genetic vulnerability marker for both unipolar and bipolar disorders, and demonstrates the power of studying biological susceptibility traits in families of patients.

CONCLUSIONS

Major depression, when defined stringently, is a heritable illness. Family members of ill persons are at significantly increased risk for developing various affective disorders compared to the general population. However, the risk of major depression in both the population and in relatives of patients varies with diagnostic criteria, age, sex, cohort, and possibly other factors. Milder disorders

Table 3. Association of Early Cholinergic REM Induction to Affective Disorders in First Degree Relatives of Patients with Early REM Induction*

	Trait Status	
Lifetime Diagnosis Status	Early REM Induction	Others
Ill	22	13
Well	8	23

χ^2 (Yates corrected) = 6.23 (1 d.f.), p = .012.

*Data from Sitaram et al (in press)

such as *DSM-III* dysthymia or RDC minor depression may not be heritable. Biological and genetic studies should focus on patients and family members who have more severe diagnoses.

Subtypes of depression based on illnesses in family members (depression spectrum disease, familial pure depressive disease, sporadic depressive disease) have not been consistently validated by independent measures. Characteristics such as early age of onset and concomitant anxiety or alcoholism may indicate a more heritable depression.

Some analyses of family data have indicated that unipolar and bipolar illness share some common genetic liability factors. Other studies do not confirm this unitary hypothesis in general, but indicate that certain subgroups of unipolar may share liability with bipolar. Single major genes that cause susceptibility to depression have not been found by analyzing the segregation pattern of the illness in families. Linkage studies have also not found any genetic marker trait chromosomally linked to a susceptibility gene for depression.

Studies of traits such as MAO and CSF metabolites have not found them to be predictive of some genetic susceptibility for depression. Abnormality on the DST also does not appear to indicate some homogeneous form of illness. However, vulnerability to increased sensitivity to cholinergic REM induction may be a marker of affective disorder.

Future studies need to continue to focus on ways of resolving the heterogeneity of major depression using clinical and biological traits. Linkage studies are now a very powerful strategy for detecting disease susceptibility genes because of the almost unlimited number of markers available. However, linkage and other biological studies need to be applied carefully. Families for analysis should be selected to have a severe form of illness. Stringent criteria should be used to classify family members as affected or unaffected because broad criteria increase the likelihood that many individuals will have a nongenetic illness. Defining a highly heritable subtype of depression using clinical, biological, or genetic marker traits remains a critical challenge to this field.

REFERENCES

American Psychiatric Association: Diagnostic and Statistical Manual of Mental Disorders, Third Edition (DSM-III). Washington, DC, American Psychiatric Association, 1980

American Psychiatric Association: Diagnostic and Statistical Manual of Mental Disorders, Third Edition, Revised (DSM-III-R). Washington, DC, American Psychiatric Association, 1987

Angst J, Dobler-Mikola A: The Zurich study, III: diagnosis of depression. Eur Arch Psychiatr Neurol Sci 1984; 234:30-37

Andreasen NC, Scheftner W, Reich T, et al: The validation of the concept of endogenous depression. Arch Gen Psychiatry 1986: 43:246-254

Asberg M, Bertilsson L, Bjorn M: CSF monoamine metabolites, depression and suicide, in Frontiers in Biochemical and Pharmacological Research in Depression. Edited by Usdin E. New York, Raven Press, 1984

Beardslee WR, Bemporad J, Keller MB, et al: Children of parents with major affective disorder—a review. Am J Psychiatry 1983; 140:825-832

Behar D, Winokur G, van Valkenburg C, et al: Clinical overlap among familial subtypes of unipolar depression. Neuropsychobiology 7:179-184, 1981

Bertelsen A, Harvald B, Hauge M: A Danish twin study of manic-depressive disorders. Br J Psychiatry 1977; 130:330-351

Bland RC, Newman SC, Orn H: Recurrent and nonrecurrent depression: a family study. Arch Gen Psychiatry 1986; 43:1085-1089

Boyd JH, Weissman MM: Epidemiology of affective disorders: reexamination and future direction. Arch Gen Psychiatry 1981; 38:1039-1046

Bucher KD, Elston RC: The transmission of manic-depressive illness, I: theory, description of the model and summary of results. J Psychiatr Res 1981; 16:53-63

Crowe RR, Namboodiri KK, Ashby HB, et al: Segregation and linkage analysis of a large kindred of unipolar depression. Neuropsychobiology 1981; 7:20-25

Crowell BA Jr, George LK, Blazer D, et al: Psychosocial risk factors and urban/rural differences in the prevalence of major depression. Br J Psychiatry 1986; 149:307-314

Decina P, Kestenbaum CJ, Farber S, et al: Clinical and psychological assessment of children of bipolar probands. Am J Psychiatry 1983; 140:548-553

Detera-Wadleigh SD, de Miguel C, Berrettini WH, et al: Neuropeptide gene polymorphisms in affective disorder and schizophrenia. J Psychiatr Res (in press)

Egeland JA, Hostetter AM: Amish Study, I: affective disorders among the Amish, 1976-1980. Am J Psychiatry 1983; 140:56-61

Elston RC, Stewart J: A general model for the genetic analysis of pedigree data, Hum Hered 21:523-542, 1971

Feighner JP, Robins E, Guze SB, et al: Diagnostic criteria for use in psychiatric research. Arch Gen Psychiatry 1972; 26:57-63

Gershon ES, Guroff JJ: Information from relatives: diagnosis of affective disorders. Arch Gen Psychiatry 1984; 41:173-180

Gershon ES, Mark A, Cohen M, et al: Transmitted factors in the morbid risk of affective disorders: a controlled study. J Psychiatr Res 1975; 12:283-299

Gershon ES, Hamovit J, Guroff JJ, et al: A family study of schizoaffective, bipolar I, bipolar II, unipolar, and normal control probands. Arch Gen Psychiatry 1982; 39:1157-1167

Gershon ES, Hamovit JR, Schreiber JL, et al: Anorexia nervosa and major affective disorder associated in families, in Childhood Psychopathology and Development. Edited by Guze SB, Earls FJ, Barrett JE. New York, Raven Press, 1983

Gershon ES, Schreiber JL, Hamovit JR, et al: Clinical findings in patients with anorexia nervosa and affective illness in their relatives. Am J Psychiatry 1984; 141:1419-1422

Gershon ES, McKnew D, Cytryn L, et al: Diagnoses in school-age children of bipolar affective disorder patients and normal controls. J Affective Disord 1985; 8:283-291

Gershon ES, Weissman MM, Guroff JJ, et al: Validation of criteria for major depression through controlled family study. J Affective Disord 1986; 11:125-131

Gershon ES, Hamovit JH, Guroff JJ, et al: Birth cohort changes in manic and depressive disorders in relatives of bipolar and schizoaffective patients. Arch Gen Psychiatry 1987; 44:314-319

Goldin LR, Gershon ES: Association and linkage studies of genetic marker loci in major psychiatric disorders. Psychiatr Dev 1983; 1:387-418

Goldin LR, Gershon ES, Targum SD, et al: Segregation and linkage analyses in families of patients with bipolar, unipolar, and schizoaffective mood disorders. Am J Hum Genet 1983; 35:274-287

Goldin LR, Cox NJ, Pauls DL, et al: The detection of major loci by segregation and linkage analysis: a simulation study. Genet Epidemiol 1984; 1:285-296

Hagnell O, Lanke J, Rorsman B, et al: Are we entering an age of melancholy: depressive illness in a prospective epidemiological study over 25 years: the Lundby Study, Sweden. Psychol Med 1982; 12:279-289

Janowski DS, El-Yousef K, Davis J, et al: A cholinergic-aminergic hypothesis of mania and depression. Lancet 1972; 2:6732-6735

Kety SS, Rosenthal D, Wender PH, et al: Mental illness in the biological and adoptive families of adopted individuals who have become schizophrenic: a preliminary report based on psychiatric interviews, in Genetic Research in Psychiatry. Edited by Fieve RR, Rosenthal D, Brill H. Baltimore, Johns Hopkins University Press, 1975

Kidd KK: Research design considerations for linkage studies of affective disorders using recombinant DNA marker. J Psychiatr Res (in press)

Klerman GL, Lavori PW, Rice J, et al: Birth-cohort trends in rates of major depressive disorder among relatives of patients with affective disorder. Arch Gen Psychiatry 1985; 42:689-693

Leckman JF, Weissman MM, Merikangas KR, et al: Panic disorder and major depression: increased risk of depression, alcoholism, panic, and phobic disorders in families of depressed probands with panic disorder. Arch Gen Psychiatry 1983; 40:1055-1060

Mazure C, Gershon ES: Blindness and reliability in lifetime psychiatric diagnosis. Arch Gen Psychiatry 1979; 36:521-525

Merikangas KR, Weissman MM, Pauls DL: Genetic factors in the sex ratio of major depression. Psychol Med 1985; 15:63-69

Murphy GE, Wetzel RD: Suicide risk by birth cohort in the United States. Arch Gen Psychiatry 1980; 37:519-523

Nurnberger JI Jr, Sitaram N, Gershon ES, et al: A twin study of cholinergic REM induction. Biol Psychiatry 1983; 18:1161-1173

Oxenstierna G, Edman G, Iselius L, et al: Concentrations of monoamine metabolites in the cerebrospinal fluid of twins and unrelated individuals: a genetic study. J Psychiatr Res 1986; 20:19-29

Perris C, Eisemann M, Ericsson U, et al: Personality characteristics of depressed patients classified according to family history. Neuropsychobiology 1983; 9:99-102

Price RA, Kidd KK, Pauls DL, et al: Multiple threshold models for the affective disorders: the Yale–NIMH collaborative family study. J Psychiatr Res 1985 19:256-259

Reich T: The familial association of bipolar and non-bipolar affective disorders. Paper presented at the annual meeting of the American College of Neuropsychopharmacology. Washington, DC, December 12, 1986

Reich T, James JW, Morris CA: The use of multiple thresholds in determining the mode of transmission of semi-continuous traits. Ann Hum Genet 1972; 36:163-184

Rice JP, Endicott J, Knesevich MA, et al: The estimation of diagnostic sensitivity using stability data: an application to major depressive disorder. J Psychiatr Res (in press)

Robins LN, Helzer JE, Weissman MM, et al: Lifetime prevalence of specific psychiatric disorders in three sites. Arch Gen Psychiatry 1984; 41:949-958

Sedvall G, Fryo B, Gullberg B, et al: Relationships in healthy volunteers between concentrations of monoamine metabolites in cerebrospinal fluid and family history of psychiatric morbidity. Br J Psychiatry 1980; 136:366-374

Sitaram N, Nurnberger JI Jr, Gershon ES, et al: Cholinergic regulation of mood and REM sleep: potential model and marker of vulnerability to affective disorder. Am J Psychiatry 1982; 139:571-576

Sitaram N, Dube S, Keshavan M, et al: The association of supersensitive cholinergic REM-induction and affective illness within pedigrees. J Psychiatr Res (in press)

Smeraldi E, Negri F, Heimbuch RC, et al: Familial patterns and possible modes of inheritance of primary affective disorders. J Affective Disord 1981; 3:173-182

Spitzer RL, Endicott J, Robins E: Research Diagnostic Criteria: rationale and reliability. Arch Gen Psychiatry 1978; 35:773-782

Strober M, Katz J: Depression in the eating disorders: a review and analysis of descriptive, family, and biological findings, in Diagnostic Issues in Anorexia Nervosa and Bulimia Nervosa. Edited by Garner DM, Garfinkel PE. New York, Bruner/Mazel (in press)

Tanna VL, Go RCP, Winokur G, et al: Possible linkage between group-specific component (Gc protein) and pure depressive disease. Acta Psychiatr Scand 1977; 55:111-115

Tanna VL, Go RCP, Winokur G, et al: Possible linkage between alpha-haptoglobin (Hp) and depression spectrum disease. Neuropsychobiology 1979; 5:102-113

Thompson WD, Weissman MM: Quantifying lifetime risk of psychiatric disorder. J Psychiatr Res 1981; 16:113-126

Thomson G: A review of theoretical aspects of HLA and disease associations. Theor Popul Biol 1981; 20:168-208

Torgersen S: Genetic factors in moderately severe and mild affective disorders. Arch Gen Psychiatry 1986; 43:222-226

Tsuang MT, Winokur G, Crowe RR: Morbidity risks of schizophrenia and affective disorders among first degree relatives of patients with schizophrenia, mania, depression and surgical conditions. Br J Psychiatry 1980; 137:497-504

Tsuang MT, Bucher KD, Fleming JA, et al: Transmission of affective disorders: an application of segregation analysis to blind family study data. J Psychiatr Res 1985a; 19:23-29

Tsuang MT, Faraone SV, Fleming JA: Familial transmission of major affective disorders: is there evidence supporting the distinction between unipolar and bipolar disorders? Br J Psychiatry 1985b; 146:268-271

van Praag HM, de Haan S: Central serotonin metabolism and frequency of depression. Psychiatry Res 1979; 1:219-224

von Knorring A, Cloninger CR, Bohman M, et al: An adoption study of depressive disorders and substance abuse. Arch Gen Psychiatry 1983; 40:943-950

von Knorring L, Perris C, Oreland L, et al: Morbidity risk for psychiatric disorders in families of probands with affective disorders divided according to levels of platelet MAO activity. Psychiatry Res 1985; 15:271-279

Weissman MM: Psychopathology in the children of depressed parents: direct interview studies, in Relatives at Risk for Mental Disorders. Edited by Dunner DS, Gershon ES. New York, Raven Press (in press)

Weissman MM, Kidd KK, Prusoff BA: Variability in rates of affective disorders in relatives of depressed and normal probands. Arch Gen Psychiatry 1982; 39:1397-1403

Weissman MM, Gershon ES, Kidd KK, et al: Psychiatric disorders in the relatives of probands with affective disorders: the Yale University–National Institute of Mental Health collaborative study. Arch Gen Psychiatry 1984a; 41:13-21

Weissman MM, Leaf PJ, Holzer CE III, et al: The epidemiology of depression: an update on sex differences in rates. J Affective Disord 1984b; 7:179-188

Weissman MM, Wickramaratne P, Merikangas KR, et al: Onset of major depression in early adulthood. Arch Gen Psychiatry 1984c; 41:1136-1143

Weissman MM, Merikangas KR, John K, et al: Family-genetic studies of psychiatric disorders: developing technologies. Arch Gen Psychiatry 1986a; 43:1104-1116

Weissman MM, Merikangas KR, Wickramaratne P, et al: Understanding the clinical heterogeneity of major depression using family data. Arch Gen Psychiatry 1986b; 43:430-434

Weitkamp LR, Pardue LH, Huntzinger RS: Genetic marker studies in a family with unipolar depression. Arch Gen Psychiatry 1980; 37:1187-1192

Wender PH, Kety SS, Rosenthal D, et al: Psychiatric disorders in the biological and adoptive families of adopted individuals with affective disorders. Arch Gen Psychiatry 1986; 43:923-929

Winokur G, Behar D, van Valkenburg C, et al: Is a familial definition of depression both feasible and valid? J Nerv Ment Dis 1978; 166:764-768

Winokur G, Tsuang MT, Crowe RR: The Iowa 500: affective disorder in the relatives of manic and depressed patients. Am J Psychiatry 1982; 139:209-212

Winokur G, Scharfetter C, Angst J: A family study of psychotic symptomatology in schizophrenia, schizoaffective disorder, unipolar depression, and bipolar disorder. Eur Arch Psychiatr Neurol Sci 1985; 234:295-298

Zimmerman M, Coryell W, Pfohl BM: Importance of diagnostic thresholds in familial classification. Arch Gen Psychiatry 1985; 42:300-304

Zimmerman M, Coryell W, Pfohl B: Validity of familial subtypes of primary unipolar depression. Arch Gen Psychiatry 1986; 43:1090-1096

Chapter 8

Biological Aspects of Depression: Implications for Clinical Practice

by James C. Ballenger, M.D.

The affective disorders have been the object of the most active psychiatric research over the past two decades. This is especially true for the biological aspects of these disorders. This chapter provides a brief and selective review of some of the most well established biological findings in depression, with an emphasis on those areas which promise to be the most clinically relevant. For more extensive information, the interested reader is referred to recent reviews (Post and Ballenger, 1984; van Praag et al, 1981).

SLEEP

Insomnia has long been recognized as a central symptom of depression. Recent studies utilizing polysomnographic electroencephalogram (EEG) sleep recordings have demonstrated specific abnormalities in the sleep of most depressed patients. These abnormalities represent some of the best established biological observations in depression.

Abnormalities of Sleep in Depression

Sleep in normals is divided into rapid eye movement (REM) sleep and nonREM sleep (Stages I to IV), in which sleep progresses from Stage I and II into Stages III and IV (delta sleep) later in the night. The first REM period generally occurs 70 to 90 minutes after sleep onset, and there are usually 3 to 5 REM periods during the night, occurring approximately every 90 minutes. REM periods average 20 to 30 minutes, increasing in length with successive REM periods during the night. In contrast, depressed individuals tend to enter their first REM period unusually early, a phenomenon which has been labelled "shortened REM latency." They also have poor sleep which is shallow, reduced in length, and less "efficient." "Shallow" sleep refers to the reduced amount of delta sleep or slow-wave sleep (Stages III and IV). Sleep of depressed patients is said to be inefficient because they awaken frequently during the night and in the early morning. The number of hours of sleep appears to be especially reduced in unipolar, agitated young depressives. However, approximately nine percent of depressed patients are actually hypersomniac. More "intense" REM sleep (an increased number of eye movements per minute) has also been reported, but less consistently, across studies. Although sleep studies of remitted depressed patients are limited, it appears that at least some of these abnormalities persist on clinical remission.

Etiology of Sleep Abnormalities

Various models for understanding the observed abnormalities in the sleep of depressed patients have been advanced, but this remains a controversial area of research. Considerable evidence suggests that the observed REM changes are related to abnormalities of biological rhythms (see next section). That is, short REM latency may represent an advance of the circadian rhythm for REM sleep relative to sleep onset and clock time. Attempts to explain the sleep abnormalities have been a major focus and stimulus for most theories of biological rhythm abnormalities in depression. Vogel and his colleagues proposed a model in which they hypothesized that sleep of depressed patients is similar to the extended sleep of normal volunteers; that is, the sleep beyond the sixth to eighth hour of sleep (Vogel et al, 1980). Similarly, Gillin (Gillin et al, 1984) has hypothesized that depressed patients are in a state of sleep satiety, providing a rationale for why depressed patients take longer to fall asleep during the day as well as a rationale for the value of sleep deprivation. As reviewed below, both the shortened REM latency and other sleep changes observed in depression can be induced by increasing brain cholinergic activity. A less well-developed line of research suggests that depletion of brain norepinephrine is associated with shortened REM latency.

Use in Diagnosis

Some studies report that REM latency is most reduced in more severely depressed patients, and that REM latency differentiates primary from secondary depression (Foster et al, 1976). Shortened REM latency seems to be associated with primary and endogenous depression and has been used diagnostically to differentiate subgroups of depressed patients. However, short REM latency also appears to be present in certain other pathological conditions (for example, narcolepsy), and even at times in normals. Interestingly, short REM latency appears to be present in those depressed patients who demonstrate nonsuppression on the dexamethasone suppression test (DST), and therefore shares with the DST both potential usefulness as a biological marker and the same lack of specificity to depression demonstrated by the DST (see below). However, utilizing discriminant analysis, Gillin and colleagues (Gillin et al, 1984) analyzed 115 subjects who were either normal, depressed, or insomniac. Utilizing total recording, total sleep time, and sleep efficiency, they were able to correctly identify 83.6 percent of the subjects: 100 percent of 41 normals, 69.6 percent of 56 depressed subjects, and 88.9 percent of the 18 insomniac subjects. In a subsequent study they were able to correctly identify 17 out of 18 depressed patients using the parameters generated in the first study. Kupfer and colleagues (utilizing only REM latency and REM density) reported similar discrimination, including the ability to separate patients with primary from secondary depressions, and patients who have delusions of guilt (Coble et al, 1976).

Prediction of Antidepressant Response

These sleep abnormalities have also been utilized in attempts to predict differential treatment responses. Kupfer and associates (Kupfer et al, 1980) have reported the provocative finding that depressed patients who show greater REM sleep suppression during the first two nights of amitriptyline treatment are more likely to have an antidepressant response. Other studies have demonstrated that the antidepressant drugs, including the tricyclics, the monoamine oxidase inhibitors, and lithium, either increase REM latency or phase delay the REM state relative to the onset of sleep, or completely eliminate REM sleep. Also, sleep deprivation or specific REM deprivation has been demonstrated in some studies to have antidepressant activity. The studies of biological rhythm abnormalities (see below) in depression have suggested that the amount or timing of REM sleep is critical for therapeutic response to the antidepressants, but work in this area remains limited. As is discussed in Chapter 10 on somatic treatment, it recently has been found that short REM latency may be a predictor of relapse following recovery from an episode of depression (Giles et al, 1986).

Conclusion

The observed sleep abnormalities in depressed patients are among the most consistent and important biological findings in depression. Although they are not specific to depression, their consistent presence supports the hypothesis that there *is* a biology of depression and provides clues to the underlying pathophysiology of depression. While sleep studies are not yet practical for routine clinical use, the sleep abnormalities described provide strong support for the diagnosis of depression, and early data suggest that sleep parameters may be useful in the prediction of treatment response. If replicated, the finding that early changes in sleep parameters predict eventual response to tricyclics could be of considerable clinical importance if it allowed correct initial treatment choices, thereby shortening the time to recovery from depressive episodes.

BIOLOGICAL RHYTHMS AND DEPRESSION

Certain features of depressive illness suggest that abnormalities in biological rhythms may play a significant role in their pathophysiology. Characteristic daily circadian mood variations and the appearance of certain regular biological rhythms that appear to be abnormal in these patients (for example, advanced REM rhythm, menstrual cycles, and so on) implicate circadian abnormalities in depression. Certain affective disorder patients and patterns of affective disturbance are most suggestive of rhythm abnormalities. These include the rare 48-hour cycling patients who shift between depression and mania on a 24-hour basis. Also, those patients who have both depressions and manic episodes with predictable yearly or seasonal rhythms are highly suggestive of a link between affective episodes and external events. The recent observation that tricyclic antidepressants and sometimes the monoamine oxidase inhibitors (MAOIs) can accelerate the affective rhythm or induce rapid cycling (Wehr and Goodwin, 1979) has underlined the importance of this area. The sleep–wake changes in affective illness provide perhaps the most compelling reason to study potential changes in the circadian system; for example, the dramatic changes in sleep between depression and mania, and the observations of shortened REM latency. Although much of this research concerns bipolar patients, this area of research is pertinent to unipolar patients as well.

Circadian Rhythms

Many normal rhythms exhibit a 24-hour variation including sleeping, waking, body temperature, endocrine functions, and neural activity. They are endogenous and persist even in the absence of external cues, although circadian rhythms generally are entrained to environmental cycles, principally the light/dark transitions of dawn and dusk. The characteristics and neural substrates of the circadian system are currently under extensive study. The suprachiasmic nucleus of the hypothalamus functions as the "biological clock" or pacemaker of these rhythms in humans. Current research suggests the human circadian system utilizes at least two subsystems that can oscillate independently: one regulating the sleep/wake cycle and the second regulating body temperature, cortisol secretion, and REM sleep propensity. Although beyond the scope of this review, certain features of the depressive process and even its potential etiology have been hypothesized to involve changes in the relative relationships of these oscillating systems. The most common hypothesis has been that the rhythms are phase advanced; that is, shifted earlier in the 24-hour cycle. This could perhaps account for the early distribution of REM sleep and shortened REM latency. Research in this area is both complicated and limited to a few laboratories, and although controversial, remains quite promising.

Clinical Studies

Two promising preliminary clinical findings have emerged from this work. First, Wehr and colleagues at the National Institute of Mental Health (NIMH) (Wehr et al, 1979) have been able to demonstrate that shifting the time of waking several hours earlier causes some patients to switch out of depression, sometimes into mania. Further, the observation that a subset of patients has a yearly or seasonal incidence of depression seems to implicate a photoperiodic mechanism in these depressions. Theoretically, their winter depressions would be caused by a perceived reduction of the interval between dawn and dusk (shortening of the day). This has led several groups (Lewy et al, 1987; Rosenthal et al, 1985; Wehr et al, 1986) to utilize bright light to induce remissions in winter depressions, although the mechanism remains controversial. Lewy and colleagues (Lewy et al, 1987) provide biochemical support for these hypotheses with observations that depressed patients tend to have a later onset of melatonin secretion and that melatonin secretion of bipolar patients was "hypersensitive" to light; that is, less intense light was required to completely suppress melatonin secretion. This appeared to be a "trait marker" in that it was present during the depressed and well state. Lewy's recent work (Lewy et al, 1987) suggests that early morning light "resets" an abnormal phase delay in depressed patients, but Wehr's data is somewhat contradictory, finding that the timing of bright light is not critical (Wehr et al, 1986). Although neither phase advance techniques nor bright light therapy is sufficiently understood to be utilized clinically outside research settings, both are promising as unique approaches to the treatment of depression.

NEUROENDOCRINE STUDIES IN DEPRESSION

Cortisol

Numerous studies have now shown dysregulation of the hypothalamic-pituitary-adrenal axis (HPA) manifest primarily by cortisol hypersecretion, disinhibition of nocturnal secretion of cortisol, and loss of the normal circadian variation. Cortisol hypersecretion is probably the best established biochemical abnormality in depression. In certain studies, urinary free cortisol (UFC) is able to differentiate between depressed (both bipolar and unipolar) and manic patients and normal volunteers (Rubinow et al, 1984). In some studies urinary and plasma cortisol values appear to correlate with the amount of depression, and the highest values are in psychotic depression (Rubinow et al, 1984). Cortisol measures appear also to correlate with cognitive abnormalities and ventricular enlargement on computerized axial tomography (CAT) scans in depressed patients (Kellner, et al, 1983). Recent basic studies utilizing the newly sensitized hypothalamic corticotropin-releasing hormone (CRH) have documented a blunted adrenocorticotropin hormone (ACTH) response to CRH (despite hypercortisolism), providing evidence that the defect in depression is at the hypothalamus, not the pituitary or adrenal (Gold et al, 1984).

DEXAMETHASONE SUPPRESSION TEST. Certainly the dexamethasone suppression test (DST) has been the most widely utilized and studied biological test in psychiatry. The initial enthusiasm associated with the DST was based on the hope that it would be the first genuine diagnostic test in psychiatry. This initial enthusiasm has given way to more critical and cautious utilization and study of the DST (Arana et al, 1987). Many of the recent advances in research in this area involve refinement of the sensitivity and specificity of the DST and utilization of concomitant dexamethasone levels (Arana et al, 1984).

Sensitivity: Sensitivity of a diagnostic test is defined as the percentage of patients with the disorder in question (in this case, major or melancholic depression) who have a positive result. As generally performed (see below), the sensitivity of the DST has been reported to vary between 30 and 70 percent (Arana et al, 1987; Carroll et al, 1981). Although the presence of melancholic features do not consistently affect sensitivity, hospitalized melancholic patients demonstrate rates of nonsuppression (a positive DST) of 50 to 60 percent, but outpatients with less severe depressions often have rates of abnormal DSTs of 40 percent or less.

As would be expected, sensitivity varies with technique, with more patients escaping when the 1 mg dexamethasone is utilized rather than 2 mg. Also, when more postdexamethasone cortisol samples are performed, sensitivity is increased. If samples are taken at 4 P.M. and 11 P.M., sensitivity is increased approximately 20 percent over sampling at 4 P.M. alone. Since only approximately 25 percent of the patients who have abnormal DSTs at 4 P.M. or 11 P.M. are abnormal at 8 P.M., the 8 A.M. sample is generally useful only to demonstrate that suppression did occur and that the dexamethasone was ingested. Although studies utilizing criterion for nonsuppression below 5 mcg/dl demonstrate increased test sensitivity, there is a corresponding loss of specificity (more false positives). Utilizing the "standard" technique (1.0 mg of dexamethasone, 1–3 samples, and criterion of approximately 5.0 mcg/dl), sensitivity for the DST in a large sample of patients with major depression is approximately 45 percent (Arana et al, 1985), making it a poor test to utilize as a screening or case-finding method.

Specificity: Specificity concerns the issue of the "true negatives," and is the chance of a negative finding when the patient tested is truly free of the diagnostic condition in question. It also involves the effect of the false positive rate on the desired 100 percent "true negative" rate. The initial studies that proposed the DST as a confirmatory test for endogenous depression (Carroll et al, 1976) reported a specificity of over 90 percent. Years of subsequent research have shown that such a high rate of specificity is probably dependent upon use of the test to compare depressed patients and normals. The more clinically relevant question of whether the DST is helpful in distinguishing patients with major affective disorders from patients with other psychiatric or medical illnesses that need to be distinguished from major depression is more problematic. A large number of studies now suggest that the overall specificity is probably 80 percent with psychiatric patients with diagnoses other than major depressive disorder. Percentages of abnormal DST results comparable to those observed in depression have been reported in mania, dementia, and the eating disorders, while the rates in patients with nonmajor depressions are generally reported to fall between those observed in normals and in patients with major depression. Considerable research has documented multiple exclusion criteria, which primarily produce abnormal DSTs (see Table 1).

Recommended Procedure: It appears that most clinicians and researchers at this point are utilizing one 1.0 mg of dexamethasone at 11 P.M. with samples drawn at 8 A.M., 4 P.M., or 11 P.M. the next day. Most clinicians probably restrict sampling to 4 P.M. and 11 P.M. or just 4 P.M. in outpatients and settle for the relatively small loss (20 percent) in sensitivity. Although most utilize the criteria of 5 mcg/dl as abnormal, this can and should depend on the assay utilized. The most commonly used assays are competitive protein binding or the various radio-immunoassays (RIAs). It is important for each laboratory to recognize that both assays require considerable attention to obtain accurate results in the low concentrations that are necessary for psychiatric use. Clinicians need to work with and be aware of the quality of the assays of the laboratory they utilize. Most of the current research would suggest that test results between 4 and 7 mcg/dl should be interpreted cautiously. The DST is so profoundly affected by the physiologic status of the patient that all patients should be medication-free for the initial DST. Drugs that increase the metabolism and clearance of dexamethasone (for example, barbiturates, anticonvulsants) can influence the validity of the DST for several weeks, as can heavy use of alcohol. However, in routine clinical practice, keeping patients medication free is difficult, and therefore strict attention should be given to the specific examples cited and to the exclusion criteria (Table 1).

DST As Predictor of Treatment: There are now over 18 studies following up the

Table 1. Factors Potentially Interfering with the Validity of the DST

Those Resulting in False Positives:
Medical; Significant medical disorders such as cardiac, renal or hepatic disease, cancer, Cushing's, diabetes mellitus, hypothyroidism or those conditions resulting in physiologic instability such as infections with fever, dehydration, nausea and vomiting, weight loss
Drugs: Barbiturates, anticonvulsants (phenytoin, carbamazepine), meprobamate, glutethimide, recent withdrawal of drugs, especially alcohol
Other: Stress of hospitalization, recent circadian change (e.g., long trip), recent seizure, brain tumor, electroconvulsive therapy
Those That May Produce a False Negative:
Drugs: High doses of benzodiazepines, tricyclic antidepressants, l-tryptophan, methylphenidate, indomethacin, isoniazid, steroids
Other: Addison's disease and hypopituitarism

initial suggestion that an abnormal DST could predict response to antidepressant treatment, perhaps even which antidepressant. If possible, this would represent an important advance. However, subsequent research has failed to replicate a significant difference in response rate between DST positive and DST negative patients, when patients are treated with adequate doses of antidepressants. It appears that the DST does not substantially improve the clinician's ability to determine who should receive antidepressant treatment. The clinical features of depression are still the most important predictor of response, whether the DST is positive or negative. Also, the DST has not yet demonstrated its utility to the clinician in predicting which patient will respond to antidepressants when the decision is not clear on clinical grounds. This is an important clinical question but requires future research.

One of the most promising areas of DST research concerns whether persistence of an abnormal DST can predict clinical outcome. There are 10 reports suggesting that when the DST normalized from an initial nonsuppression, only 17 percent had a poor clinical outcome. In marked contrast, in those patients who continued to have an abnormal DST or redeveloped an abnormal DST, 78 percent experienced a poor clinical outcome (Arana et al, 1987). These reports concern patients who appeared to be clinically recovered after one to three months of acute, in-hospital treatment, as well as some patients one to six months after recovery and discharge from the hospital. As discussed by Prien (Giles et al, 1986) in Chapter 10, this area of research suggests one of the most valuable current and future uses for the DST; that is, as a predictor of patients who will relapse (Thase et al, 1985), need hospitalization or continued treatment, or even those who will attempt suicide.

Current Recommendations: Extensive research now suggests a more restricted utilization of the DST in psychiatry. Given the limited sensitivity for major affective disorder, a negative DST has little clinical significance. The DST has limited specificity and therefore limited diagnostic utility when patients with major depression are compared to those with nonmajor affective disorders or other severe acute psychiatric illnesses. However, it may prove to have differential ability in other conditions that may respond to antidepressants (for example, stroke patients, pain patients). Overall, its utility is limited when the clinical presentation makes it likely or unlikely that the patient has a major affective disorder. However, the "confirmation" provided by a positive DST is useful to some depressed patients, making it easier for them to accept antidepressant treatment. The clinician must realize that a positive DST does not predict an improved response rate to antidepressants, nor should a negative DST discourage a trial of treatment if clinical symptoms support such a decision. Perhaps one of the most important areas for clinical use as well as future research are the indications that a persistently abnormal DST, or one that reverts to abnormal after the patient has clinically recovered, is associated with a high risk of relapse.

Thyroid Abnormalities

Classical endocrinology has demonstrated clear psychiatric abnormalities, including depression with both frank hypothyroidism and hyperthyroidism. More recently, Gold and colleagues (Gold et al, 1981) have also suggested that a subset (5–10 percent) of patients with depression or anergia could be said to have Grade II or III hypothyroidism. These patients would have been considered euthyroid if they had been worked up by traditional methods. This subclinical hypothyroidism is demonstrated only by basal increases in thyroid-stimulating hormone (TSH) or in an abnormal TSH response to thyrotropin-releasing hormone (TRH). These patients often have detectable levels of antimicrosomal thyroid antibodies, and Nemeroff (Nemeroff et al, 1985) has recently demonstrated that 20 percent of depressed patients admitted consecutively to a psychiatric hospital had antithyroid antibodies. Furthermore, lithium may induce antithyroid antibodies, and those patients developing the antithyroid antibodies are more likely to develop overt hypothyroidism when given lithium. However, at this point it is difficult to define the stages of subclinical hypothyroidism, how to integrate these results with the data of blunted TSH responses (see below), or how both relate to psychiatric symptoms and treatment issues.

TRH TEST. *Procedure:* It has now been demonstrated in multiple studies that the TSH response to exogenous doses of TRH is reduced or "blunted" in approximately 25 percent of depressed patients (Loosen, 1985; Loosen and Prange, 1982). That is, if given a dose of TRH that in normals would produce a maximal rise in TRH, some depressed patients show a "blunted" (smaller) response. The TSH response is generally studied in medication-free patients by administering 500 mcg of synthetic TRH over 30 seconds through an indwelling catheter. Samples are obtained at baseline and 15, 30, 60, and 90 minutes after the TRH infusion. The maximal TSH response, called the delta TSH (change from baseline), is generally considered to be low or "blunted" if it is less than five microinternational units per millimeter of serum, although criteria vary and some groups utilize other thresholds (for example, 7 microIU/ml) for a positive test.

Proposed Pathophysiology: Certain evidence suggests that this abnormality may be related to the chronicity of the depressive process or may be a "state" marker of depression. Some patients demonstrate this abnormality only while depressed, but preliminary evidence suggests that some patients have it before, during, and after a depressive episode and that it therefore may represent a "trait" marker. The pathophysiology of this abnormality is currently unknown. Since TRH release is under central nervous system (CNS) control of neurotransmitters implicated in the depressive process (including norepinephrine, serotonin, and dopamine), it has been hypothesized that the observation of blunted TRH responses is related to neurotransmitter abnormalities. Certain data suggest that unipolar patients with abnormal TRH tests have serotonin overactivity and/or norepinephrine hypoactivity, but the data are preliminary and contradictory, and multiple combinations of neurotransmitter abnormalities are consistent with the available data.

Preliminary evidence from other studies suggests that these findings may reflect a dysfunction of the HPA axis. The 24-hour secretion of TSH and the nighttime rise in TSH have both been observed to be decreased in major depression, suggesting abnormalities in the relationship of hypothalamic TRH and pituitary TSH secretion. Since TSH has also been observed to be an active CNS neuromodulator, other theories suggest an abnormality in that area.

Potential Diagnostic Uses: Probably the most clinically promising line of research in this area suggests that a blunted TRH test may help differentiate major unipolar depression from the similar-appearing, nonmajor depressions in which the TRH is within normal limits. This might assist in making the decision as to whether somatic treatments are indicated for these depressions. There is similar, but more controversial, evidence suggesting that TRH blunting is not observed in bipolar depressions. This may prove to be of considerable clinical utility with the recent observations that the tricyclic and MAOI antidepressants may actually worsen the overall course of bipolar illness by inducing mania or increasing the frequency of rapid cycling in a significant portion of bipolar patients (Wehr and Goodwin, 1979). There is some suggestion that the TRH test is actually augmented in bipolar depressed patients and therefore might help identify "false unipolar" depressed patients before they develop identifying manic episodes. Similarly, preliminary evidence suggests that the TRH test may be clinically useful when the clinical presentation seems to conflict with the biological test; for example, when the depression seems minor and characterologic, but the TRH is abnormal. In such a situation, it may prove to be that the biological test might better predict response to somatic treatments than the clinical presentation.

The clinical question of whether the TRH test can identify a group of patients who are more likely to respond to treatment or respond to specific treatments also remains preliminary and somewhat controversial. Langer and colleagues (1984) reported that a blunted TRH test is predictive of a positive response to tricyclic antidepressants. As is discussed in Chapter 10 on somatic treatment (Giles et al, 1986), similar to the DST utilization to predict potential relapse, failure of the TRH to normalize with apparent clinical recovery may be predictive of relapse after various treatments of depression, including antidepressants (Kirkegaard et al, 1977), sleep deprivation (Kvist and Kirkegaard, 1980), and electroconvulsive therapy (Kirkegaard and Faber, 1981).

Conclusion: As with the DST, preliminary results with the TRH test certainly promise future clinical utility and provide hints as to the pathophysiology of depression. However, the research is early, limited, and somewhat contradictory.

NEUROTRANSMITTER ABNORMALITIES

Norepinephrine

Certainly the modern study of the biological aspects of depression began with the catecholamine hypothesis of affective disorders in the mid-1960s. Most simply stated, this hypothesis proposed that at least some depressions were associated with a functional deficiency of norepinephrine (NE) at important synapses of the brain, whereas mania was hypothesized to involve increases in NE. The earliest evidence was indirect, following the observations that the MAO inhibitor antidepressants blocked an important pathway for NE metabolism, and the tricyclic antidepressants prevented the metabolism of NE by blocking its reuptake into the presynaptic nerve terminal.

NERVOUS SYSTEM ANATOMY. The widespread projection of the CNS NE system should allow it to have important and diverse behavioral and emotional effects. Cell bodies for NE-containing neurons are found in the mid-brain, primarily in the bilateral nuclei, the locus coerulei. Neurons from these nuclei project both to the limbic system and to the cortex and produce 70 percent of the NE in the brain. Attempts to demonstrate abnormalities in this system in depressed patients have primarily utilized peripheral measures putatively related to CNS NE turnover. These have included studies of cerebrospinal fluid (CSF) NE and its principal metabolite MHPG, plasma NE and MHPG, and urinary measures of these catecholamines, as well as various challenge strategies. Considerable animal work in primates and rodents suggests that each of these methods "reflects" brain NE activity to at least some extent. However, a direct measure of CNS NE turnover is still lacking, and each of these methods has its own limitations and restrictions.

CEREBROSPINAL FLUID. Whereas limited evidence suggests increases in NE and MHPG in manic patients, less than one-half of the studies report lower levels of MHPG in depressed patients.

URINARY MEASURES. Urinary MHPG is certainly the most widely studied measure and is thought to reflect CNS NE metabolism at least in part. In bipolar patients, levels of urinary MHPG do appear to be lower during depression and higher during mania or hypomania. Further, bipolar depressed patients appear to have lower levels of MHPG than both normals and nonbipolar depressed patients.

Unipolar depressed patients appear to have a wide range of urinary MHPG levels that overlap considerably with the range in normals. Some research allows subtyping of depressed patients into low, normal, and high urinary MHPG (compared to normals). Only the subtype with low pretreatment urinary MHPG levels is thought to have low CNS NE output. Low MHPG may identify bipolar patients who have not yet had their first manic or hypomanic episode, an important clinical distinction. Some studies report a subgroup of very severely depressed (unipolar) patients whose urinary MHPG and urinary free cortisols are both quite high. Perhaps in this subgroup increased cholinergic activity may be the primary defect with secondary MHPG and UFC changes (see below).

Goodwin and colleagues (1977) have reported a provocative finding that patients with high urinary MHPG tend to have low CSF levels of the serotonin metabolite 5-HIAA, lending support to the hypothesis that there are "noradrenergic" and "serotonergic" depressions.

Schildkraut and colleagues (1978) have utilized multiple urinary measures in a multivariate discriminant function analysis, and using this equation report preliminary findings that low scores provide reliable discrimination between bipolar and unipolar depressions and nonendogenous chronic characterologic depressions. Although currently impractical for clinical use, this technique appears to fulfill several of the requirements for a reliable biological diagnostic test.

Prediction of Antidepressant Response: Depressed patients with low pretreatment urinary MHPG levels (versus high) have been found to respond more favorably to antidepressants active in the noradrenergic system (for example, imipramine, desipramine, nortriptyline, or maprotiline). Furthermore, some studies have found that depressed patients with "high" pretreatment MHPG levels respond better to amitriptyline than patients with lower MHPG levels. Perhaps most interesting was the single report that patients with low pretreatment urinary MHPG levels responded more rapidly to relatively low doses of maprotiline, a relatively specific NE drug. Those with more elevated MHPG levels required significantly higher doses and longer periods for response. The clinician's hope that urinary MHPG levels could predict both good response to antidepressants and response to specific antidepressants has been dampened, unfortunately, as recent studies have failed to confirm these early promising results.

This same strategy has been extended to other biological measures. For example, Sabelli and colleagues (1983) reported that 24-hour urinary excretion of phenylactate, the major metabolite of the amino acid phenylalanine, was significantly lower in unipolar patients. However, one subsequent study (Karoum et al, 1984) failed to observe this difference.

RECEPTOR STUDIES. Adrenergic receptors have been studied by utilizing receptors on red cells, white cells, and platelets and have involved estimates of receptor number, binding affinity, and coupling of receptors to their functions. Although it is unknown what relationship these receptors have to CNS adrenergic receptors, there is at least some evidence that they share certain characteristics, and their availability make them valuable research tools. Changes in neurotransmitter receptor function have been postulated to be central to both the pathophysiology of depression and to the response to therapeutic agents. Some studies suggest decreased beta-adrenergic function and others a deficiency in the coupling between the alpha 2-adrenergic receptors and the adenylate cyclase in the platelets of unipolar depressed patients. Recent studies have utilized direct binding to alpha-adrenergic receptors of labeled ligands such as dihydroergocriptine, yohimbine, and clonidine and have demonstrated increased yohimbine and clonidine binding on platelets of depressed patients when compared to normals (Garcia-Sevilla et al, 1981). Kafka and colleagues (1980) observed increased binding of dihydroergocriptine to platelets of depressed patients.

Challenge tests: In an effort to gain a valuable "window" on membrane function, challenge tests have become increasingly utilized. This involves stimulating a system of known receptor type and measuring an available end product of that system, for example, the growth hormone response to the alpha-adrenergic agonist clonidine. The decreased or "blunted" growth hormone response to clonidine in some depressed patients is felt to be evidence of decreased sensitivity of these receptors (Jimerson and Post, 1984).

The findings with clonidine are supported by growth hormone responses to other adrenergic challenges including desmethylimipramine, insulin, and L-dopa, and all demonstrate blunting of the growth hormone response. These studies provide evidence of decreased postsynaptic alpha receptor responsivity and, when coupled with observations of high urinary MHPG in unipolar patients, suggest that these receptors desensitize because of exposure to higher than normal levels of NE. In depressed patients, MHPG levels ranging from low to above normal are consistent with the hypothesis that some depressed patients (particularly bipolar) show evidence of decreased noradrenergic function and have increased receptor responsivity. However, others (notably unipolar) are thought to have increased NE availability with decreased receptor responsivity, or inconstant or dysregulated NE availability. Although these studies do not yet allow a definitive picture of adrenergic function in depression, they have added an important new level of observation to the field.

Use in Diagnosis: Some data suggest that these blunted clonidine responses discriminate endogenous depression from other forms of depression. The blunted growth hormone response to D-amphetamine also reportedly distinguishes endogenous depression from other types of depression (Langer et al, 1976). Early studies reported that a transient mood improvement in depressed patients when they were given amphetamines predicted subsequent response to imipramine. Although this study was subsequently replicated in 5 of 10 studies, and evidence suggests it could predict response to particular antidepressants (Goff, 1986), the stimulant-challenge tests have surprisingly failed to influence research or clinical practice to any significant extent.

Dopamine

While most of the original interest in the catecholamine theory of depression as well as more recent studies have centered largely on NE, there is increasing neurochemical and pharmacological evidence that functional dopamine activity (DA) may be reduced in some depressed patients and increased in manic patients. PHARMACOLOGICAL EVIDENCE. The initial pharmacological evidence implicating involvement of DA in depression involved studies demonstrating modest antidepressant effects with the DA precursor L-dopa. It was particularly provocative that pretreatment levels of the principal DA metabolite homovanillic acid (HVA) in cerebrospinal fluid predicted a favorable response to L-dopa. The recently developed relatively specific postsynaptic DA agonists have demonstrated even more clear antidepressant activity for these agents. In a double blind trial with piribedil, Post and colleagues reported antidepressant effects in 12 of 16 patients, and again a low pretreatment level of CSF HVA predicted greater clinical improvement (Post et al, 1978). Subsequent trials with piribedil and bromocriptine (Silverstone, 1984) also reported antidepressant responses and occasional shifts into mania. Certainly, the recent trials demonstrating clear efficacy in large clinical trials of nomifensine and bupropion, which have prominent effects on DA systems, have further implicated the DA system in depression. CEREBROSPINAL FLUID STUDIES. The majority of studies of CSF HVA in medication-free patients demonstrates reduced CSF HVA in patients when compared to controls (Goodwin et al, 1973), and limited family data suggest it may be a trait marker. Roy and colleagues (1985) suggest that CSF HVA differentiates melancholic major depression from nonmelancholic depressive episodes or dysthymic disorder.

Conversely, evidence of increased DA turnover, such as increased CSF HVA, has been observed in delusional or psychotic depression (Agren and Terenius, 1985). NEUROENDOCRINE STUDIES. Multiple studies of prolactin and growth hormone responses to DA agonists have failed to demonstrate differences between depressed patients and normals. However, these neuroendocrine challenge tests presumably reflect postsynaptic DA receptor function in the tubero-infundibular pathway rather than the mesolimbic or mesocortical dopamine pathways presumably of importance in depression.

Serotonin

Interest in the potential role of serotonin (5-HT) abnormalities in the biochemistry of affective disorders has been second only to the catecholamines. Available evidence suggests that decreased 5-HT activity may either increase the vulnerability to depression or, in fact, be a causative factor. Its wide distribution in the brain and interaction with multiple other neurotransmitters permit it to function as an inhibitory influence on neuronal mechanisms and on behavior. Considerable evidence suggests that it is involved in those processes which appear to be abnormal in depression, for example, mood, insomnia, short REM latency, disturbed circadian rhythms, abnormal neuroendocrine function, and sexual abnormalities. Several animal models of depression are also consistent with a hyposerotonergic hypothesis of depression, as are the studies in man reported below.

CEREBROSPINAL FLUID 5-HYDROXYINDOLEACETIC ACID (5-HIAA). Although several studies (Vestergaard et al, 1978; Roy et al, 1985; Banki et al, 1981) have failed to observe any differences in CSF 5-HIAA between depressed patients and controls, two of the best recent studies (Agren, 1980; Asberg et al, 1984) reported significantly reduced levels in unipolar (and bipolar) depressed patients compared to normal controls. One study reported that CSF 5-HIAA increased after recovery in those patients whose pretreatment levels were low (Traskman-Bendz et al, 1984). Some studies have shown correlations between 5-HIAA and depressive symptoms and considerable work suggests low 5-HIAA may identify a subgroup of depressed patients prone to suicide.

PLASMA TRYPTOPHAN. In a series of 25 studies of free plasma tryptophan, one-half of the studies report significantly lower levels in depressed patients, suggesting that decreased availability of tryptophan in brain may contribute to a deficiency of CNS 5-HT in depression (Meltzer et al, in press, 1987). Low plasma tryptophan has been correlated with severity of depression and response to L-tryptophan but not to tricyclic antidepressants (Meltzer, in press). Lower plasma tryptophan after oral and intravenous tryptophan suggests significant metabolic differences resulting in lower serum levels in depressed patients.

SEROTONIN UPTAKE AND IMIPRAMINE BINDING IN PLATELETS. Many studies have reported decreased platelet 5-HT uptake in depressed patients (Suranyi-Cadotte et al, 1985) secondary to a decrease in the number of uptake sites (V_{max}). However, 5-HT uptake into platelets did not predict response to zimelidine or desipramine (Aberg-Wistedt, 1982). Platelet imipramine binding has been reported to be decreased in depressed patients (Paul et al, 1981; Meltzer et al, 1984). This is secondary to a decrease in the number of imipramine binding sites (B_{max}) which modulate 5-HT uptake into the platelet. Both the V_{max} changes and B_{max} changes may represent adaptive attempts to normalize serotonin function.

NEUROENDOCRINE RESPONSE. The cortisol response to oral DL-5-HTP has been reported to be increased in depressed and manic patients (Meltzer et al, 1984) and inversely correlated with CSF 5-HIAA levels, suggesting that the enhanced cortisol response is secondary to supersensitivity of 5-HT receptors. Conversely, intravenous L-tryptophan results in a reduced prolactin (PRL) response in depressed patients compared to normals (Heninger et al, 1984), but this normalizes on recovery.

PHARMACOLOGICAL EVIDENCE. Although tryptophan alone has not been observed to be as effective as standard antidepressants, considerable evidence now suggests that it can potentiate the action of tricyclic antidepressants or MAO inhibitors (Baldessarini, 1984). Also, a series of studies suggests that L-5-HTP is effective in converting previously refractive depressed patients when added to tricyclic antidepressants. Lithium's ability to convert inadequate antidepressant responses provides further support for serotonergic mechanisms in depression (Blier and deMontigny, 1985).

Despite the clear evidence that so-called specific 5-HT reuptake blockers are effective in depression, paradoxically, this effectiveness has not provided further evidence of a role for serotonin in depression. Therapeutic responses have not been generally specific to the 5-HT reuptake blockers, and these agents clearly have effects on other critical neurotransmitters.

CLINICAL PREDICTORS. Unfortunately, both low and high CSF 5-HIAA levels have been reported to predict clinical response to antidepressants. However, Maas and colleagues (1982) reported that low CSF 5-HIAA predicted good clinical response to imipramine but not to amitriptyline, and Aberg-Wistedt and colleagues (1982) reported that it predicted response to zimelidine, a 5-HT uptake blocker. Van Praag and colleagues (1972) demonstrated that low 5-HIAA predicted both acute and prophylactic response to 5-HTP. Dahl and colleagues observed no correlation of 5-HIAA to clinical response of femoxetine, a new serotonin uptake blocker (Dahl et al, 1982). However, Lingjaerde (1983) did observe positive correlations between platelet 5-HT uptake and clinical improvement on zimelidine and not desipramine; however, this failed to be replicated in a subsequent study (Aberg-Wistedt, 1982).

CONCLUSIONS. These studies have provided increasing biochemical and pharmacological evidence for the hyposerotonergic hypothesis of depression. These and other studies have moved us closer to understanding potential defects in the 5-HT system in depression. Decreased availability of tryptophan in the brain for conversion to 5-HT, decreased 5-HT firing secondary to autoreceptor supersensitivity, increased reuptake, and decreased postsynaptic receptor responsivity all appear to be viable candidates for biochemical abnormalities in the serotonin system of depressed patients.

Acetylcholine

Janowsky and colleagues, in 1972, focused attention on the cholinergic system when they hypothesized that affective disturbances could be related to relative imbalances between the brain adrenergic and cholinergic systems. They postulated that depression represented a relative cholinergic predominance, with mania thought to be an illness of relative adrenergic predominance. Most of the subsequent evidence has supported this model, and suggests at least some involvement of the cholinergic system in depression.

CNS ANATOMY. Although it has been technically difficult to map the CNS acetylcholine (Ach) system accurately, cholinergic activity in the primate brain appears to be primarily located in the basal ganglia, amygdala, hippocampus, superior and inferior caliculi, frontal, perifrontal, and cerebellar cortices, the inferior olive, medulla oblongata, cervical cord, locus coeruleus, and the lateral hypothalamus. Its prominent innervation of limbic areas and the locus coeruleus is certainly consistent with an involvement in regulation of affective states.

In multiple animal models of depression including the learned helplessness, chronic stress, hypoactivity, and behavioral despair (or forced swim) models, all seem to involve the cholinergic system. Centrally active cholinomimetic drugs consistently produce lethargy, hypoactivity, and decrease self-stimulation, which are all felt to be analogous to depressive symptoms. Recent selective breeding studies for increased cholinergic sensitivity in rats are consistent with an important role for cholinergic mechanisms in depression.

HUMAN STUDIES. Certainly the most direct evidence that Ach is involved in depression stems from the observations that agents which increase central cholinergic activity can rapidly induce a depressed mood. Multiple research groups have now demonstrated increases in depression in depressed or manic patients and normals given physostigmine or arecoline (Janowsky et al, 1973; Risch et al, 1983).

Many of the symptoms of depression appear consistent with central cholinergic hyperactivity or "supersensitivity." Cholinergic agonists generally shorten REM latency and result in an increase in REM density similar to the sleep abnormalities observed in depressed patients. Sitaram and colleagues (1982) have also shown that induction of muscarinic upregulation by the withdrawal of chronic scopolamine results in a shortening of REM latency and an increase in REM density. In addition, they have observed that REM latency was significantly shortened following arecoline infusions in patients both when they are depressed and after remission of their depressive episode. This suggests that the change in the cholinergic system either predisposes individuals to develop depression or is a result of past episodes of depression. Interestingly, this more rapid induction of REM sleep is also observed in volunteers with a family history of affective disorders.

Intriguingly, there is evidence from a range of studies that cholinomimetic drugs elevate serum cortisol, ACTH, and can promote resistance to dexamethasone, all observed neuroendocrine abnormalities in depression.

Certainly the observations in manic patients are consistent with this model, in which increases in CNS cholinergic activity have been observed to decrease manic symptoms. Following Janowsky's original observation that physostigmine caused a dramatic but brief reduction in hypomanic or manic symptoms, multiple other groups have provided supportive evidence for the antimanic efficacy of cholinomimetic agents. It remains somewhat unclear whether the effects are primarily on mood and motor activity and not on manic thought disorder.

MUSCARINIC RECEPTORS. Although several recent studies have suggested differences in muscarinic receptor binding between affective patients and normals, this remains a controversial area. Nadi and colleagues (1984) reported that fibroblasts grown in culture from affective disorder patients and their relatives had more muscarinic cholinergic (QNB) binding sites than normals. Further, Meyerson and colleagues (1982) reported increased muscarinic receptor binding activity in the brains of patients dying from suicide as compared to those dying from other causes. However, recent studies from multiple groups have failed to find evidence of increased muscarinic binding either in the brain or peripheral measures in suicides.

CONCLUSION. Some of the available evidence is consistent with the hypothesis that Ach could be involved in the etiology or expression of affective disorders. Although there is little available direct biological evidence, certainly the pharmacological data are suggestive that acetylcholine may be involved in the induction of the symptoms of depression and perhaps some of the biological abnormalities (cortisol, sleep, and so on) observed in depression. It is even more likely that changes in the Ach system may either cause or interact with perturbations in other systems, most notably the noradrenergic system. The recent findings of enhanced cholinergic REM induction in volunteers with a family history of affective illness and the persistence of that abnormality in remitted patients suggests important genetic factors, and that cholinergic abnormalities may result in a predisposition to depression rather than being actively involved in "causing" depression. The Ach system interacts at an anatomic as well as a pharmacological level with the NE system to probably "modulate" changes in the adrenergic system. Muscarinic hypersensitivity might predispose to the development of depression in response to changes in the NE system secondary to adverse life experiences. This type of model is certainly more consistent with a growing data base suggestive of the involvement of multiple brain neurotransmitters in depression, and evidence suggesting that biological deficits in depression may be related to defective regulatory processes.

CONCLUSIONS

This chapter provides a selective review of various biological investigations in depression with a particular emphasis on those findings which might have current or future clinical relevance. There is no coherent "biology" of depression at this point, nor is it likely that there will be in the near future. Research has tended to focus on one area to the exclusion of others, and this, coupled with the inherent complexity of the work, has prevented definitive elucidation of even single mechanisms; certainly coherent relationships among areas of research have been impossible to date. However, as research in this area has expanded, areas of consensus have been formed and are touched on in this chapter.

As work on various neurotransmitters has evolved from the simplistic to the more complex, interactions among the four most widely studied neurotransmitters (NE, DA, 5-HT, and Ach) have become more clear. Certainly there is considerable evidence for important interactions between the NE and 5-HT systems, as well as the NE, 5-HT, and Ach systems. Hypotheses have moved from the initial "too much–too little" type to those involving interactions between pertinent neurotransmitter systems; for example, that removal of the 5-HT inhibition of the Ach system results in depression secondary to Ach overactivity. This promise of convergence of findings also extends to the best developed areas of research, for example, implicating low 5-HT in the failure of cortisol to suppress to dexamethasone. Similarly, evidence of hyposerotonergic function has been implicated in the well-replicated findings of insomnia and decreased REM latency seen in depression.

While such hints of convergence and basic explanations of biological mechanisms in depression are exciting, more definitive understanding of these mechanisms probably awaits decades of further research. The practical and widespread use of biological factors clinically is probably also relegated to the future. Despite increasing confidence in certain findings, particularly sleep changes, HPA axis abnormalities, and certain of the urinary and CSF measures, none is ready for routine use by the clinician. The early relatively uncritical use of DST reflected both the great need for external and easily obtained measures, as well as the difficulties of moving these biological measures into routine practice.

REFERENCES

Aberg-Wistedt A: A double-blind study of zimelidine, a serotonin uptake inhibitor, and desipramine, a noradrenaline uptake inhibitor, in endogenous depression, I: clinical findings. Acta Psychiatr Scand 1982; 66:50-65

Aberg-Wistedt A, Ross SB, Jolstell K-G, et al: A double-blind study of zimelidine, a serotonin uptake inhibitor, and desipramine, a noradrenaline uptake inhibitor, in endogenous depression, II: biochemical findings. Acta Psychiatr Scand 1982; 66:66-82

Agren H: Symptom patterns in unipolar and bipolar depression correlating with monoamine metabolites in the cerebrospinal fluid, I: general patterns. Psychiatry Res 1980; 3:211-224

Agren H, Terenius L: Hallucinations in patients with major depression. J Affective Disord 1985; 9:25-34

Arana GW, Workman R, Baldessarini RJ: Association between low plasma levels of dexamethasone and elevated levels of cortisol in psychiatric patients given dexamethasone. Am J Psychiatry 1984; 141:1619-1620

Arana GW, Baldessarini RJ, Ornsteen M: The dexamethasone suppression test for diagnosis and prognosis in psychiatry: commentary and review. Arch Gen Psychiatry 1985; 42:1193-1204

Arana GW, Baldessarini RJ, Brown WA, et al: The dexamethasone suppression test: an overview of its current status in psychiatry. Task Force Report for the American Psychiatric Association. Washington, DC, American Psychiatric Association, 1987

Asberg M, Bertilsson L, Martensson B, et al: CSF monoamine metabolites in melancholia. Acta Psychiatr Scand 1984; 69:201-219

Baldessarini RJ: Treatment of depression by altering monoamine metabolism: precursors and metabolic inhibitors. Psychopharmacol Bull 1984; 20:224-239

Banki CM, Vojnik M, Molnar G: Cerebrospinal fluid amine metabolites, tryptophan and clinical parameters in depression, part I: background variables. J Affective Disord 1981; 3:81-89

Blier P, deMontigny C: Short-term lithium administration enhances serotonergic neurotransmission: electrophysiological evidence in the rat CNS. Eur J Pharmacol 1985; 113:69-77

Carroll BJ, Curtis GC, Mendels J: Neuroendocrine regulation in depression, II: discrimination of depressed from nondepressed patients. Arch Gen Psychiatry 1976; 33:1051-1058

Carroll BJ, Feinberg M, Greden JF, et al: A specific laboratory test for the diagnosis of melancholia: standardization, validation, and clinical utility. Arch Gen Psychiatry 1981; 38:15-22

Coble P, Foster FG, Kupfer DJ: Electroencephalographic sleep diagnosis of primary depression. Arch Gen Psychiatry 1976; 33:1124-1127

Dahl L-E, Lunden L, LeFevre HP, et al: Antidepressant effect of femoxetine and desipramine and relationship to the concentration of amine metabolites in cerebrospinal fluid. Acta Psychiatr Scand 1982; 66:9-17

Foster FG, Kupfer DJ, Coble P, et al: Rapid eye movement sleep density: an objective indicator in severe medical-depressive syndromes. Arch Gen Psychiatry 1976; 33:1119-1123

Garcia-Sevilla JA, Zis AP, Hollingsworth PJ, et al: Platelet alpha-2-adrenergic receptors in major depressive disorder. Arch Gen Psychiatry 1981; 38:1327-1333

Giles DE, Jarrett RB, Roffwarg HP, et al: Monthly longitudinal study of remitted depression, in Scientific Program, Annual Meeting of the Society of Biological Psychiatry. Washington, DC, May, 1986

Gillin JC, Sitaram N, Wehr T, et al: Sleep and affective illness, in Neurobiology of Mood Disorders. Edited by Post RM, Ballenger JC. Baltimore, Williams & Wilkins, 1984

Goff DC: The stimulant challenge test in depression. J Clin Psychiatry 1986; 47:538-543

Gold MS, Pottash ALC, Extein I: Hypothyroidism and depression: evidence from completed thyroid function evaluation. JAMA 1981; 245:1919-1925

Gold PW, Chrousos G, Kellner C, et al: Psychiatric implications of basic and clinical studies with corticotropin-releasing factor. Am J Psychiatry 1984; 141:619-627

Goodwin FK, Post RM, Dunner DL, et al: Cerebrospinal fluid amine metabolites in affective illness: the probenecid technique. Am J Psychiatry 1973; 130:73-79

Goodwin FK, Rubovitz R, Jimerson DC, et al: Serotonin and norepinephrine "subgroup" in depression: metabolite findings and clinical pharmacological correlations. Scientific Proceedings of the American Psychiatric Association 1977; 130:108-131

Heninger GR, Charney DS, Sternberg DE: Serotonergic function in depression. Arch Gen Psychiatry 1984; 41:398-402

Janowsky DS, Risch SC: Role of acetylcholine mechanisms in the affective disorders, in Psychopharmacology, the Third Generation of Progress. Edited by Meltzer HY, Bunney WE, Coyle J, et al. New York, Raven Press (in press)

Janowsky DS, El-Yousef MK, Davis JM, et al: A cholinergic-adrenergic hypothesis of mania and depression. Lancet 1972; 2:6732-6735

Janowsky DS, El-Yousef MK, Davis JM, et al: Parasympathetic suppression of manic symptoms by physostigmine. Arch Gen Psychiatry 1973; 28:542-547

Jimerson DC, Post RM: Psychomotor stimulants and dopamine agonists in depression, in Neurobiology of Mood Disorders. Edited by Post RM, Ballenger JC. Baltimore, Williams & Wilkins, 1984

Kafka MS, van Kammen DP, Kleinman JE, et al: Alpha-adrenergic receptor function in schizophrenia, affective disorder, and some neurological diseases. Communication Psychopharmacology 1980; 4:477-486

Karoum F, Potkin S, Chuang L, et al: Phenylacetic acid excretion in schizophrenia and depression: the origins of PAA in man. Biol Psychiatry 1984; 19:165-178

Kellner CH, Rubinow DR, Gold PW, et al: Relationship of cortisol hypersecretion to brain CT scan alterations in depressed patients. Psychiatry Res 1983; 8:191-197

Kirkegaard C, Faber J: Altered serum levels of thyroxine, triiodothyronines and diiodo-thyronines in endogenous depression. Acta Endocrinologica 1981; 96:199-207

Kirkegaard C, Bjorum N, Cohn D, et al: Studies on the influence of biogenic amine stimulation test in endogenous depression. Psychoneuroendocrinology 1977; 2:131-136

Kupfer DJ, Spiker DG, Coble PA, et al: Depression, EEG sleep, and clinical response. Compr Psychiatry 1980; 21:212-220

Kvist J, Kirkegaard C: Effect of repeated sleep deprivation on clinical symptoms and TRH test in endogenous depression. Acta Psychiatr Scand 1980; 62:494-502

Langer G, Heinze G, Reim B, et al: Reduced growth hormone responses to amphetamine in "endogenous" depressive patients: studies in normal, "reactive" and "endogenous" depressive schizophrenic, and chronic alcoholic subjects. Arch Gen Psychiatry 1976; 33:1471-1475

Langer G, Resch F, Aschauer MS, et al: TSH response patterns to TRH stimulation may indicate therapeutic mechanisms of antidepressant and neuroleptic drugs. Neuropsychobiology 1984; 11:213-218

Lewy AJ, Sack RL, Miller LS, et al: Antidepressant and circadian phase-shifting effects of light. Science 1987; 235:352-354

Lingjaerde O: The biochemistry of depression. Acta Psychiatr Scand 1983; 302 (suppl):36-51

Loosen PT: The TRH-induced TSH response in psychiatric patients: a possible neuroendocrine marker. Psychoneuroendocrinology 1985; 10:237-260

Loosen PT, Prange AJ: The serum thyrotropin (TSH) response to thyrotropin-releasing hormone (TRH) in depression: a review. Am J Psychiatry 1982; 139:405-416

Maas JW, Kocsis JH, Bowden CL, et al: Pre-treatment neurotransmitter metabolites and response to imipramine or amitriptyline treatment. Psychol Med 1982; 12:37-43

Meltzer HY: The serotonin hypothesis of depression, in Psychopharmacology, the Third Generation of Progress. Edited by Meltzer HY, Bunney WE, Coyle J, et al. New York, Raven Press (in press)

Meltzer HY, Umberkoman-Wiita B, Roberton A, et al: Effect of 5-hydroxytrophan on serum cortisol levels in major affective disorders, I: enhanced response in depression and mania. Arch Gen Psychiatry 1984; 41:366-374

Meyerson LR, Wennogle LP, Abel MS, et al: Human brain receptor alterations in suicide victims. Pharmacol Biochem Behav 1982; 17:159-163

Nadi, NS, Nurberger JL, Gershon ES: Muscarinic cholinergic receptors on skin fibroblasts in familial affective disorder. N Engl J Med 1984; 311:225-230

Nemeroff CB, Simon JS, Haggerty JJ, et al: Antithyroid antibodies in depressed patients. Am J Psychiatry 1985; 142:840-843

Paul SM, Rehavi M, Skolnick P, et al: Depressed patients have decreased binding of tritiated imipramine to platelet serotonin "transporter." Arch Gen Psychiatry 1981; 38:1315-1317

Post RM, Ballenger JC (Eds): Neurobiology of Mood Disorders. Baltimore, Williams & Wilkins, 1984

Post RM, Gerner RH, Carman JS, et al: Effects of a dopamine agonist piribedil in depressed patients. Arch Gen Psychiatry 1978; 35:609-615

Risch SC, Siever LJ, Gillin JC: Differential mood effects of arecoline in depressed patients and normal volunteers. Psychopharmacol Bull 1983; 19:696-698

Rosenthal NE, Sack DA, Carpenter CJ, et al: Antidepressant effects of light in seasonal affective disorder. Am J Psychiatry 1985; 142:606-608

Roy A, Pickar D, Linnoila M, et al: Cerebrospinal fluid monoamine and monoamine metabolite concentrations in melancholia. Psychiatry Res 1985; 15:281-292

Rubinow DR, Post RM, Gold PW, et al: The relationship between cortisol and clinical phenomenology of affective illness, in Neurobiology of Mood Disorders. Edited by Post RM, Ballenger JC. Baltimore, Williams & Wilkins, 1984

Sabelli HC, Fawcett J, Gusovsky F, et al: Urinary phenyl acetate: a diagnostic test for depression? Science 1983; 220:1187-1188

Schildkraut JJ, Orsulak PJ, LaBrie RA, et al: Toward a biochemical classification of depressive disorders, II: application of multivariate discrimination function analysis to data on urinary catecholamines and metabolites. Arch Gen Psychiatry 1978c; 35:1436-1439

Sitaram N, Nurnberger J, Gershon ES: Cholinergic regulation of mood and REM sleep: potential model and marker of vulnerability to affective disorder. Am J Psychiatry 1982; 139:571-576

Silverstone T: Response to bromocriptine distinguishes bipolar from unipolar depression. Lancet 1984; 1:903-904

Suranyi-Cadotte BE, Quiron R, Nair NPV, et al: Imipramine treatment differentially affects platelet ^{3}H-imipramine binding and serotonin uptake in depressed patients. Life Sci 1985; 36:795-799

Thase ME, Frank E, Kupfer DJ: Biological processes in major depression, in The Handbook of Depression: Treatment, Asssessment, and Research. Edited by Beckham EE, Leber WR. Homewood, IL, Dorsey Press, 1985

Traskman-Bendz L, Asberg M, Bertilsson L, et al: CSF monoamine metabolites of depressed patients during illness and after recovery. Acta Psychiatr Scand 1984; 69:333-342

van Praag HM, Korf J, Dols LCW, et al: A pilot study of the predictive value of the probenecid test in application of 5-hydroxytryptophan as antidepressant. Psychopharmacologia 1972; 25:14-21

van Praag HM, Lader MH, Rafealsen OJ, et al (Eds): Handbook of Biological Psychiatry, part IV: Brain Mechanisms and Abnormal Behavior. New York, Marcel Dekker, 1981

Vestergaard P, Sorensen T, Hoppe E, et al: Biogenic amine metabolites in cerebrospinal fluid of patients with affective disorders. Acta Psychiatr Scand 1978; 58:88-96

Vogel GW, Vogel F, McAbee RS, et al: Improvement of depression by REM sleep deprivation. Arch Gen Psychiatry 1980; 37:247-253

Wehr TA, Goodwin FK: Rapid cycling in manic depressives induced by tricyclic antidepressants. Arch Gen Psychiatry 1979; 36:555

Wehr TA, Wirz-Justice A, Goodwin FK, et al: Phase advance of the circadian sleep–wake cycle as an antidepressant. Science 1979; 206:210-213

Wehr TA, Jacobsen FM, Sack DA, et al: Phototherapy of seasonal affective disorder. Arch Gen Psychiatry 1986; 43:870-875

Chapter 9

Diagnostic Issues and Clinical Course of Unipolar Illness

by *Martin B. Keller, M.D.*

OVERVIEW

The concept of unipolar illness began with Kraepelin, who, by the end of the 19th century, included unipolar and bipolar affective disorders in his definition of manic-depressive illness. In 1962, Leonhard and colleagues proposed the separation of manic-depressive psychosis into a bipolar group (those depressed patients with a history of manic episodes), and a unipolar group (those patients who have had only episodes of depression).

Although there is familial/genetic, neurophysiological, biochemical, personality, and clinical evidence to support the bipolar–unipolar distinction (Wolpert, 1980), etiological evidence is lacking (Krauthammer and Klerman, 1978). Nonetheless, the differential treatment response of unipolar and bipolar patients and marked differences in phenomenology and course warrant distinguishing these two groups for clinical and research purposes. However, there are many theoretical and practical questions which point to substantial heterogeneity within the category of unipolar depressive illness, and much of this chapter will be devoted to discussing such issues.

There is a long history of changing nosology with regard to unipolar depression that is still active. For example, terms such as melancholia, neurotic depression, and endogenous depression have been dropped and added to major systems of classification over the years. A detailed account of this shifting nomenclature is beyond the scope of this chapter, which will use the revised third edition of the *Diagnostic and Statistical Manual of Mental Disorders (DSM-III-R)* (American Psychiatric Association, 1987) as the basis for definition and differential diagnosis. However, many terms which are not in *DSM-III-R*, but which have been in common usage, will be discussed.

Unless otherwise specified in this chapter, unipolar depression refers to conditions without any known organic etiology. Chapter 12, by Dr. Cassem, is devoted to depression secondary to organic conditions. Although it will not be discussed further in this chapter, it is critical to emphasize at the outset that depressive symptoms and syndromes should always lead the clinician to look for the presence of an organic etiologic agent.

DEFINITION AND DESCRIPTION

In the *DSM-III-R*, the affective disorders are subgrouped into major affective disorders, other specific affective disorders, and atypical affective disorders. The

The author would like to acknowledge the excellent assistance of Ms. Fran Sessa, B.A., in all phases of the planning, writing, and editing of this chapter.

major affective disorders, bipolar disorder and major depression, require a full affective syndrome and are distinguished by the occurrence or nonoccurrence of a manic episode. The other specific affective disorders require a less severe syndrome with at least two years' duration, and include cyclothymia and dysthymia. The atypical group ("bipolar disorder not otherwise specified" and "depressive disorder not otherwise specified") includes those syndromes that cannot be classified into the major and other categories.

Major Depression

The broad range of depressive states subsumed under the category of major depression includes: psychotic depressive disorder, psychoneurotic depressive reaction, and nonbipolar forms of recurrent manic-depressive insanity, melancholia, depression with psychotic features, and "situational" depression.

"The essential clinical feature is a dysphoric mood usually experienced consciously as a depression. The disturbance of mood is prominent, persistent, and associated with other symptoms. However, it is necessary to recognize that all individuals who are diagnosed as having a major depressive episode do not have to report being subjectively depressed" (Cancro, 1985, p. 761).

DSM-III-R defines a "major depressive syndrome" as the presence of at least five of the following symptoms, simultaneously, nearly every day for at least two weeks:

1. persistent depressed mood most of the day
2. loss of interest or pleasure in all or almost all activities (anhedonia) [at least one of the five requisite symptoms must be persistent dysphoric mood or anhedonia]
3. significant weight loss or weight gain in the absence of dieting or binge-eating, or decreased or increased appetite
4. insomnia or hypersomnia
5. psychomotor agitation or retardation
6. fatigue or loss of energy (anergia)
7. feelings of worthlessness or excessive or inappropriate guilt
8. diminished ability to think, concentrate, or make decisions
9. thoughts that he or she would be better off dead, or suicidal ideation or a suicide attempt (*American Psychiatric Association, 1987*).

According to DSM-III-R, the diagnosis of a major depressive episode would not be made if the etiology of the disturbance is organic, or if it is a normal reaction to the loss of a loved one. The normal reaction to the loss of a loved one would be diagnosed as "uncomplicated bereavement." However, if the depressive symptoms associated with the grief are morbidly severe and prolonged, the diagnosis of bereavement complicated by major depression should be made.

Other *DSM-III-R* exclusion criteria for the diagnosis of major depression include the presence of delusions or hallucinations for as long as two weeks in the absence of prominent mood symptoms, or the superimposition of the depressed episode in schizophrenia, schizophreniform disorder, or delusional disorder.

Several nonsymptom features are included in the criteria, such as an absence of significant personality disturbance prior to the first major depressive episode, and prior good response to specific and adequate somatic antidepressant therapy.

A detailed comparison between *DSM-III-R* and the affective disorders categories in the Research Diagnostic Criteria (RDC) (Spitzer et al, 1985) is beyond the scope of this chapter. However, since the RDC is widely used in research and appears very frequently in many of the articles currently published in psychiatric journals, it is noted here that the criteria for major depression are essentially identical, with the exception that the RDC requires evidence of functional impairment.

The *DSM-III-R* criteria for major depression are the subject of controversy. Most previous nomenclatures and common clinical usage in Western Europe make the distinction between the endogenous/psychotic and the neurotic forms of depression as coded in ICD-9. Since this distinction is based on presumed etiology rather than clinical psychopathology and symptoms it is not included in *DSM-III-R*. Psychodynamically oriented psychiatrists tend to be dissatisfied with the elimination of "neurotic depression," and the atheoretical discussion of each of the affective disorders. Biological psychiatrists typically view the criteria as too broad, the symptom set too general, and the criterion of two weeks' duration of symptoms too brief. They tend to strongly advocate subtyping major depression. In addition, the biologic viewpoint holds that many patients diagnosed as having "major depression" are experiencing states of demoralization and/or having transient responses to situational stress and/or to chronic adverse social circumstances, such as poverty, or persistent marital discord, rather than a "true—that is, biological—depression." In keeping with this objection, Gershon, Angst, and others have proposed a more stringent impairment criteria requiring some evidence of hospitalization, or occupational role impairment (Klerman et al, 1987).

Dysthymic Disorder

Dysthymic disorder is a chronic nonpsychotic disturbance involving depressed mood or a loss of interest or pleasure in all or almost all usual activities and pastimes, and the associated symptoms must not be of sufficient severity to meet the criteria for major depression. A duration of one year is required for children and two years for adults, during which time the symptoms must either be sustained or intermittent. The disorder may begin at any age, often without a clear onset. Patients meeting *DSM-III-R* criteria for dysthymia have frequently been diagnosed as having a neurotic depression, depressive personality, or characterologic depression. Symptom levels fluctuate, and may range from moderate to severe, allowing patients to maintain some degree of occupational, family, and community roles. However, their emotional distress often has an impact on families, co-workers, and friends, with serious impairment in social functioning being commonly observed (Klerman, 1980).

Diagnosis for *DSM-III-R* dysthymia cannot be made if the patient has a major depressive episode within the first two years of the disorder, and the patient must have been in full remission from any previous episodes of major depression for at least six months prior to developing dysthymia. After the two-year duration for dysthymia has been met, major depressive episodes can be superimposed on the chronic condition.

Similar to the *DSM-III-R* classification of dysthymia are the RDC categories of chronic and intermittent depression and chronic minor depression of two years' duration.

Atypical Depression

In *DSM-III-R*, this is a residual category for individuals whose depressive symptoms do not meet the severity or duration of major depression or dysthymia.

There is considerable confusion about this diagnostic category, which appears to be used in at least three ways:

1. to refer to patients with depressive features, who do not meet the criteria of intensity of symptoms and/or duration and/or impairment; this use is similar to terms such as "sub-clinical" or "borderline" depression
2. to refer to the presence of mixed symptoms and clinical course
3. to refer to a specific constellation of signs and symptoms, often considered to be responsive to monoamine oxidase (MAO) inhibitors (Klerman et al, 1987)

It is this latter use that has the greatest clinical and research precedence and has led to the following working definition: "prominent symptoms of anxiety or hysteria; excessive sleep (hypersomnia); excessive eating (hyperphagia, bulimia); and mood responsiveness (the patient may be temporarily cheered by pleasant environmental stimuli)" (Lehmann, 1985, p. 796).

An historical account of the use of the term atypical depression is given by Dr. Prien in Chapter 10. This review is consistent with what is described above, but is more detailed and focused on the utility of this category for differential therapeutics. Prien considers atypical depression as essentially synonymous with nonendogenous depression and suggests that either MAOI or TCA are indicated, unless panic attacks, anxiety, or hysteroid dysphoria are prominent, in which case MAOI should be given primary consideration.

CLASSIFICATION OF UNIPOLAR ILLNESS

Whether depression is a single disease that varies from mild to severe along a continuum or whether it represents subtypes that differ in phenomenology, pathophysiology, and etiology has been a longstanding topic of debate among clinicians and researchers (Eysenck, 1970; Kendell, 1976). However, there is now strong agreement that major depression is a very heterogeneous condition or group of conditions. Subtyping depression in order to reduce this heterogeneity would be of assistance in making more accurate predictions about prognosis and likely response to treatment.

Clinical experience and research has led to a variety of systems for subclassifying major depression. However, efforts to validate subtypes of major depressive disorder have made only minimal contributions to our power to predict familial background, the presence of precipitating factors, course and outcome, laboratory findings, or response to treatment. Despite this lack of "scientific" success in validating these subtypes, many of them remain in widespread clinical use and researchers continue to make vigorous efforts at validation. This section discusses the most commonly used subtypes of unipolar depression and what is known to date about the value of delineating them as separate entities.

Primary/Secondary Distinction

Robins and Guze (1972) proposed the primary/secondary distinction based on chronology of illness onset which was agnostic to etiology. A primary depression is defined as one that has not been preceded by and is not associated with any other nonaffective psychiatric disorder. "Complicated" depression (Grove et al, 1986, unpublished manuscript) refers to depressive disorders in patients whose first psychiatric disturbance was a major depression that was followed by a nonaffective psychiatric disorder, that was later followed by another major depressive episode.

Research indicates that the primary/secondary distinction has some value for unipolar depression, but that bipolar I and bipolar II disorders cannot be usefully subdivided into primary and secondary groups (Grove et al, 1986, unpublished manuscript).

Psychomotor retardation is the only depressive symptom that has been found to be more common in primary depression (Brim et al, 1984). It has been reported that secondary depressives experience an earlier onset of depressive symptoms and describe the depression as a worsening of the baseline state rather than as a distinctly different condition (Weissman et al, 1977; Clayton, 1983). Secondary patients more often attempt suicide and make more suicide attempts per patient (Reveley and Reveley, 1981). Data showing some differential value in predicting time to recovery and time to relapse from the major depressive episode, based on the primary/secondary distinction, will be discussed in the section entitled "Course and Outcome."

Overall, data have given only moderate support to the primary/secondary or the "complicated" subtype of unipolar depression as relatively pure diagnostic groups. There appears to be value for treatment planning in recognizing the nonaffective syndrome, but it is as yet questionable as to whether these subtypes represent different disease entities.

Endogenous Depression

The concept of an endogenous subtype has a long history in psychiatry (Kendell, 1976) with many different meanings (Klerman, 1980; Young et al, 1986). Depressions precipitated by biological factors rather than stress, and depressions that are not responsive to the environment but that are responsive to somatotherapy, are a few of the conceptual definitions differentiating between endogenous and nonendogenous depressions (Young et al, 1986). In keeping with its atheoretical philosophy, *DSM-III-R* uses the term "melancholia" to remove any presumption of etiology from the diagnosis of "endogenous depression."

The *DSM-III-R* criteria for specifying the melancholic subtype of major depression require five of the following symptoms: 1) loss of interest or pleasure in all or almost all activities; 2) lack of reactivity to usually pleasurable events; 3) mood worse in the morning; 4) terminal insomnia; 5) psychomotor agitation or retardation; 6) significant weight loss; 7) no significant personality disturbance prior to first major depressive episode; 8) one or more prior episodes of major depression followed by complete or nearly complete recovery; and 9) prior good response to somatic antidepressant therapy (American Psychiatric Association, p.224).

As is described by Drs. Goldin and Gershon in Chapter 7, family studies using the *DSM-III* criteria for melancholia or the RDC criteria for endogenous depression have provided inconsistent evidence for increased familial aggregation of depression among relatives of patients diagnosed with melancholia or endogenous depression (Andreasen et al, 1986; Leckman et al, 1984). These findings are surprising in view of the assumption made by most psychiatrists that, among all the subtypes of depression, patients with melancholia or endogenous depression would be most likely to show a "constitutional" basis with a genetic/familial pattern of transmission (Klerman et al, 1987). In addition, as will be discussed further in the section, "Course and Outcome," there is minimal difference in time to recovery and relapse when comparing patients with endogenous and nonendogenous depressions. Differential treatment response is discussed in detail in Chapter 10, on somatic treatment, by Dr. Prien. Here, the weight of evidence is that the melancholic/endogenous depressions do respond particularly well to tricyclic antidepressants (TCAs) or to electroconvulsive therapy (ECT); and, although TCAs will also often be effective in nonendogenous depression, the monoamine oxidase inhibitors (MAOIs) may be more effective in those states, especially if anxiety features are prominent. However, as explained in Chapter 10, the presence of panic attacks in patients with an endogenous depression makes it likely that MAOIs will be effective. Therefore, the presence of anxiety, rather than endogenicity, may be the variable which leads to differential treatment response in depressed patients.

Research aimed at validating the endogenous or melancholic subtypes or similarly defined categories, such as an "endogenomorphic" subtype proposed by Klein (1974), Nelson and colleagues' (1980) criteria for endogenous depression, and the Newcastle endogenous criteria (Carney et al, 1965), have all met with only minimal success. However, the "endogenous" concept still retains enormous popularity, and in all likelihood will remain in widespread usage, with continued efforts being made at validation.

Situational Depression

The concept of depression occurring in reaction to environmental stress has also been endorsed by most psychiatrists. Depression and most other psychiatric disorders were deemed reactions in *The Diagnostic and Statistical Manual of Mental Disorders, First Edition (DSM-I)* (Hirschfeld, 1981). Although subsequent revisions of the *DSM* no longer maintain this distinction, it is still commonly accepted that depressions can be differentiated by the presence or absence of a precipitant, especially interpersonal loss (Hirschfeld et al, 1985).

Situational depression is not defined as a separate entity in *DSM-III-R*. However, in the RDC, situational depressions are stress-induced depressions that may or may not have symptomatology commonly associated with endogenous depression. Thus, a patient can be diagnosed simultaneously with endogenous and situational depression. This is different from the use of the term reactive depression, which means that associated endogenous symptoms cannot be present.

Hirschfeld (1981) has described differences between situational and nonsituational episodes of depression. They include measures of current symptomatology, with situational depressives having more suicidal ideas and behavior, more manic features, more current alcohol and drug abuse, more miscellaneous psychopathology, and higher levels of both subjective and overt anger and self-pity. In addition, situational depressives have a somewhat more severely depressed mood, although no significant differences emerge in impairment in functioning, level of psychopathology, or even differences in levels of psychosocial stress levels between situational and nonsituational depressives. Furthermore, although situational depressives do recover from their depressive episodes somewhat more quickly than nonsituational depressives, the two groups show similar overall recovery rates.

Despite the differences described above, there are insufficient data to warrant validation of the situational/nonsituational distinction. However, the popularity of the notion of a situational depression remains strong. This probably reflects a deeply held assumption that situational depressions are psychologically rather than biologically caused. For these reasons it appears likely that this term will be used for quite some time, regardless of the lack of empirical data to support its validity. Although this will be discussed further in Chapter 10, it is strongly recommended here that the distinction of premorbid stressors not be used to assign treatment, since research indicates good response to somatotherapy in a high proportion of patients with situational depression (Tyrer et al, 1980).

Psychotic Depression

Klerman and colleagues (1987) have reviewed the different applications of the concept of psychotic depression. Criteria for psychotic depression relying exclusively on cross-sectional psychopathology have most commonly been based on the presence or absence of delusions, hallucinations, and confusion. The psychoanalytic view (Fenichel, 1945) has defined psychosis on the basis of level of regression and impairment of ego functions. More biologically oriented clinicians and researchers have used the term "psychotic" synonymously with "endogenous" to imply a biological etiology. Finally, many American clinicians typically have used the term "psychotic" to mean "severely ill" because they have equated psychotic depression with severe impairment. The RDC category of "incapacitating depression" attempts to separate the American notion of psychotic depression from depression with delusions and hallucinations (Klerman et al, 1987).

The *DSM-III-R* subcategory of major depression with psychotic features relies exclusively on evidence of the presence of delusions or hallucinations, either mood-congruent or mood-incongruent.

There now appears to be agreement that the hallmarks of psychotic depression are the presence of hallucinations, delusions, thought disorder, or grossly inappropriate behavior (Lehmann, 1985). The literature indicates that while depressed patients with mood-incongruent psychotic features should not as a group be included with schizophrenics, controversy exists as to whether patients with mood incongruent delusions should be classified separately (as schizoaffective-depressed) from patients with major depressive disorder who are psychotic (Brockington et al, 1980).

There are good data that outcome differences between psychotic and nonpsychotic depression vary over time (Coryell et al, 1984). Depressed patients with psychotic features have episodes that are more disabling, and they are slower to recover in the first six months after seeking treatment. However, the eventual likelihood of recovery is similar to that of patients with nonpsychotic depression (Coryell et al, 1984). Moreover, as mentioned by Goldin and Gershon, there does not appear to be an increased rate of psychosis in relatives of psychotically depressed probands compared to nonpsychotically depressed probands (Winokur et al, 1985).

As described in detail by Prien, there is evidence that the combination of an antidepressant and antipsychotic drug is the treatment of choice for psychotic depression with mood congruent delusions, and that ECT should be considered when patients do not respond to this combination.

Depressive Spectrum Disease

This approach to classifying unipolar depression was put forth in 1978 by Winokur and colleagues, who posited subtypes based on different familial constellations of illness. It is presented here because the approach of beginning with familial background is a departure from the traditional system of starting with symptom differences and then using familial aggregation as a validating variable.

The subtypes are familial pure depressive disease, sporadic depressive disease, and depressive spectrum disease. Familial pure depressive disease occurs when the family history shows only unipolar depression. Sporadic depressive disease occurs in families in which no other psychiatric disorder exists. Depressive spectrum disease occurs in families in which alcoholism, antisocial personality, and depression exist (Winokur, 1985).

Differences between the clinical profile and precipitating factors of these three groups exist. However, the largest differences occur in the areas of personal problems, personality, and course of illness (van Valkenburg et al, 1977; Klerman, 1980). Depressive spectrum disease patients are more likely to recover completely than are pure depressive disease patients; are less likely to experience loss of interest in usual activities; and are more likely to have a history of sexual problems, divorce, or separation (van Valkenburg et al, 1977; Klerman, 1980). Furthermore, depressive spectrum disease patients are commonly described as irritable, and to have a history of prior episodes of depression.

As with the preceding subtypes, the concept of depressive spectrum disease has some utility but still awaits further validation.

DIFFERENTIAL DIAGNOSIS

There are a number of conditions that create problems in the differential diagnosis of major depression. These include: schizoaffective disorder, bipolar disorder (particularly bipolar II disorder), personality disorders, and uncomplicated grief. In addition, dementia, adjustment disorder with depressed mood, and masked depression must be considered when diagnosing major depression.

Schizoaffective Disorder

The term schizoaffective was introduced by Kasanin in 1933. In the 1950s, schizoaffective disorder appeared in the United States and international nomenclatures, and has since been a source of controversy as to whether it is a form of affective disorder, a variant of schizophrenia, or an independent disorder (Klerman, 1980).

In DSM-III-R, schizoaffective disorder is labeled as Psychotic Disorder not Elsewhere Classified. Criteria for schizoaffective-depressive disorder include the concurrent existence of symptoms of schizophrenia and a major depressive episode (with no history of mania); the presence of delusions or hallucinations in the absence of affective symptoms for at least two weeks; and the absence of a diagnosis of schizophrenia or organic mental disorder.

Despite many variations in the definition of this condition, the literature consistently shows (with a few exceptions) that in comparison to patients with depression, schizoaffective-depressed patients have a poorer outcome and a higher morbid risk for schizophrenia among relatives; and in comparison to schizophrenics, schizoaffectives have a better outcome and a higher morbid risk for affective disorder among relatives (Coryell et al, 1984).

In summary, current knowledge suggests that there is prognostic, clinical, and research value in differentiating schizoaffective-depression from major depression, with and without psychosis. However, these distinctions may not be as valid when considering bipolar disorder and schizoaffective-mania.

Bipolar Disorder

There is particular interest in trying to clarify the relationship of bipolar II disorder to bipolar I disorder and to recurrent unipolar disorder. Although current knowledge is not conclusive, data have emerged recently on prior course, characteristics of the index episode, diagnostic stability, and familial aggregation of patients with bipolar II disorder that support separating bipolar II disorder from patients with bipolar I disorder and those with recurrent unipolar disorder. Despite these data, many investigators still hold the viewpoint that the relationship between recurrent unipolar depression and bipolar disorder is not yet resolved.

Research on genetic and family studies suggesting a continuum among bipolar, unipolar, and schizoaffective disorders has been reported by Gershon and colleagues (1982). In contrast, there is evidence from Winokur (1984) that does not support the concept of a continuum of multifactorial vulnerability. This fundamental question is currently unresolved, and is discussed by Drs. Goldin and Gershon in Chapter 7.

In terms of clinical practice and research, the marked differences in the phenomenology, demographics, and course of depressed patients with and without mania or hypomania seem to warrant maintaining the bipolar I, bipolar II, and recurrent unipolar distinction.

Personality

The differential diagnosis of unipolar illness (in the form of dysthymia) and a variety of personality disturbances is a considerable problem. There is a body of opinion that most chronic, early onset, low-grade depressions should be thought of as personality or character disorders, and an equally strong opinion that such conditions more likely represent "subsyndromal" primary affective disorders.

Patients with dysthymia are often considered to have "characterologic depressions" because of the early age of onset of this disorder and/or the enduring quality of their problems with self-esteem, guilt, and poor interpersonal relations. In most instances, it is the theoretical orientation of the researcher or the clinician that will determine the extent to which chronic low-grade depression is viewed as either a subsyndromal affective disorder or as a personality disorder. Although empirical data do not support definitively either dichotomy, the reader is referred to a recent article by Keller and colleagues (1987) for a more in-depth discussion of this issue.

Approximately 40 percent of patients who meet the criteria for *DSM-III* major depression also have an Axis II diagnosis (Shea, 1983). *DSM-III-R* addresses this issue by encouraging simultaneous diagnoses of Axis I and Axis II disorders. Dependent, avoidant, borderline, or narcissistic personality disorders are the most common Axis II diagnoses made in conjunction with major depression. The relationship between personality factors and depressions other than dysthymia will be considered in the section entitled, "Personality Factors Related to Unipolar Depression."

Uncomplicated Grief

Uncomplicated grief is differentiated from major depression even when it is associated with the full depressive syndrome. However, if the grief reaction is unduly severe or prolonged, the diagnosis can be changed to major depression (American Psychiatric Association, 1980). This determination is usually the subjective judgment of the clinician.

Researchers have used different criteria for the diagnosis of uncomplicated bereavement. Weissman and Myers (1978) suggest that a normal grief reaction begins within three months of the death of a close relative and can last up to one year (Clayton, 1982). In the Schedule for Affective Disorders and Schizophrenia (SADS), an uncomplicated bereavement is diagnosed if the depressive syndrome does not last for more than six months, no suicide attempt was made, hospitalization was not required, and marked retardation, morbid preoccupation with guilt or self-worth, and excessive suicidal ideation were not present.

Most people recover from uncomplicated grief (Clayton, 1982); and although they often seek medical attention and may be in great distress, most societies do not regard the grieving person as having an illness, which is consistent with the *DSM-III-R* category of "complicated grief" (Klerman et al, 1987).

Other Differential Diagnoses of Unipolar Illness

ADJUSTMENT DISORDER WITH DEPRESSED MOOD. Adjustment disorder with depressed mood is used to describe "patients who, following some life event, have a degree of depressed mood that exceeds the limits of normal in terms of either subjective distress or role dysfunction, but who do not meet the full syndromal criteria of a major depression" (Glass, 1985, p. 1126). The ascertainment of precipitants is necessary to make this diagnosis, which Hirschfeld and colleagues (1985) note to be an extremely common disorder in outpatient settings in both psychiatry and primary care (Glass, 1985).

MASKED DEPRESSION. Large numbers of patients seen in general hospitals and outpatient clinics with recurrent diagnosed medical complaints who are called hypochondriacs or crocks, often have unrecognized intermittent or chronic depressions. Over time, this population has come to use their bodily complaints as a means of gaining entrance to the health care system (Klerman, 1980). They are usually middle-aged and elderly patients, although Carlson and Cantwell (1980) have reported the presence of masked depression in children.

The diagnosis of masked depression is common in the United States, and masked depressions have been found to represent 10 percent of all depressive conditions in Europe based on a survey of European general practitioners (Lehmann, 1985).

DEMENTIA. The presence of disorientation, apathy, difficulty concentrating, and memory loss may make it difficult to distinguish either primary degenerative or multi-infarct dementia from major depression in the elderly. This differential diagnosis is mentioned here because of the very high prevalence of depression secondary to dementia. Further discussion appears in Chapter 12.

COMORBIDITY OF UNIPOLAR DEPRESSION WITH OTHER NONAFFECTIVE PSYCHIATRIC DISORDERS

It has long been observed that patients who are depressed also suffer from a variety of nondepressive symptoms. Until 5 to 10 years ago, there was a very strong tendency to consider the coexistence or "comorbidity" of the "other" symptoms as depressive equivalents or nonaffective manifestations of depression, which were in some way related to the depressive disorder. In particular, the RDC was heavily weighted in the direction of having the depressive syndromes subsume other coexisting disorders such as the various anxiety states.

Data from family and genetic studies, a more active neo-Kraepelian adherence to descriptive phenomenology, and the search for specific somatic and psychosocial treatments has led many teams of investigators to reconsider the relationship between depression and other coexisting syndromes. The term "comorbidity" implies that the concurrent presence of symptoms of affective and nonaffective syndromes may mean that two separate disorders are present.

Alcoholism

From 33 to 59 percent of alcoholics in treatment have a clinical depression (Cadoret, 1981), and there is a high incidence of suicidal behavior associated with both affective disorder and alcoholism (Schuckit, 1979). Moreover, family studies have demonstrated a high incidence of alcoholism in families of patients with affective disorder (Taylor et al, 1974), and a high incidence of affective disorder in the families of alcoholics (Schuckit, 1983).

Several investigators have suggested that a depressed premorbid personality type leads to alcoholism, whereby the individual tries to self-medicate the depressive symptomatology with alcohol (Tahka, 1966). With this supposition, it seems that the course of alcoholism may be secondary to the course of depressive symptoms and episodes (Clark et al, 1985). The contrasting view is that the depressive symptoms of alcoholics are attributed to the chronic intoxication, physical withdrawal symptoms, or the lifestyle of the alcoholic (Kielholz, 1969; Schuckit, 1983; Clark et al, 1985).

In summary, although there is a high rate of comorbidity of alcoholism and depression, the etiologic relationship of these disorders is unknown, and their transmission seems to be independent of each other genetically. However, the presence of one of these disorders does predispose individuals to the other; and, they appear to have an additive or even synergetic effect in worsening outcome. Therefore, clinicians need to search carefully for a history of both alcoholism and depression when an individual presents with either condition, and should be prepared to institute treatment targeted at each disorder.

Eating Disorders

There is substantial evidence suggesting a link between eating disorders and affective illness. Depressive symptoms and syndromes are common in patients diagnosed as having bulimia and anorexia nervosa. Johnson and colleagues (1982) found that 62 percent of *DSM-III* bulimic women described themselves as either often or always depressed, and Hudson and associates (1983) found that 60 percent of their bulimic subjects had a lifetime diagnosis of major depression. Similarly, a number of studies have reported that from 33 to 56 percent of anorexic patients are also currently diagnosed as having a depressive syndrome (Herzog, 1984).

The fact that numerous neuroendocrine abnormalities, common to depressed patients, have been noted in anorexic and bulimic patients (Gwirtsman and Gerner, 1981; Hudson et al, 1983; Biederman et al, 1984) and the fact that antidepressants are the most frequently used psychotropic agents in the treatment of eating disorders in the United States, has added to the thinking that there may be similarities in the underlying physiology and phenomenology of these disorders (Herzog and Copeland, 1985).

Herzog and colleagues (in press) have demonstrated the highly pernicious effect on the depression of the comorbidity of bulimia and depression. They found a 24 percent rate of recovery from depression in patients with an underlying bulimia after 6 months. This is compared to a 62 percent rate of recovery by 6 months in patients with a major depressive disorder without an eating disorder.

Despite the high rate of coexisting symptoms and syndromes in patients with eating disorders and depression and the similarity of neuroendocrine abnormalities, familial association, and treatment response, the nature of the association among these conditions remains an area of controversy and is the subject of active interest on the part of researchers and clinicians. Clinicians should look carefully for depression in patients with an eating disorder, and be aware of the pernicious course of patients in whom these syndromes exist.

Anxiety

The considerable overlap between anxiety and depressive syndromes, drug efficacy research, and family/genetic studies have contributed to the belief that there is a strong association between anxiety states and depression (Breier et al, 1985). Therefore, clinicians often do not know whether a patient should be classified as suffering from "depression with secondary anxiety" or as "anxiety with associated depression." There has been a tradition, especially in the United States, of including anxiety states within the affective disorders and for creating a single continuum from anxiety to depression. Although many patients with depression are also anxious and many anxious patients suffer depressive symptoms, in the past few years evidence has become available that certain types of anxiety states and depressive syndromes should be thought of as separate disorders, even when they occur at the same time.

The temporal occurrence of generalized anxiety disorder, panic disorder, and depression over an individual's life indicates that they probably are not symptomatic variants of one disorder. In addition, specific symptoms have been identified as distinguishing features between depression and anxiety. Depressed mood, early awakening, suicidal ideation, and psychomotor retardation are more characteristic of depressed patients (Gurney et al, 1972; Mountjoy and Roth, 1982), while panic attacks, agoraphobia, and compulsive features best characterize patients with anxiety disorder (Breier et al, 1985). Evidence is now accumulating that panic disorder, but not generalized anxiety, can be separated from major depression on the basis of symptoms and signs (Gurney et al, 1972; Mountjoy and Roth, 1982; Breier et al, 1985).

In summary, the available data support the existence of anxiety (and panic attacks in particular) and depression as two distinct groups of illnesses.

RELIABILITY AND STABILITY OF DIAGNOSIS

When experienced clinicians are well versed in diagnostic criteria, the reliability of diagnosing major depression has been shown to be very good based on a series of interrater and test-retest reliability studies (Andreasen et al, 1981; Mazure et al, 1986).

Between 10 and 15 percent of unipolar patients will have subsequent episodes that will involve manic or hypomanic symptoms, at which point they should be reclassified as having a bipolar disorder. This occurs less frequently as patients become older and have an increased number of depressive episodes (Perris, 1966; Angst, 1973; Grof et al, 1973; Clayton, 1981; Keller, 1985). Additional factors that predict which unipolar patients are most likely to develop a bipolar disorder include: a previous history of mild hypomanic swings, a family history of bipolar illness in first-degree relatives, and a hypomanic response to tricyclic and MAO medication (Akiskal, 1981; Klerman et al, 1987). The size of the risk of developing bipolar disorder in response to medication is not known because it is difficult to separate the effect of the medication from the inherent tendency of patients with unipolar depression to develop hypomania or mania (Keller et al, 1986). Patients who only evince manic or hypomanic disorder after the use of antidepressant medication have been classified as having bipolar II disorder by Klerman (1981).

NATURAL COURSE OF UNIPOLAR ILLNESS

In the past 5 to 10 years clinicians and researchers have become increasingly aware that although most patients recover from episodes of major depression, a substantial proportion do not, and enter a chronic course. This awareness, combined with recent methodologic research advances to describe, classify, and treat patients with major depression, has led to extensive work describing the natural course of this disorder.

In order to understand properly the data available on longitudinal course, it is necessary to recognize that essentially all of the prospective studies' published rates of recovery, recurrence, chronicity, and predictors of outcomes were gleaned from patients who sought treatment at university medical centers. These data are not necessarily generalizable to the entire population of depressed patients since a substantial proportion of people have depressive episodes which remit spontaneously and for which they never seek treatment, or for which they are treated in nonmedical or nonpsychiatric settings. In addition, much of the information available on course has been collected in naturalistic studies in which the patients' treatment was not under the control of investigators. These studies do report that a high proportion of depressive patients received either minimal or no somatic treatment in the community and after they seek treatment at university medical centers (Keller et al, 1982a; Keller et al, 1986).

Recovery

TIME TO RECOVER. Eighty to 90 percent of patients with an episode of major depression recover within 5 years. Of the 10 to 20 percent of patients with episodes of major depression who go on to have a course marked by long-term chronicity, it has been found that the likelihood of recovery decreases substantially the longer they remain depressed after initially seeking treatment or after they first enter into clinical research studies. For example, data from the NIMH Collaborative Depression Study (Katz and Klerman, 1979), show that, after 6 months of follow-up, 65 percent of the patients are likely to recover; after 12 months, 76 percent are likely to recover; after 18 months, 78 percent are likely to recover (Keller et al, 1982b); by 24 months only 79 percent are likely to recover (Keller et al, 1982b); and by 5 years, the cumulative probability of recovery is 90 percent (Keller and Lavori, unpublished data). Expressed in terms of interval-specific probabilities of recovery: 64 percent of patients will recover after 6 months; of those not recovered by 6 months, 28 percent can be expected to recover within the next 6 months; of those not recovered by 1 year, 15 percent will recover in the next 6 months; and if not recovered by 18 months, only 10 percent will recover in the following 6 months.

PREDICTORS OF RECOVERY. The acuteness of onset and severity of major depressive disorder in patients without an underlying dysthymia are highly significant predictors of recovery (Keller et al, 1982b). Protracted illness prior to seeking treatment has been found to be the most powerful predictor of a slow time to recovery and a higher rate of chronicity (Keller et al, 1982b). The primary/secondary distinction also has predictive value for the course of unipolar depression. Keller and colleagues (1984) found that patients with secondary unipolar depression followed a more chronic course (23 percent rate of recovery) than patients with primary unipolar depression (90 percent rate of recovery) after 2 years of follow-up.

Relapse/Recurrence

TIME TO RELAPSE/RECURRENCE. Between 50 and 85 percent of patients with one major depressive episode who seek treatment at university medical centers will have at least one subsequent episode of depression in their lifetimes (Keller, 1985). It has been reported that the mean number of lifetime episodes in patients with unipolar depression is five to six (Angst, 1973; Grof et al, 1973).

The highest rate of relapse into an affective disorder occurs in the first few months after recovery from an episode of major depressive disorder, and the probability of relapse declines steadily during the course of the prospective follow-up. For example, the NIMH Collaborative Depression Study found that 40 percent of their unipolar depressed patients relapsed by 1 year, 54 percent by 2 years, 64 percent by 3 years, 70 percent by 4 years, and 76 percent by 5 years (unpublished data).

PREDICTORS OF RELAPSE/RECURRENCE. The best predictor of relapse is the number of previous affective episodes; Keller and colleagues (1982c) have found that three or more previous affective episodes predicted an increased rate of relapse. Of patients who are suffering from their first episode of depression, those who are older are more likely than those who are younger to relapse sooner, as are patients whose depression is secondary to a nonaffective psychiatric disorder (Keller et al, 1983b).

Well Interval

Although there are no published reports defining the average length of a well interval, data on relapse rates indicate that patients with three or more prior episodes of depression have higher relapse rates and shorter well intervals (Keller et al, 1983). Furthermore, it is now commonly observed that a high proportion of patients have some residual symptoms and psychosocial impairment in the intervals between episodes, which is a departure from Kraepelin's writings that most patients returned to their "premorbid" level of functioning after recovery.

Chronicity

It has been reported that between 10 and 20 percent of all patients diagnosed as having a major depression will have a chronic course (Robins and Guze, 1972; Murphy, 1974). The NIMH Collaborative Depression Study found that 19 percent of nonbipolar depressed patients remained chronically depressed after 2 years of follow-up and that 10 percent were still chronically ill after 5 years (unpublished data).

Suicide and Mortality

Although an entire section of this volume is devoted to suicide, it is important to mention that suicides and accidents account for almost all excess mortality in unipolar illness (Tsuang and Woolson, 1978). This phenomenon is primarily manifest within the first decade of follow-up, and the lifetime rate of suicide has been reported to stabilize at approximately 15 percent across a large number of studies (Guze and Robins, 1970).

Dysthymia

RECOVERY. Several studies have found significant differences in the recovery rates of patients with low-grade chronic versus major depressive disorders. Gonzales and colleagues (1985) found a 43 percent recovery rate for intermittent depressives compared to a 75 percent rate for patients with a major depression; and Barrett (1984) found a 37 percent rate of improvement among chronic depressives compared to a 72 percent rate for patients with a major depression, based on self-reports at 2 years.

RELAPSE. Gonzales and colleagues (1985) found a one-year relapse rate of 33 percent for chronic and intermittent depressed patients compared to a 31 percent relapse rate for patients with a major depression.

CHRONICITY. Rounsaville and associates (1980) found an average duration of chronic and intermittent depression of 5.5 years with a range of from 2 to 20 years among chronically ill depressed outpatients. Keller and Shapiro (1982) report similar findings.

Double Depression

The term double depression refers to the clinical state wherein a major depressive episode is superimposed on a dysthymic disorder that preceded the onset of the major depression by at least two years (Keller and Shapiro, 1982).

RECOVERY. The two-year recovery rates from major depression in patients with a double depression are significantly higher (97 percent) than the recovery rates from major depression alone (79 percent) in patients without an underlying chronic disorder. This does not mean that patients with a double depression become healthier than those with a major depression alone; rather, it is easier to return to a state of chronic or intermittent minor depression than to a usual self characterized by no depression at all (Keller and Shapiro, 1982).

RELAPSE. Patients with a double depression who recover from the major depression have a significantly shorter time before relapse than patients without an underlying dysthymic disorder. In addition, patients with a double depression have a significantly faster cycle time for their major depression over a period of two years (Keller, 1985).

CHRONICITY. In patients with a double depression, the longer the patient remains chronically ill after recovering from the major depression, the greater the likelihood that relapse will preempt complete recovery from both the major depression and the chronic depression. Keller and colleagues (1983) report that after six months, almost all patients with a double depression will relapse into an episode of major affective disorder before they recover from their chronic depression.

Nosologic Subtypes of Major Depression as Predictors of Clinical Course

Several investigators have described the predictive value of nosologic subtypes to the clinical course of major depression.

Coryell and associates (1984) report clear trends showing a faster time to recovery for patients with psychotic depression after six months of follow-up. However, they found that the recovery rates for psychotic and nonpsychotic patients tend to resemble each other after two years of follow-up.

Keller and colleagues (1982a) found that secondary major depression (particularly depression secondary to alcoholism) predicted a more chronic course than primary depression after one year of follow-up.

Data on the endogenous/nonendogenous distinction are conflicting. Several researchers report that patients with endogenous depression have a better course (Kay et al, 1969; Paykel et al, 1974), while others indicate that patients with endogenous depression show a poorer outcome (Endicott and Spitzer, 1979).

Results from the NIMH Collaborative Depression Study (unpublished data) indicate that the situational subtype of major depression has little predictive validity for describing clinical course.

PERSONALITY FACTORS RELATED TO UNIPOLAR ILLNESS

The relationship between personality and depression has mainly been postulated in four different ways (Akiskal et al, 1983). First, there may be personality features that predispose an individual to depression. In their review of the literature, Akiskal and associates (1983) conclude that although a constellation of personality attributes are commonly cited as predisposing factors, only introversion in unipolar patients can be implicated as a predisposing characterologic trait for depressive illness based on research done to date.

Second, it has been hypothesized that certain personality features influence the course of unipolar depression. Examples of this include studies which showed that high neuroticism scores in depressed patients correlated with poor outcome (King, 1977), "unstable" characterologic traits were the strongest predictor of unfavorable social outcome in affective disorders (Akiskal et al, 1978) and that particular personality traits affect the expression of depressive symptomatology in hospitalized depressed women (Lazare and Klerman, 1968). Third, it has been suggested that enduring personality features represent attenuated expressions of affective illness. Historically, this concept was posed by the works of Kraepelin (1921), Schneider (1958), and Kretschmer (1936); and current data support the notion that cyclothymic, hyperthymic and, to a degree, dysthymic personalities represent attenuated forms of major affective disorders (Akiskal et al, 1983).

Finally, it has been posited that postdepressive personality characteristics exist, and "it is conceivable that these disturbances represent accentuation of premorbid traits, or the incorporation of episode-related affective experiences into the interepisodic phase of the illness" (Akiskal et al, 1983, p. 805).

Although these theories are of great interest, research has not yet been able to validate these alternatives, largely because validation requires premorbid personality assessments that have not been biased by retrospective reports.

UNIPOLAR ILLNESS IN CHILDREN AND ADOLESCENTS

In the past decade, there has been renewed interest in childhood depression. Most of the methodologic advances that were developed by researchers working with adults are now being used by investigators studying affective disorders in children.

Clinical Profile

According to *DSM-III-R*, the essential features of a major depressive episode are similar in infants, children, adolescents, and adults, but there are differences in the associated features. In prepubertal children separation anxiety may develop, causing the child to cling to parents. In adolescent boys, negativistic or antisocial behavior is common.

Other associated features similar to those found in depressed adults have been observed in depressed children and adolescents (McConville and Bruce, 1985). Low self-esteem, social withdrawal, poor peer relations, and impaired schoolwork are common. Fantasy material is frequently reduced (McConville and Bruce, 1985). In addition, initial sleep disturbances are more common than middle or terminal disturbances, differing from depressed adults, for whom early morning awakening is the most typical form of sleep disturbance (McConville and Bruce, 1985).

The *DSM-III-R* criteria for diagnosis of dysthymia is the same for adults, children, and adolescents, with the exception that the disorder must last for at least one year, compared to two, in children and adolescents. Kovacs (1985) found that the course of dysthymia in childhood is similar to that in adults, and also that episodes of superimposed major depression (double depression) were diagnosed in at least 70 percent of her depressed cohort within a five-year follow-up.

Differential Diagnosis with Other Affective and Nonaffective Disorders

ANXIETY, ATTENTION/CONDUCT DISORDERS, SUBSTANCE ABUSE. An ongoing project at the Massachusetts General Hospital has found that 53 percent of the children with a diagnosis of major depression also had a history of at least one other major childhood disorder [such as panic/anxiety disorders (8 percent), attention/conduct disorders (18 percent)—or substance use (5 percent)—unpublished data]. Kovacs and colleagues (1984) found that 33 percent of their depressed cohort had a concurrent diagnosis of anxiety disorder; Puig-Antich and associates (1978) reported similar findings. Thirty-two percent of the depressed children in Carlson's and Cantwell's (1980) study met *DSM-III* criteria for conduct or attention deficit disorder; and Puig-Antich (1982) found that 37 percent of his prepubertal boys with major depression had a diagnosable conduct disorder.

BIPOLAR DISORDER. In a 3- to 4-year prospective follow-up, 20 percent of the adolescents diagnosed with primary major depression developed manic episodes and had to be rediagnosed with bipolar disorder (Strober, 1985). Rapid episode onset, psychosis and psychomotor retardation, and increased familial loading and multigenerational transmission of affective illness were the best predictors of bipolar outcome (Strober, 1985). Akiskal and colleagues (1983) report similar predictors of outcome.

ADJUSTMENT DISORDER WITH DEPRESSED MOOD. Adjustment disorder with depressed mood can be diagnosed in children before puberty with high reliability (Kovacs, 1985). Its prognosis is much better than dysthymia or major depressive disorder; children with adjustment disorder with depressed mood are less likely to have recurrences, have shorter episodes, and have a low likelihood of developing dysthymia or major depressive disorder (Kovacs, 1985; Klerman et al, 1987).

Course

Long-term prospective follow-up studies of large groups of depressed children have not yet been done. However, similar to the course of affective illness in adults, the available evidence suggests that depression developing in adolescence often has a severe and chronic course, and that a high proportion of those who recover have symptoms and impaired psychosocial functioning in the intervals between episodes.

RECOVERY. Current evidence suggests that episodes of major depression in children last about 7½ months (Kovacs, 1985; Strober, 1985), and the younger the child when he or she first manifests a major depression, the more prolonged the episode will be (Kovacs, 1985). Rates of recovery of between 86 percent by 3 years (Strober, 1985) and 92 percent by 18 months (Kovacs, 1985) closely parallel the rates reported for adult major depressives by Keller and colleagues

(1982b), and document the slow rates of recovery and the substantial proportion of children who go on to have a chronic course.

RECURRENCE/RELAPSE. The diagnosis of major depressive disorder in childhood is associated with a high risk of relapse. Within 5 years after the onset of the first episode, there is a 72 percent probability of a second episode of major depression (Kovacs, 1985). The presence of an underlying dysthymic disorder has been found to increase the risk for a recurrent major depression (Kovacs et al, 1984).

SUICIDE. In the last three decades, there has been a dramatic increase in the rate of suicide in children and adolescents and it is the third leading cause of death among adolescents and young adults (Monthly Vital Statistics Report of the National Center for Health Statistics, 1985). The relationship between childhood depression and suicide attempts will not be presented here; however, the reader is referred to in Chapter 17, in the section on suicide, in this volume.

Conclusion

The emerging data on childhood depression reveal that unipolar disorder occurs with a greater frequency than previously believed. Although significant strides have been made to describe the presentation, severity, and course of depression in children and adolescents, further research is needed. The application of the recent research advances made by investigators of adult depression to studies of child and adolescent depression will advance this important area of research.

SUMMARY

Although etiological evidence is not yet available, there are substantial family, neurophysiological, biochemical, and clinical data to support the distinction between unipolar and bipolar disorder as proposed by Leonhard in 1962. Of particular relevance for clinical practice are the differences that have been reported in prognosis, response to treatment, and familial aggregation. Similarly, most research on affective disorder, be it biological or clinical, also requires that subjects be classified as unipolar or bipolar.

Unipolar depression, as is true of mania or hypomania, is often secondary to medical illness, and the presence of depression should always lead the clinician to search for an organic etiology, as is discussed in detail in Chapter 12.

Depression that does not have an organic etiology is a highly prevalent condition which encompasses an extremely broad.range of disorders with substantial heterogeneity in terms of clinical profile, course, familial aggregation, response to treatment, and neurophysiological and biological correlates. Depression sufficient to meet *DSM-III-R* criteria ranges from states of mild to moderate severity with little impairment in functioning, to episodes in which there is psychosis and extreme inability to function. The course of depression may be brief without recurrence, may be chronic lasting for many years, or may have a course marked by brief episodes with frequent recurrences.

It is presumed that there are multiple, diverse etiologies for episodes of unipolar depression. These may include: external precipitants (such as loss of one's job or becoming physically ill, which would disturb most people regardless of their intrapsychic functioning or genetic vulnerability); depressive states with no clear-cut situational triggers, which seem to be primarily psychological in origin (probably secondary to trauma and deficiencies in childhood or adolescent psychosexual or cognitive development) and a wide variety of physiological and biochemical abnormalities that are primarily genetic in origin. Understanding the etiology of depressive disorders remains a major quest for psychiatry and is beyond the realm of this chapter.

The focus of this chapter has been on describing the classification, differential diagnosis, comorbidity, and course of the widest possible spectrum of depressive disorders, without regard to etiology. In order to make this material meaningful for clinical practice and research, the approach has been to emphasize the heterogeneity of depression by discussing the evidence available for different ways of subtyping depression, and by presenting data on course and outcome that include information on subtypes and comorbidity whenever possible.

The basic *DSM-III-R* structure of classifying depression on Axis I into major depressive episodes, less severe depression of at least two years' duration, and depressions which are "not otherwise specified" creates several very broad groups whose clinical and biological boundaries often merge together. Furthermore, it may well be that a common etiology could result in any of these different phenotypes. Recognition of this is necessary to prevent premature closure in diagnosis and the search for causality and more effective treatments.

Subtyping patients with major depression into dichotomies such as endogenous/nonendogenous, primary/secondary, situational/nonsituational, and psychotic/nonpsychotic has been a widespread practice for many years. Although several of these distinctions are very useful descriptively and have some value for prognosis and treatment planning, none of them has been validated as a distinct clinical entity. However, each of these approaches to categorization remains popular in clinical practice, and the search for validation remains an active target of research.

Despite the broad scope of disorders subsumed under the heading of major depression, research demonstrates that there is considerable value in careful efforts to make a differential diagnosis between major depression and a variety of other psychiatric disorders, including: schizoaffective depression, bipolar II disorder, uncomplicated grief, and many of the personality disorders that have depressive features. Each of these conditions is distinguished from major depression in the domains of phenomenology, course, familial aggregation, biologic correlates, or treatment response. Nonetheless, there is a reasonably high proportion of patients in whom these distinctions are extraordinarily difficult to make with precision, and some patients may truly be on the boundaries among several such conditions.

It has been observed for many years that depressed patients often also have a variety of other nonaffective symptoms, such as anxiety, alcoholism, or eating disorders. Common practice has been either to consider these conditions, particularly anxiety, as part of the depressive syndrome, or to see disorders such as alcoholism and eating disorders as "attempts to treat one's depression," or as manifestations of the underlying depressive disorder. There is evidence from genetic studies, longitudinal clinical research, and biologic findings that anxiety syndromes, substance abuse, and eating disorders may coexist with depression as separate syndromes. These disorders should usually be diagnosed separately and their presence conceptualized as the comorbidity of at least two different conditions.

Although 80 to 90 percent of patients with major depression do recover, a substantial proportion of them will have at least one subsequent episode, and many will have an average of 5 to 6 subsequent episodes. The complete recovery rates for patients with dysthymia are considerably lower than those for patients with major depression.

The acuteness of onset, severity of illness, number of prior episodes, and presence of an underlying chronic depression (double depression) are of prognostic importance when assessing the course of unipolar depression.

The relationship between personality and unipolar depression, particularly dysthymic disorder, is a controversial topic. Research cannot yet provide a definitive description of the association between depression and personality. Hypotheses about their association are as follows: premorbid personality features predispose an individual to depression; personality characteristics affect the course of unipolar depression; certain personality traits represent attenuated forms of depression; and postmorbid personality features appear following an episode of depression. Until researchers are able to assess "true" baseline personality measurements, the relationship between personality and depression will remain uncertain.

Although much less is known about the presentation and course of unipolar depression in children than in adults, the disorder is more prevalent in children and adolescents than once thought. The clinical features of childhood unipolar depression are similar to those of adult depression, and the emerging data on the natural course and differential diagnosis of the disorder in children parallel those found in adults.

REFERENCES

Akiskal HS: Subaffective disorders: dysthymic, cyclothymic, and bipolar II disorders in the "borderline" realm. Psychiatr Clin North Am 1981; 4:25-46

Akiskal HS, Bitar AH, Puzantian VR, et al: The nosological status of neurotic depression: a prospective three- to four-year follow-up examination in light of the primary–secondary and unipolar–bipolar dichotomies. Arch Gen Psychiatry 1978; 35:756-766

Akiskal HS, Hirschfeld RMA, Yerevanian BI: The relationship of personality to affective disorders: a critical review. Arch Gen Psychiatry 1983; 40:801-810

American Psychiatric Association: Diagnostic and Statistical Manual of Mental Disorders, Third Edition (DSM-III). Washington, DC, American Psychiatric Association, 1980

American Psychiatric Association: Diagnostic and Statistical Manual of Mental Disorders, Third Edition, Revised (DSM-III-R). Washington, DC, American Psychiatric Association, 1987

Andreasen NC, Grove WM, Shapiro RW, et al: Reliablity of lifetime diagnosis: a multicenter collaborative perspective. Arch Gen Psychiatry 1981; 38:400-405

Andreasen NC, Scheftner W, Reich T, et al: The validation of the concept of endogenous depression. Arch Gen Psychiatry 1986; 43:246-254

Angst J: The course of monopolar depression and bipolar psychoses. Psychiatrie, Neurologie et Neurochirurgie 1973; 76:489-500

Barrett JE: Naturalistic change after 2 years in neurotic depressive disorders (RDC categories). Compr Psychiatry 1984; 25:404-418

Biederman J, Rivinus TM, Herzog DB, et al: Platelet MAO activity in anorexia nervosa patients with and without a major depressive disorder. Am J Psychiatry 1984; 141:1244-1247

Breier A, Charney DS, Heninger GR: The diagnostic validity of anxiety disorders and their relationship to depressive illness. Am J Psychiatry 1985; 142:787-797

Brim J, Wetzel RD, Reich T, et al: Primary and secondary affective disorder, part III: longitudinal differences in depressive symptoms. J Clin Psychiatry 1984; 45:64-69

Brockington IF, Kendell RE, Wainwright S: Depressed patients with schizophrenic or paranoid symptoms. Psychol Med 1980; 10:665-675

Cadoret RJ: Depression and alcoholism, in Evaluation of the Alcoholic: Implications for Research, Theory, and Treatment. Research Monograph No. 5. Edited by Meyer RE, Glueck BC, O'Brien J, et al. Rockville, Maryland, National Institute on Alcohol Abuse and Alcoholism, 1981

Cancro R: Affective disorders, in Comprehensive Textbook of Psychiatry/IV, vol 1, fourth edition. Edited by Kaplan HI, Sadock BJ. Baltimore, Williams & Wilkins, 1985

Carlson GA, Cantwell DP: Unmasking masked depression in children and adolescents. Am J Psychiatry 1980; 137:445-449

Carney MWP, Roth M, Garside RF: The diagnosis of depressive syndromes and the prediction of ECT response. Br J Psychiatry 1965; 111:659-674

Clark DC, Gibbons RD, Fawcett J, et al: Unbiased criteria for severity of depression in alcoholic inpatients. J Nerv Ment Dis 1985; 173:482-487

Clayton PJ: The epidemiology of bipolar affective disorder. Compr Psychiatry 1981; 22:31-43

Clayton PJ: Bereavement, in Handbook of Affective Disorders. Edited by Paykel ES. New York, Guilford Press, 1982

Clayton PJ: A further look at secondary depression, in Treatment of Depression: Old Controversies and New Approaches. Edited by Clayton PJ, Barrett JE. New York, Raven Press, 1983

Coryell W, Lavori PW, Endicott J: Outcome in schizoaffective, psychotic and nonpsychotic depression: course over a six- to twenty-four month follow-up. Arch Gen Psychiatry 1984; 41:787-791

Endicott J, Spitzer RL: Use of research diagnostic criteria and the schedule for affective disorders and schizophrenia to study affective disorders. Am J Psychiatry 1979; 136:52-56

Eysenck HJ: The classification of depressive illnesses. Br J Psychiatry 1970; 117:241-250

Fenichel O: The Psychoanalytic Theory of Neurosis. New York, Norton, 1945

Gershon E, Hamovit J, Guroff J, et al: A family history of schizoaffective bipolar I, bipolar II, unipolar and normal control probands. Arch Gen Psychiatry 1982; 39:1157-1167

Glass RM: Situational and neurotic-reactive depression. Arch Gen Psychiatry 1985; 42:1126-1127

Gonzales LR, Lewinsohn PM, Clarke GM: Longitudinal follow-up of unipolar depressives: an investigation of predictors of relapse. J Consult Clin Psychol 1985; 53:461-469

Grof P, Angst J, Haines T: The clinical course of depression: practical issues, in Classification and Prediction of Outcome of Depression. Edited by Angst J, Stuttgart J. New York, FK Schattauer Verlag, 1973

Gurney C, Roth M, Garside RF, et al: Studies in the classification of affective disorders: the relationship between anxiety states and depressive illness. Br J Psychiatry 1972; 121:162-166

Guze SB, Robins E: Suicide and primary affective disorders. Br J Psychiatry 1970; 117:437-438

Gwirtsman HE, Gerner RH: Neurochemical abnormalities in anorexia nervosa: Similarities to affective disorders. Biol Psychiatry 1981; 16:991-995

Herzog DB: Are anorexic and bulimic patients depressed? Am J Psychiatry 1984; 141:1594-1597

Herzog DB, Copeland PM: Eating disorders. N Engl J Med 1985; 313:295-303

Herzog DB, Keller MB, Lavori PW, et al: Short term prospective study of recovery in bulimia. Psychiatry Res (in press)

Hirschfeld RMA: Situational depression: validity of the concept. Br J Psychiatry 1981; 139:297-305

Hirschfeld RMA, Klerman GL, Andreasen NC, et al: Situational major depression disorder. Arch Gen Psychiatry 1985; 42:1109-1114

Hudson JI, Pope HG, Jonas JM, et al: Phenomenologic relationship of eating disorders to major affective disorder. Psychiatry Res 1983; 9:345-354

Johnson CL, Stuckey MK, Lewis LD, et al: Bulimia: a descriptive survey of 316 cases. International Journal of Eating Disorders 1982; 2:3-16

Kasanin J: Acute schizo-affective psychoses. Am J Psychiatry 1933; 90:97-126

Katz MM, Klerman GL: Introduction: overview of the clinical studies program. Am J Psychiatry 1979; 136:49-51

Kay DWK, Garside RF, Roy JR, et al: Endogenous and neurotic syndromes of depression: a 5 to 7 year follow-up of 104 cases. Br J Psychiatry 1969; 115:389-399

Keller MB: Chronic and recurrent affective disorders: incidence, course, and influencing factors, in Chronic Treatments in Neuropsychiatry. Edited by Kemali D, Recagni G. New York, Raven Press, 1985

Keller MB, Shapiro RW: "Double depression": superimposition of acute depressive episodes on chronic depressive disorders. Am J Psychiatry 1982; 139:438-442

Keller MB, Klerman GL, Lavori PW, et al: Treatment received by depressed patients. JAMA 1982a; 248:1848-1855

Keller MB, Shapiro RW, Lavori PW, et al: Recovery in major depressive disorder. Arch Gen Psychiatry 1982b; 39:905-910

Keller MB, Shapiro RW, Lavori PW, et al: Relapse in major depressive disorder. Arch Gen Psychiatry 1982c; 39:911-915

Keller MB, Lavori PW, Endicott J, et al: "Double depression": two-year follow-up. Am J Psychiatry 1983a; 140:689-694

Keller MB, Lavori PW, Klerman GL: Predictors of relapse in major depressive disorder. JAMA 1983b; 250:3299-3304

Keller MB, Klerman GL, Lavori PW, et al: Long-term outcome of episodes of major depression. JAMA 1984; 252:788-797

Keller MB, Lavori PW, Coryell W, et al: Differential outcome of pure manic, mixed/cycling and pure depressive episodes in patients with bipolar illness. JAMA 1986; 255:3138-3142

Keller MB, Sessa FM, Jones LP: Chronic depressive disorders, in Handbook of Outpatient Treatment of Adults. Edited by Thase MA, Edelstein BA, Hersen M. New York, Plenum Press, 1987

Kendell RE: The classification of depression: a review of contemporary confusion. Br J Psychiatry 1976; 129:15-28

Kielholz P: Alcohol and depression. British Journal of the Addictions 1969; 65:187-193

King D: Pathological and therapeutic consequences of sleep loss: a review. Diseases of the Nervous System 1977; 38:873-879

Klein DF: Endogenomorphic depression: a conceptual and terminological revision. Arch Gen Psychiatry 1974; 341:447-454

Klerman GL: Affective disorders, in Comprehensive Textbook of Psychiatry/III, vol 2, third edition. Edited by Kaplan HI, Sadock BJ. Baltimore, Williams & Wilkins, 1980

Klerman GL: The spectrum of mania. Compr Psychiatry 1981; 22:11-20

Klerman GL, Keller MB, Fawcett JA, et al: Major depression and related affective disorders, in Diagnosis and Classification in Psychiatry: A Critical Appraisal of DSM-III. Edited by Tischler G. New York, Cambridge University Press, 1987

Kovacs M: The natural history and course of depressive disorders in childhood. Psychiatric Annals 1985; 15:387-389

Kovacs M, Feinberg TL, Crouse-Novak MA, et al: Depressive disorders in childhood, I: a longitudinal prospective study of characteristics and recovery. Arch Gen Psychiatry 1984; 41:229-237

Kraepelin E: Manic-depressive Illness. Edinburgh, E&S Livingstone, 1921

Krauthammer CD, Klerman GL: Secondary mania: manic syndromes associated with antecedent physical illness or drugs. Arch Gen Psychiatry 1978; 35:1333-1339

Kretschmer E: Physique and Character. Translated by Miller E. London, Kegan Paul, Trench, Trubner and Co, 1936

Lazare A, Klerman G: Hysteria and depression: the frequency and significance of hysterical personality features in hospitalized depressed women. Am J Psychiatry 1968; 124:48-56

Leckman JF, Weissman MM, Prusoff BA, et al: Subtypes of depression. Arch Gen Psychiatry 1984; 41:833-838

Lehmann HE: Affective disorders: clinical features, in Comprehensive Textbook of Psychiatry/IV, vol 1, fourth edition. Edited by Kaplan HI, Sadock BJ. Baltimore, Williams & Wilkins, 1985

Leonhard K, Korff I, Shultz H: Die temperamente in den familien der monopolaren und bipolaren phasischen psychosen. Psychiatry and Neurology 1962; 143:416

Mazure C, Nelson C, Price LH: Reliability and validity of the symptoms of major depressive illness. Arch Gen Psychiatry 1986; 43:451-456

McConville BJ, Bruce RT: Depressive illnesses in children and adolescents: a review of current concepts. Can J Psychiatry 1985; 30:119-129

Mountjoy CQ, Roth M: Studies in the relationship between depressive disorders and anxiety states. J Affective Disord 1982; 4:149-161

Murphy GE: Variability of the clinical course of primary affective disorder. Arch Gen Psychiatry 1974; 30:757-761

Nelson JC, Charney DS, Quinlan DM: Characteristics of autonomous depression. J Nerv Ment Dis 1980; 168:637-643

Paykel ES, Klerman GL, Prusoff BA: Prognosis of depression and the endogenous-neurotic distinction. Psychol Med 1974; 4:57-64

Perris C: A study of bipolar (manic depressive) and unipolar recurrent depressive psychoses. Acta Psychiatr Scand 1966; 42:Suppl 194

Puig-Antich J: Major depression and conduct disorder in prepuberty. J Am Acad Child Psychiatry 21:118-128, 1982

Puig-Antich J, Blau S, Marx N, et al: Prepubertal major depressive disorders: a pilot study. J Am Acad Child Psychiatry 17:695-707, 1978

Reveley AM, Reveley MA: The distinction of primary and secondary affective disorders: clinical implications. J Affective Disord 1981; 3:273-279

Robins E, Guze SB: Classification of affective disorders: the primary-secondary, the endogenous, and the neurotic-psychotic concepts, in Recent Advances in the Psychobiology of Depressive Illness. Edited by Williams TA, Katz MM, Shield JA. Washington, DC, Department of Health, Education and Welfare, 1972

Rounsaville BJ, Sholomskas D, Prusoff B: Chronic mood disorders in depressed outpatients: diagnosis and response to pharmacotherapy. J Affective Disord 1980; 2:73-88

Schneider K: Psychopathic Personalities. Translated by Hamilton MW. London, Cassell Ltd, 1958

Schuckit MA: Drug and Alcohol Abuse. New York, Plenum Press, 1979

Schuckit MA: Alcoholic patients with secondary depression. Am J Psychiatry 1983; 140:711-714

Shea T: Report presented at the Society for Psychotherapy Research. Bristol, England, June 1983

Spitzer RL, Endicott J, Robins E: Research Diagnostic Criteria (RDC) for a Selected Group of Functional Disorders. New York, New York State Psychiatric Institute, 1985

Strober M: Depressive illness in adolescence. Psychiatric Annals 1985; 15:375-378

Tahka V: The Alcoholic Personality. Helsinki, Finnish Foundation for Alcohol Studies, 1966

Taylor MA, Gaztanage P, Abrams R: Manic-depressive illness and acute schizophrenia: a clinical, family history, and treatment-response study. Am J Psychiatry 1974; 131:678-682

Tsuang MT, Woolson RF: Excess mortality in schizophrenia and affective disorders. Arch Gen Psychiatry 1978; 35:1181-1185

Tyrer PJ, Lee I, Edwards JG, et al: Prognostic factors determining response to antidepressant drugs in psychiatric outpatients and general practice. J Affective Disord 1980; 2:149-156

van Valkenburg C, Lowry M, Winokur G, et al: Depression spectrum disease versus pure depressive disease. J Nerv Ment Dis 1977; 165:341-345

Weissman MM, Pottenger M, Kleber H, et al: Symptom pattern in primary and secondary depression. Arch Gen Psychiatry 1977; 34:854-862

Weissman MM, Myers J: Affective disorders in a U.S. urban community: the use of Research Diagnostic Criteria in an epidemiological study. Arch Gen Psychiatry 1978; 35:1304-1311

Winokur G: Psychosis in bipolar and unipolar affective illness with special reference to schizo-affective disorder. Br J Psychiatry 1984; 145:236-243

Winokur G: The validity of neurotic-reactive depression: new data and reappraisal. Arch Gen Psychiatry 1985; 42:1116-1122

Winokur G, Behar D, van Valkenburg C, et al: Is a familial definition of depression both feasible and valid? J Nerv Ment Dis 1978; 166:764-769

Winokur G, Scharfetter C, Angst J: A family study of psychotic symptomatology in schizophrenia, schizoaffective disorder, unipolar depression, and bipolar disorder. Eur Arch Psychiatr Neurol Sci 1985; 234:295-298

Wolpert EA: Major affective disorders, in Comprehensive Textbook of Psychiatry/III, vol 2, third edition. Edited by Kaplan HI, Sadock BJ. Baltimore, Williams & Wilkins, 1980

Young MA, Scheftner WA, Klerman GL, et al: The endogenous sub-type of depression: a study of its internal construct validity. Br J Psychiatry 1986; 148:257-267

Chapter 10

Somatic Treatment of Unipolar Depressive Disorder

by Robert F. Prien, Ph.D.

This chapter deals with research findings, issues, and strategies pertaining to the somatic treatment of unipolar depression and is organized into four sections according to categories of treatment: 1) acute therapy; 2) continuation therapy; 3) preventive therapy; and 4) treatment of chronicity.

TERMINOLOGY

Unipolar Disorder

Although unipolar depressive disorder is a popular term in the therapeutic literature, it was not adopted into the *Diagnostic and Statistical Manual of Mental Disorders, Third Edition (DSM-III)* (American Psychiatric Association, 1980) because of the diversity of diagnostic criteria that have been used to define the disorder and the heterogeneity of conditions that such diagnostic criteria can represent. A summary of the issues and controversies in the classification of unipolar depression are found in Chapter 9, by Dr. Keller. For the purposes of this chapter, the term "unipolar disorder" refers to a depressive disorder with no history of a manic or unequivocal hypomanic episode, and with no known organic etiology.

Purposes of Treatment

ACUTE AND CONTINUATION TREATMENTS. The interconnected concepts of acute therapy and continuation therapy took root in the early 1960s. Clinicians, alarmed by the high relapse rate that occurred when antidepressant medication was withdrawn immediately following control of major depressive symptoms, stressed the importance of continuing treatment for several months after the disappearance of symptoms to make sure that the episode had run its course (Seager and Bird, 1962; Oltman and Friedman, 1964). The term "acute therapy" was applied to treatment directed at the initial control of major depressive symptoms. The term "continuation therapy" was adopted to describe the continuation of drug treatment after control of major depressive symptoms for the purpose of maintaining control over the episode. The differentiation of acute from continuation therapy is based upon the assumption that antidepressant drugs can suppress symptoms of a major depressive episode without immediately correcting the postulated biological process or pathophysiology underlying the episode. This distinction is supported by several placebo controlled studies (see this chapter's section on continuation treatment) and is considered relevant not only for treatment with antidepressant drugs but for lithium, ECT, and other somatic treatments for affective disorders.

PREVENTIVE TREATMENT. Interest in long-term maintenance treatment for preventive purposes was generated by reports by Hartigan (1963) and Baastrup (1964), suggesting that lithium was effective in preventing or attenuating recurrences of depressive and manic episodes in patients with a history of frequent attacks. Evidence for the preventive efficacy of antidepressant drugs for recurrent major depression was provided a decade later (Prien et al, 1973). In this chapter, the term "preventive treatment" will refer to the use of long-term treatment to modify the course of recurrent major depression through reduction in the frequency and/or severity of recurrences. It reflects current thinking that maintenance drug treatment may modify the course of illness by either preventing the occurrence of a new episode or by dampening an emerging episode sufficiently to avoid a full-blown attack.

TREATMENT OF CHRONICITY. This category refers primarily to the treatment of so-called "subacute" depressive disorders such as dysthymia and other chronic disorders that do not meet the prevailing criteria for major depression. In the current revision of the *Diagnostic and Statistical Manual of Mental Disorders, Third Edition, Revised DSM-III, DSM-III-R*, (American Psychiatric Association, 1987), chronic depression also includes major depressive episodes that persist for at least two years without a full remission for longer than two months.

The aforementioned categories may overlap or be blurred in clinical practice. The boundary between acute and continuation therapy may be blurred by a waxing and waning of symptoms following initial recovery or a less than full remission. Continuation therapy may become preventive therapy once the episode has run its course. Preventive therapy may serve the dual purpose of preventing new episodes while resolving chronic interepisode psychopathology. Despite the potential for overlap or blurring, these categories are useful for evaluating the purposes of both short-term and long-term treatment.

Relapse and Recurrence

The differentiation between continuation and preventive therapies led investigators to coin the term "relapse" to refer to worsening of an ongoing episode and "recurrence" to represent the occurrence of a new episode (Klerman, 1978). An arbitrary but common convention is that worsening that occurs within six months following remission of the previous episode constitutes a relapse, whereas worsening occurring thereafter is a recurrence (Quitkin et al, 1976).

ACUTE TREATMENT

Discussion of acute treatment will focus on four prominent subtypes of major depressive disorder: 1) major depression with melancholic or endogenous features; 2) major depression with atypical features; 3) major depression with mood congruent psychotic features; and 4) situational depression.

Depression with Melancholic/Endogenous Features

DIAGNOSTIC CRITERIA. Recent studies focusing on melancholic or endogenous depression have used the Research Diagnostic Criteria (RDC) (Spitzer et al, 1978) or the *DSM-III* to diagnose the disorder. The RDC diagnosis specifies four symptoms in group A (distinct quality of mood, lack of reactivity to pleasurable environmental stimuli, mood worse in morning, and pervasive anhedonia) and six in group B (guilt, middle or terminal insomnia, psychomotor retardation or agitation, poor appetite, weight loss, and pervasive or nonpervasive anhedonia). A definite diagnosis of endogenous depression requires at least six symptoms, including at least one from group A. In the *DSM-III*, the eight criteria used to diagnose melancholia are also part of the RDC. The major difference between the two criteria sets is that the *DSM-III* melancholics must exhibit pervasive or near pervasive anhedonia and exhibit lack of reactivity to pleasurable environmental stimuli. The *DSM-III-R* adds three criteria to the list: a history of at least one major depressive episode with complete recovery; a prior good response to somatic therapy; and no personality disorder preceding the initial major depression.

SOMATIC TREATMENT. Tricyclic antidepressants (TCAs) are the treatments of choice for major depressive episodes with melancholic/endogenous features and without psychosis. Most of the published clinical studies showing the superior efficacy of TCAs over placebo were conducted with severely depressed patients with endogenous symptoms. Although most of these studies were conducted prior to the development of current diagnostic criteria, most of the patients probably would have satisfied the RDC and *DSM-III* criteria for endogenous or melancholic depression. Recovery rates with TCAs are typically 70 to 80 percent compared to 20 to 40 percent for placebo (Klein et al, 1980).

Reviews of predictors of response suggest that the TCAs are most effective in endogenous depression compared to other subtypes of depression. Symptoms that are most predictive of good response to TCAs are psychomotor retardation, anhedonia, appetite and weight loss, early morning awakening, and lack of reactivity (Bielski and Friedel, 1976; Nelson and Charney, 1981; Avery et al, 1983). Results suggest that the strongest clinical predictor for TCAs is psychomotor change, with retardation being a predictor of good response, and agitation a predictor of poor response (Nelson and Charney, 1981).

There is little justification for selecting one TCA over another in terms of clinical efficacy. Determining factors in choice of drug are the patient's medication history, the pattern of side effects, and the physician's familiarity with selected antidepressants. Antidepressant drugs marketed in the United States are listed in Table 1.

Electroconvulsive therapy (ECT) remains the most rapid and effective treatment for severe melancholic or endogenous depression. Recovery rates average 80 to 90 percent (Klein et al, 1980). Indicators for ECT as a first treatment are a history of good response to ECT, a history of poor response to antidepressants, and an urgent need for rapid resolution of symptoms (for example, because of high risk for suicide). Otherwise, ECT is regarded as an alternate treatment for severely ill patients who are refractory to or cannot tolerate standard antidepressant drugs.

Monoamine oxidase inhibitors (MAOIs) usually are not employed to treat melancholic or endogenous depression, even in cases refractory to TCAs. Studies evaluating the effectiveness of MAOIs in endogenous depression are generally negative (Paykel, 1979). However, some clinicians regard the issue as unsettled because the early trials used relatively low doses (Davis, 1985). Robinson and

Table 1. Antidepressant Drugs Available in the United States

Tricyclics		Monoamine Oxidase Inhibitors		Miscellaneous	
Drug	Usual Therapeutic Range (mg/day)	Drug	Usual Therapeutic Range (mg/day)	Drug	Usual Therapeutic Range (mg/day)
Tertiary Amines		Phenelzine	45–90	Amozapine	250–600
Amitriptyline	75–300	Tranylcypromine	20–60	Maprotiline	75–250
Imipramine	75–300	Isocarboxazid	20–30	Trazodone	150–400
Doxepine	50–300			Lithium	600–1800
Trimipramine	50–300				
Secondary Amines					
Nortriptyline	50–150				
Desipramine	75–300				
Protriptyline	15–60				

colleagues (1985) and McGrath and associates (1986) provide results suggesting that the MAOIs are as effective as the TCAs with melancholic patients. In addition, the findings by Robinson and colleagues (1985) suggest that melancholic patients with panic attacks respond even better to MAOIs than to TCAs. The latter is an important finding because the incidence of panic disorder in patients with major depression without atypical features is reported to range from 15 to 37 percent (Robinson et al, 1985). There is need for further study of the value of MAOIs in endogenous or melancholic depressive disorders.

The possibility that antidepressants other than TCAs and MAOIs are effective for endogenous/melancholic depression has not been carefully explored. A large multicenter study comparing trazodone, amoxapine, and maprotiline reports that all three drugs produced recovery rates consistent with expected rates in TCA trials (Robinson et al, 1984).

In summary, TCAs constitute the usual treatment of choice for endogenous depression without psychosis. However, ECT may be given preference if there is a history of poor response to antidepressant drugs or a critical need for rapid control of symptoms. MAOIs should be considered if there is a history of panic attacks.

Depression with Atypical Features

DIAGNOSTIC CONSIDERATIONS. During the past 30 years, the term "atypical depression" has been used to describe a number of conditions. Most of the definitions have been developed in the context of studies evaluating MAOI therapy in nonendogenous depression. The term was first employed by British investigators in the late 1950s to refer to patients without endogenous symptoms who responded well to the MAOI, iproniazid, and poorly to ECT (West and Dally, 1959). The MAOI-responsive syndrome was characterized by prominent anxiety and phobic features, emotional overreactivity, hysterical features, fatigue, initial insomnia, and reversed diurnal variation of mood.

Pollit (1965) separated the anxiety component of atypical depression from the pattern of depression symptoms. He argued that the term "atypical" as used by West and Dally may refer to two syndromes. It may describe patients with marked anxiety and phobic symptoms in addition to depression; or it may describe a pattern of "reversed" vegetative symptoms opposite to those characterizing endogenous depression (for example, hyperphagia rather than anorexia, hypersomnia rather than insomnia, and symptoms worse in the evening than in the morning). Davidson and colleagues (1982) independently arrived at the same conclusion several years later, noting that failure to differentiate the two syndromes accounts for much of the confusion regarding findings for atypical or nonendogenous depression.

A recent approach to defining atypical depression was developed by Liebowitz and coworkers (1984) who merged the earlier British concepts with work on mood reactivity (Ravaris et al, 1980) and hysteroid dysphoria (Klein et al, 1980) to construct a set of operational criteria for use in clinical studies. The core characteristics are mood reactivity to pleasurable environmental stimuli while depressed, reversed vegetative symptoms, and hypersensitivity to rejection. The DSM-III-R diagnostic criteria for atypical depression are similar to those described above, and are defined in Chapter 9.

Panic attacks may play an even more critical role in atypical depression than they play in melancholic depression. As will be discussed in the next section, results from pharmacologic studies suggest that atypical depression associated with panic attacks constitutes an important subtype in terms of treatment response. Investigators report that between one-third and one-half of study patients with atypical or nonendogenous depression have a history of panic attacks (Quitkin et al, 1984; Liebowitz et al, 1985; Robinson et al, 1985).

SOMATIC TREATMENT. Attempts to target MAOIs to specific constellations of atypical or nonendogenous symptoms have met with mixed success. Several studies report that MAOIs provide greater improvement among atypical depressives than among endogenous depressives (West and Dally, 1959; Ravaris et al, 1976; Davidson et al, 1982; Liebowitz et al, 1984). Other studies indicate no particular advantage with MAOIs in atypical depression (Ravaris et al, 1980; Giller et al, 1982; Zisook et al, 1985). The lack of a commonly accepted definition of atypical depression and the considerable heterogeneity of nonendogenous depressions make it difficult to develop general treatment recommendations from these trials.

Further problems arise when MAOIs are compared to TCAs in populations in which the MAOIs have demonstrated special effectiveness. Ravaris and co-workers (1976) compared the MAOI, phenelzine, with a placebo in patients with major depression and found that phenelzine was most effective in nonendogenous depression characterized by significant anxiety, phobic symptoms, hysterical personality, fatigue, and initial insomnia. However, in a subsequent comparison of phenelzine to a TCA (amitriptyline), the features associated with the positive MAOI response in the earlier trial failed to predict differences in outcome between the two drugs (Ravaris et al, 1980). Thus, the specificity of MAOIs compared to TCAs remains unvalidated.

A major finding from recent studies is the importance of panic attacks for response to MAOIs and TCAs. Liebowitz and colleagues (1984) compared phenelzine with a TCA (imipramine) in a placebo-controlled study of 120 atypical depressives using the operational criteria specified in the previous section, and found that phenelzine produced better results than the TCA and placebo. A particularly important finding was that patients with a history of panic attacks responded well to phenelzine, moderately well to imipramine, and very poorly to placebo. Patients without panic attacks responded moderately well to each of the treatments, indicating the absence of a specific drug effect with this subgroup. This finding was corroborated by Robinson and associates (1985) in a trial comparing phenelzine with imipramine in 169 patients with major depression. The investigators found no significant difference in improvement between the two treatments. However, phenelzine showed significantly greater improvement than imipramine in patients with a history of panic attacks. When data were analyzed separately for atypical depression and melancholic depression, the same pattern of improvement held true. With both subtypes, patients with panic attacks improved more than those without panic attacks. Davidson and co-workers (1986) also found that panic attacks contribute to differences in efficacy between MAOIs and TCAs.

Two other factors that warrant further study as predictors of MAOI response in atypical depression are prominent anxiety (Ravaris et al, 1980; Paykel et al, 1982; McGrath et al, 1984) and hysteroid dysphoria, a syndrome characterized by rejection sensitivity, extreme fatigue, and atypical vegetative symptoms (Liebowitz et al, 1984; Kayser et al, 1985).

In summary, available evidence suggests that patients with atypical depression or nonendogenous depression warrant a trial with either an MAOI or a TCA. However, in the presence of panic attacks, prominent anxiety, or, possibly, hysteroid dysphoria, the MAOI should be given primary consideration.

Major Depression with Mood Congruent Psychotic Features

DIAGNOSTIC CRITERIA. In the *DSM-III* and *DSM-III-R*, the category of major depressive episode with mood congruent features is characterized by delusions or hallucinations in which content is consistent with the typical depressive themes of personal inadequacy, guilt, disease, death, nihilism, or deserved punishment. Depressive stupor is a criterion in the *DSM-III* but not in the *DSM-III-R*.

Over the years, mood congruent psychotic disorder has been viewed in one of two ways—as a severe form of major depressive disorder (Guze et al, 1975; Quitkin et al., 1978) or as a separate clinical entity (Glassman and Roose, 1981). Available evidence from therapeutic, biological, family history, and course of illness studies tends to support the view of psychotic depression as a clinical entity distinct from nonpsychotic depression (Brotman et al, 1987). However, more definitive data are needed before final conclusions can be drawn.

SOMATIC TREATMENT. Spiker and co-workers (1986) recently conducted a review of the literature on the pharmocologic treatment of depressed patients with mood congruent delusions. The review focused on reports from 16 studies evaluating the clinical efficacy of TCAs. Only 32 percent of the 377 delusional depressives in these studies responded positively to the TCAs. The response rate was similar for imipramine and amitriptyline and there were no documented diagnostic or demographic characteristics that differentiated responders from nonresponders. Nine of the studies reported response rates for control groups of nondelusional depressives: 66 percent of the 620 nondelusional patients responded favorably to TCAs compared to only 34 percent of the 300 delusional depressives.

There are several uncontrolled trials and one controlled study that report that the combination of a TCA and an antipsychotic drug is more effective than a TCA alone in the treatment of psychotic depressives (Kaskey et al, 1980). The controlled trial (Spiker et al, 1986) found that the combination of amitriptyline and perphenazine produced a response rate of 78 percent compared to 41 percent for amitriptyline alone and 19 percent for perphenazine alone. The authors reported that the combination was significantly superior even after analyses controlled for the plasma level of the TCA.

ECT provides a response rate similar to that obtained with the combination drug treatment. In three studies (Hornden et al, 1963; Glassman et al, 1977; Avery et al, 1979), 105 (82 percent) of 127 patients with delusional depression that was refractory to TCAs responded to ECT. However, the relapse rate following withdrawal of ECT reportedly is quite high, even for patients who receive continuation treatment with a TCA (Klein et al, 1980).

Another treatment approach, based on results from small sample trials, is the addition of lithium either to a single antidepressant or to the combination of a

TCA and antipsychotic drug (Price et al, 1983). Although promising, the value of this approach requires scientific verification.

In summary, available evidence indicates that the combination of an antidepressant and antipsychotic drug is the treatment of choice for psychotic depression with mood congruent delusions. There is a subgroup that appears to respond well to an antidepressant alone, but there are no established predictors for identifying these patients. ECT is a viable second line treatment for patients who do not respond to the combination.

Situational Depression

DIAGNOSTIC CONSIDERATIONS. The classification of situational depression continues to enjoy popularity despite its absence in the last two editions of the *Diagnostic and Statistical Manual (DSM-II* and *DSM-III)*. The popularity of the classification is based, in large measure, on the presumption that depression can be subdivided on the basis of the presence or absence of an environmental precipitant, such as marital disruption or financial reversals. Situational depression remains a classification in the RDC, representing "situations in which the episode almost certainly would not have developed at that time, in the absence of the external events" (Spitzer et al, 1978). The diagnosis does not require the presence or absence of any specific depressive symptoms (for example, endogenicity) but is based entirely on the clinician's judgments about the causal relationship between the psychosocial stressor and onset of the depressive episode. Thus, a patient may receive a diagnosis of both situational depression and endogenous depression.

As discussed in Chapter 9, there is insufficient data to validate situational depression as a distinct clinical entity separate from nonsituational depression. However, as Hirschfeld and co-workers (1985) point out, there is continued need for further research in this field, using alternatives to the clinician's judgment in identifying stress related depression.

SOMATIC TREATMENT. Theoretical considerations have led some clinicians to view situational depressions as "nonbiological," and, therefore, relatively unresponsive to pharmacotherapy (Comstock, 1977). However, research evidence shows that patients with well defined situational depression tend to respond as positively to antidepressant drug treatment as those with nonsituational depression. Garvey and co-workers (1984), using the RDC definition of situational depression, failed to find a significant difference in treatment outcome after four and six weeks between patients classified as situational depressives and those classified as nonsituational depressives. Both groups showed significant improvement. Tyrer and associates (1980), in a survey of treatment outcome with 200 patients, found that the presence of a precipitant was associated with as good an antidepressant drug response as absence of a precipitant. Prusoff and colleagues (1980) also report positive findings with antidepressants in both patients with situational and nonsituational major depressive disorder. These findings strongly indicate that clinicians should not deny antidepressant drug treatment to patients with major depression merely because a significant situational event preceded the onset of the episode.

Approaches to Treatment Resistant Depression

ISSUES. Despite advances in treating depressive disorders during the past decade, a considerable number of patients are characterized as treatment resistant or refractory. The extent of the problem is difficult to determine because of differing definitions of treatment resistant depression. One definition describes treatment resistant depression as "an ongoing and unremitting depressed state in a patient who has been adequately treated with at least two different anti-depressants or an antidepressant and a course of ECT" (Ayd, 1983). Another definition describes treatment resistant depression as an episode which, once established, does not respond to TCAs, MAOIs, or ECT (Shaw, 1977). A more conservative set of criteria requires a treatment resistant major depression of at least two years' duration with a documented history of failure to respond to either TCAs or MAOIs (Feighner et al, 1985).

A World Psychiatric Association report on treatment refractory depression (Ayd, 1983) makes a distinction between "absolute" and "relative" treatment resistance. Absolute resistance is defined as failure to respond to a course of "adequate treatment" and relative resistance as failure to respond to an "inadequate treatment." The report concludes that only a minority of patients categorized as treatment resisters are absolute resisters, and that the majority of relative resisters can be helped substantially by appropriate treatment with a TCA, MAOI, or ECT. Two studies in which so-called treatment resistant patients were referred to affective disorders clinics report that two-thirds of the patients responded with marked improvement to an adequate regimen of a TCA or an MAOI (Remick et al, 1983; Schatzberg et al, 1983).

There are certain conditions that must be met before a patient can be described as refractory to a specific treatment. Although there are many dosage guidelines for antidepressant drugs, the most comprehensive is the *Imipramine Administration Manual* by Fawcett and Epstein (submitted for publication), developed for the Treatment of Depression Research Program Collaborative Study coordinated by the National Institute of Mental Health (NIMH). The dosage schedule for outpatients assures that each patient is exposed to a minimum of 200 mg/day of imipramine by the third week unless the patient manifests severe side effects that appear dose related. Over the ensuing weeks, dosage may be increased to a maximum of 300 mg/day based upon the patient's response. If dosage is held at a lower level because of side effects, an attempt is made to increase the dosage to the therapeutic range. With inpatients, the rate of increase to maximum dose may be increased. Plasma levels may be a helpful guide in determining further need for increase in dosage if patients fail to respond at usual therapeutic levels.

Adequate duration of treatment usually is defined as a minimum of three to four weeks at the adequate dose, although arguments can be made for a minimum five- to six-week trial (Klein et al, 1980; Prien and Levine, 1984).

An often neglected contributor to nonresponse is patient noncompliance with the medication schedule. Surveys suggest that 25 to 50 percent of patients being treated for affective disorders discontinue medication, reduce dosage, or otherwise fail to take medication as prescribed (Prien and Caffey, 1977). Klein and co-workers (1980) and Shaw (1986) elaborate on the reasons for noncompliance and discuss means for improving acceptance of the treatment program and adherence to the therapeutic schedule.

TREATMENT STRATEGIES FOR NONRESPONDERS. Even with therapeutic dose levels, adequate trial duration, and good compliance, a certain proportion of patients with major depressive episodes either fail to improve acceptably on their initial treatment or cannot tolerate side effects of adequate doses (10 to 25 percent are frequently cited estimates). However, a failure on one antidepressant treatment does not mean that the patient will be resistant to other somatic treatment approaches.

Numerous systematic approaches involving sequences of second-, third-, and even fourth-line treatments have been recommended for nonresponsive disorders. The following is a listing of general approaches described in the literature for patients who fail to respond to therapeutic doses of a TCA.

STRATEGIES FOR TCA NONRESPONDERS. There are a series of steps that may be followed, but not necessarily in the order indicated:

Step 1. If the patient is not receiving the maximum dose of the TCA and is showing no significant adverse reactions at the current level, consider increasing the dose to maximum level (for example, 300 mg of imipramine per day).

Step 2. Patients who fail to improve after aggressive treatment may warrant a reassessment of diagnosis, together with a repeat of physical and laboratory examinations to exclude medical illness. The clinician should also look for possible psychosocial or situational factors that may be contributing to the poor response.

Step 3. Six alternatives may be considered if the first two steps fail:

a) If the disorder is severe or incapacitating or has a high potential for suicide, consider a course of ECT.

b) If the disorder is rediagnosed as psychotic, consider either ECT or the combination of a TCA and antipsychotic drug. Amitriptyline plus perphenazine is the most well documented combination (Spiker et al, 1986).

c) If the disorder is nonendogenous or atypical, or associated with panic attacks or prominent anxiety, consider a change to a MAOI. MAOIs may also be effective for endogenous depression that fails to respond to a TCA or to ECT.

d) A change to another TCA with a dissimilar mode of action or different profile of side effects may be beneficial, but is often a futile exercise unless adverse reactions are a problem with the initial TCA. One of the second generation antidepressants (for example, trazodone) may also be considered.

e) If standard antidepressant treatments are ineffective and the patient has a family history or course of illness suggesting a latent or undiagnosed bipolar disorder, lithium is worth a trial. Akiskal (1985) defines characteristics of a lithium responsive "soft bipolar spectrum" that may be overlooked in diagnosing major depressive disorder.

f) Lithium may be used as a supplement to the TCA. Lithium is presumed to potentiate TCA response by facilitating presynaptic serotonergic neurons in the presence of a postsynaptic supersensitivity associated with the TCA (DeMontigny et al, 1983). The treatment is fast and safe but of unpredictable effectiveness.

Step 4. Other alternatives that have been used to treat TCA-resistant depression include supplements to the TCA of l-triiodothyronine (T_3) (Prange and Loosen, 1980; Goodwin et al, 1982), psychostimulants (Rabkin et al, 1983) or reserpine (Ayd, 1985). Despite some positive results, the efficacy of these supplements remains unproven. Supplementary T_3 is the most promising of the three alternatives, but requires further study. The combination of a TCA and an MAOI also has the potential for good response (Feighner et al, 1985; Klein et al, 1980). However, it is unclear whether or not the combination provides substantial gains over aggressive use of either drug alone. Care should be taken in mixing a TCA and an MAOI (Ananth and Luchins, 1977). For example, an MAOI can be added to a TCA but the reverse probably should not be attempted. The procedures for combining a TCA and an MAOI and for replacing a TCA with an MAOI or vice versa are summarized elsewhere (Klein et al, 1980; Baldessarini, 1985).

STRATEGIES FOR MAOI NONRESPONDERS. As with TCA nonresponders, there should be reassessment of the adequacy of dose level and examination of the possible contribution of biological and psychosocial factors to the poor response. A change to a TCA may be considered. However, care should be taken not to introduce the TCA too soon after withdrawal of the MAOI because of increased risk of adverse reactions, including convulsions and cerebral hemorrhage. Change to another MAOI may be beneficial if the first MAOI is unacceptable to the patient. For example, tranylcypromine may be less objectionable than phenelzine in terms of sedation and weight gain. However, tranylcypromine's stimulant action may cause troublesome restlessness or insomnia (Pare, 1985). A small number of case reports suggests that initiating one MAOI less than 10 to 14 days after discontinuing another may produce hypertensive or hyperthermic crises (Baldessarini, 1985). Although this is not a well established finding, it nonetheless should generate caution in switching MAOIs.

CONTINUATION TREATMENT

Need for Continuation Treatment

There is ample evidence from placebo controlled studies to support the need for continuation treatment following initial control of the symptoms of acute depression (summarized in Prien and Kupfer, 1986). In each study, an antidepressant or lithium was used to control symptoms of major depression, after which approximately one-half of the sample was switched, double blind, to a placebo, and the other one-half continued to receive the drug. The treatments evaluated were amitriptyline, imipramine, lithium, phenelzine, and the combination of imipramine and lithium. In all studies, the relapse rate for patients receiving placebo was significantly greater than that for patients who continued on active treatment. Overall, approximately 50 percent of the placebo-treated patients developed symptoms that met criteria for an episode of major depression, compared to only about 20 percent receiving medication. Most of these episodes occurred relatively rapidly, within one week to three months following withdrawal of the active treatment. The rapidity of these episodes of depression following substitution of placebo suggests that they represent a worsening of the previously controlled episode rather than the occurrence of a new episode. As defined earlier, although not yet empirically validated, there is evidence to suggest that the former be considered a relapse and the latter be thought of as a recurrence.

Duration of Continuation Treatment

One problem facing the clinician is that when continuation treatment is effective in suppressing acute symptoms, it may be difficult to determine when the episode is over and the drug is no longer required. The problem is complicated by the fact that it is not known whether antidepressants primarily suppress symptoms until the episode runs its natural course, or whether they actually shorten the episode.

To be safe, continuation treatment should be maintained for as long as the episode would be expected to last if left untreated. However, if there are no symptoms to serve as a guide to episode length (that is, if continuation treatment is effective in suppressing symptoms), the clinician may either withdraw medication prematurely, thereby subjecting the patient to a high likelihood of relapse, or prolong treatment unnecessarily. There are risks associated with unnecessary continuation of treatment. Advocates of relatively short periods of continuation treatment argue that the risk of adverse reactions and the potential for misuse of medication accompanying prolonged use of potent antidepressant drugs may be more harmful than an emerging relapse, and that by withdrawing continuation medication slowly and reinstating therapeutic dosage at the first sign of returning symptoms, a full blown relapse can be avoided in the majority of cases (Klein et al, 1980). This strategy is not without risk. There is evidence suggesting that reinstating a discontinued drug tends to provide less rapid and effective control of symptoms than increasing an established maintenance dose (Prien and Caffey, 1977).

There have been two avenues of research in estimating episode length during continuation treatment. One involves work with possible biological markers of episode length (that is, state dependent markers). A study evaluating the relationship between electroencephalogram (EEG) sleep and vulnerability to relapse suggests that short REM latency may be a predictor of relapse (Giles et al, 1986). Studies of neuroendocrine parameters also suggest that the persistence of residual abnormalities, such as dexamethasone nonsuppression or blunted thyrotropin response to thyroid releasing hormone, may identify patients at high risk for relapse (Thase et al, 1985). However, none of these findings is at a stage in which they can be translated into guidelines for clinical practice. A more in-depth discussion of the physiologic mechanisms underlying each of these predictors of a propensity for greater relapse may be found in Chapter 8.

The second approach for estimating episode length during continuation therapy involves comparison of patient subgroups with different levels of symptom suppression during continuation treatment. Results from a multicenter collaborative study on maintenance therapy coordinated by NIMH (Prien and Kupfer, 1986) indicate that withdrawal of continuation treatment following a major depressive episode is safe only after the patient has been free of significant symptoms or has returned to his or her usual level of interepisode functioning for at least four months. A patient was considered to be free of symptoms if he or she manifested no more than minimal or transient symptoms as defined by the Global Assessment Scale (Endicott et al, 1976). The importance of the presence of residual symptoms in predicting relapse when continuation treatment is withdrawn is supported by results from a multicenter study conducted by the Medical Research Council in England (Mindham et al, 1973).

In summary, the presence and severity of residual symptoms during continuation treatment provide guidelines for determining when it is safe to withdraw medication. However, there is still the need for a valid and easily measured biological or psychopathological state dependent marker. Theoretically, such a marker could serve three functions: 1) determining when drug treatment can be safely discontinued; 2) identifying an incomplete remission that requires more aggressive treatment; and 3) serving as a prodrome of an impending recurrence.

PREVENTIVE TREATMENT

There is general agreement that drugs such as lithium can be effective preventive treatments for certain patients. Major issues are: who should receive treatment; what drug(s) should be employed; what dosage is required; and how long treatment should be maintained.

Who Should Receive Preventive Treatment

Several factors determine whether or not treatment should be initiated: 1) the likelihood of a recurrence in the near future; 2) the severity and abruptness of prior episodes and the potential impact of a new episode on patient functioning; 3) the patient's willingness to participate in the therapeutic program; 4) response to prior treatment regimens; and 5) potential contraindications to treatment. These factors cannot easily be quantified into a formula. However, for a key factor, the likelihood of a recurrence in the near future, there is guidance from the literature. Most clinicians who have published an opinion on the topic recommend that there should be at least two or three well defined major episodes before preventive treatment is administered. Patients who have only a single episode, mild episodes, or long intervals between episodes (for example, longer than five years) should probably not receive preventive treatment. The exception is the patient for whom a second episode would be life threatening or highly disruptive to career or family functioning.

Studies on the natural course of depressive illness clearly demonstrate the relationship between episode frequency and risk of recurrence (Angst et al, 1973; Perris, 1976; Angst, 1981; Keller et al, 1983). Cycle length (the period between the onset of one episode and the onset of the next) tends to decrease with each successive episode. Angst and colleagues (1973) found that cycle length decreased from an average of three years after the initial episode to two years after the second, to 1½ years after the third. Angst (1981) further indicates that after a patient has had two major depressive episodes within five years, there is a 70 percent probability of having two or more episodes during the subsequent five years.

Choice of Drug

Pivotal studies evaluating the preventive efficacy of TCAs and lithium (Baastrup et al, 1970; Prien et al, 1973; Kane et al, 1982; Glen et al, 1984; Prien et al, 1984) were reviewed at the *Consensus Development Conference on Mood Disorders: Pharmacologic Prevention of Recurrences,* organized by the NIMH and the NIH in 1984. The Conference Report (NIMH/NIH Consensus Development Conference Statement, 1985) concluded that both the TCAs and lithium are effective preventive treatments for unipolar recurrent depression, each with advantages for certain patients. The TCAs have a logistic advantage over lithium. Because most acute unipolar depressions are treated with an antidepressant rather than with lithium, continuation of the antidepressant for preventive treatment avoids the decisions and problems as to how and when to switch the patient from an antidepressant to lithium. Furthermore, evidence from a multicenter collaborative study indicates that the TCAs are more effective than lithium in preventing severe depressive episodes (Prien et al, 1984).

Lithium's advantage stems from its potent antimanic properties. The Conference Report notes that 10 to 15 percent of patients with a diagnosis of unipolar disorder subsequently develop a manic episode. Because of the serious consequences of an unexpected manic episode, it is recommended that lithium preventive therapy be considered when there is suspicion of a previously undiagnosed or latent bipolar disorder. In cases in which there is a higher than usual risk for developing a bipolar disorder, lithium is sometimes added to the antidepressant drug regimen. Factors increasing the risk of bipolar disorder are early age at onset of depression (under 25), bipolar family history, and a history of affective disorders in consecutive generations (Akiskal, 1985). The risk diminishes with increasing age and the number of depressive episodes.

Alternatives to lithium and TCAs for preventive treatment have not been evaluated. This raises the question of what one uses for preventive treatment when the acute episode is treated successfully with a drug other than a TCA or lithium. Taking away a drug that is producing a good response and substituting a TCA or lithium for preventive therapy can post logistical, ethical, and compliance problems as well as possible loss of control over symptoms during and after the substitution. There is also the possibility that the patient may have failed to respond or had adverse reactions to prior treatment with TCAs or lithium. Unless the original drug presents special risks when used on a long-term basis, or has not been adequately tested for safety for long-term use, the advantages of continuing the original drug would seem to outweigh the disadvantages. The most cautionary statements regarding long-term use are for amoxapine because of the risk of tardive dyskinesia and extrapyramidal symptoms, and for the MAOIs in patients who may fail to follow dietary restrictions. Comprehensive reviews of the long-term side effects of lithium and the various classes of antidepressants are provided by Klein and colleagues (1980), Pare (1985), and Siris and Rifkin (1983).

Dosage of Preventive Treatment

For lithium, the maintenance dose of 0.6 to 1.2 mEq/L recommended in the package insert is based primarily on trial and error experiences of individual investigators with bipolar patients (Prien and Caffey, 1977). Although there are no published guidelines for unipolar disorder, there is no evidence to suggest that effective levels are dissimilar to those used in the treatment of bipolar disorders. Some investigators recommend a higher minimum level of 0.7 to 0.8 mEq/L (Prien and Caffey, 1977). Others recommend more conservative levels of 0.4 to 0.6 mEq/L (Hullin, 1980). In general, levels below 0.6 mEq/L should be reserved for elderly patients, patients with compromised renal or cardiovascular function, and patients who have a history of disruptive side effects at levels as high as 0.6 mEq/L. Higher levels (for example, above 0.8 mEq/L) generally are reserved for patients who have a history of failure at lower levels.

The dosage for preventive treatment with TCAs has received even less attention than the dosage for lithium. Most experienced clinicians maintain patients on a dose equivalent to 75 to 150 mg/day of imipramine. Clinicians who employ the lower end of the dose range often do so with the expectation of rapidly increasing the dose at the first sign of an emerging recurrence, a strategy that has not been adequately studied. The value of using doses of TCAs exceeding the equivalent of 150 mg of imipramine also requires study.

Duration of Preventive Treatment

Although there is no evidence that preventive therapy cures recurrent major depression, recurrences may cease spontaneously after many years. Angst and Grof (1976) found that one of three patients over 65 years of age who had been free of abnormal mood swings for several years no longer required medication. However, other studies in which long-term treatment was withdrawn after years of stable mood report a high incidence of recurrences (Baastrup et al, 1970). The only way to determine whether or not the patient still requires preventive treatment is to discontinue the drug and carefully follow the patient for early signs of recurrence. The physician and patient must weigh the likelihood and consequences of a recurrence against the risk of continued medication. Patients with a history of suicide attempts, hospitalization for depression, or serious disruption of career or family life should have medication withdrawn only if there is reasonable assurance that subsequent episodes can be detected quickly enough to prevent a full blown episode.

In summary, several studies demonstrate the value of TCAs and lithium in the preventive treatment of major recurrent depression. However, there is a need to evaluate a wider range of antidepressants. There is a particular need to test the notion that if a drug is effective for acute and continuation treatment for a given patient, it will also be effective as a preventive treatment. The MAOIs and second generation antidepressants warrant special attention in this regard. More research is also required to establish meaningful guidelines for dosage and duration of treatment.

TREATMENT OF CHRONICITY

Diagnostic Issues

Recent therapeutic research on chronic depression generally has used RDC or DSM-III criteria to identify the disorders. Patients are considered to be chronically depressed if they satisfy the RDC diagnosis for chronic and intermittent depressive disorder or the DSM-III diagnosis of dysthymic disorder. Both diagnoses represent disorders of at least two years' duration characterized by a persistent or intermittent syndrome that is not of sufficient severity or duration to satisfy the criteria for a major depressive episode. *DSM-III-R* has made changes in the diagnosis of dysthymic disorder. The most significant is the separation of late onset chronicity following a major depressive episode from early onset chronicity that typically develops in childhood or adolescence, often in the context of characterologic and personality disturbances. This is a distinction that should aid subsequent therapeutic research on dysthymic disorder.

Dysthymic disorder is often unrecognized or misdiagnosed. As Weissman and Klerman (1977) point out, many practitioners, including psychiatrists, tend to equate affective disorders with an episodic and acute course and are unaccustomed to making a diagnosis of dysthymic disorder or chronic depression. Researchers also tend to focus on the more florid phases of affective illness, despite accumulating evidence that dysthymic disorder is a significant public health problem. The Epidemiologic Catchment Area Program indicates that four percent of women and two percent of men suffer from dysthymic disorder (Robins et al, 1984). The disorder can cause significant disruption in the patient's interpersonal functioning and life activities, and places the patient at high risk for multiple recurrences of major depression (Keller et al, 1983; Kovacs et al, 1984).

Somatic Treatment

Trials that include patients with dysthymic disorder suggest that the disorder may respond positively to antidepressants (Rounsaville et al, 1980; Paykel et al, 1982; Akiskal, 1985). However, the criteria for patient selection vary significantly among studies, making it difficult to compare findings and establish guidelines for treatment. The only published controlled clinical trial dealing exclusively with dysthymic disorder is a 25-patient study (Kocsis et al, 1985), which reports that imipramine is effective in controlling both major depressive symptoms and a preexisting dysthymic disorder. Some clinicians suggest that the combination of an antidepressant and psychotherapy may be beneficial in treating dysthymic disorder and other chronic depressions (Weissman and Akiskal, 1984), but there are no definitive data indicating which combination of treatments will work with which patients.

There is definite need for developing treatment strategies for alleviating or managing dysthymic disorder. One problem is that the RDC and *DSM-III* classifications of the disorder subsume too heterogeneous a group of depressive conditions to provide adequate guidelines for selection of patients for specific long-term treatments. The high comorbidity of dysthymic disorder with other Axis I disorders (notably major depression, anxiety disorders, and substance abuse), Axis II disorders, and medical conditions creates further problems in obtaining homogeneous samples. Weissman (1986) reports that more than three-fourths of the patients with a *DSM-III* diagnosis of dysthymic disorder identified in the Epidemiologic Catchment Area Program had another Axis I disorder.

To adequately study treatment in dysthymic disorder, it will be necessary to develop distinct subtypes of chronic depression defined by clinical course, symptom pattern, biological features, or coexisting Axis I or Axis II disorders and, then, investigate the differential response of the subtypes to various treatment interventions.

One of the more promising classification systems is proposed by Akiskal (1985), who differentiates chronic depression into four subtypes, two of which are reported to be responsive to somatic and psychosocial treatments. Among the treatment responsive subtypes is a late onset chronicity that typically occurs after age 40 in patients with no significant premorbid psychopathology who fail to recover from episodes of major depression. According to Akiskal, the recommended therapy is a heterocyclic antidepressant to alleviate vegetative and psychomotor disturbances, and interpersonal or cognitive psychotherapy to attenuate impairment in coping capacity and social functioning. A second treatment responsive subtype is an early onset dysthymia labeled "subaffective primary depression," often characterized by miniepisodes of depression lasting for days or weeks, a positive family history of primary affective disorder, hypersomnolence, shortened REM latency, and the potential for TCA generated hypomania. The suggested treatment is lithium and/or MAOIs combined with social skills training. This subtype may represent a precursor to subsequent severe chronic primary affective illness. Nonresponsive subtypes are an early onset characterologic depression and a depression secondary to a preexisting nonaffective disorder.

In summary, antidepressant drugs appear to be effective in treating some patients with dysthymic disorder, but the results are inconsistent and do not provide the basis for planning a comprehensive treatment program. The heterogeneity of the symptoms and course of illness of patients who satisfy the criteria for dysthymic disorder, coupled with the high comorbidity of dysthymic disorder and other psychiatric disorders, makes it difficult to identify treatment responsive subtypes. Akiskal's subtypes are attractive but need to be validated in a controlled therapeutic trial.

CONCLUDING COMMENTS

Research on the effectiveness of somatic therapy for depressive disorders has provided significant guidance to the practitioner for selected areas of treatment. TCAs have been established as the treatment of choice for major depression with melancholic features. MAOIs are emerging as a preferred treatment for nonendogenous depressions with atypical features such as panic attacks, marked anxiety, and rejection sensitivity. The combination of a TCA and a neuroleptic has proven to be an effective treatment for mood congruent psychotic depression, and ECT is a valuable alternative treatment for severe melancholic depression and depression with mood congruent psychotic features. Antidepressant drug therapy appears to be useful for situational depression as well as nonsituational depression.

The need for continuation treatment is firmly established and TCAs and lithium are regarded as effective preventive treatments for recurrent major depression. TCAs appear to be more advantageous than lithium in preventing or attenuating severe recurrences, whereas lithium's potent antimanic properties make it an especially attractive treatment when there is evidence of a latent or undiagnosed bipolar disorder. Finally, although there is no established treatment for dysthymic disorder or other chronic depressions, there are ongoing efforts to identify subtypes that are responsive to antidepressant agents alone or in combination with psychotherapy.

However, there are many questions that remain unanswered. In general, therapeutic research on drugs other than the TCAs and lithium has been limited to short-term (three to six week) trials of acute treatment. There appears to be an inherent assumption in these short-term studies that a drug capable of initially controlling acute symptoms is also effective for the longer term treatment. This assumption tends to be supported in the literature by open trials and case history reports, but has not been systematically evaluated. Controlled studies evaluating continuation and preventive treatment or treatment of chronicity are relatively few in number. Even with lithium and the TCAs, questions remain regarding appropriate dosage and duration of long-term maintenance treatment. For example, most textbooks recommend that the clinician use the lowest effective dose of lithium or TCAs for preventive treatment but fail to specify how this can be achieved without exposing the patient to a relapse or a recurrence. Also, long-term trials with TCAs or lithium usually focus on patients with major recurrent depression with uncomplicated melancholic features and a course characterized by complete or nearly complete recovery between episodes. The long-term treatment of psychotic depression, nonendogenous atypical depression, chronic disorders, and depressions associated with nonaffective psychiatric disorders remains relatively uncharted.

There is a need for longitudinal designs that extend beyond the acute treatment phase with treatments other than the TCAs and lithium in disorders other than recurrent major endogenous depression. Until there are concentrated research efforts in these areas, the practitioner will continue to operate with less than optimal information on the efficacy, safety, and proper procedures for managing the heterogeneous group of depressive disorders requiring treatment.

There is a caveat for both researchers and clinicians. The NIMH Collaborative Depression Study evaluating the naturalistic course of affective illness at five university medical centers (Keller et al, 1986) suggests that there is a large gap between knowledge about efficacy of available treatment and its actual use. The investigators conclude that a substantial proportion of depressives seeking help in the community receive inadequate levels of treatment and that after entering the study centers, a majority continue to be undertreated even when there are established standards regarding drug, dosage, and duration. The task of translating research findings into clinical practice constitutes one of the most important challenges facing the research and clinical communities and is a subject for research in and of itself.

REFERENCES

Akiskal H: The clinical management of affective disorders, in Psychiatry, Vol 7. Edited by Cavenar JO, Michels R, Brody HKH, et al. Philadelphia, J.B. Lippincott, 1985

American Psychiatric Association: Diagnostic and Statistical Manual of Mental Disorders, Third Edition (DSM-III). Washington, DC, American Psychiatric Association, 1980

American Psychiatric Association: Diagnostic and Statistical Manual of Mental Disorders, Third Edition, Revised (DSM-III-R). Washington, DC, American Psychiatric Association, 1987

Ananth F, Luchins D: A review of combined tricyclic and MAOI therapy. Compr Psychiatry 1977; 18:221-230

Angst J: Clinical indications for a prophylactic treatment of depression, in Depressive

Illness—Biological Issues. Edited by Mendlewicz J, Coppen A, van Praag HM. Basel, S Krager, 1981

Angst F, Baastrup PC, Grof P, et al: The course of monopolar depression and bipolar psychoses. Psychiatrie Neurologie et Neurochirurgie (Amst) 1973; 76:489-500

Angst J, Grof P: The course of monopolar depressions and bipolar psychosis, in Lithium in Psychiatry: A Synopsis. Edited by Villeneuve A. Quebec, Canada, Les Presses de L'University Laval, 1976

Avery D, Lubrano A: Depression treated with imipramine and ECT: the DeCarolis study reconsidered. Am J Psychiatry 1979; 136:559-562

Avery DH, Wilson LG, Dunner DL: Diagnostic subtypes of depression as predictors of therapeutic response, in Treatment of Depression: Old Controversies and New Approaches. Edited by Clayton PJ, Barrett JE. New York, Raven Press, 1983

Ayd FJ: Treatment-resistant depression. International Drug Therapy Newsletter 1983; 18:25-27

Ayd FJ: Reserpine therapy for tricyclic-resistant depressions. International Drug Therapy Newsletter 1985; 20:17-20

Baastrup PC: The use of lithium in manic-depressive psychosis. Compr Psychiatry 1964; 5:396-408

Baastrup PC, Poulson JC, Schou M, et al: Prophylactic lithium: double-blind discontinuation in manic-depressive and recurrent disorders. Lancet 1970; 2:326-330

Baldessarini RJ: Chemotherapy in Psychiatry: Principles and Practice. Cambridge, Harvard University Press, 1985

Bielski RJ, Friedel RO: Prediction of tricyclic antidepressant response. Arch Gen Psychiatry 1976; 33:1479-1489

Brotman AW, Falk WE, Gelenberg AJ: Pharmacologic treatment of acute depressive subtypes, in Psychopharmacology: A Generation of Progress, second edition. New York, Raven Press, 1987

Comstock BS: Outpatient management of depressive disorders, in Phenomenology and Treatment in Depression. Edited by Fann WE. Jamaica, New York, Spectrum Publications, 1977

Davidson JT, Pelton S: Forms of atypical depression and their response to antidepressant drugs. Psychiatry Res 1986; 17:87-95

Davidson JT, Miller RD, Turnbull CD, et al: Atypical depression. Arch Gen Psychiatry 1982; 39:527-534

Davis JM: Antidepressant drugs, in Comprehensive Textbook of Psychiatry, vol. 4. Edited by Kaplan HI, Sadock BJ. Baltimore, Williams & Wilkins, 1985

DeMontigny C, Cowinoyer G, Marissette R, et al: Lithium carbonate addition in tricyclic antidepressant resistant unipolar depression. Arch Gen Psychiatry 1983; 40:1327-1334

Endicott J, Spitzer RL, Fleiss JL: The Global Assessment Scale: a procedure for measuring overall severity of psychiatric disturbance. Arch Gen Psychiatry 1976; 33:766-771

Feighner JP, Herbstein J, Damlouju N: Combined MAOI, TCA, and direct stimulant therapy of treatment resistant depression. J Clin Psychiatry 1985; 46:206-209

Garvey MJ, Schaffer CB, Tuason VB: Comparison of pharmacological treatment response between situational and non-situational depressions. Br J Psychiatry 1984; 145:363-365

Giles DE, Jarrett RB, Roffwarg HP, et al: Monthly longitudinal study of remitted depression, in Scientific Program, Annual Meeting of the Society of Biological Psychiatry. Washington, DC, May 1986

Giller E, Bialos D, Riddel M, et al: Monoamine oxidase inhibitor responsive depression. Psychiatry Res 1982; 6:41-48

Glassman AH, Roose SP: Delusional depression: a distinct clinical entity? Arch Gen Psychiatry 1981; 38:424-427

Glassman AH, Perel JM, Shostak M, et al: Clinical implications of imipramine plasma levels for depressive illness. Arch Gen Psychiatry 1977; 34:197-204

Glen AIM, Johnson AL, Shepherd M: Continuation therapy with lithium and amitriptyline in unipolar depressive illness: a randomized double-blind controlled trial. Psychol Med 1984; 14:37-50

Guze SB, Woodruff RA, Clayton PJ: The significance of psychotic affective disorders. Arch Gen Psychiatry 1975; 32:1147-1150

Goodwin F, Prange A, Post R, et al: Potentiation of antidepressant effects by L-triiodothyronine in tricyclic nonresponders. Am J Psychiatry 1982; 139:34-38

Hartigan CP: The use of lithium salts in affective disorders. Br J Psychiatry 1963; 109:810-814

Hirschfeld RMA, Klerman GL, Andreasen NC, et al: Situational major depressive disorder. Arch Gen Psychiatry 1985; 42:1109-1114

Hornden A, Holt NF, Burt CG, et al: Amitriptyline in depressive states: phenomenology and prognostic considerations. Br J Psychiatry 1963; 109:815-825

Hullin RP: Minimum serum lithium levels for effective prophylaxis, in Handbook of Lithium Therapy. Edited by Johnson FN. Lancaster England, MTP Press, 1980

Kane JM, Quitkin FM, Rifkin A, et al: Lithium carbonate and imipramine in the prophylaxis of unipolar and bipolar II illness. Arch Gen Psychiatry 1982; 39:1065-1069

Kaskey GB, Nasr S, Meltzer HY: Drug treatment in delusional depression. Psychiatry Res 1980; 1:267-277

Kayser AK, Robinson DS, Nies A, et al: Response to phenelzine among depressed patients with features of hysteroid dysphoria. Am J Psychiatry 1985; 142:486-488

Keller MB: Chronic and recurrent affective disorders: Incidence, course and influencing factors, in Chronic Treatments in Neuropsychiatry. Edited by Kemali D, Racagni G. New York, Raven Press, 1985

Keller MB, Shapiro RW, Lavori P, et al: Double depression: two year follow-up. Am J Psychiatry 1983; 140:689-694

Keller MB, Lavori PW, Klerman GL, et al: Low levels and lack of predictors of somatotherapy and psychotherapy received by depressed patients. Arch Gen Psychiatry 1986; 43:458-466

Klein DF, Gittelman R, Quitkin FM, et al: Diagnosis and Drug Treatment of Psychiatric Disorders: Adults and Children. Baltimore, Williams & Wilkins, 1980

Klerman GL: Long-term treatment of affective disorders, in Psychopharmacology: A Generation of Progress. Edited by Lipton M, DiMascio A, Killam KF. New York, Raven Press, 1978

Kocsis JH, Frances AJ, Mann JJ: Imipramine for the treatment of chronic depression. Psychopharmacol Bull 1985; 21:698-700

Kovacs M, Feinberg TL, Crouse-Novak MA, et al: Depressive disorders in childhood. Arch Gen Psychiatry 1984; 41:643-649

Liebowitz MR, Quitkin FM, Stewart JW, et al: Phenelzine versus imipramine in atypical depression. Arch Gen Psychiatry 1984; 41:669-677

Liebowitz MR, Quitkin FM, Stewart JW, et al: Effect of panic attacks on the treatment of atypical depressives. Psychopharmacol Bull 1985; 21:558-561

McGrath PJ, Quitkin FM, Harrison W, et al: Treatment of melancholia with tranylcypromine. Am J Psychiatry 1984; 141:288-289

McGrath PJ, Stewart JW, Harrison W, et al: Phenelzine treatment of melancholia. J Clin Psychiatry 1986; 47:420-422

Mindham RHS, Howland C, Shepherd M: An evaluation of continuation therapy with tricyclic antidepressants in depressive illness. Psychol Med 1973; 3:5-17

Nelson JC, Charney DS: The symptoms of major depressive illness. Am J Psychiatry 1981; 138:1-13

NIMH/NIH Consensus Development Conference Statement. Am J Psychiatry 1985; 142:469-476

Oltman JE, Friedman S: Relapses following treatment with antidepressant drugs. Diseases of the Nervous System 1964; 25:699-701

Pare CMB: The present status of monoamine oxidase inhibitors. Br J Psychiatry 1985; 146:576-584

Paykel ES: Predictors of treatment response, in Psychopharmacology of Affective Disorders. Edited by Paykel ES, Coppen A. New York, Oxford University Press, 1979

Paykel ES, Rowan PR, Parker RR, et al: Response to phenelzine and amitriptyline in subtypes of outpatient depression. Arch Gen Psychiatry 1982; 39:1041-1049

Perris C: The course of depressive psychoses. Acta Psychiatr Scand 1968; 44:238-248

Perris C: Frequency and hereditary aspects of depression, in Depression: Behavioral, Biochemical, Diagnostic and Treatment Concepts. Edited by Gallant DM, Simpson GM. New York, Spectrum Publications, 1976

Pollitt J: Depression and Its Treatment. London, Heinemann, 1965

Prange AJ, Loosen PT: Some endocrine aspects of affective disorders. J Clin Psychiatry 1980; 41:29-34

Price LH, Conwell Y, Nelson JC: Lithium augmentation of combined neuroleptic-tricyclic treatment in delusional depression. Am J Psychiatry 1983; 140:318-322

Prien RF, Caffey EM: Long-term maintenance drug therapy in recurrent affective illness: current status and issues. Diseases of the Nervous System 1977; 38:981-992

Prien RF, Kupfer DJ: Continuation drug therapy for major depressive episodes: how long should it be maintained? Am J Psychiatry 1986; 143:18-23

Prien RF, Levine J: Research and methodological issues for evaluating the therapeutic effectiveness of antidepressant drugs. Psychopharmacol Bull 1984; 20:250-257

Prien RF, Klett CJ, Caffey EM: Lithium carbonate and imipramine in prevention of affective episodes. Arch Gen Psychiatry 1973; 29:420-425

Prien RF, Kupfer DJ, Mansky PA, et al: Drug therapy in the prevention of recurrences in unipolar and bipolar affective disorders. Arch Gen Psychiatry 1984; 41:1096-1104

Prusoff BA, Weissman MM, Klerman GL, et al: Research Diagnostic Criteria subtypes of depression: their role as predictors of differential response to psychotherapy and drug treatment. Arch Gen Psychiatry 1980; 37:796-801

Quitkin FM, Rifkin A, Klien DF: Prophylaxis of affective disorders. Arch Gen Psychiatry 1976; 33:337-341

Quitkin FM, Rifkin A, Klein DF: Imipramine response in deluded depressive patients. Am J Psychiatry 1978; 135:806-811

Quitkin FM, Liebowitz MR, Stewart JW, et al: Deprenyl in atypical depressives. Arch Gen Psychiatry 1984; 41:777-781

Rabkin JG, Klein DF, Quitkin FM: Somatic treatment of acute depression, in Schizophrenia and Affective Disorders. Edited by Rifkin A. Boston, John Wright PSG Inc., 1983

Ravaris CL, Nies A, Robinson DS, et al: A multiple-dose controlled study of phenelzine in depression-anxiety states. Arch Gen Psychiatry 1976; 33:347-350

Ravaris CL, Robinson DS, Ives JO, et al: Phenelzine and amitriptyline in the treatment of depression. Arch Gen Psychiatry 1980; 37:1075-1080

Remick RA, Barton JS, Patterson B, et al: On so-called treatment resistant depression. Reported in Ayd, FJ: Treatment-resistant depression. International Drug Therapy Newsletter 1983; 18:25-27

Robins LN, Helzer JE, Weissman MM, et al: Lifetime prevalence of specific psychiatric disorders in three sites. Arch Gen Psychiatry 1984; 41:949-958

Robinson DS, Corcella J, Feighner JP, et al: A comparison of trazodone, amoxapine and maprotiline in the treatment of endogenous depression: results of a multicenter study. Current Therapeutic Research 1984; 35:549-560

Robinson DS, Kayser A, Corcella J, et al: Panic attacks in outpatients with depression: Response to antidepressant treatment. Psychopharmacol Bull 1985; 21:562-567

Rounsaville BJ, Sholomskas D, Prusoff BA: Chronic mood disorders in depressed outpatients. J Affective Disord 1980; 2:73-88

Schatzberg AF, Cole JO, Cohen BM, et al: Survey of depressed patients who have failed to respond to treatment, in The Affective Disorders. Edited by Davis JM, Maas JW. Washington, DC, American Psychiatric Press, 1983

Seager CP, Bird R: Imipramine with electrical treatment in depression—a controlled trial. Journal of Mental Science 1962; 108:704-707

Shaw DM: The practical management of affective disorders. Br J Psychiatry 1977; 130:432-451

Shaw E: Lithium noncompliance. Psychiatry Annals 1986; 16:583-587

Siris SG, Rifkin A: Side effects of drugs used in the treatment of affective disorders, in Schizophrenia and Affective Disorders. Biology and Drug Treatment. Edited by Rifkin A. Littleton, MA, John Wright PSG, 1983

Spiker DG, Perel JM, Hanin I, et al: The pharmacological treatment of delusional depression, part II. J Clin Psychopharmacol 1986; 6:339-342

Spitzer RL, Endicott J, Robins E: Research Diagnostic Criteria: rationale and reliability. Arch Gen Psychiatry 1978; 35:773-782

Thase ME, Frank E, Kupfer DJ: Biological processes in major depression, in The Handbook of Depression: Treatment, Assessment, and Research. Edited by Beckham EE, Leber WR. Homewood IL, Dosey Press, 1985

Tyrer PJ, Lee I, Edwards JG, et al: Prognostic factors determining response to antidepressant drugs in psychiatric outpatients and general practice. J Affective Disord 1980; 2:149-156

Weissman MM: Epidemiological Catchment Area Program Results on Dysthymic Disorder. Presented at the NIMH Workshop on Dysthymic Disorder. Washington, DC, July 1986

Weissman MM, Akiskal HS: the role of psychotherapy in chronic depressions: a proposal. Compr Psychiatry 1984; 25:23-31

Weissman MM, Klerman GL: The chronic depressive in the community: under-recognized and poorly treated. Compr Psychiatry 1977; 18:523-531

West ED, Dally PJ: Effects of iproniazid on depressed syndromes. Br Med J 1959; 1:1491-1497

Zisook S, Braff DL, Click MA, et al: Monoamine oxidase inhibitors in the treatment of atypical depression. J Clin Psychopharmacol 1985; 5:131-140

Chapter 11

Psychotherapeutic Treatment of Depression

by M. Tracie Shea, Ph.D., Irene Elkin, Ph.D., and Robert M.A. Hirschfeld, M.D.

There have been considerable advances in the treatment of depression over the past 30 years. The first major developments were in psychopharmacological treatment, with the discovery of monoamine oxidase inhibitors (MAOIs) and tricyclic antidepressants (TCAs). Numerous controlled clinical trials have since demonstrated the efficacy of these somatic treatments. The past 15 years have been characterized by advances in psychotherapeutic approaches to treating depression. These developments mark a notable change in the philosophy and application of psychotherapeutic approaches in the treatment of mental disorders, which have traditionally been nonspecific with regard to symptoms or disorders. These more recent treatments have been developed or modified specifically for the treatment of depression; this is reflected in the theory, rationale, strategies, techniques, and goals of each. And like the pharmacological treatments, there is increasing evidence of their effectiveness through controlled studies.

Given the established efficacy of medication in the treatment of depression, the question of the need for or appropriateness of psychosocial treatments is sometimes raised. There are several reasons why these treatments are important as alternative or adjunctive treatments. First, some depressed patients do not respond at all to medication, and others show only a partial response. Although it is not clear whether failures with medication will be successes with psychotherapy, alternative forms of treatment for nonresponders are necessary. Second, a substantial number of patients who do respond to medication develop new episodes within the first year or two following treatment (Klerman, 1978), indicating the need for a more prophylactic treatment. Third, some patients cannot take antidepressants because of medical contraindications or because of intolerance to side effects. Also to be considered is the preference of the patient; some do not want to take medication. Finally, these treatments may be beneficial as adjuncts to treatment with medication. In this context they may be viewed as important in increasing compliance with the medication, in restoring morale, and/or in dealing more directly with certain aspects of the patient's life, such as marital, parental, or work functioning, which may be disturbed as a result of the depression or its sequelae.

This chapter will provide an overview of empirical evidence to date for three prominent psychotherapeutic treatment approaches which have been developed for the treatment of nonbipolar, nonpsychotic depression. These are cognitive therapy, behavior therapy, and interpersonal therapy. Psychodynamic approaches, although not specific either in development or in application for the treatment of depression, have sometimes been included as comparison conditions in studies investigating the more specific psychotherapies. While this approach has not yet been systematically studied, findings from such comparison conditions are reported. The questions addressed are: 1) Are these treatments effective? 2) Do they differ in effectiveness, either in eliminating depressive symptoms, or in specific, targeted domains of functioning? 3) Do these treatments have enduring effects, beyond recovery from the current episode of depression? And 4) Are there advantages in using a combination of psychotherapy and pharmacotherapy in treating depression? Studies included meet at least minimal scientific standards, with random assignment to treatment and adequately defined samples of depressed patients.

DESCRIPTION OF THE TREATMENTS

Cognitive, behavioral, and interpersonal therapy, while distinct approaches, have certain features in common. They were all developed as short-term treatments, generally ranging from 12 to 20 sessions over a period of 12 to 16 weeks, although in practice they may continue for longer durations. They are structured treatments, characterized by an active approach on the part of the therapist and by active collaboration between therapist and patient. Usually there is an emphasis on current issues and functioning. Detailed description of treatment rationales, strategies, and techniques are available in treatment manuals for each approach.

Cognitive Therapy

Cognitive therapy, developed by Aaron T. Beck and his colleagues (Beck et al, 1979), is based on the theory that faulty cognitions or patterns of thinking underlie the depressive syndrome and that associated features of depression, including affective and physical changes, are consequences of the cognitive dysfunctions. The thinking of a depressed person is described in terms of the cognitive triad, which consists of unrealistically negative views of the self, the world, and the future. These cognitions are based on relatively stable attitudes or assumptions (schemas) developed from previous experiences. The techniques of cognitive therapy are designed to identify, reality-test, and correct the distorted cognitions and underlying schemas. The goal is to alleviate the depression and to prevent its recurrence by changing the way the patient thinks. Behavioral techniques may also be used to increase the patient's activity level, particularly during the initial phase of treatment when the depression may make it difficult for the patient to engage directly in cognitive tasks.

Behavioral Approaches

The behavioral approach to depression was introduced by Ferster's proposal that depression is caused by a loss of positive reinforcement (Ferster, 1965). This loss of the usual supply of reinforcement, which may be due to events such as separation, death, or sudden environmental change, is believed to result in reduction of the entire behavioral repertoire, and to produce depressed behaviors and dysphoric feelings. Several specific behavior therapies have been developed for the treatment of depression which vary in focus and emphasis, and in frequency of use of specific techniques. There is, however, considerable overlap among these approaches, which have certain assumptions and strategies in common. For example, all view the principle of reinforcement as a crucial element in depression, and all consider changing behavior to be the most effective way to alleviate depression. Two prominent behavioral approaches include Lewinsohn's approach (Lewinsohn et al, 1980) and Rehm's self-control therapy (Rehm, 1977; Fuchs and Rehm, 1977). Lewinsohn's approach focuses on the quality and quantity of the patient's interaction with the environment, with techniques designed to increase positive and decrease negative interactions and activities. Rehm's self-control model emphasizes the importance of self-administered reinforcement and punishment, proposing that depressed persons focus on negative aspects of their experience, set unrealistically high standards for themselves, and provide themselves with too little self-reinforcement and too much self-punishment. Strategies are designed to correct such deficits in self-monitoring, self-evaluation, and self-reinforcement.

Interpersonal Therapy

Interpersonal therapy, developed by Klerman, Weissman, and associates (Klerman et al, 1984), is based on the assumption that depression occurs in an interpersonal context. Interpersonal difficulties are viewed as a possible cause and/or consequence of depression, with etiology differing among individual patients. Strategies are thus designed to help the patient deal more effectively with current interpersonal problems and to improve social functioning. While the roots of interpersonal therapy are largely psychodynamic, there are important differences. The focus of interpersonal therapy is on current interpersonal issues, and not on early developmental experiences or intrapsychic factors such as defense mechanisms or unconscious conflicts. The treatment aims at mastery of interpersonal situations, with no attempt at personality reconstruction. Examples of techniques include clarification (restructuring and feeding back the patient's communication); encouragement of affect (helping the patient to recognize and accept painful affects, and to express suppressed affects); and communication analysis (identifying maladaptive communication patterns and increasing effective communication). While the focus of interpersonal therapy tends to be on current relationships outside of the therapy, in the absence of meaningful current or past relationships in the life of the patient, the therapeutic relationship may be used as a model of the patient's interactions with others.

Psychodynamic Therapy

While psychodynamic therapies have not been developed specifically for the treatment of depression, this approach in practice is a widely used intervention for depressed patients. In recent years, several short-term approaches characterized by common psychodynamic concepts have been developed, which may be applicable to the treatment of depression. These include approaches developed by Malan (1976, 1979), Davanloo (1980), and Sifneos (1979), among others. More recently, Strupp and Binder (1984) and Luborsky (1984) have developed treatment manuals for time-limited psychodynamic approaches. In general, the goals of a psychodynamic treatment approach are to change personality structure or character, and not simply to alleviate symptoms, which are viewed as the result of unconscious conflicts. Most of the time-limited approaches are characterized by identification and emphasis on a single focal issue, or "dynamic focus." A particular issue, usually interpersonal, is selected and used as a micro-cosm for long-lasting, unconscious conflicts in the patient's life. The transference relationship is a key feature in all of these approaches. The transference refers to thoughts, feelings, or behaviors of the patient toward the therapist that are unrealistic or inappropriate in the current therapeutic situation; these are used to identify and reexperience problems and patterns that developed in important relationships early in life. Certain criteria for patient selection are advocated for many of these short-term psychodynamic approaches. These include ability to tolerate anxiety and frustration, flexibility, motivation for change, and a capacity for meaningful relationships.

EFFICACY

Studies have varied in approach to investigating the efficacy of psychosocial treatments. One approach is to include an antidepressant drug treatment as a comparison condition. The efficacy of these drugs, usually tricyclic antidepressants such as amitriptyline or imipramine, has been established in numerous placebo-controlled clinical trials. Findings of no significant differences between a psychosocial treatment and an antidepressant drug of established efficacy are generally considered as evidence for *relative* efficacy, assuming the sample size is large enough to provide adequate power (that is, a sufficiently high probability of finding true treatment differences when they exist). A finding of significant superiority of the psychosocial treatment compared to the drug is, of course, also considered as evidence of efficacy. Another method used to demonstrate efficacy is to compare the treatment with a control condition, although this approach is complicated by the difficulty of defining an adequate control treatment for psychosocial treatments (Parloff, 1986).

Table 1 summarizes results from seven studies comparing one or more psychotherapeutic treatments with an antidepressant drug comparison condition. There are a total of 10 comparisons across the seven studies. Three of these showed superiority of the psychotherapy (two cognitive therapy and one behavioral) compared to the drug, and six comparisons (four cognitive therapy and two interpersonal therapy) showed no significant differences between the psychotherapy and the drug. Only one comparison found the drug to be superior; this was in comparison with an insight-oriented psychotherapy condition.

In Table 2, findings from 10 studies including some form of control condition are summarized. In the majority of studies, the control is a waiting list or delayed treatment condition. Other control conditions include attention assessment, pill-placebo plus clinical management, relaxation training, and nonscheduled treatment. Since these latter conditions control for at least some of the "nonspecific" effects of treatment, such as attention and perhaps some expectation of improvement, they are likely to provide more stringent tests of effectiveness. Out of a total of 18 comparisons across the 10 studies, 15 showed the psychotherapy to be significantly superior to the control condition. The three exceptions were the findings of no differences between a behavioral group treatment and attention assessment control (Shaw, 1977), and between cognitive therapy and placebo plus clinical management (Elkin et al, 1986), and the finding of superiority of the control (relaxation training) condition compared to an insight-oriented psychotherapy condition (McLean and Hakstian, 1979). It is interesting to note that each of the three comparisons failing to show superiority of the psychotherapy included more "active" control conditions. This is particularly true for the NIMH Collaborative Study (Elkin et al, 1986), where the placebo plus clinical management condition served as a control both for expectations due to administration of a drug and for contact with a caring, supportive therapist (Elkin et al, 1985).

In summary, there is a fair amount of evidence that these defined psychotherapeutic treatments are efficacious in the treatment of outpatient depression. Considering the above findings by treatment approach, there is evidence of efficacy for cognitive therapy and for behavioral treatments. There is also some evidence for the effectiveness of interpersonal therapy, although this approach has been investigated in fewer studies. With regard to psychodynamic therapy, the sparse findings are mixed and should be interpreted cautiously. In no study has this approach been the focus of investigation, and in general the psychodynamic conditions are characterized by less standardization and more heterogeneity of procedures than cognitive therapy, interpersonal therapy, and behavioral therapy.

DIFFERENTIAL AND SPECIFIC EFFECTS

A more complicated and difficult question than *whether* a treatment is effective is *why* it is so. Each of the three treatment approaches with demonstrated efficacy (cognitive therapy, behavioral therapy, and interpersonal therapy) are based on different theories of depression, and are characterized by distinct strategies that address different psychological domains based on the respective theory's understanding of etiology. The fact that treatment approaches with different techniques and different "active" ingredients are effective demonstrates that no single theory is uniquely accurate and that no treatment approach is uniquely effective. A question of interest is whether these treatments are differentially effective in eliminating depressive symptomatology.

Of 14 studies including comparisons of 2 or more distinct psychotherapeutic treatments, 8 found no significant differences in outcome between the psychotherapeutic approaches studied (Comas-Diaz, 1981; Wilson et al, 1983; Gallagher and Thompson, 1982; Thompson and Gallagher, 1984; Elkin et al, 1986; Gallagher, 1981; Hersen et al, 1984; Kornblith et al, 1983). Six studies did find at least some evidence of significant superiority of one psychotherapeutic approach (Shaw, 1977; Steuer et al, 1984; Covi and Lipman, 1987; McLean and Hakstian, 1979; Fuchs and Rehm, 1977; Fleming and Thornton, 1980). With the exception of Shaw (1977), however, who found group cognitive therapy to be superior to a behavioral group, the "inferior" treatments in these studies were less clearly defined and not the focus of the study (that is, "psychodynamic," "insight-oriented," "nonspecific" group, "nondirective"). Without much information regarding the content and delivery of these treatments, it is difficult to judge the adequacy of these conditions.

Five studies have included a comparison of different strategies within a single (behavioral) approach. Two of these (Rehm et al, 1979; Fleming and Thornton, 1980) did find one behavioral approach (self-control) to be superior to another behavioral approach (social skills and cognitive modification, respectively). The other three found no significant differences in outcome (Zeiss et al, 1979; Rehm

Table 1. Summary of Studies Comparing Psychotherapy and Drug Conditions

N^a	Weeks	Psychotherapy > Drug	No Differences	Psychotherapy < Drug	Results
41	12	Rush et al. (1977)			cognitive therapy > imipramine
64	12	Blackburn et al. (1981) (general practice patients)			cognitive therapy > tricyclic[2]
64	12		Blackburn et al. (1981) (psychiatric patients)		cognitive therapy and tricyclic[2]: no difference
70	12		Murphy et al. (1984)		cognitive therapy and nortriptyline: no difference
106	12		Hollon et al. (1986)		cognitive therapy and imipramine: no difference
239	16		Elkin et al. (1986)		cognitive therapy and imipramine: no difference[3]
178	10	McLean and Hakstian (1979)			behavior therapy > amitriptyline

Table 1. Summary of Studies Comparing Psychotherapy and Drug Conditions *(continued)*

N^1	Weeks	Psychotherapy > Drug	No Differences	Psychotherapy < Drug	Results
96	16		Weissman et al (1979)		interpersonal therapy and amitriptyline: no difference[4]
239	16		Elkin et al (1986)		Interpersonal therapy and imipramine: no difference[3]
178	10			McLean and Hakstian (1979)	insight < amitriptyline

[1]N = total number of subjects in study
[2]Doctor's choice of tricyclic medication
[3]No differences at termination, although imipramine was more rapid in effect
[4]Symptomatic failure as outcome

Table 2. Summary of Studies Comparing Psychotherapy with Control

N[1]	Weeks	Psychotherapy > Control	No Differences	Psychotherapy < Control	Control Condition
Cognitive					
32	4	Shaw (1977) (group)			1. attention assessment 2. waiting list assessment
26	4	Comas-Diaz (1981)[2]			waiting list assessment
25	8	Wilson et al (1983)[2]			no treatment
37	12	Thompson and Gallagher[3] (1984)			delayed treatment
239	16	Elkin et al (1986)			placebo + clinical management
Behavioral					
25	8	Wilson et al (1983)[2]			no treatment
63	8	Brown and Lewinsohn (1984)			delayed treatment
32	4	Shaw (1977) (group)			waiting list assessment
32	4		Shaw (1977) (group)		attention assessment
37	12	Thompson and Gallagher (1984)[3]			delayed treatment
178	10	McLean and Hakstian (1979)			relaxation training

Table 2. Summary of Studies Comparing Psychotherapy with Control *(continued)*

N[1]	Weeks	Psychotherapy > Control	No Differences	Psychotherapy < Control	Control Condition
28	6	Fuchs and Rehm (1977)[2]			waiting list
49	7	Rehm et al (1981)[2]			waiting list
Interpersonal					
96	16	Weissman et al[4] (1979)			nonscheduled treatment
239	16	Elkin et al[5]			placebo + clinical management
Psychodynamic					
37	12	Thompson and Gallagher (1984)[3]			delayed treatment
				McLean and Hakstian (1979)	relaxation therapy

[1]N = total number of subjects in study

[2]Volunteers

[3]Geriatric patients

[4]Symptomatic failure as outcome

[5]Recovery criterion as outcome

et al, 1981; Fleming and Thornton, 1980). Overall, the most consistent finding from these comparative studies of psychotherapeutic treatments is that comparisons of well-defined psychosocial treatments will yield comparable outcome in the treatment of depression.

Even if results of different treatments are similar with regard to improvement in depressive symptomatology, one might still predict differences in specific areas of functioning that are related to the distinctive rationales, strategies, and techniques of the various treatments. A number of studies have addressed this possibility. Five of these have reported results of investigations of possible treatment-specific or differential effects of cognitive therapy. In their study of cognitive therapy and imipramine, Rush and colleagues (1981) reported that cognitive symptoms and mood improved before vegetative and motivational symptoms for patients in cognitive therapy, while patients in the imipramine condition showed no consistent pattern in timing of specific symptom improvement. In a later article that reported results from the same study, the authors noted greater improvement in hopelessness, and a trend for more improvement in self-concept for cognitive therapy patients in comparison to imipramine patients (Rush et al, 1982). As these latter results parallel the general pattern of outcome findings reported in the original study (Rush et al, 1977), however, it is not clear to what extent these findings reflect specific, treatment-targeted effects versus the general effects of improvement. Blackburn and Bishop (1983) reported on target measures for two samples of depressed patients treated with cognitive therapy, antidepressant drugs, or a combination of cognitive therapy and antidepressant drugs. In both samples, changes in cognitive measures (views of self, world, and future) paralleled changes in mood and severity of depression, and the authors concluded that there was no evidence for specific effects, either at termination or throughout the course of treatment.

Simons and colleagues (1984) reported similar findings for comparisons of patients treated with cognitive therapy or nortriptyline. Patients in both conditions showed the same change on all measures, including cognitive measures, and in general, change in cognitive processes appeared to be more directly associated with clinical improvement than with the course of cognitive therapy. The authors concluded that cognitive change may more accurately be viewed as a part of improvement than as the primary cause of improvement.

A study including cognitive and behavioral treatments (Wilson et al, 1983) found that both of these treatments had a comparable impact at termination on treatment-related target areas, although cognitive therapy was superior to the behavioral treatment on some cognitive measures at the midpoint of treatment.

An investigation of specific effects of cognitive therapy in the NIMH Treatment of Depression Collaborative Research Program (Elkin et al, 1985; Imber et al, 1986) found cognitive therapy to be superior to imipramine and to interpersonal therapy on one of two factors (need for social approval) from the Dysfunctional Attitude Scale (DAS). There were no differences among any of the treatments on the other DAS factor (perfectionism), or on two secondary target measures for cognitive therapy at termination from treatment. Also, there were no differences in DAS total scores for cognitive therapy at earlier points (4, 8, or 12 weeks) in treatment (Watkins et al, 1986).

Three additional studies comparing behavioral treatments with another treatment approach have included results on measures tapping specific treatment-related domains. Two of these report some evidence of superiority of the behavioral treatment on measures of social skills, despite equivalent effects on depressive symptomatology. One study compared the behavioral treatment with supportive group therapy in a sample of elderly depressed patients (Gallagher, 1981); the other compared behavioral (social skills) conditions (combined with amitriptyline or placebo) with amitriptyline alone and dynamic therapy plus placebo conditions (Bellack et al, 1983). In contrast, McLean and Hakstian (1979) found little evidence for specificity of treatment effects. They reported that while their behavioral treatment was superior to amitriptyline on social measures, it was also superior on measures of mood. The drug was marginally better than insight psychotherapy on social outcome, a finding also similar in direction to overall outcome, and in the opposite direction of predicted specific effects. The authors interpret their findings as contrary to the specific effects hypothesis.

Three additional studies investigated possible differences in outcome on overall and target measures among specific strategies within behavioral approaches. Rehm and colleagues (1979) compared a self-control behavior treatment with a behavioral assertion training program. Assertion training subjects showed greater gains on social skill variables, while the self-control subjects improved more on self-control measures as well as on behavioral and self-report indices of depression. In contrast, Zeiss and associates (1979) found no differences on any target measures related to three behavioral strategy conditions, each with a distinct focus (social skills, cognitions, and increase in pleasant events). Similar findings of no differences on target measures were reported by Kornblith and co-workers (1983), who compared comprehensive self-control, self-monitoring plus self-evaluation, self-control principles without homework, and dynamic group therapy conditions.

Investigations of specific effects of interpersonal therapy have been reported from three separate studies. In one study of maintenance treatment, a factorial design was used with high contact psychotherapy (the forerunner of interpersonal therapy) and low contact psychotherapy, each crossed with amitriptyline, placebo, or no medication. The drug and the psychotherapy conditions did seem to have their strongest impact on different areas of functioning. Main effects for psychotherapy appeared after eight months of maintenance treatment on measures of social functioning (Weissman et al, 1974); in contrast, the drug conditions were more effective than the no-drug conditions in preventing relapse and symptom recurrence (Klerman et al, 1974; Paykel et al, 1975). These differential effects were no longer detectable, however, at one year following completion of the maintenance treatment (Weissman et al, 1976). In a separate study of acute treatment of outpatient depression, amitriptyline, interpersonal therapy, amitriptyline plus interpersonal therapy, and nonscheduled treatment were compared. Although not present at termination from treatment, main effects for interpersonal therapy on social functioning were found at one year following treatment (Weissman et al, 1981). In addition, there were differences in temporal pattern of symptom change. Main effects for interpersonal therapy on anxiety/depression and apathy were present early in treatment; for the drug, early main effects appeared for vegetative symptoms, particularly sleep (DiMascio et al, 1979).

Initial investigations from the NIMH Collaborative Study have found no evidence of specific effects for interpersonal therapy, either at termination from treatment (Imber et al, 1986) or at earlier evaluation points (Watkins et al, 1986).

In conclusion, while there is some suggestion of specific effects for behavior therapy and interpersonal therapy, particularly in the area of social functioning, and perhaps for cognitive therapy in self-concept and one aspect of dysfunctional attitudes, the majority of studies have yielded negative findings, at least when assessed at termination from treatment. It is possible that investigations very early in treatment (that is, before four weeks) or at later follow-up points might be more successful in uncovering specific effects. The only acute treatment study investigating this question at follow-up (Weissman et al, 1981) did find evidence of specific effects.

FOLLOW-UP STUDIES

Although the primary goals of the psychotherapeutic treatments described in the current chapter are to alleviate the symptoms of depression, the techniques and strategies of each are designed to help patients develop more effective coping mechanisms, enabling them to deal more effectively with their lives. Such benefits might be helpful in preventing the recurrence of depressive symptoms or future episodes of depression. Thus, compared to nonactive comparison or control conditions, or to time-limited pharmacotherapy, the psychotherapeutic treatments should result in more lasting effects.

Findings have been reported from six follow-up studies of cognitive therapy. In each, there has been at least some suggestion of long-term effectiveness. Kovacs and colleagues (1981) reported on the status of patients at one year following treatment with cognitive therapy or imipramine (Rush et al, 1977). Cognitive therapy patients were significantly less depressed on a self-report measure (Beck Depression Inventory) than were imipramine patients. Fifty-six percent of the cognitive therapy patients, compared to 35 percent of the imipramine patients, were in remission throughout the year; this difference was not statistically significant.

A one-year follow-up (Simons et al, 1986) of a study (Murphy et al, 1984) in which patients were treated with cognitive therapy, nortriptyline, cognitive therapy plus nortriptyline, or cognitive therapy plus placebo showed that of those patients who had responded to treatment, patients in the cognitive therapy conditions (with or without drug) had a significantly lower frequency of relapse (that is, return of symptoms within six months following treatment termination) than patients who received pharmacotherapy alone. In contrast, patients who had received medication had a significantly higher rate of relapse than those who had not received medication.

Blackburn and colleagues (1986) followed patients who responded to treatments with cognitive therapy alone, pharmacotherapy alone, or combined cognitive therapy and pharmacotherapy, for two years after treatment. For the first six months, patients received maintenance treatment (the same treatment received during the study, with the exception that cognitive therapy was reduced to one session every six weeks). The rest of the follow-up period was naturalistic. A significantly greater number of the patients in the drug maintenance group relapsed during the six-month maintenance phase compared to the combined treatment group and to the two cognitive therapy groups considered together.

The proportion of patients becoming depressed again at any point during the two-year follow-up (that is, relapse or recurrence) was significantly higher in the pharmacotherapy group than in either of the cognitive therapy groups.

Evans and colleagues (1985) also followed patients for two years following response to 12 weeks of acute treatment. Patients in this study were treated with cognitive therapy, imipramine with posttreatment maintenance (throughout the entire follow-up phase), imipramine without maintenance, or cognitive therapy plus imipramine without maintenance (Hollon et al, 1986, unpublished manuscript). Patients in the two cognitive therapy conditions were combined with patients in the imipramine with maintenance condition and compared with patients in the imipramine without maintenance condition. This combined group of treatment responders had significantly lower rates of relapse/recurrence (that is, return of symptoms at any point in the two years following treatment termination), compared to the responders in the imipramine without maintenance condition.

In a nine-month follow-up study of patients treated with group cognitive therapy, group cognitive therapy plus imipramine, or traditional dynamic group therapy, Covi and associates (1987) found patients in the two cognitive therapy conditions to be doing significantly better at the time of follow-up than patients in the traditional group treatment. Finally, Gallagher and Thompson (1982) followed elderly depressed patients for one year after completion of treatment with cognitive therapy, behavior therapy, or insight therapy. Although there were no differences at termination, cognitive therapy and behavior therapy patients were significantly less depressed at the time of follow-up than insight therapy patients on self-report and clinician-rated measures of depression. One out of the nine patients (11 percent) in each of the cognitive therapy and the behavior therapy conditions was diagnosed as currently in an episode of major depression, compared to four of nine patients (44 percent) for the insight condition. This difference was not statistically significant.

Two follow-up reports are available for interpersonal therapy. One reported on the status of patients one year following completion of eight months of maintenance treatment with high or low contact psychotherapy, each combined with either amitriptyline, placebo, or no pill (Weissman et al, 1976). There were no main effects for interpersonal therapy or the medication on clinical status or any aspect of social functioning. One consideration, as the authors note, is that the patients were initially treated with drugs alone, and only drug responders were included in the maintenance study. A different finding was reported from a one-year follow-up of patients receiving acute treatment of interpersonal therapy alone, interpersonal therapy combined with amitriptyline, amitriptyline alone, or nonscheduled treatment. While there were no differential long-term effects of the treatments on clinical status or symptoms throughout the follow-up period or at the time of follow-up, patients who received interpersonal therapy (with or without drugs) were significantly better on measures of social functioning at the one-year follow-up (Weissman et al, 1981)

COMBINED TREATMENT

Another important question concerns the possible advantage of combined psychotherapy and pharmacotherapy in the treatment of depression. The possible mechanisms of interaction of these two treatment modalities are numerous and complex, as is outlined by Klerman (1986) in his summary of issues involved in research on combined treatments. Here the focus will be on the following possible outcomes: no effect (the effects of combined treatment are no greater than the single treatment alone); positive effects (combined treatment is more effective than the individual treatment); and negative effects (combined treatment results in a poorer outcome than the individual treatment). Table 3 summarizes results of existing studies in terms of two questions: 1) Does the addition of psychotherapy to pharmacotherapy result in better outcome, compared to pharmacotherapy alone? and 2) Does the addition of pharmacotherapy to psychotherapy result in better outcome, compared to psychotherapy alone? Outcome considered here is related to symptoms of depression.

With regard to the first question, seven acute treatment studies and one maintenance treatment study have included comparisons of combined treatment and drug-alone conditions. Four of these have found the combination to be superior, while four studies found no differences between combined treatment and pharmacotherapy alone. Three out of four studies that included cognitive therapy found the combination to be superior to the drug alone (Blackburn et al, 1981; Teasdale et al, 1984; Hollon et al, 1986, unpublished manuscript); one (Murphy et al, 1984) reported no differences. One study of interpersonal therapy in the acute treatment of depression (Weissman et al, 1979) reported that rates of symptomatic failure were lower in the combined condition than in the drug-alone condition. The other interpersonal therapy study was of maintenance treatment, and reported no advantage of the combination compared to the drug alone in preventing symptom relapse (Klerman et al, 1974). Only one study has investigated the combination of a behavioral treatment with pharmacotherapy (Hersen et al, 1984); no differences were found between the combination and the drug-alone condition.

Eleven studies have made comparisons of combined treatment with a psychotherapy-alone condition (nine acute treatment and one maintenance treatment) or with psychotherapy plus placebo (acute treatment). Eight of these found no differences, two found the combination to be superior to the psychotherapy alone, and one (Blackburn et al, 1981) found the combination to be superior for a sample of psychiatric outpatients, but not for a separate sample of general practice patients. Cognitive therapy again was the most frequently studied psychotherapy. Of seven comparisons in six studies including cognitive therapy, two found the combination to be superior (Blackburn et al, 1981; Hollon et al, 1986, unpublished manuscript); the other five did not find significant differences. Of the two interpersonal therapy studies, the acute treatment study found the combination to result in significantly lower rates of symptomatic failure compared to interpersonal therapy alone, while the maintenance study reported no differences in relapse rates (Klerman et al, 1974). Two studies of behavior therapy also reported no differences between combined treatment and behavior therapy alone (Roth et al, 1982; Wilson et al, 1982). In addition, Hersen and colleagues (1984) found no differences between a behavioral treatment plus placebo and the behavioral treatment combined with amitriptyline.

In summary, the current data do not provide strong support for an advantage of combined psychotherapy and pharmacotherapy over either modality alone, at least with regard to outcome of depressive symptoms. These findings should be interpreted with caution, however, as the sample sizes are frequently small, and thus may sometimes not provide the necessary sensitivity or power to detect possible real treatment differences, particularly since the comparison conditions (the single modalities) are themselves quite effective. A recent review of studies of combined psychotherapy and drug compared to single modalities in the treatment of nonpsychotic depressed outpatients (Conte et al, 1986) is relevant here. Based on findings from a meta-analysis approach that weighted studies in terms of quality of research design, these authors concluded that the combination of psychotherapy and pharmacotherapy is more effective than either drug or psychotherapy alone, but that the effect is a modest one. A second consideration concerns the possible advantage of combined treatment compared to psychotherapy alone in terms of rapidity of treatment effects, as there is some evidence that the beneficial effects of pharmacotherapy may become apparent earlier than the effects of psychotherapy (Watkins et al, 1986). Of the studies summarized here, two found combined treatment with behavioral therapy and pharmacotherapy to result in significantly more rapid improvement compared to the behavioral treatment alone (Roth et al, 1982; Wilson, 1982). Finally, most of the combined treatment studies restricted comparisons to measures of depression, and there are almost no data regarding other areas of outcome, such as social functioning. In the maintenance study of interpersonal therapy and amitriptyline cited earlier (Klerman et al, 1974), significant main effects for interpersonal therapy were shown on measures of social adjustment (Weissman et al, 1974), while main effects for amitriptyline were found on symptom measures (Paykel et al, 1975). Although these findings are not from direct comparisons of combined versus single modality treatments, considered together they suggest an advantage of combined treatment when a broader domain of outcome is considered.

SUMMARY AND COMMENT

Although the evidence suggests that the specific psychotherapeutic treatments are effective, we know little about *why* they are effective. Superiority of these treatments in comparison with delayed treatment or assessment controls rules out the influence of time or assessment alone in producing results; however, the absence of differential effectiveness in eliminating depression or in targeted domains of functioning prevents conclusions regarding the specific techniques as the "active" ingredients. This applies not only to studies of depression, but characterizes the field of psychotherapy outcome research as a whole (Smith et al, 1980; Luborsky et al, 1975). Two hypotheses are most frequently offered in explanation of these findings: 1) common or "nonspecific" factors are responsible for improvement; and 2) methodological limitations are responsible for the failure to find differential effects. Frank (1971) originally developed the common factors hypothesis, proposing that the specific content of various techniques or interventions is less important than the belief system, characterized by positive expectation and the reversal of demoralization, that they create. Frances and colleagues (1985) provide an extensive and critical review of the evidence for and against the specific effects position.

Here we will comment on one methodological factor that we believe is particularly important to consider in interpreting the evidence presented in this chap-

Table 3. Summary of Studies Including Comparisons of Combined Psychotherapy and Pharmacotherapy with Single Modalities[1]

N[2]	Number of Weeks	Drug	Psychotherapy	Combined versus Drug Alone (No. studies = 8)		Combined versus Psychotherapy Alone (No. studies = 11)	
				Combined > Drug Alone	No Differences: Combined versus Drug Alone	Combined > Psychotherapy Alone	No Differences: Combined versus Psychotherapy Alone
70	14	imipramine	cognitive therapy (group)				Covi and Lipman, 1987
64	12	tricyclic[3]	cognitive therapy	Blackburn et al (1981) (general practice and psychiatric patients)		Blackburn et al (1981) (psychiatric patients)	Blackburn et al (1981) (general practice patients)
70	12	nortriptyline	cognitive therapy		Murphy et al (1984)		Murphy et al (1984)
39	12	antidepressant[3]	cognitive therapy				Rush and Watkins (1981)
34	15	antidepressant[3]	cognitive therapy	Teasdale et al (1984)			
33	12	amitriptyline	cognitive therapy	Hollon et al (1986, unpublished manuscript)		Hollon et al[4] (1984, unpublished manuscript)	
106	12	imipramine	cognitive therapy				Beck et al (1985)

Table 3. Summary of Studies Including Comparisons of Combined Psychotherapy and Pharmacotherapy with Single Modalities[1] (*continued*)

N[2]	Number of Weeks	Drug	Psychotherapy	Combined versus Drug Alone (No. studies = 8)		Combined versus Psychotherapy Alone (No. studies = 11)	
				Combined > Drug Alone	No Differences: Combined versus Drug Alone	Combined > Psychotherapy Alone	No Differences: Combined versus Psychotherapy Alone
120	12	amitriptyline	behavior therapy		Hersen et al (1984)		Hersen et al (1984)[5]
26	12	desipramine	behavior therapy (group)				Roth et al (1982)[6,7]
64	8	amitriptyline	behavior therapy		Wilson (1982)		Wilson (1982)[5,6]
96	16	amitriptyline	interpersonal therapy	Weissman et al (1979)		Weissman et al (1979)	
150	32	amitriptyline	interpersonal therapy		Klerman et al (1974)[8]		Klerman et al (1974)[8]

[1]Outcome for depressive symptoms
[2]N = Total number of subjects in study
[3]Doctor's choice
[4]Trend
[5]Psychotherapy plus placebo
[6]Conditions equal at termination, although combined treatment more rapid in effect
[7]Volunteers
[8]Maintenance treatment

ter. This concerns sample size and the resulting power of the statistical tests (probability of finding a treatment difference if it exists). The strength of a conclusion of no difference rests directly upon the power of the study to detect such differences should they exist, yet it is not clear in most studies what the power is. This makes findings of no differences among different psychotherapeutic treatments difficult to interpret when sample sizes are small (as they are in many of the studies reviewed), since power is heavily dependent on sample size. The power and sample size issue becomes even more salient when the treatments being compared are both likely to result in change (Kazdin, 1986). The same point is relevant to investigations of relative efficacy in studies comparing psychotherapies with antidepressant drug conditions, and to studies of combined treatments compared with single modalities.

There are a number of other important questions that remain to be answered. While findings from existing follow-up studies, at least of cognitive therapy, are promising, more work is needed to determine whether these treatments have prophylactic effects, and to determine which patients are most vulnerable to relapse and recurrence. With a few exceptions (for example, Simons et al, 1985), little can be said about patient characteristics important to treatment response for any of these approaches. Similar to findings from pharmacotherapy studies, each of these treatments has a nonresponder rate of up to 20 to 30 percent of patients treated. We need to learn more about who these patients are, and how they can best be treated.

Very little is known about the role of psychotherapeutic treatments in dysthymic disorder, despite recent epidemiological reports of up to a four percent prevalence rate for women (Robins et al, 1984). There are no completed controlled studies focusing exclusively on this disorder, although one study of social skills training is now in progress (Becker and Heimberg, unpublished manuscript).

Finally, controlled studies of psychodynamic therapy in the treatment of outpatient depression are needed. This approach requires the same systematic and careful study that has been applied to the more recently developed treatments, particularly given the widespread use of psychodynamic approaches in clinical practice.

REFERENCES

Beck AT, Rush AJ, Shaw BF, et al: Cognitive therapy of depression. New York, Guilford Press, 1979

Beck AT, Hollon SD, Young JE, et al: Treatment of depression with cognitive therapy and amitriptyline. Arch Gen Psychiatry 1985; 42:142-148

Bellack AS, Herson M, Himmelhoch JM: A comparison of social-skills training, pharmacotherapy and psychotherapy for depression. Behav Res Ther 1983; 21:101-107

Blackburn IM, Bishop S: Changes in cognition with pharmacotherapy and cognitive therapy. Br J Psychiatry 1983; 143:609-617

Blackburn IM, Bishop S, Glen AIM, et al: The efficacy of cognitive therapy in depression: a treatment trial using cognitive therapy and pharmacotherapy, each alone and in combination. Br J Psychiatry 1981; 139:181-189

Blackburn IM, Eunson KM, Bishop S: A two-year naturalistic follow-up of depressed patients treated with cognitive therapy, pharmacotherapy and a combination of both. J Affective Disord 1986; 10:67-75

Brown RA, Lewinsohn PM: A psychoeducational approach to the treatment of depression:

comparison of group, individual and minimal contact procedures. J Consult Clin Psychol 1984; 52:774-783

Comas-Diaz L: Effects of cognitive and behavioral group treatment on the depressive symptomatology of Puerto Rican women. J Consult Clin Psychol 1981; 49:627-632

Conte HR, Plutchik R, Wild KV, et al: Combined psychotherapy and pharmacotherapy for depression. Arch Gen Psychiatry 1986; 43:471-479

Covi L, Lipman RS: Cognitive behavioral group psychotherapy combined with imipramine in major depression: a pilot study. Psychopharmacol Bull 1987; 23:173-176

Davanloo H: Short-term dynamic psychotherapy, vol. 1. New York, Jason Arenson, 1980

DiMascio A, Weissman MM, Prusoff BA, et al: Differential symptom reduction by drugs and psychotherapy in acute depression. Arch Gen Psychiatry 1979; 36:1450-1456

Elkin I, Parloff MB, Hadley SW, et al: NIMH Treatment of Depression Collaborative Research Program: background and research plan. Arch Gen Psychiatry 1985; 42:305-316

Elkin I, Shea MT, Watkins J, et al: NIMH Treatment of Depression Collaborative Research Program: major outcome findings. Paper presented at the 129th Annual Meeting of the American Psychiatric Association, Washington, DC, May 1986

Evans MD, Hollon SD, DeRubeis RJ, et al: Accounting for relapse in a treatment outcome study of depression. Paper presented at the annual meeting of the Association for the Advancement of Behavior Therapy, November 1985

Ferster CB: Classification of behavioral pathology, in Research in Behavior Modification. Edited by Krasner L, Ullmann LP. New York, Holt, Rinehart and Winston, 1965

Ferster CB: A functional analysis of depression. Am Psychol 1973; 10:857-870

Fleming BM, Thornton DW: Coping skills training as a component in the short-term treatment of depression. J Consult Clin Psychol 1980; 48:652-654

Frances A, Sweeney J, Clarkin J: Do psychotherapies have specific effects? Am J Psychother 1985; 39:159-174

Frank JD: Therapeutic factors in psychotherapy. Am J Psychother 1971; 25:350-361

Fuchs CZ, Rehm LP: A self-control behavior therapy program for depression. J Consult Clin Psychol 1977; 45:206-215

Gallagher DE: Behavioral group therapy with elderly depressives: an experimental study, in Behavioral Group Therapy, vol 3. Edited by Upper D, Ross S. Champaign, IL, Research Press, 1981

Gallagher DE, Thompson LW: Treatment of major depressive disorder in older adult outpatients with brief psychotherapies. Psychotherapy: Theory, Research and Practice 1982; 19:482-490

Hersen M, Bellack AS, Himmelhoch JM, et al: Effects of social skills training, amitriptyline, and psychotherapy in unipolar depressed women. Behav Ther 1984; 15:21-40

Imber SD, Pilkonis PA, Sotsky SM, et al: The differential effects of three brief treatments for major depression: interpersonal therapy, cognitive behavior therapy and pharmacotherapy. Paper presented at the 139th Annual Meeting of the American Psychiatric Association, Washington, DC, May 1986

Kazdin AE: Comparative outcome studies of psychotherapy: methodological issues and strategies. J Consult Clin Psychol 1986; 54:95-105

Klerman GL: Long-term treatment of affective disorders, in Psychopharmacology: A Generation of Progress. Edited by Lipton MA, DiMascio A, Killam KF. New York, Raven Press, 1978

Klerman GL: Drugs and psychotherapy, in Handbook of Psychotherapy and Behavior Change: An Empirical Analysis, second edition. Edited by Garfield SL, Bergin AE. New York, Wiley, 1986

Klerman GL, DiMascio A, Weissman MM, et al: Treatment of depression by drugs and psychotherapy. Am J Psychiatry 1974; 131:186-191

Klerman GL, Weissman MM, Rounsaville BJ, et al: Interpersonal Psychotherapy of Depression. New York, Basic Books, 1984

Kornblith SJ, Rehm LP, O'Hara MW, et al: The contribution of self-reinforcement training and behavioral assignments to the efficacy of self-control therapy for depression. Cognitive Therapy Research 1983; 6:499-528

Kovacs M, Rush AJ, Beck AT, et al: Depressed outpatients treated with cognitive therapy or pharmacotherapy: a one-year follow-up. Arch Gen Psychiatry 1981; 38:33-38

Lewinsohn PM, Sullivan JM, Grosscup SJ: Changing reinforcing events: an approach to the treatment of depression. Psychotherapy: Theory, Research and Practice 1980; 17:322-334

Luborsky L: Principles of Psychoanalytic Psychotherapy. New York, Basic Books, 1984

Luborsky L, Singer B, Luborsky L: Comparative studies of psychotherapies: is it true that everyone has won and all must have prizes? Arch Gen Psychiatry 1975; 32:995-1008

Malan DH: The Frontier of Brief Psychotherapy. New York, Plenum Press, 1976

Malan DH: Individual Psychotherapy and the Science of Psychodynamics. London, Butterworths, 1979

McLean PD, Hakstian AR: Clinical depression: comparative efficacy of outpatient treatments. J Consult Clin Psychol 1979; 47:818-836

Murphy GE, Simons AD, Wetzel RD, et al: Cognitive therapy and pharmacotherapy: singly and together in the treatment of depression. Arch Gen Psychiatry 1984; 41:33-41

Parloff MB: Placebo controls in psychotherapy research: a sine qua non or a placebo for research problems? J Consult Clin Psychol 1986; 54:79-87

Paykel ES, DiMascio A, Haskell D, et al: Effects of maintenance amitriptyline and psychotherapy on symptoms of depression. Psychol Med 1975; 5:67-77

Rehm LP: A self-control model of depression. Behavior Therapy 1977; 8:787-804

Rehm LP, Fuchs CZ, Roth DM, et al: A comparison of self-control and assertion skills treatments of depression. Behavior Therapy 1979; 10:429-442

Rehm LP, Kornblith SJ, O'Hara MW, et al: An evaluation of major components in a self-control behavior therapy program for depression. Behav Modif 1981; 5:459-490

Robins LN, Helzer JE, Weissman MM, et al: Lifetime prevalence of specific psychiatric disorders in three sites. Arch Gen Psychiatry 1984; 41:949-958

Roth D, Bielski R, Jones M, et al: A comparison of self-control therapy and combined self-control therapy and antidepressant medication in the treatment of depression. Behavior Therapy 1982; 13:133-144

Rush AJ, Watkins JT: Group versus individual cognitive therapy: a pilot study. Cognitive Therapy Research 1981; 5:95-104

Rush AJ, Beck AT, Kovacs M, et al: Comparative efficacy of cognitive therapy and pharmacotherapy in the treatment of depressed outpatients. Cognitive Therapy Research 1977; 1:17-37

Rush AJ, Kovacs M, Beck AT, et al: Differential effects of cognitive therapy and pharmacotherapy on depressive symptoms. J Affective Disord 1981; 3:221-229

Rush AJ, Beck AT, Kovacs M, et al: Comparison of the effects of cognitive therapy and pharmacotherapy on hopelessness and self-concept. Am J Psychiatry 1982; 139:862-866

Shaw BF: Comparison of cognitive therapy and behavior therapy in the treatment of depression. J Consult Clin Psychol 1977; 45:543-551

Sifneos PE: Short-term Dynamic Psychotherapy Evaluation and Technique. New York, Plenum, 1979

Simons AD, Garfield SL, Murphy GE: The process of change in cognitive therapy and pharmacotherapy for depression. Arch Gen Psychiatry 1984; 41:45-51

Simons AD, Lustman PJ, Wetzel RD, et al: Predicting response to cognitive therapy of depression: the role of learned resourcefulness. Cognitive Therapy Research 1985; 9:79-89

Simons AD, Murphy GE, Levine FL, et al: Cognitive therapy and pharmacotherapy for depression: sustained improvement over one year. Arch Gen Psychiatry 1986; 43:43-48

Smith ML, Glass G, Miller T: The Benefits of Psychotherapy. Baltimore, Johns Hopkins University Press, 1980

Steuer JL, Mintz J, Hammen CL, et al: Cognitive-behavioral and psychodynamic group psychotherapy in treatment of geriatric depression. J Consult Clin Psychol 1984; 52:180-189

Strupp HH, Binder JL: Psychotherapy in a New Key. New York, Basic Books, 1984

Teasdale JD, Fennell MJV, Hibbert GA, et al: Cognitive therapy for major depressive disorder in primary care. Br J Psychiatry 1984; 144:400-406

Thompson LW, Gallagher DE: Efficacy of psychotherapy in the treatment of late-life depression. Advances in Behavior Research Therapy 1984; 6:127-139

Watkins JT, Leber UR, Imber SI, et al: Temporal course of symptomatic change. Paper presented at the 139th Annual Meeting of the American Psychiatric Association, Washington DC, May 1986

Weissman MM, Klerman GL, Paykel ES, et al: Treatment effects on the social adjustment of depressed patients. Arch Gen Psychiatry 1974; 30:771-778

Weissman MM, Kasl SV, Klerman GL: Follow-up of depressed women after maintenance treatment. Am J Psychiatry 1976; 133:757-760

Weissman MM, Prusoff BA, DiMascio A, et al: The efficacy of drugs and psychotherapy in the treatment of acute depressive episodes. Am J Psychiatry 1979; 136:555-558

Weissman MM, Klerman GL, Prusoff BA, et al: Depressed outpatients: results one year after treatment with drugs and/or interpersonal psychotherapy. Arch Gen Psychiatry 1981; 38:51-55

Wilson PH: Combined pharmacological and behavioural treatment of depression. Behav Res Ther 1982; 20:173-184

Wilson PH, Goldin JC, Charbonneau-Powis M: Comparative effects of behavioral and cognitive treatments of depression. Cognitive Therapy Research 1983; 7:111-124

Zeiss AM, Lewinsohn PM, Munoz RF: Nonspecific improvement effects in depression using interpersonal, cognitive, and pleasant events focused treatments. J Consult Clin Psychol 1979; 47:427-439

Chapter 12

Depression Secondary to Medical Illness

by Edwin H. Cassem, M.D.

By definition, depression is secondary to medical illness when it appears after the medical illness has been diagnosed. The distinction between primary and secondary affective disorder arose at Washington University in St. Louis in the 1950s as a result of the work of Robins, Guze, and Winokur (Clayton and Lewis, 1981). Although medical illnesses were considered by Robins and colleagues, their major interest focused on secondary affective disorder that arose after another psychiatric disorder had been diagnosed. Although secondary affective disorder has not been as studied as primary affective disorder, some consistent generalizations have emerged from the literature.

DEPRESSION SECONDARY TO PSYCHIATRIC DISORDERS

The symptom picture in secondary depression (depression secondary to another *psychiatric* disorder) is clinically indistinguishable from that of primary depression—the insomnia, anhedonia, psychomotor, and other symptoms look to the examiner the way they look in primary depression. Moreover, the syndrome of secondary depression is common. In general, in every five patients with a diagnosis of depression, two have a secondary depression. How do these patients differ from primary depressed patients? The secondary depressive patient is more likely to be younger at the time of study, with an earlier onset of depression, and more likely to be male. The most likely primary diagnosis is alcoholism, with hysteria, sociopathy, drug abuse, and anxiety neurosis also common preexisting syndromes. There is more likely to be a family history of alcoholism. Weissman and colleagues (1977) found the symptom patterns of primary and secondary depressives to be similar, although the secondary group's symptoms were less severe. It was initially believed that biological markers could distinguish primary from secondary depressives; but when secondary depressives were matched with primary depressives for age and severity, sleep electroencephalogram (EEG) measurements revealed decreased rapid eye movement (REM) latency and increased REM density to be present in both groups (Thase et al, 1984).

DEPRESSIONS ARISING IN THE MEDICALLY ILL

What, then, of the depression that arises in the presence or aftermath of a serious or life-threatening illness? Klerman (1981) was a strong advocate for the retention of a diagnositc category for depression secondary to serious medical illness. With Krauthammer (1978) he established secondary mania as an important clinical entity among medically ill patients. Interest in major depression among medical patients has increased greatly in recent years, but much less is known about it than about depression secondary to other psychiatric disorders. In a recent review, Rodin and Voshart (1986) ascribed the lack of progress to unclear definitions of depression, absence of standardized assessment measures, sample selection bias, hererogeneity of subjects, and absence of appropriate control groups. A lucid, comprehensive, and practical review by Cohen-Cole and Stoudemire (1987) provides essentially state-of-the-art information on diagnosis and biological treatment of major depression in the medically ill.

Epidemiology

No adequate prevalence studies of depression secondary to medical illness have been done. Depression is often seen in general medical practice, and studies estimate that of all medical inpatients, between 20 and 32 percent show at least mild depression (Stewart et al, 1965; Schwab et al, 1967; Moffic and Paykel, 1975; Cavanagh, 1984).

Kathol and Petty (1981) reviewed five studies of depression in medical illness, concluding that an association exists but that the existing research has inadequately described family incidence, course of the disease, and response to treatment.

One difficulty with the prevalence estimates is that in most studies the diagnosis of depression has been based on a rating scale such as the Beck Depression Inventory (BDI) or the Hamilton Depression Scale (HAM-D). As a clinical diagnosis, major depression requires a psychiatric examination, with application of Research Diagnostic Criteria (RDC) or *Diagnostic and Statistical Manual of Mental Disorders, Third Edition, Revised (DSM-III-R)* (American Psychiatric Association, 1987) criteria.

Another way to estimate overall prevalence is to look at studies that have focused on specific subpopulations of the medically ill. Among patients hospitalized with cancer, for example, in a multicenter study, *Diagnostic and Statistical Manual of Mental Disorders, Third Edition (DSM-III)* (American Psychiatric Association, 1980) major depression was found in approximately 20 percent (Derogatis et al, 1983). In a random sample of 62 hospitalized cancer patients, Bukberg and colleagues (1984) found a higher percentage (42 percent) who met standard *DSM-III* criteria for major depression; although when they modified the criteria to eliminate anorexia and fatigue, and looking at a more severely depressed group, the incidence was 24 percent of the total sample. Data on family and past history of depression were not reported, but depression correlated with severity of physical disability as measured by the Karnovsky scale. In a study of 83 North Carolina women with cervical, endometrial, or vaginal cancer consecutively admitted to the gynecological tumor service, 23 percent met *DSM-III* criteria for major depression (Evans et al, 1986).

In a carefully selected sample of patients with end-stage renal disease, Hong and associates (1987) found that 18 of 60 (30 percent) met *DSM-III* criteria for one or more episodes of major depression, although one patient had a single episode prior to the onset of renal disease and none thereafter. A family history of major depression was no more prevalent in this group than in the nondepressed group of patients.

Certain subpopulations have been carefully studied for the incidence of major depression (such as patients with stroke), in whom direct brain alerations are present and the incidence of depression is much higher than it is in other medically ill populations. Here the cause–effect relationship between illness and depression seems much clearer; and for this reason depression in stroke and other special conditions is discussed below.

In a very early and excellent study, Stewart and colleagues (1965) compared a "severely ill" group (judged by their physicians to have an illness likely to be fatal within a period of one to two years), a less severely medically ill control group, and a manic-depressive group. The authors rejected the use of insomnia, anorexia, and fatigue as symptoms of depression because of their common presence in medical conditions, but using an extensive clinical examination still made a firm diagnosis of depression in 8 of 30 severely ill patients, selected for study by their grim prognosis—a life expectancy of less than one or two years. Five of these patients related their depressive symptoms primarily to their illnesses. The authors concluded that their data supported a significant association between severe medical illness and depression, were impressed with the clear-cut association between the patients' fear of death or disability and their depression, and noted that these patients had a lower incidence of depressive illness in family and past histories. None of the medical patients had seriously thought of suicide or attempted it, as opposed to 9 out of 20 manic-depressive controls. They concluded that the depression in the medically ill probably was closer to the concept of "psychogenic depression" or "reactive depression."

Little further study was devoted to depression in the medically ill; and despite this early interest, Andreasen and Winokur (1979) concluded that depression secondary to medical illness was "a concept . . . so broad as to be meaningless: consequently, the disorder should probably be defined as secondary only to psychiatric disorder" (p. 62).

Winokur and colleagues, in a paper not yet published, has fortunately returned to the study of depression in the medically ill, comparing three groups of secondary depressives: to substance abuse, to somatoform/anxiety/personality disorder, and to medical illness. All patients studied were taken from consecutive admissions to the University of Iowa Psychiatric Hospital. Medical illnesses were considered only if they predated or paralleled the depression and were considered severe or life threatening. The psychiatric diagnosis of depression was made according to the Feighner criteria (Feighner et al, 1972). Compared to the primary psychiatric disorder patients, the medically ill depressives had a later age of onset, were about evenly represented by males and females, were less likely to have suicidal thoughts and prior suicide attempts, had more memory and other organic difficulties, were more likely to be married at the time of admission (possibly a function of older age), and had less alcoholism in their family history. Compared to the combined groups of depressives secondary to psychiatric disorder, the medically ill patients showed a significantly greater number with marked improvement as a result of treatment (50 as opposed to 38 percent) and a greater number who did not relapse (66 as opposed to 49 percent). The authors concluded that depression secondary to medical illness better fit a concept of a "reactive" depression, occurring later in life with no prior psychiatric difficulties. These findings are similar to those of the study by Stewart and colleagues (1965). The question of genetic loading remains unanswered, but 36 percent of the medically ill depressed patients had a family history of depression (one-half of these included alchoholism), certainly higher than the expected incidence in the normal population.

DIAGNOSING DEPRESSION IN THE MEDICALLY ILL

Protest can still legitimately be lodged that depression secondary to medical illness is not the same entity as primary depression. Clinically, however, diagnosis is made and treatment selected in the same manner as it is for primary depression. The *DSM-III-R* diagnostic criteria are the same. Antidepressants effective for primary depression are effective for secondary depression as well. However, when depression appears within the context of active medical illness, characteristic difficulties arise in confidently making the diagnosis and safely prescribing antidepressants. Beyond these potentially confusing complexities, the search continues for differences between the depressive episode secondary to medical illness and the primary depressive episode.

Failure to treat depression in the medically ill leaves the patient at even higher risk for further complications and death. Proceeding to cardiac surgery while in a state of major depression, for example, is known to increase the chances of a fatal outcome (Tufo et al, 1970). Even in depressed outpatients the risk of death, chiefly due to cardiovascular disease, is more than doubled (Rabins et al, 1985). Moreover, there remains a clinical sense that any seriously ill person who has neurovegetative symptoms and has given up, wishing he or she were dead, is going to fare less well than a seriously ill person who has hope and is motivated to recover. Some investigators have been able to demonstrate that the immune defenses, specifically lymphocyte function, become defective with the onset of depression (Schleifer et al, 1985; Kronfol et al, 1985). Major depression, even if the patient were healthy in every other way, is misery requiring treatment.

DSM-III-R in the Medical Setting

DSM-III-R does not provide for a distinction between primary and secondary depression. Major depression almost always requires drug treatment or, occasionally, electroconvulsive therapy (ECT). Since this is the case, the first question becomes: What is *major* depression in the medically ill and how is it diagnosed? *DSM-III-R* (1987) criteria for major depression should be applied to the patient with medical illness in the same way that they are applied to the patient with psychiatric disorder. This immediately creates an academic difficulty, since one of the exclusion criteria in *DSM-III-R*, that the dysphoria not be due to any organic mental disorder, could be interpreted as excluding a diagnosis of major depression in any patient with a preexisting medical illness. A stroke in the left hemisphere, for example, is commonly followed by a syndrome clinically indistinguishable from major depression (Robinson et al, 1985). According to the earlier distinction between primary and secondary depression, such a patient could be diagnosed as having a *secondary* depression. (That is, the depressive episode occurred later in time than the stroke and is therefore termed "secondary.") Since this distinction is not available in *DSM-III-R*, what does one do? One could call it organic affective disorder, particularly in the case of a stroke, where a cause–effect relationship is rather clear. Nevertheless, a patient does not have to meet the full criteria for major depression in order to be diagnosed as having organic affective disorder (only two or more of the same eight criteria need be met instead of four or more). Hence, minor depressions also qualify for this diagnosis, leaving the clinician without a label appropriate to the severity of the disorder. This dilemma is further confused when no cause–effect relationship is clear—as in a case where a patient sustains a myocardial infarction (MI) and later develops the syndrome of major depression. My recommendation is to represent the clinical reality as accurately as possible by the diagnosis. Therefore, when the patient meets full criteria for major depression, this diagnosis should be entered on Axis I.

The Symptoms of Major Depression

Faced with a cancer patient who describes anorexia, is one to ascribe this to the malignancy or to a depressive state? First of all, the patient must have a pervasive dysphoria or loss of interest and pleasure for a period of two weeks. The subtleties of establishing this are discussed below. Medical illness may play a significant role in the production of the other symptoms that are part of the DSM-III-R diagnosis of major depression. Of the following eight symptoms of major depression—appetite or weight disturbance; sleep disturbance; psychomotor agitation or retardation; loss of sexual interest or libido; loss of energy or fatigue; feelings of worthlessness, self-reproach, or excessive guilt; diminished ability to think, concentrate, or make decisions; and recurrent thoughts of death or suicide—disturbance in weight and energy level seem particularly vulnerable to medical illness, and other symptoms may result from the concomitant physical effects of pain and sickness. In this diagnostic dilemma there are four ways of enhancing clinical confidence that depression is genuinely present.

First, the dilemma is exaggerated by a certain anti-mental illness bias in the entire population, both lay and physician. On the one hand, those with this attitude fail to appreciate that major depression is a devastating disorder with phsyical manifestations, its sufferers emaciated, exhausted, and unable to think clearly; some who suffer from major depression are as unable to sit still as sufferers of akathisia, and they are devoid of responsiveness to anything—small wonder that many of them do not care if they fall asleep at night never to awaken again. Silver (1987) has emphasized that physical distress is part of the core depressive syndrome. Although not the defining symptoms of the disorder, a plethora of other somatic symptoms commonly accompany depression. It is enough to make one regret that "depression" is such a common word, as easily passed off by many as "the blues" or other minor mood fluctuation. On the other hand, let the patient suffer a distinct medical disorder such as cancer and depression is said to be "appropriate"—the poor fellow lost a lung and has less than a year to live; who would not be "depressed"? If the same patient were to become septic and thereafter hypotensive, would we say that his state of shock was, after all, "appropriate," because his Foley catheter induced urosepsis, causing shock? This is a devastating complication: it can be referred to as "possible" or perhaps, more accurately, "feared," but not "appropriate." Major depression is best regarded as a *dread* complication of a medical illness.

Medically ill patients are no exceptions to the pervasive anti-mental illness bias. Many welcome a physician who understands what is wrong with them and has a treatment for it. Others will have florid DSM-III-R symptomatology and do their best to prevent the psychiatrist from making the diagnosis of depression. This label is often viewed as signifying some inner loss of courage or motivation, often with the fear that the patient's physician asked for psychiatric consultation because the symptoms were thought to be "in my head" or even the result of malingering. Some patients who readily recognize a feeling such as sadness mistakenly assume that they should know automatically when they are depressed, a state they erroneously equate with a more severe sadness. This is no more logical than the assumption that one should know, in the presence of multiple, vague, systemic symptoms, that one has systemic lupus erythematosus. (Moreover, some individuals lack awareness of even simple feelings such as sadness.) The somatic manifestations of depression (insomnia, restlessness, anhedonia, and so on) may even be construed as proof by patients that they have no "psychic" illness. "No, doctor, no way am I depressed; if I could just get rid of this exhaustion everything would be fine." Persistence and aggressive questioning are required to elicit the presence or absence of the eight symptoms.

Depression—one of those words used by most to describe even minor and transient mood fluctuations—shares the misfortune of other overused words: it is seen everywhere, often thought to be normal, and therefore is likely to be dismissed even when it is serious. This is all the more true in a patient with serious medical illness: the man has cancer, therefore his depression is appropriate. Depression here denotes the disorder of major depression. It is a seriously disabling condition, endangering the patient's life, and is never appropriate.

One way to enhance diagnostic accuracy in the presence of medical illness is to emphasize the psychological symptoms in the criteria, symptoms that are more clearly the result of major depression, such as the presence of self-reproach ("I feel worthless"), the wish to be dead, or psychomotor retardation (few medical illnesses of themselves produce psychomotor retardation: hypothyroidism and Parkinson's disease are two of them). Insomnia or hypersomnia can also be useful indicators, although the patient may have so much pain, dyspnea, or frequent clinical crises that sleep is impaired by these events. Although libidinous interests may not be high in an intensive care unit patient, some form of interest can usually be assessed—as when talk gets around to children or grandchildren, key interests or people—do they still find that their interest quickens, or is it blunted? The ability to think or concentrate, like the other functions, needs to be specifically asked about in every case.

The group at Rush Medical College collected most enlightening data on depressive symptomatology in Beck Depression Inventory (BDI) scales of 335 medically ill patients, compared with BDI scales of over 100 *DSM-III* diagnosed major depressives and 100 normals, in order to discriminate symptoms uniquely related to severity of depression in both depressed groups (Clark et al, 1983; Cavanaugh et al, 1983). This group concluded that there were six symptoms for depressive severity that successfully discriminated both medically ill depressives and psychiatric depressives from normals and hence may not be confounded by the physical illness or its attendant distress: sense of failure, loss of social interest, feeling punished, suicidal ideation, dissatisfaction, and indecision (in descending order). Although crying did not discriminate depressive severity in the psychiatric population, it was significant in discriminating depressive severity in the medical sample. One must remember that prominent crying can also signify neurologic disease, especially when it is inappropriate to context, push-button in response, and stereotyped (Green et al, 1987). All of these symptoms apply to the *DSM-III-R* criteria for major depression.

Another method for discriminating the presence of depression associated with a medical illness arises from the clinical impression of two distinct conditions existing within the same patient, just as the patient who undergoes a bowel resection may develop a postoperative pneumonia that retards recovery. The primary illness, for example, an MI, has its own course and trajectory of expected complications and normal recovery. Notes in the chart often specify mood and behavior changes in the patient, and a careful reading may reveal an approximate time of onset and rather distinctive progression. If the current examination establishes the presence of six of the eight criteria for a major depressive episode, one must make a judgment whether there is anything in the treatment of the primary medical condition that can be improved. Of course, when the consultee requested psychiatric consultation, the patient's symptoms were probably judged to have been in excess of the effects of the disease process. Sometimes the consultee will put in the consultation without being confident of this, but hoping that the consultant can locate some psychiatric symptomatology which can be treated, thereby relieving the patient of distress that current treatment has been unable to alter. Moreover, depression is a relatively common disorder (roughly one in five) in serious medical illness, if the preliminary prevalence data are any indication. The threshold for making the diagnosis should be low rather than high.

An additional method of clarifying with relative ease and safety whether major depression is present is to use a psychostimulant. Strictly speaking, this is a probe for responsiveness of depressive symptomatology, since stimulant response is not an absolute guarantee of the presence of major depression (Goff, 1986). Dextroamphetamine (not the sustained release preparation) or methylphenidate can be used. The starting dose of dexedrine in medically ill patients is usually 5 or 10 mg, given once in the morning before breakfast. It is given once because the half-life varies between 7 and 30 hours; late administration can cause insomnia. Methylphenidate's starting dose for the same type of probe is also 5 to 10 mg., but it should be given at least twice a day, for example at 8 A.M. and 2 P.M. The half-life is short, from two to four hours, and in some cases the patient may benefit from a third dose. When there is concern that the stimulant might in some way worsen the patient's condition—for example, specifically elevate the blood pressure of a hypertensive patient (as in the depressed renal failure patient with a pressure of 230/110 despite antihypertensive medications) or aggravate cardiac conduction in a patient with arrhythmias—one can start with an initial dose of 2.5 mg of either drug and carefully check vital signs over the next four hours. When successful the test is quite dramatic: nurses, family, and sometimes even patients comment on how much better they feel. Failure should not be pronounced until the dose has been successively increased (for example, 5 mg the first day, 10 mg the second, 15 mg the third) to the point that recognizable effects are reported by the patient, such as "I feel nervous and on edge today but not better." A further examination of psychostimulants appears below.

Cohen-Cole and Stoudemire (1987) succinctly summarize the four approaches to diagnosing depression in medical illness. The *inclusive* approach takes into account all symptoms of depression, even though either depression or the primary medical problem could have caused them. The *etiologic* approach takes into account a depressive symptom only if it is not "caused" by the primary illness (the decision rule for the Diagnostic Interview Scale [DIS], although the way in which one determines the causality is of course not known). The *substitutive* approach suggests changing the criteria for major depression in medical illness; and the *exclusive* approach eliminates certain symptoms that may be common to the primary illness (see the section on cancer, later in this chapter). Cohen-Cole and Stoudemire suggest the inclusive approach, with its higher reliability and sensitivity. This is strongly recommended here as well.

States Commonly Mislabeled "Depression"

Up to one-third of patients referred for depression will, on clinical examination, have neither major nor minor depression. By far the most common diagnosis found among these mislabeled patients at the Massachusetts General Hospital has been an organic mental syndrome. A quietly confused patient often looks depressed. The patient with dementia or with a frontal lobe syndrome due to brain injury can lack spontaneous initiative and thus appear depressed. Sleep apnea, which may occur in as many as one-third of elderly men, is commonly associated with depressive symptoms, but is easily diagnosed by asking the patient and spouse about insomnia, excessive daytime sleepiness, and snoring (McNamara et al, 1987). Male patients with prolactin-secreting tumors of the pituitary commonly present with apathy as a clinical feature (Cohen et al, 1984). Only the complete physical and mental status examinations reveal the telltale abnormalities specific for organic mental syndrome.

Although much less common, mental retardation may also be mistaken for depression, especially when failure to grasp or comply with complex instructions make no sense to those caring for the patient ("He seems not to care"). Retardation may be suggested by the school history, or verified if family is available and able to confirm it.

Another state sometimes termed depression by the patient, though easier for the psychiatrist to recognize for what it is, is anger. The patient's physician, realizing that the patient has been through a long and difficult illness, may perceive reduction in speech, smiling, and small talk on the patient's part as depression. The patient may thoroughly resent the illness, be irritated by therapeutic routines, and be fed up with the hospital environment, but, despite interior fuming, remains reluctant to discharge overt wrath in the direction of the physician or nurse.

Excluding Organic Causes of Depression

When clinical findings confirm that the patient's symptoms are fully consistent with major depression, the consultant is still responsible for the differential diagnosis of this syndrome. Could the same constellation of symptoms be due to medical illness or its treatments? The psychiatrist functions here as the last court of appeal. Should the patient's symptoms be due to an as yet undiagnosed illness, the last physician with the chance of detecting it is the consultant.

Throughout the evaluation, it is helpful to have in mind a systematic schema for the exclusion of organic disorder. Ludwig (1980) has provided an excellent comprehensive list that has been expanded somewhat in Table 1. This 13-category list, carried on a 3" × 5" card in one's pocket, permits one a leisurely but brief review of all possible disease categories otherwise possibly forgotten.

Table 1. Differential Diagnosis of Medical Illnesses Capable of Causing Depressive Symptoms*

General Etiology	Specific Etiologies
Vascular	Hypertensive encephalopathy; cerebral arteriosclerosis; intracranial hemorrhage or thromboses; circulatory collapse (shock); systemic lupus erythematosus; polyarteritis nodosa; thrombotic thrombocytopenic purpura
Infectious	Encephalitis; meningitis; general paresis
Neoplastic	Space-occupying lesions such as gliomas, meningiomas, abscesses
Degenerative	Senile and presenile dementias such as Alzheimer's or Pick's dementia, Huntington's chorea
Intoxication	Chronic intoxication or withdrawal effect of sedative-hypnotic drugs such as bromides, opiates, tranquilizers, anticholinergics, dissociative anesthetics, anticonvulsants
Congenital	Epilepsy; postictal states; aneurysm
Traumatic	Subdural and epidural hematomas; contusion; laceration; postoperative trauma; heat stroke
Intraventricular	Normal pressure hydrocephalus
Vitamin	Deficiencies of thiamine (Wernicke-Korsakoff), niacin (pellagra), B_{12} (pernicious anemia)
Endocrine-Metabolic	Diabetic coma and shock; uremia; myxedema; hyperthyroidism, parathyroid dysfunction; hypoglycemia; hepatic failure; porphyria; severe electrolyte or acid/base disturbances; remote side-effect of carcinoma; Cushing's or Addison's syndrome; sleep apnea
Metals	Heavy metals (lead, manganese, mercury); carbon monoxide; toxins
Anoxia	Hypoxia and anoxia secondary to pulmonary or cardiac failure, anesthesia, anemia
Depression–Other	Depressive pseudodementia; hysteria; catatonia

*Ludwig's differential diagnosis of the confusion-delirium-dementia-coma complex

Table 2 presents drugs most commonly associated with the production of a depressive syndrome.

A check on the medications that the patient is currently receiving will generally tell the phsyician whether or not the patient is receiving something that might cause a change in mood. Ordinarily one would like to establish that a relationship between the depressive symptoms' onset and either the start of or a change in the medication did in fact occur. If such a connection can be established, the simplest course would be to stop the agent and monitor the patient for improvement. In cases in which the patient requires continued treatment, as, for example, in the case of hypertension, the presumed offending agent can be changed—with the hope that the change to another antihypertensive will be followed by resolution of depressive symptoms. When this fails or when clinical judgment warrants no change in medication, it may be necessary to start an antidepressant along with the antihypertensive drug.

Table 2. Drugs Associated with Depressive Syndromes

Antihypertensives	Cimetidine, ranitidine
reserpine	Barbiturates
methyldopa	Benzodiazepines
thiazides	Beta-blockers
spironolactone	especially propranolol
clonidine	Metoclopramide
Oral contraceptives	Cocaine
Steroids and adrenocorticotropin hormone	Amphetamine
(ACTH)	

Table 3. Basic Laboratory Values in a Depressed Medical Inpatient

Blood count: hematocrit, WBC and diff, MCV, ESR

Blood chemistries: glucose, electrolytes, Ca, P, albumin, BUN/creatinine, Ammonia and LFT's Thyroxin (T^4), T3Uptake, TSH

Drug levels: toxic screen/toxic level

Urinalysis

B_{12}, folate

Serum test for syphilis

HIV antibody (received blood, 1977–1983)

Electrocardiogram

Arterial blood gases (where hypoxia possible)

Optional additional tests: CT, EEG, LP, heavy metal and thiamine levels, LE prep, ANA, urinary PBG

Abnormal laboratory values should never be missed and may provide the clues to an undiagnosed abnormality responsible for the depressive symptoms. A workup is not complete if the evaluation of thyroid and parathyroid function is not included. Table 3 outlines the basic laboratory values that one would be likely to see in a depressed medical inpatient.

Medical Illnesses Specifically Linked to Depression

Many medical illnesses have been associated with depressive symptoms. The list is extensive and for all practical purposes can be fused with the list of medical illnesses that can cause delirium. For more than 50 years (Yaskin, 1923) carcinoma of the pancreas has been noted to show frequent association with psychiatric symptoms, especially depression, which in some cases seems to be the first manifestation of the disease. Using a group of gastric cancer patients as the control, Holland and colleagues (1986), in a prospective study, demonstrated that pancreatic cancer patients reported significantly greater psychiatric disturbance, depression included, than did gastric cancer patients. *DSM-III* criteria were not used. Whether the increase in psychiatric symptoms is due to the grim prognosis of pancreatic cancer (though depression has often been demonstrated before the patient or physician knew the diagnosis) or to a humoral process initiated by the malignancy is unclear. Pomara and Gershon (1984) reported a case of treatment-resistant, dexamethasone suppression test (DST) -positive depression, in which the patient was eventually diagnosed to have pancreatic carcinoma. After excision, the response to antidepressants was improved and the DST normalized. Although the ability of pancreatic cancer to induce major depression still awaits scientific confirmation, the clinical lore justifies its inclusion in the differential diagnosis for organic causes of psychiatric symptoms. Patients with hereditary pancreatitis, inherited by autosomal dominance, are predisposed to develop cancer of the pancreas, so that if a person with this family history were to become depressed, gastrointestinal symptoms and pathology would be an essential subject of inquiry.

STROKE.   Direct injury to the brain can produce regular changes of affect that progress to a full syndrome of major depression. One model for this is the cerebrovascular accident (CVA), now shown by Robinson and co-workers (Robinson et al, 1985; Lipsey et al, 1984) and others to be followed often by major depression. According to these studies, when the stroke is unilateral, major depression will occur in approximately 60 percent of the patients with a left hemisphere lesion and in approximately 15 percent of patients with a right hemisphere lesion. The depression will appear within the acute period in approximately two-thirds of the patients destined to suffer it, with the remainder developing depression by the sixth month. If left untreated, this severe depression will last at least eight to nine months. Moreover, the severity of the depression is directly related to the distance of the injury from the frontal pole (correlation for left = -0.92, for right = $.76$). That is, the closer the insult to the left frontal pole, the more depressed the patient will be. This is not a function of aphasia, which can exist without depression, just as depression can be found in the absence of aphasia. The authors also found that the relationship between severity and location remained strong when intellectual and physical impairment, quality of social supports, and age were taken into account. Further work by the same group established the same relationship between location of injury and severity of depression in patients with traumatic brain injury other than stroke, patients with bilateral brain injury, and even in left-handed patients with similar lesions.

Right hemisphere lesions deserve special diagnostic attention. As noted above, the closer the lesion is to the occipital pole, the more likely the patient is to be depressed. But when the lesion is in the right anterior location, the mood disorder tends to be an apathetic, indifferent state associated with "inappropriate cheerfulness." The patient, however, seldom *looks* cheerful, and may have complaints of loss of interest or even worrying. This disorder was found in 6 of 20 patients with single right hemisphere strokes (and none of 28 patients with single left hemisphere lesions) (Ross and Rush, 1981).

Prosody is also at risk in right hemisphere injury. Ross and Rush (1981) focused clinical attention on the presentation of *aprosodia* (lack of "prosody," or inflection, rhythm, and intensity of expression) when the right hemisphere is damaged. Such a patient could appear quite depressed and be so labeled by staff and family, but simply lacks the neuronal capacity to express and/or recognize emotion. These authors compared aprosodias to the aphasias that occur when corresponding sites in the left hemisphere are damaged. If one stations oneself out of the patient's view, selects a neutral sentence (for example, "The book is red."), asks the patient to identify the mood as mad, sad, frightened, or elated, and then declaims the sentence with the emotion to be tested, one should be able to identify those patients with a receptive aprosodia. Next the patient is presented with facial portrayals of the same emotions and asked to identify them (thereby separating visual from auditory clues). The patient can then be asked to portray facial or vocal expressions for the same emotions in order to test for the presence of an expressive aprosodia. There is no reason that a stroke patient cannot suffer from both aprosodia and depression, but there are separate diagnostic criteria and clinical examinations to diagnose each one.

Because stroke is among the most disabling of injuries, the danger of labeling major depression associated with it as "appropriate" is extremely high since, when it is so labeled, one can almost assume that treatment of the depression with antidepressants will not occur.

When depressed stroke patients are treated with appropriate drugs they respond well. In a randomized, double blind study of depressed stroke patients, Lipsey and colleagues (1984) demonstrated a significant response to therapeutic plasma levels of nortriptyline after six weeks of treatment. Without treatment the depression is quite likely not to remit for nine months, if at all.

MULTI-INFARCT DEMENTIA.   Cummings and associates (1987) applied *DSM-III* diagnostic criteria to 45 consecutive patients referred for dementia, 30 with Alzheimer's dementia, and 15 with multi-infarct dementia (MID). Four of 15 MID patients, as opposed to none of 30 Alzheimer's patients, were diagnosed as having had major depressive disorder. They speculated that the increased incidence of this disorder may be of the same etiology as that seen in stroke patients, but subcortical lesions could produce the same symptoms.

THE SUBCORTICAL DEMENTIAS.   Parkinson's disease and Huntington's disease commonly include major depression within their symptomatology. In as many as one-half of the cases of Huntington's disease, a major depression prior to the onset of either chorea or dementia may represent the first appearance of the disease (Folstein et al, 1983). Diagnosis is made clinically, as described above.

In Parkinson's disease depression is the most frequent mental change, and major depressive episodes occur in 40 percent or more of patients (Mayeux et al, 1986). As in Huntington's disease, in a substantial proportion of patients depression antedates the appearance of motor and/or cognitive symptoms. Antidepressants are required and are beneficial. Some reports note that as depression is treated in the patient with Parkinson's disease, the parkinsonian symptoms will also improve, and may do so before the depressive symptoms subside (Asnis, 1977). This is especially striking in case reports in which ECT was used (Holcomb et al, 1983), although the same improvement has been reported after tricyclic antidepressants.

Treatment of major depression in either disease may increase the comfort of the patient and is always worth a try. Huntington's patients may be sensitive to the anticholinergic side effects of tricyclics (though not invariably) so that less anticholinergic drugs should be tried first.

Another subcortical dementia that has drawn increased interest recently is Binswanger's encephalopathy, a state of white matter demyelination presumably based on arteriosclerosis, presenting with an abulic withdrawn state and a paucity of focal neurologic findings. Antidepressant medication has produced striking relief for depressive symptoms in this supposedly rare condition (Summergrad, 1985). Fewer than 50 cases of Binswanger's disease with pathological findings have been reported in the world literature. It was a disease in which hypertension was a hallmark. Today a mislabeled epidemic of Binswanger cases is being reported because computerized tomography (CT) and magnetic resonance imaging (MRI) are able to detect deep white matter lesions in the geriatric population. These lesions appear to be related to cognitive impairment and reflex/motor changes in these patients. Some but not all of these changes can be related to cerebral infarcts and hypertension. Hachinski and colleagues (1987) have coined a new term to describe these white matter changes in the elderly: *leuko-araiosis* (literally, white matter rarefication). Mood changes associated with these changes must be studied, but involvement of neurotransmitter systems that are important in affective disorder is likely.

MULTIPLE SCLEROSIS. Using the Schedule for Affective Disorders and Schizophrenia–Lifetime (SADS-L) to make the RDC diagnosis of affective disorder in a consecutive sample of 100 patients with multiple sclerosis, Joffe and associates (1987) found a lifetime prevalence of 38 percent with unipolar major depression and 13 percent with bipolar disorder. Not only is the unipolar depression rate higher, but that for bipolar disorder is 13 times the expected rate. Moreover, degree of disability, as measured by the Kurtzke scale, was correlated neither to the presence nor severity of mood disorder. Strong evidence for an epidemiological association between multiple sclerosis (MS) and bipolar disorder was also found by Schiffer and colleagues (1986).

HUMAN IMMUNODEFICIENCY VIRUS (HIV). The encephalopathy caused by HIV, particularly in its earlier manifestations, produces a syndrome that verges on and often becomes major affective disorder. Depression can exist, as can mania or hypomania, in more advanced stages of the infection or with some of the opportunistic infections suffered by patients with AIDS-related complex (ARC) or Acquired Immunodeficiency Syndrome (AIDS). The subtle impairment of concentration and attention is often the first sign noticed by the sufferer of the illness, but these symptoms will be followed by mild memory impairment, lethargy, loss of libido, and social withdrawal. Marked psychomotor retardation may be present (Snider et al, 1983; Shaw et al, 1985; Ho et al, 1985; Holland and Tross, 1985; Navia et al, 1986). At least in the earlier stages and often in the more advanced instances of infection, whether with the HIV itself or with one of the opportunistic infections of the central nervous system (CNS), a dramatic response can occur to antidepressive treatment. Our current recommendation is to start with dextroamphetamine, 5 to 10 mg, once in the morning. Table 4 presents the CNS complications of AIDS. Any one of these complications can produce devastating mental status changes, some of them appearing quite rapidly. Since the patient with AIDS is at high risk for all complications, even a mood change must raise a question of some newly acquired process.

Table 4. Central Nervous System Complications of AIDS*

Infectious Complications
  Viral
    cytomegalovirus
    herpes simplex I and II
    herpes zoster
    papovavirus (progressive multifocal leukoencephalopathy)
    HIV dementia
  Bacterial
    mycobacterium avium intracellulare
    mycobacterium tuberculosis hominis
    nocardia
    listeria monocytogenes
  Fungal
    candida
    cryptococcus neoformans
    histoplasma capsulatum
    coccidioides immitis
    aspergillus
    blastomycetic dermatitis
  Protozoa
    toxoplasma gondii

Noninfectious Complications
  Neoplasms
    primary CNS lymphoma
    Kaposi's sarcoma
    metastatic lymphoma
  Vascular
    marantic endocarditis
    cerebral hemorrhage
  peripheral neuropathy
  retinopathy
  reactive versus induced depression

*Adapted from Harris AA, Segreti J, Levin S: Central nervous system infections in patients with acquired immune deficiency syndrome (AIDS). Clin Neuropharmacol 1985; 8:201-210

CUSHING'S SYNDROME. Although careful prospective studies had shown a strikingly high incidence of major affective disturbance in patients with Cushing's syndrome (Starkman et al, 1981; Kelly et al, 1983), Haskett (1985) used the SADS-L to diagnose affective disorder episodes in 30 patients sequentially admitted to a clinical research unit. Twenty-four met critiera for major affective disorder— 16 for unipolar depression and 8 for bipolar affective disorder. Two of these patients were psychotically depressed. In all patients the affective disorder preceded the diagnosis of Cushing's disease by one to six years.
    Investigators have evidence that there are other medical illnesses that regu-

larly produce depressive symptoms, such as temporal lobe epilepsy or complex partial seizures (Schiffer and Babigian, 1984; Mendez et al, 1986). As with stroke, HIV, Parkinson's disease, or reserpine, there is an implication of true cause–effect between these diseases or drugs and major depression. Therefore one could not call these "reactive" depressions, a word which implies no direct pathophysiological link between events (for example, a loss and a depressed state).

Winokur and co-workers (in submission) continue to see depression secondary to medical illness as "reactive" for the most part. When asked about relationships such as that between stroke and depression, Winokur said they would be better referred to as "induced" depressions, indicating the more clear causal relationship (personal communication, Oct. 8, 1985). In medical illness the distinction between reactive and induced is not clinically important when a diagnosis of major depression has been made. A threatening disorder in itself, depression is likely to increase the morbidity of the primary medical illness as well and must be treated.

CHOOSING APPROPRIATE ANTIDEPRESSANT TREATMENT

Although there has been concern that medically ill depressed patients will not respond well to antidepressants (Popkin et al, 1985), our experience, like that of the Iowa group (Winokur et al, in submission) is encouraging. Whenever major depression is diagnosed, effort to alleviate the clinical symptoms almost always includes somatic treatments. The consultant who understands the interactions of the antidepressants with illness and other drugs is best prepared to prescribe these agents effectively (Jefferson, 1985). Detailed instructions for the prescription of antidepressants for the depressed medically ill can be found elsewhere (Cassem, 1987; Cohen-Cole, Stoudemire, 1987).

Electroconvulsive therapy remains the single most effective somatic treatment for depression, often the treatment of choice for medically ill patients with severe depression (Welch, 1987).

REFERENCES

American Psychiatric Association: Diagnostic and Statistical Manual of Mental Disorders, Third Edition (DSM-III). Washington, DC, American Psychiatric Association, 1980

American Psychiatric Association: Diagnostic and Statistical Manual of Mental Disorders, Third Edition, Revised (DSM-III-R). Washington, DC, American Psychiatric Association, 1987

Andreasen NC, Winokur G: Secondary depression: familial, clinical, and research perspectives. Am J Psychiatry 1979; 136:62-66

Asnis G: Parkinson's disease, depression, and ECT: a review and case study. Am J Psychiatry 1977; 134:191-195

Bradford BA, Jordan BD, Price RW: The AIDS dementia complex, I: clinical features. Ann Neurol 1986; 19:517-524

Bukberg J, Penman D, Holland JC: Depression in hospitalized cancer patients. Psychosom Med 1984; 46:199-212

Cassem NH: Depression, in Massachusetts General Hospital Handbook of General Hospital Psychiatry, second edition. Edited by Hackett TP, Cassem NH. Littleton, MA, PSG Publishing Co, 1987

Cavanaugh S: Diagnosing depression in the hospitalized patient with chronic medical illness. J Clin Psychiatry 1984; 45:13-16

Cavanaugh S, Clark DC, Gibbons RD: Diagnosing depression in the hospitalized medically ill. Psychosomatics 1983; 24:809-815

Clark DC, Cavanaugh SV, Gibbons RD: The core symptoms of depression in medical and psychiatric patients. J Nerv Ment Dis 1983; 171:705-713

Clayton PJ, Lewis CE: The significance of secondary depression. J Affective Disord 1981; 3:25-35

Cohen LM, Greenberg DB, Murray GB: Neuropsychiatric presentation of men with pituitary tumors (the 'four As'). Psychosomatics 1984; 25:925-928

Cohen-Cole SA, Stoudemire A: Major depression and physical illness. Psychiatr Clin North Am 1987; 10:1-17

Cummings JL, Miller B, Hill MA, et al: Neuropsychiatric aspects of multi-infarct dementia and dementia of the Alzheimer type. Arch Neurol 1987; 44:389-393

Derogatis LR, Morrow GR, Fetting J, et al: The prevalence of psychiatric disorders among cancer patients. JAMA 1983; 249:751-757

Evans DS, McCartney CF, Nemeroff CB, et al: Depression in women treated for gynecological cancer: clinical and neuroendocrine assessment. Am J Psychiatry 1986; 143:447-452

Feighner J, Robins E, Guze S, et al: Diagnostic criteria for use in psychiatric research. Arch Gen Psychiatry 1972; 26:57-63

Folstein SE, Abbott MH, Chase GA, et al: The association of affective disorder with Huntington's disease in a case series and in families. Psychol Med 1983; 13:537-542

Goff DC: The stimulant challenge test in depression. J Clin Psychiatry 1986; 47:538-543

Green RL, McAllister TW, Bernat JL: A study of crying in medically and surgically hospitalized patients. Am J Psychiatry 1987; 144:442-447

Hachinski VC, Potter P, Merskey H: Leuko-Araiosis. Arch Neurol 1987; 44:21-23

Harris AA, Segreti J, Levin S: Central nervous system infections in patients with the Acquired Immune Deficiency Syndrome (AIDS). Clin Neuropharmacol 1985; 8:201-210

Haskett RF. Diagnostic categorization of psychiatric disturbance in Cushing's syndrome. Am J Psychiatry 1985; 142:911-916

Ho DD, Rota TR, Schooley RT, et al: Isolation of HTLV-III from cerebrospinal fluid and neural tissues of patients with neurologic syndromes related to the Acquired ImmunoDeficiency Syndrome. N Engl J Med 1985; 313:1493-1497

Holcomb HH, Sternberg DE, Heninger GR: Effects of electroconvulsive therapy on mood, Parkinsonism, and tardive dyskinesia in a depressed patient: ECT and dopamine systems. Biol Psychiatry 1983; 18:865-873

Holland JC, Tross S: The psychosocial and neuropsychiatric sequelae of the Acquired Immunodeficiency Syndrome and related disorders. Ann Intern Med 1985; 103:760-764

Holland JC, Korzun AH, Tross S, et al: Comparative psychological disturbance in patients with pancreatic and gastric cancer. Am J Psychiatry 1986; 143:982-986

Hong BA, Smith MD, Robson AM, et al: Depressive symptomatology and treatment in patients with end-stage renal disease. Psychol Med 1987; 17:185-190

Jefferson JW: Biologic treatment of depression in cardiac patients. Psychosomatics 1985; 26:31-38

Joffe RT, Lippert GP, Gray TA, et al: Mood disorder and multiple sclerosis. Arch Neurol 1987; 44:376-378

Kathol RG, Petty F: Relation of depression to medical illness. J Affective Disord 1981; 3:111-121

Kelly WF, Checkley SA, Bender DA, et al: Cushing's syndrome and depression—a prospective study of 26 patients. Br J Psychiatry 1983; 142:16-19

Klerman GL. Depression in the medically ill. Psychiatr Clin North Am 1981; 4:301-317

Krauthammer C, Klerman GL: Secondary mania. Arch Gen Psychiatry 1978; 35:1333-1339

Kronfol Z, Nasrallah HA, Chapman S, et al: Depression, cortisol metabolism and lympho-cytopenia. J Affective Disord 1985; 9:169-173

Lipsey JR, Robinson RG, et al: Nortriptyline treatment of post-stroke depression: a double-blind study. Lancet 1984; 1:297-300

Ludwig AM: Principles of Clinical Psychiatry. New York, The Free Press, 1980

Mayeux R, Stern Y, Williams JBS, et al: Clinical and biochemical features of depression in Parkinson's disease. Am J Psychiatry 1986; 143:756-759

McNamara ME, Southwick SM, Fogel BS: Sleep apnea and hypothyroidism presenting as depression in two patients. J Clin Psychiatry 1987; 48:164-165

Mendez MF, Cummings JL, Benson DF: Depression in epilepsy. Arch Neurol 1986; 43:766-770

Moffic HS, Paykel ES: Depression in medical in-patients. Br J Psychiatry 1975; 126:346

Navia BA, Jordon BD, Price RW: The AIDS dementia complex, I: clinical features. Ann Neurol 1986; 19:517-524

Pomara N, Gershon S: Treatment-resistant depression in an elderly patient with pancreatic carcinoma: case report. J Clin Psychiatry 1984; 45:439-440

Popkin MK, Callies AL, Mackenzie TB: The outcome of antidepressant use in the medically ill. Arch Gen Psychiatry 1985; 42:1160-1163

Rabins PV, Harvic K, Koven S: High fatality rates of late-life depression associated with cardiovascular disease. J Affective Disord 1985; 9:165-167

Robinson RG, Lipsey JR, Price TR: Diagnosis and clinical management of post-stroke depression. Psychosomatics 1985; 26:769-778

Rodin G, Voshart K: Depression in the medically ill: an overview. Am J Psychiatry 1986; 143:696-705

Ross ED, Rush AJ: Diagnosis and neuroanatomical correlates of depression in brain-damaged patients. Arch Gen Psychiatry 1981; 38:1344-1354

Schiffer RB, Babigian HM: Behavioral disorders in multiple sclerosis, temporal lobe epilepsy, and amyotrophic lateral sclerosis. Arch Neurol 1984; 41:1067-1069

Schiffer RB, Wineman NM, Weitkamp LR: Association between bipolar affective disorder and multiple sclerosis. Am J Psychiatry 1986; 143:94-95

Schleifer SJ, Keller SE, Siris SG, et al: Depression and immunity: lymphocyte function in ambulatory depressed patients, hospitalized schizophrenic patients, and patients hospi-talized for herniorrhaphy. Arch Gen Psychiatry 1985; 42:129-133

Schwab JJ, Bialow M, Brown JM, et al: Diagnosing depression in medical inpatients. Ann Intern Med 1967; 67:695-707

Shaw GM, Harper ME, Hahn BH, et al: HTLV-III infection in brains of children and adults with AIDS encephalopathy. Science 1985; 227:177-182

Silver H: Physical complaints are part of the core depressive syndrome: evidence from a cross-cultural study in Israel. J Clin Psychiatry 1987; 48:140-142

Snider WD, Simpson DM, Nielsen S, et al: Neurological complications of Acquired Immune Deficiency Syndrome: analysis of 50 patients. Ann Neurol 1983; 14:403-418

Starkman MN, Schteingart DE, Schork MA: Depressed mood and other psychiatric mani-festations of Cushing's syndrome: relationship to hormone levels. Psychosom Med 1981; 43:3-18

Stewart JA, Drake F, Winokur G: Depression among medically ill patients. Diseases of the Nervous System 1965; 26:479-485

Summergrad P: Depression in Binswanger's encephalopathy responsive to tranylcypro-mine: case report. J Clin Psychiatry 1985; 46:69-70

Thase ME, Kupfer DJ, Spiker DG: Electroencephalographic sleep in secondary depression: a revisit. Biol Psychiatry 1984; 19:805

Tufo HM, Ostfeld AM, Shekelle R: Central nervous system dysfunction following open-heart surgery. JAMA 1970; 212:1333

Welch CA: Electroconvulsive therapy in the general hospital, in The Massachusetts General Hospital Handbook of General Hospital Psychiatry. Edited by Hackett TP, Cassem NH. Littleton, MA, PSG Publishing Co. 1987

Weissman MM, Pottenger M, Kleber H, et al: Symptom patterns in primary and secondary depression. Arch Gen Psychiatry 1977; 34:854-862

Woods S, Tesar GE, Murray GB, et al: Psychostimulant treatment of depressive disorders secondary to medical illness. J Clin Psychiatry 1986; 47:12-15

Yaskin JD: Nervous symptoms at earliest manifestations of carcinoma of the pancreas. JAMA 1923; 96:1664-1668

Afterword

by Martin B. Keller, M.D.

Unipolar depression has been discussed in depth in this section. The heaviest concentration has been on epidemiology, familial and genetic models of transmission, biology, differential diagnosis and clinical course, somatic and psychosocial treatment, and depression secondary to medical illness. Depression is a multidimensional and multifaceted disorder that interfaces with most areas of psychiatric theory, practice, and research and is far too broad a condition to be covered comprehensively in this volume. Other sections in this volume cover critically important topics related to depression such as suicide, comorbidity with anxiety states, cognitive therapy, and electroconvulsive therapy (ECT). What is covered in this volume must be put into perspective by pointing out that many important aspects of depression have been left untouched or given only the briefest mention. For example, entire sections could be devoted to: psychoanalytic, interpersonal, and behavioral theories about the etiology, pathogenesis, and treatment of depression; depression in the elderly; depression in children and adolescents; the relationship between personality and depression; culturally determined components of depression throughout history and in other societies; and basic science research on molecular physiology, neuroendocrine regulatory mechanisms, and neurotransmitters.

I will highlight a few of the major findings from the chapters in this section and point out new areas of research that are needed to augment the depth and breadth of knowledge in each of these domains.

Drs. Goldin and Gershon have thoroughly covered the genetic epidemiology of major depressive illness by reviewing epidemiologic, family, twin, and adoption studies, and by examining research concerning the mode of transmission of depression and the relationship of depression and genetic marker traits and biologic traits. They cite data that are consistent with a genetic etiology for depression, namely that unipolar major depression is more common in relatives than in the general population, and that monozygotic twins are more often concordant for depression than dizygotic twins.

Although there is variability, the weight of the evidence from epidemiologic studies indicates that the prevalence of depression is twofold higher in women than in men, with the most recent lifetime estimates for DSM-III major depression in the United States varying from 5 to 9 percent in women and from 2 to 4 percent in men.

Perhaps the most intriguing and alarming finding from epidemiologic research in the past decade has been the identification of the birth cohort effect, which indicates that successive cohorts defined by decade of birth, starting around 1940, have significantly higher rates of depression and earlier age of onset than earlier born cohorts. Although possible artifacts such as differential reporting in older and younger individuals, earlier mortality in older individuals with a history of depression, or decreased memory in older people may partially explain this phenomenon, most investigators are of the opinion that individuals from more recent decades have a greater susceptibility for depression and that we may indeed be in the midst of an era of melancholia. Regardless of the explanation, the cohort effect must be accounted for in genetic studies, which in the past have simply pooled different birth cohorts for risk estimates.

Family studies strongly support the heritability of unipolar major depression with concordance rates ranging from 45 to 54 percent in monozygotic twins compared to 22 to 24 percent in dizygotic twins; however, such heritability has not yet been demonstrated for dysthymia or major depression with marked hysterical personality features. Similarly, several adoption studies also suggest that more severe depression is heritable but that milder depression is not. However, these studies are not as definitive in demonstrating heritability as were the adoption studies of schizophrenia. In addition, there are now several excellent studies that have found an increased frequency of major and minor affective disorder in children of parents with a major depression compared to children of controls, a finding which supports a genetic etiology but does not in any way rule out environmental factors. Regardless of the mode of transmission, these findings should alert adult and child psychiatrists to look carefully for the earliest manifestations of depression in the children of depressed parents. An overview of family studies indicates that whereas certain subgroups of unipolar patients may share liability with bipolar patients, many researchers do not confirm a unitary liability model for unipolar and bipolar patients.

Efforts to demonstrate genetically heterogeneous subtypes of unipolar depression have not yet yielded consistently positive findings based on categorizing subtypes according to severity of depression (the endogenous/nonendogenous or the psychotic/nonpsychotic subtype), or for subclassifying patients according to clinical characteristics based on different familial histories of depression that were proposed by Winokur.

Drs. Goldin and Gershon take the position that although several studies are consistent with multifactorial models and that single gene locus models are usually rejected, this does not rule out single locus inheritance. This may be due to the relatively low power of these models to detect major depression in complex diseases, particularly if affective disorders are genetically heterogeneous. The association of genetic linkage of unipolar depression to a genetic marker locus has not yet demonstrated evidence for a single gene susceptibility. However, since unipolar depression is likely to be heterogeneous, and since there is such a large number of variations in DNA sequences, the authors recommend that linkage studies be conducted in families with a well defined depressive illness, as has been done with bipolar disorder.

The search for biologic traits that have been examined in relation to genetic susceptibility has included the investigation of dexamethasone suppression, platelet monoamine oxidase activity, cerebrospinal fluid (CSF) monoamine metabolites, and cholinergic inductions of rapid eye movement (REM) sleep cycles. Of these traits, only a vulnerability to increased sensitivity to cholinergic REM induction has shown any promise of being a marker for affective disorders, and even here, further confirmatory studies are necessary.

In conclusion, issues that Drs. Goldin and Gershon believe are still unresolved by genetic studies are: 1) the genetic relationship between unipolar and bipolar illness; 2) evidence for the heterogeneity of depression based on patterns of family illness or clinical characteristics; 3) whether the mode of inheritance is a single gene or polygenic trait; 4) the association or linkage with genetic marker traits; and 5) the underlying biologic risk factors.

Dr. Ballenger's chapter presents a comprehensive and scholarly account of the most well established biological findings organized into four substantive areas: sleep, biologic rhythms, neuroendocrine studies, and neurotransmitter abnormalities. The fundamentals of this biological knowledge base should be accessible to all practicing psychiatrists and mental health practitioners, since each of these areas has at some point either been thought to be of great theoretical or clinical relevance, or currently holds such promise for the future. An underlying theme of Dr. Ballenger's chapter is that there is, as yet, no coherent "biology" of depression, nor is there likely to be in the future; however, areas of consensus have emerged and the discussion of these data form the substance of his chapter.

Although sleep abnormalities are not specific to depression, their consistent presence provides clues to the underlying pathophysiology of depression and strongly supports the hypothesis that there is a biology of depression. Sleep abnormalities that are described may aid the diagnosis of depression and the prediction of treatment response; however, such tests are not yet practical for routine clinical use.

Among the most fascinating biological findings are those which suggest that abnormalities in characteristic daily circadian mood variations, and regular biologic rhythms such as REM rhythms and menstrual cycles and yearly or seasonal rhythms, may be associated with certain features of depressive illness and be related to the pathophysiology of depression. These observations tend to be more pronounced in bipolar patients, but they are also observed in unipolar patients. Although not yet sufficiently understood to be clinically useful outside research settings, there is optimism that such findings may lead to future advances in our understanding and treatment of depression.

Neuroendocrine studies that have generated the most widespread interest and promise in the past 5 to 10 years involve the cortisol system and the dexamethasone suppression test (DST), and the thyroid regulatory system and the tests for thyroid releasing hormone (TRH). Dr. Ballenger concludes that despite the tremendous enthusiasm generated by the DST, its limited sensitivity and specificity for major affective disorder means that a negative DST has little clinical significance and minimal diagnostic utility when patients with major depression are compared to those with nonmajor affective disorder or other severe, acute psychiatric illness. Moreover, a positive DST does not predict an improved response rate to antidepressant medication, nor should a negative DST discourage a trial of treatment. Currently the most promising area for clinical use and future research is the indication from several studies that an abnormal DST following clinical improvement is associated with a high risk of relapse.

Many investigations have now demonstrated that the response of thyroid stimulating hormone (TSH) to TRH is reduced in approximately 25 percent of depressed patients. What is very intriguing about this finding is that preliminary evidence suggests it may be a trait marker that is present before, during, and after a depressive episode and not just a "state" marker of depression. There is also some evidence that a reduced TRH response may help differentiate major unipolar depression from nonmajor, secondary, or characterologic depression.

Whether the TRH test is useful in predicting treatment response is still controversial; however, similar to the DST, the failure of TRH to normalize with clinical recovery may be predictive of an increased risk for subsequent relapse.

An in-depth discussion of neurotransmitter abnormalities is organized into the norepinephrine (NE), dopamine (DA), serotonin (5-HT), and acetylcholine (Ach) systems. Dr. Ballenger emphasizes important interactions among all four systems, in particular those between the NE and 5-HT systems, as well as the 5-HT and Ach systems. The shift from hypotheses that emphasized "too much–too little" theories to those involving more complex interactions among these systems are some of the more exciting and promising findings in the area of biologic mechanisms of depression.

Despite the tremendous progress and promise of "the biology" of depression, Dr. Ballenger closes with a conservative caution that a more definitive understanding of these mechanisms is probably decades away, as is the practical clinical use of biological measures.

In my chapter, I began by stating that although etiological evidence is still lacking, there is substantial data to support the clinical and research utility of distinguishing between unipolar and bipolar disorder. The organic etiology of depression is the subject of Dr. Cassem's chapter; however, any discussion of diagnostic issues must begin and end by emphasizing the necessity of always searching for a "primary" medical illness in depressive patients. The heterogeneity of the clinical profile, course, familial aggregation, biology, neurophysiology, and treatment response of depression that meets *Diagnostic and Statistical Manual of Mental Disorders, Third Edition, Revised (DSM-III)* (American Psychiatric Association, 1987) criteria for major depression must always be in the forefront of the mind of clinicians and researchers, and the quest to reduce depressive disorders to more homogeneous subgroups remains one of the major challenges in this field. Subtyping patients into dichotomies such as endogenous/nonendogenous, primary/secondary, psychotic/nonpsychotic, and situational/nonsituational is appealing descriptively and has had some value for prognosis and treatment planning, but has not yet resulted in the validation of distinct subclassifications. Despite these "facts," the popularity and widespread use of such distinctions is likely to persist in the hearts and vocabularies of most practitioners.

Recognizing that the coexistence with depression of symptoms of alcoholism, eating disorders, and anxiety states may represent the presence of at least two distinct syndromes and is not just the "multiple faces" of depression is one of the more significant advances made by clinical psychiatry in the past five years. Even more complex and controversial is the relationship between depression and personality, particularly dysthymic disorder. I have touched very briefly on this topic which was covered thoroughly by Dr. Robert M.A. Hirschfeld in a section on personality disorders in *Psychiatry Update: The American Psychiatric Association Annual Review*, Volume 5 (Frances and Hales, 1986).

In the last 5 to 10 years it has become recognized that depression in children and adolescents is far more prevalent than once thought, which may be related to the birth cohort phenomenon discussed by Drs. Goldin and Gershon. It is especially "depressing" that several research studies are finding that the clinical course of childhood depression appears to be as severe and chronic as adult depression. These findings and others warrant careful attention and have encouraged a burgeoning interest and activity in research on childhood depression.

Finally, data on the course of patients who are not in systematic treatment protocols gathered by different research groups are forging a consensus that depressive disorders in many patients should be thought of as lifetime conditions and not isolated episodes. Rates of chronicity after 2–5 years are as high as 10–20 percent, and a substantial proportion of patients who recover go on to a course marked by multiple recurrences with substantial interepisode symptoms and psychosocial impairment. Fortunately, clinically useful predictors that identify those patients likely to suffer a severe and chronic course are emerging, and there is an increasing availability of more specific and effective treatments for unipolar depression that are reviewed thoroughly in the chapters on somatic therapy and psychosocial treatment.

Dr. Prien's chapter on somatic treatment is creatively organized according to acute, continuation, preventive, and chronic treatment. This approach blends smoothly with the chapter on the diagnosis and natural history of depression and meets the dual heuristic role of teaching about the underlying course of depression while describing its treatment. Dr. Prien's experience in developing and coordinating several large-scale collaborative research programs and research consortiums on the treatment of affective disorder is evident in his systematic review of the field, and his recommendations are also consistent with the recent NIMH Consensus Development Statement on the treatment of recurrent mood disorders (NIMH/NIH Consensus Development Conference Statement, 1985). Dr. Prien uses a balanced approach in describing the treatment strategies known to be effective and also in delineating the many unanswered questions in the field. The use of tricyclic antidepressants (TCAs) as the treatment of choice for major depression with melancholic features, monoamine oxidase inhibitors (MAOIs) as the preferred treatment of nonendogenous depression with atypical features such as panic and severe anxiety, the combination of a TCA and a neuroleptic for mood congruent psychotic depression, and the use of ECT as an alternative for severe melancholic depression and depression with mood congruent psychotic features are all well established, as is the utility of continuation treatment for most patients. There is a valuable discussion of the advantages of TCAs over lithium in attenuating or preventing severe recurrences of depression, versus the comparative advantage of lithium when there is evidence of a latent bipolar disorder. The major gaps in our knowledge concern the paucity of controlled trials that last longer than six weeks with a consequent lack of more definitive information on the most effective approach for continuation therapy, preventive treatment, and the treatment of chronic major depression and dysthymic disorder. In particular, more precise data are needed to guide us in the critical issue of balancing the lowest effective dose for preventive treatment and unduly exposing the patients to an increased risk of new episodes.

Drs. Shea, Elkin, and Hirschfeld have done a masterful job of synthesizing the advances that have been established for the psychotherapeutic treatment of depression over the past 15 years. The authors articulate a view of the value of using psychosocial treatments for depression that is consistent with the review of somatic treatment in Dr. Prien's chapter. This includes the reality that some patients respond minimally or not at all to antidepressant medication; the high rate of relapse and recurrence following treatment, and the lack of sufficient studies on the value of antidepressant medication for the prophylactic and continuation of treatment of depression; the inability of some patients to tolerate the side effects of medication or contraindications to medical illness; and the refusal of some patients to take medication. Even when medication is accepted and is effective, there is evidence that successful psychotherapy may result in additional improvement in overall morale, occupational functioning, and in one's interpersonal functioning with friends, children, and spouse.

Although findings are reported on psychodynamic psychotherapy, which is the most widely used psychosocial treatment in clinical practice, research on this approach is limited and it has primarily been studied as a comparison condition in research studies on the more structured and time-limited psychotherapies. The main focus of the chapter is on the three modalities that have undergone the greatest empirical research: cognitive, behavioral, and interpersonal therapy. While these therapies are designed to be distinctive from each other, they have many common features, including being short-term and structured; emphasizing current issues and functioning; having an active role for the therapist and an active collaboration between the therapist and the patient; and having treatment manuals with detailed descriptions of treatment, rationale, strategies, and techniques. Evidence is reviewed that demonstrates the efficacy of these three specific treatments for outpatients with unipolar major depression. Despite these findings on beneficial efficacy and the very different theories and techniques that characterize these three therapies, most studies attempting to discern specific effects for the individual treatments have been negative—the exception being the area of social functioning for behavior therapy and interpersonal therapy and in self-concept for cognitive therapy. As with antidepressant medication, there is a paucity of follow-up studies measuring the longer-term effects of these treatments, and research in this area is sorely needed. Contrary to prevailing wisdom, the empirical evidence only shows a modest advantage for the combination of psychotherapy and pharmacotherapy compared to either psychotherapy or drug alone; however, there are two studies which show that pharmacotherapy plus psychotherapy leads to a more rapid response compared to psychotherapy alone.

Areas in which our knowledge is still lacking have to do with understanding why these three psychotherapies are effective. Competing hypotheses are that "nonspecific" or common factors account for improvement versus the view that methodologic limitations are responsible for the failure to find differential effects. Little is known about patient characteristics that are important to response to psychotherapy, particularly for the 20 to 30 percent of patients who are nonresponders, and there are essentially no data on the psychotherapeutic treatment of dysthymia. As is correctly emphasized by the authors, there is a dire need for controlled studies of psychodynamic therapy, since in the United States that is currently the most widely practiced psychosocial intervention.

In his scholarly and comprehensive chapter on depression secondary to medical illness, Dr. Cassem skillfully details how to put on the "white coat" of the internist or surgeon in order to diagnose multiple medical illnesses and identify toxic agents that cause depression, and how to take these factors into account when treating the depressive symptoms and syndrome. At the same time, he vividly conveys the necessity of empathizing with our patients, whether operating from the vantage point of the general medical diagnostician or from the perspective of the treating clinical psychiatrist.

An example of how Dr. Cassem "brings the reader to the bedside" of the medically ill patient is conveyed by his creative categorization of the causes of a depressive syndrome into four groups: 1) the effect of the illness or its treatment on the central nervous system (CNS), such as a left hemisphere stroke; 2) the effect of the illness on the patient's mind ("the subjective CNS"), exemplified by the "patient who becomes convinced that he is 'washed up' after a myocardial infarction"; 3) the "pure" creation of mind, as the patient who lies that he is depressed or exhibits fictitious grief; and 4) the result of interactions between the sick person and the environment of family, as seen in the patient who looks fine and has no complaints until the family arrives, and then becomes sad and withdrawn. An awareness that all factors may be playing some role must drive the clinician to begin by thoroughly understanding the disease of the patient. Dr. Cassem begins by giving us a systematic schema for excluding medical illness and then discusses several of the most common organic syndromes in greater detail. The discussion of how to treat depression in the medically ill is equally vivid, comprehensive, and systematic with a special emphasis on the side effects of tricyclic antidepressants and monamine oxidase inhibitors in patients who have a compromised cardiovascular system.

Among the myriad of Dr. Cassem's thoughtful discussions is a section on the use of psychostimulants such as dextroamphetamine and methylphenidate as the treatment of choice for many patients in whom TCAs or MAOIs are contraindicated or ineffective.

This well crafted approach to the diagnosis and treatment of depression in the medically ill should be an indispensable handbook for the practitioner who primarily treats outpatients as well as for the consultation/liaison psychiatrist who works in a hospital setting.

In summary, depression is perhaps the best understood of the major psychiatric disorders. However, several areas in which substanitally more work needs to be done must be emphasized. The opening chapter on genetics and family studies emphasized that the likelihood of future success in this area will be greatly enhanced by the resolution of the heterogeneity of major depression by clinical and biologic traits. This challenge for the field was also prominently discussed in most of the other chapters in this section. Therefore, it is clear that the quest for understanding the genetics, course, biology, and treatment of depression will be far more successful when valid homogeneous subtypes of major depression are delineated.

In conclusion, depression is the most widespread of all the major mental illnesses, with epidemiologic studies estimating an annual point prevalence of between four and six percent and a cumulative lifetime incidence of two to four percent for men and five to nine percent for women. Paradoxically, despite the in-depth available knowledge about depression, its high frequency in the general population, the misery and suffering inherent in being depressed, the potential morbidity and lethality of depression, and a diversity of effective somatic and psychosocial treatments, depression is often underrecognized, underdiagnosed, and undertreated. Estimates place the rate of failure to recognize or seek treatment for any given episode of major depression in the United States to be as high as 65 to 75 percent. As is discussed in the chapter by Dr. Prien, even after individuals seek treatment, rates of inadequate or inappropriate prescription or treatment compliance may be as high as 75 percent for psychiatric outpatients and 60 percent for patients who are hospitalized. In response to this sobering and sorrowful reality, in December 1985, the National Institute of Mental Health initiated a large-scale public health program entitled Depression Awareness, Recognition, and Treatment (DART). It is hoped that this educational campaign, which is modeled after successful public awareness programs in hypertension and breast cancer, will lead to more frequent recognition of depression, more rapid help-seeking behavior, and more effective early interventions by generalists in the health care profession and more regular referrals to mental health specialists. The goal of the chapters in this section is to ensure that psychiatrists and other mental health practitioners are armed with the most up-to-date and state-of-the-art knowledge on the epidemiology, genetics, course, biology, and treatment of this disorder. The ultimate objective is that this wisdom will result in a large pool of expert diagnosticians and clinicians who will teach and disseminate this knowledge to colleagues in the health care field, and that this will lead to more consistent and effective treatment of depressed patients.

REFERENCES

American Psychiatric Association: Diagnostic and Statistical Manual of Mental Disorders, Third Edition, Revised. Washington, DC, American Psychiatric Association, 1987

Frances AJ, Hales RE (Eds.): Psychiatry Update: The American Psychiatric Association Annual Review, vol. 5. Washington, DC, American Psychiatric Press, Inc., 1986

NIMH/NIH Consensus Development Conference Statement: Mood disorders: pharmacologic prevention of recurrences. Am J Psychiatry 142:469-476, 1985

III

Suicide

Section III

Suicide

Foreword

by J. John Mann, M.D., and Michael Stanley, Ph.D.,
Section Editors

I'll change my state with any wretch,
Thou canst from gaol or dunghill fetch;
My pain's past cure, another hell,
I may not in this torment dwell!
Now desperate I hate my life,
Lend me a halter or a knife;
All my griefs to this are jolly,
Naught so damn'd as melancholy.

Robert Burton (1652)

The pain of melancholia is commonly associated with suicidal thoughts, and the risk of suicide in melancholia is 80 times greater than it is in the general population. However, suicide appears to be only poorly correlated with the severity of the depressive illness. Why does a moderately ill patient commit suicide, and yet another, severely ill, patient not attempt suicide? How can the clinician distinguish the patient who will make a serious or successful suicide attempt from the patient who will not? Having identified the patient who appears to be at high risk, what kind of therapeutic intervention is likely to succeed? This section is dedicated to answering these questions.

The section begins at the point where Durkheim inaugurated the modern era of research into the causes of suicide; namely, by reviewing the application of the classical epidemiological research strategies to the study of suicide. In Chapter 13, Dr. Lee N. Robins and Dr. Pamela A. Kulbok describe advantages and limitations of the epidemiological approach. The goal of the approach is not merely to quantify the extent of the problem, but to identify potentially correctable social environmental risk factors. For the reasons given by Robins and Kulbok, the conclusions that can be drawn from the work of Durkheim and later investigators regarding risk factors for suicide are more modest than those stated by Durkheim, but are still of great importance.

A closer description of the risk factors for suicide and suicide attemptors is provided by Dr. Robert M.A. Hirschfeld and Dr. Lucy Davidson in Chapter 14. They generate a psychosocial profile that describes most patients who attempt or complete suicide. Unfortunately, this profile also describes a far *greater* number of patients who never attempt suicide. Thus, as a diagnostic tool, this clinical profile has high sensitivity but poor specificity. Some additional probe was needed to detect those at higher risk, and a potential breakthrough came from the area of psychobiological research.

In Chapter 15, Dr. Michael Stanley and Dr. J. John Mann describe how a correlation between reduced serotonergic function and violent suicidal acts (as an offspring of the neurobiological studies of despressive disorders) became apparent. Together with evidence that there is a genetic risk for suicide, the evidence that there are biological correlates of violent suicidal acts creates the hope that biological tests will permit more precise identification of high-risk patients and that a biological treatment to reduce suicide risk, regardless of diagnosis, will become possible.

The process of identification of the at-risk patient must be followed by treatment. The management of suicidal patients is discussed by Dr. David Brent and colleagues in Chapter 16, with a focus on the associated psychiatric disorder that is present in almost all cases. The authors emphasize that the associated psychiatric disorder requires specific treatment, as does the suicidal tendency.

The special problem of suicidal behavior among children and adolescents is addressed by Dr. Cynthia Pfeffer in Chapter 17. Suicide was and is rare in prepubertal children. In contrast, an alarming increase in the suicide rate in the 15–24-year-old age group (actually in males younger than 40) has occurred over the last 20 years. Although the rate of increase in youth suicide has slowed substantially and has been small in the last five years, suicide is now the second most common cause of death in this age group. Why has this increase occurred? Why is the rate of suicide so low in prepubertal children? Dr. Pfeffer addresses these questions, which have immense theoretical and practical implications for understanding the factors that increase and decrease the risk for suicide.

Ultimately, prevention of illness is the basic goal of medicine. Nowhere is this goal more important than in the case of suicide, which is such a major cause of death and in which 1 in 10 attempts are fatal. Unfortunately, suicide prevention centers and hot lines have not been shown to reduce suicide rates, probably because patients at risk for suicide usually do not turn to these centers for help. Dr. George E. Murphy reviews this difficult area and highlights alternative prevention approaches in Chapter 18.

Chapter 13

Epidemiologic Studies in Suicide

by Lee N. Robins, Ph.D., and Pamela A. Kulbok, D.N.Sc.

This chapter provides an epidemiologic approach to the understanding of suicide. Unlike psychiatric disorders—in which there are many unrecorded cases as well as recorded cases that are missed because they are in the files of various non-psychiatrist physicians, welfare agencies, and criminal justice agencies—suicide is uniquely suited to epidemiologic study because it is universally recorded on death certificates. The only missing cases are those that are misclassified, and the small number for which no corpse is ever found. The availability of total rosters of suicides in the Department of Vital Statistics records allows for the comparison of suicide rates across countries and geographic regions, and allows for the investigation of changes in rates over time and across demographic groups. Death records can also be linked to other records to study a broader set of correlates.

While the study of suicide has unique advantages, it also has unique disadvantages. Interviews with the suicide victim are obviously impossible after the fact. The suicide victim's survivors may be able to recall immediate precursors of the event as well as earlier personal history, but in order to obtain information from the perpetrator, the study design must be prospective. Since suicide is a rare and not very predictable event, prospective studies of suicide require enormous samples from the general population and sizeable samples from the population who seem to be at high risk for suicide.

This chapter, then, reviews the results obtained by the following approaches to the study of suicide: ecological analyses (achieved by comparing data from death records with census data); analysis of individual correlates (achieved by relating the various types of data found on death records); the extension of individual analyses (achieved by linking death records to other records); interviews with the suicide victim's survivors; and prospective interviews with general populations or persons at high risk.

STUDIES BASED ON DEATH CERTIFICATES

An ecological study calculates suicide rates for populations by using the number of death certificates in which suicide is listed as the cause of death as the numerator, and by using an estimate of the population at risk for suicide as the denominator. Rates may be compared across population groups that are distinguished by their geographical boundaries or by any characteristics that are known for both populations, such their economic systems or their religious preferences, or by demographic parameters such as age, race, and sex distributions. Sometimes ecological studies attempt to explain the difference in rates in two

This work was supported in part by Research Grant MH 31302, Research Scientist Award MH 00334, and Research Training Grant in Psychiatric Epidemiology and Biostatistics MH 17104.

geographically defined populations by differences in their religious, economic, or demographic characteristics. Such explanations are dubious, however, because those who commit suicide may not share the characteristics that distinguish the populations from which they come. Since suicide is atypical behavior in all populations, it would not be surprising to find that those who commit suicide have age, sex, racial, marital, or occupational patterns very different from those of the general population.

Ecological studies also attempt to explain changes in the same population over time by correlating them with historical changes affecting the base population. Again, such conclusions are dubious because these changes may not have affected the small group of persons who committed suicide.

Death certificates are useful for studies of individuals as well as for ecological studies. For example—by comparing the demographic characteristics recorded on the death certificates of suicide victims with the characteristics recorded on the death certificates of those dying by other causes, or by comparing the demographic characteristics of suicide victims with characteristics of survivors in the parent population—one can learn which demographic characteristics are risk factors for suicide. Death certificates can, in principle, be linked to other types of records to learn, for example, how many felons or welfare recipients eventually commit suicide. They can be the starting point for selecting a consecutive series of suicides for retrospective interviewing of their survivors. And they can be the end-point for the long-term prospective follow-up of a general population or a high risk sample.

Variation Across Groups and Areas

As an example of an ecological study, we have the World Health Organization's (1982) comparison of suicide rates for 1975–1980 in 24 European countries. Hungary ranked first, with a rate of 45.2 per 100,000. Czechoslovakia, Denmark, Austria, Finland, Germany, Sweden, and Switzerland followed, with reported rates above 24 per 100,000. France, Poland, and Bulgaria reported rates of 15–24 per 100,000. If the United States had been included, it would have ranked 15th, with a suicide rate of 12 per 100,000. In the same range were the Netherlands, Norway, Scotland, England, and Wales, where the rates are between 10 and 12 per 100,000. Italy, Spain, and Northern Ireland reported rates of 5–8, and Greece was lowest of all the countries studied, with a rate of 4.1 per 100,000.

The rate for the United States has remained approximately the same since it was estimated to be 11.8 per 100,000 in 1984 (Centers for Disease Control, 1985). Not all countries have shown such stable rates over time. Rates in England and Wales have declined, while those in Belgium, the Netherlands, and Ireland have sharply risen (Diekstra, 1985).

The striking differences between suicide rates in various countries and the rates in particular countries over time are in marked contrast to prevalence rates of schizophrenia, for example, which show great cross-national and cross-era stability. This variation encourages speculation that suicide may be influenced by local cultures and historical events. If this is the case, there is reason to believe that suicide rates should be influenced by prevention strategies. However, before coming to this conclusion, there are a number of cautions that researchers have stressed. For example, there is reason to question the comparability of suicide rates across countries and across time. Since suicide is extremely rare before the age of 15, it is to be expected that rates will be low in countries with high fertility rates. And since rates for white males increase with age, health standards that protect against early deaths from natural causes are associated with a greater number of persons surviving into ages at which the risk for suicide is high. Clearly, then, suicide rates should not be compared across countries without standardization for age and adjustment for the frequency of competing causes of death.

It is also suspected that variations in ascertainment procedures account for a good deal of the variation in rates. When more cases are referred to coroners and more autopsies performed, more suicides will be discovered. And when the coroners accept less definitive evidence of suicide, more of the questionable cases will be labeled as such. Coroners have considerable discretionary power in determining whether a suicide has occurred, because no standard criteria have yet been adopted to guide this determination. Clearly, a high suicide rate in a country with high rates of autopsy, and with coroners under no political or religious pressure to minimize the number of suicides ascertained, does not necessarily mean that there is something in that culture conducive to suicide; it may mean only that a very high proportion of all true suicides are being reported.

Variation over Time

Trends over time need to be examined cautiously, not only because ascertainment procedures may change over time with change in law, medical examiner personnel, or local custom with respect to ordering autopsies, but because a change in the international system for listing causes of death in 1968 probably had some effect on suicide rates. A "cause–undetermined" category was added, so that there was no longer a forced choice between accident and suicide in doubtful cases. This should have decreased the suicide rate somewhat, although it probably decreased the accident rate more, since it is generally believed that in every country doubtful decisions tend to go against suicide.

When, despite these opportunities for artifactual influences, a common time trend across countries is found, one tends to believe that it is correct. One such trend appears to be widespread: In 11 countries studied, suicide rates in the 15–24-year-old age group have been rising. Between 1970 and 1980 in the United States there was a 50 percent increase in rates for males in the 15–24-year-old age group (WHO, 1982). In white males 15–19 in 1970, the suicide rate had been 9 per 100,000; in 1984, the rate was 16 per 100,000, almost double. The increase seemed to slow in about 1980, but since then, the trend is still upward. Lower but still alarming increases in young male suicide rates (13–32 percent) were reported in European countries between 1973 and 1980 (Diekstra, 1985). In the United States, rates for black males and for black and white females were initially lower than the rates for white males. There has been a modest rise in suicide rates for black males and virtually no change over time in suicide rates for females of either race.

How Age, Sex, and Rates of Suicide Have Changed over Time in the United States

This observation of a rapidly increasing rate for young people in the United States needs to be seen in the context of stability of the total rate. This stability implies two important facts: first, that rates for older men in the United States have been declining—this good news tends to be overlooked in the concern over rising suicide rates among the young; and second, that these very large increases in the suicide rate among youths have occurred in a group that had an almost negligible rate 40 years ago—so that while the percentage of increase is large, youths still contribute relatively little to the overall rate. Interestingly, this pattern of rising rates among the young and falling rates among the elderly have also been found in England (Sainsbury and Jenkins, 1982).

Figure 1 shows these time trends dramatically for white males in the United States. Rates are presented by 10-year age brackets between 1950 and 1982 (National Center for Health Statistics, 1984). For the final three years repre-sented, annual rates were available; before that, rates were available only by decade. In 1950, suicide rates were strongly and positively associated with age for white males, increasing steadily with age from only 6 per 100,000 for those aged 15–24, to 10 times that rate for those aged 75 or older. Since then, suicide rates have fallen for all age groups above 44. Despite these changes, the ratio of rates for those aged 75 or older remains approximately double the rate for those aged 45–54. The decline seems to have ended in 1970 for those aged 75 and over, but has continued into the present for others over age 44.

There has been little or no change in suicide rates over this period for persons aged 35–44, while rates for the young have been increasing. As a result, the range has narrowed. In 1970, the rates were still perfectly correlated with age, but the ratio of rates for the oldest to youngest had dropped from 10:1 to 3.6:1. In the succeeding 12 years, as the suicide rates of the elderly declined and the rates of the young rose, the 25–34-year-olds' suicide rate became as high as the rate of the 55–64-year-olds.

Women and black males showed much less variation by age in 1950 and have shown less dramatic changes since then. Figure 2 illustrates the suicide rates

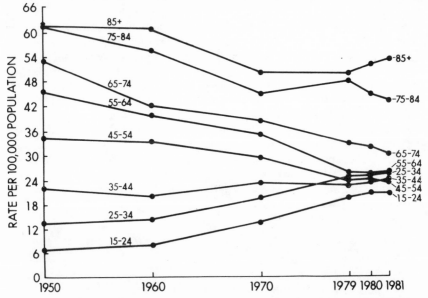

Figure 1. Suicide in white males, aged 15 and older, in the United States—1950–1981

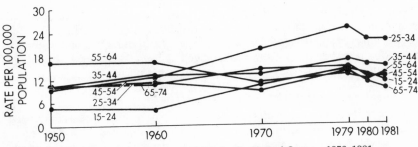

Figure 2. Suicide in black males, aged 15–74, in the United States—1950–1981

for black males. In 1950, while the youngest group had the lowest rate, there was no clear relationship with age overall. However, deaths in young black males have paralleled the sharply rising rates in young white males, so that by the 1980s, the 25–34-year-olds had the highest rates among black males.

These results, divided by age, sex, and race, show the degree to which findings of a stable rate over time for the United States population can hide the patterns for subpopulations. These fascinating, but so far uninterpretable, results are achieved by using death certificates as a source not only for the fact of suicide, but for the age, race, and sex of the suicide victim. This allows for the calculating of suicide rates for specific groups categorized by age, race, or gender. Use of these demographic variables on death certificates overcomes much of the skepticism about the validity of ecological comparisons across areas or nations, or even across time within a single nation. While ways to calculate suicide rates may vary across nations or may have changed over time, it is not obvious that they would change differentially by age, race, or gender within a single country.

It is not that analyses contrasting rates by age, sex, or racial groups within a single country are proof against artifacts. If, for example, older white males shifted from guns and hanging to pills as their means of suicide, or stopped writing suicide notes, the apparent decline in their suicide rates might be due only to a lower proportion ascertained. However, we have no reason to believe that there have been such shifts. But there may be reason to suspect some improved ascertainment among blacks. Part of the rise in black suicides might be only apparent, because the black migration from the rural South to cities throughout the country in the 1940s and 1950s probably exposed their sudden deaths to a more standardized set of procedures and greater opportunities for autopsy. However, the fact that an increase in youthful suicide has been found for both races, and for males more than females, suggests that migration of blacks is not the sole explanation.

While blacks have had a greater shift from rural to urban living than has the rest of the population, there has been a general urbanization of America since the 1940s. If urbanization has meant a general improvement in ascertainment, the fact that the overall suicide rate has been stable over this time span must imply a true decline in suicide.

Our capacity to follow changes over time, not only in total rates but in particular age, sex, and racial groups, has been created by the computerization of death certificates. In theory, it should be possible to follow changes in rates according to other variables as well, since on United States death certificates there is also a place to enter place of birth, marital status, veteran status, usual occupation, and place of residence. These variables could be used to study the possible effect of social class, marital status, geographical region, and history of migration on suicide. So far, little advantage has been taken of these items, in part, no doubt, because they are less frequently and reliably filled in.

Variation across Small Geographic Areas

One item that appears on death certificates—place of residence—has been used to see whether variations in community types are associated with differences in suicide rates. However, small area studies are particularly liable to the effects of local coroners' practices. To learn how great such effects might be, Nelson and colleagues (1978) studied the practices of 191 coroners in 11 Western states with respect to certifying suicides. They found extensive variation in the educational backgrounds of coroners, in professional resources available to them, in the statutes under which they function, and in their procedures. For example, 30 percent of the coroners reported that autopsies were almost always performed if suicide was suspected; the remainder rarely performed autopsies under these circumstances. The authors cite the work of Litman, who found that the frequency with which death from a self-inflicted gunshot wound was determined to be suicide varied among local jurisdictions from 50 to 95 percent.

Much of this local variation could probably be eliminated by the adoption of standards for the investigation and reporting of suicide, and by the adoption of uniform training requirements for coroners. But uniform codes would not entirely overcome some modicum of underreporting that is to be expected because family members would prefer some other assignment of cause of death when there is a reasonable doubt—a negative bias that is likely to be enhanced when the coroner is locally elected. In addition to bias caused by a general disinclination to make a determination of suicide, there are cases missed for other reasons: when no body is found, in which case no death certificate is filed, even if the circumstantial evidence of suicide is persuasive; when suicide occurs in a person with a known preexisting illness that could have been directly responsible for the death; or in a drug addict whose tolerance results in drug blood levels likely to be interpreted by a coroner, unaware of the addiction, as sufficient to explain accidental death by overdose.

Testing for the Severity of Ascertainment Artifacts

Because it seems so reasonable that ascertainment practices could bias estimates of suicide rates, it is interesting to see whether that bias appears to be so serious as to invalidate comparisons across nations or coroners' jurisdictions.

COMPARING NATIVES WITH EMIGRANTS. Barraclough alone (1973), with Sainsbury (Sainsbury and Barraclough, 1968), and with Jenkins (Sainsbury and Jenkins, 1982) used two ingenious methods to see whether the large differences across nations previously noted were simply artifacts of differential ascertainment. First, he compared the rank order of rates by nation with the rank order of suicide rates of immigrants from those countries to the United States. It was presumed that in the United States ascertainment would not be correlated with the nation of origin. Therefore, if the rank order within the United States corresponded with the ranks among their countries of origin, the explanation for the variation must lie in the culture or in the biology of the national group, not in ascertainment procedures. The rank order correlation between rates in native countries and among immigrants from those countries was very high. In addition, the spread of rates across countries of origin was little reduced from the spread in the homelands. Similar results were obtained by Lester (1972) for immigrants in Australia.

ADDING DEATHS FROM UNDETERMINED CAUSES. Barraclough's (1973) second method was to compare ranks for suicide rates with ranks for suicide plus undetermined causes across countries. He argued that if the difference in rates across countries was only due to the fact that some countries were using much more rigid criteria than others, there should be much less variation in rates of suicide plus undetermined causes than in suicide rates alone. He found a very high correlation between ranks for suicide alone versus suicide plus undetermined cause (0.89 in 1968 for 22 countries, and 0.96 for 19 countries in 1970–1973). On the basis of these findings, he concluded that national differences were real.

Similarly, Malla and Hoenig (1983), asking whether the low rate of suicides in Newfoundland as compared with the rest of Canada could be due to ascertainment problems, combined cases that were termed suicides with unexplained and undetermined deaths. The resulting suicide rate in Newfoundland (6.36 per 100,000) was still less than one-half the overall Canadian rate of 14. They, too, concluded that underreporting alone could not account for the lower rate.

Each of these attempts to show that local variations in suicide rates were artifacts of ascertainment procedures failed. These demonstrations help to convince us that national and regional differences are real. However, they do not tell us what the true rate of suicides is in these localities. There remains the unknown proportion of suicides that appear on death certificates as accidents, homicides, and natural deaths. It is difficult to see how these misclassified suicides can be recovered to correct our estimates, short of sampling deaths from *all* causes over a short period during which a special independent effort would be made to correctly assign them according to well specified criteria. Such an exercise could be extremely helpful in estimating what the actual undercounting is, by comparing the trial period with statistics from matched control areas and from the test areas themselves shortly before the trial. Such a study would yield a "correction factor" that could be applied to our normal data collection from the Department of Vital Statistics, and enable us to put standard errors around our national estimates.

Explaining Variation across Site and Time

ECOLOGICAL CORRELATES. The finding in the studies just mentioned—that variation in suicide rates across time and place is not an artifact of ascertainment methods—convinces us that there are real variations in rates, but we still would like to understand why these variations occur.

A more complex form of ecologic analysis is needed to test hypotheses about social, economic, religious, and political factors that may contribute to suicide rates. The classic work of Durkheim (1951) is an excellent example of ecologic analysis that tests causal hypotheses.

Durkheim explored differences in rates in rural and urban areas, in and out of the military, by age and marital status, by the dominant religion and ethnic affiliation, by occupation, and by climate. He concluded that suicide mortality varies with social integration, social structure, and social change (Selkin, 1983). While his work still stimulates research, it has also been cited as a prime example of the dangers of ecologic fallacy (Kleinbaum et al, 1982). Having found that predominantly Protestant provinces in Western Europe had higher suicide rates than predominantly Catholic provinces, Durkheim concluded that Protestants were more likely to commit suicide than Catholics. While probably correct, this inference cannot be made with certainty so long as there are both Catholics and Protestants in all provinces. In predominantly Protestant provinces it could have been the Catholics who were taking their own lives. The risk of ecological fallacy exists whenever the composition of each group in the analysis is not homogeneous with respect to the study factor.

If Durkheim had had access to a computerized system such as the National Death Register, he might have been able to do individual rather than ecological analyses, and thus have had a more definitive result. While religion does not appear on our death certificates, the name of the undertaker does—and there is a strong tendency for undertakers to specialize in Jewish, Protestant, or Catholic funerals. Knowing the funeral directors thus makes possible an inference about the deceased's religion. But even now, Durkheim would have trouble obtaining access to the National Death Register for these purposes. It can be used by researchers doing follow-up studies, who have identifiers such as name, birth date, and social security number to submit. If a match to the identifiers is located, researchers are told in what state the death certificate is filed, and they can arrange to get a copy from that state office. Only then do they learn the cause of death. But most investigators cannot use the National Death Register to test hypotheses about relationships among variables on the death certificate. For the present, we must rely on the staff of the Department of Vital Statistics to pursue these questions, since only they have access to the Register.

Even if the Register's data tapes were to become accessible to the public, there would be some problems with using them. Sometimes there is no knowledgeable informant to provide items such as usual employment, marital status, and place of birth. Furthermore, the completed items may be misleading. For example, Monday has been found to be the day of the week with the largest proportion of suicides. While one might think that this means that it is depressing to have to return to work after the weekend, it may actually only mean that Monday is the day for *discovering* suicides committed over the weekend, because a search begins when the suicide victim does not appear on the job (MacMahon, 1983). LINKING RATE CHANGES TO SOCIAL AND HISTORICAL EVENTS. A number of studies have attempted to relate changes in suicide rates to concomitant historical changes. As an example, Henry and Short (1954) related changes in suicide rates to fluctuations in official crime statistics in a sample of cities. They found an inverse relationship between suicide and homicide, which they believed substantiated the psychoanalytic theory that suicide and homicide are alternative ways of expressing aggression; that is, that suicide is aggression turned inward. Assuming that the amount of aggression in the population is constant, according to this theory, as homicide increases, suicide should decrease.

Holinger and Klemen (1982) extended the span of years to 1975 and included the total United States. They found a direct rather than an inverse relationship between suicide and homicide that held for all racial and gender groups, a finding consistent with the earlier work of Brenner (1979) that indicated that suicide and homicide increase in parallel when unemployment rises, and consistent with clinical studies that find high rates of suicidal behavior in violent patients.

A high rate of suicide associated with unemployment has been observed with considerable regularity (Platt, 1984; Wasserman, 1984; Platt and Kreitman, 1985) both in ecological studies showing correlations between rates of unemployment and suicide across geographic areas, and in studies noting that the rate of joblessness on death certificates of suicides is well above the concurrent population rate.

However, the ecological finding that local unemployment and suicide rates are positively correlated might have other explanations. Communities with high unemployment often have many of the other features that Durkheim summarized as "social disorganization"—crime, broken families, secularism. It might be these factors rather than unemployment that explains the suicide rate. The finding of a high frequency of unemployment on death certificates of suicides might also be misleading. The unemployment may only reflect the impairment in function brought about by psychiatric disorder, which in turn was the actual cause of the suicide.

More convincing evidence for a causal relationship would be the finding that a national increase in unemployment is regularly followed by an increase in suicide rate, an increase which is reversed when the employment picture improves. The effect of employment on suicide over time must be studied in the nation as a whole rather than in smaller geographic areas, because changes in local rates might simply show that the local area is changing character due to migration in or out.

There was an increase in suicides during the Great Depression, but it has been difficult to show a consistent relationship with less dramatic fluctuations in employment, in part, perhaps, because there is no agreement about what the proper lag time is between changes in employment levels and changes in suicide rates. An interesting technique was developed by Wasserman (1984), who used the average length of unemployment rather than the number unemployed as the indicator of a depressed economy, and found a significant increase in suicide nine months after the beginning of an economic depression.

Wars are unique, datable historical events that have been found to be related to a drop in suicide rates. The drop has sometimes been attributed to participation in a shared national goal and consequent greater sense of self-worth and integration into the community. Because movement from peace to war and from war to peace are events over which the individual has no control, the advent of war and peace appear to offer many of the advantages of an experiment in which the subject is randomly assigned to the experimental or control condition by the investigator. However, effects of a "natural experiment" such as war must be scrutinized to be sure that its apparent effects are not spurious. Unlike a true experiment in which all changes are controlled by the experimenter, in the case of war and suicide the drop in deaths designated as suicides might be only apparent if ascertainment declines as medical examiners depart for war-related jobs, or if suicides in the military are misreported as combat deaths.

CHANGES IN RATES WITH SHIFTS IN OPPORTUNITY. Other historical events that can lead to a change in suicide rates are shifts in medical practice toward prescription of less lethal sedatives (for example, the shift from barbiturates to benzodiazepines (Oliver and Hetzel, 1973), or the enactment of laws that markedly change access to common means of suicide, such as restrictions on the sale of guns or the removal of carbon monoxide from cooking gas (Lester and Murrell, 1980; Kreitman, 1976). If it can be assumed that nothing has changed except access to the means of committing suicide, then changes in suicide rates following these events can be attributed to them. When a sustained drop in rates follows restriction of a single important means, as occurred in England, Vienna, and Brisbane when cooking gas was detoxified, it demonstrates that intervention is worthwhile, because barring suicide by one means does not simply lead to the substitution of some other method.

We still need to be sure that the cause of the drop in suicide rates when the means are reduced is not a coincidence. Brown (1979) offered two observations in support of the effect of detoxifying cooking gas that addressed the possibility of such a spurious relationship. First, there was the essential temporal order—the detoxification of cooking gas clearly preceded the decline in the British suicide rate. Second, the total decline in suicides was numerically equivalent to the decline in suicide mortality from carbon monoxide during the relevant period. Though not absolute proof, this showed that the two events probably were related, and it was not merely that the law was passed at a time when the rate of suicide happened to be declining independently.

When historical changes happen gradually rather than at a fixed date, the causal argument is more difficult to make. In the United States, the number of handguns in private possession has been rising sharply, but there is no date on which they can be said to have become common. Boyd (1983) used a similar line of argument to that used for cooking gas, to show that the increased availability of guns had caused the rise in suicide. First, he showed that the increasing rate of suicide by firearms from 1953 to 1978, from 4.9 per 100,000 to 7.1 per 100,000, paralleled the increase in the overall suicide rate during this 25-year period. Next, Boyd showed that nonfirearm suicides did not increase during this period. Finally, he showed that accidental deaths by firearms did not increase during this period, so that one could conclude that the effect was specific to suicides, not just a general increase in gun deaths. Lester and Murrell (1980) tested the same hypothesis by comparing suicide rates in states that differed in the strictness of their gun control laws. States with stricter laws had lower male suicide rates during the period from 1969 to 1971. The fact that only males were affected was consistent with (although not definitive proof of) the argument that the availability of guns explained the difference, because men are twice as likely as women to use firearms as their method of suicide. Markush and Bartolucci (1984) examined regional United States suicide rates in the mid-1970s and also found a statistically significant correlation between gun and pistol prevalence and suicide rates. Farmer and Rohde (1980) examined methods of suicide and self-injury in 11 countries from 1969 to 1973. They compared total suicide rates with suicide rates excluding the use of firearms and hangings. Excluding these methods reduced the variation across countries, showing that the availability of firearms could play an important role in determining suicide rates.

Each of these demonstrations, while consistent with the argument that the increased availability of firearms leads to a rise in suicides, is also consistent with the view that violent people buy guns, vote against laws restricting their ownership, *and* commit suicide. The association is clear; the causal argument remains uncertain.

CHANGING SUICIDE RATES AND PREVENTIVE ACTIVITIES. The opening, in the 1960s, of suicide prevention centers over much of the United Kingdom and the United States and their continued operation since that time provides the closest parallel between epidemiological assessment and a true experiment. All that is lacking is the random assignment of prevention centers to some areas while others are left alone. Still, suicide rates could be compared before and after the centers were opened. If a decline were found, there would still be a need to be sure it was not attributable to other changes in the same period. However, the issue of how to interpret a decline has become moot, since there was no decline after the prevention movement began (Miller et al, 1984). One probable explanation for the prevention movement's lack of impact on suicide rates seems to be that prevention centers have attracted primarily young white female clients, a demographic group with a high rate of suicide attempts but a low rate of suicide completions.

Linking Death Records to Other Records

Another way in which to use death certificates to study suicide is to link death records with records from other rosters. For areas in which there are cancer registers that can be assumed to offer reasonably complete coverage, for example, the effect of knowing that one has a life-threatening disease on suicide risk can be studied by comparing the rates of suicide among cancer registrants with rates of suicide for the general population, standardized to the cancer registrants by age, sex, and race. When names in a tumor registry were linked with vital statistics records, a twofold increase in the risk of suicide was found for the cancer patients (Marshall et al, 1983).

Linking the 16-year accumulation of records in the Monroe County, New York, psychiatric register to death records (Kraft and Babigian, 1976) allowed researchers to ascertain the proportion of suicide victims who had been psychiatric patients within that 16-year period (45 percent had been) or in the 30 days before death (one-half as many were). Record linkage provided two sets of controls for the treated suicides—untreated suicides and nonsuiciding patients. Comparing the treated suicides to these two groups shows how vital the choice of control subjects is, since the two control samples differed from the treated suicides in diametrically opposed directions. As compared to the untreated suicide controls, a higher proportion of suicide victims who had received psychiatric treatment were young, female, black, and of low social class. As compared with the other psychiatric patients, a higher proportion of patients who committed suicides were old, white, male, and of higher social status. Thus, psychiatric patients as a group have a very different demographic profile from suicide victims as a group, and patients who commit suicide fall between the two.

Record linkage studies of suicide are rare in the United States because there are so few rosters other than those available through the Department of Vital Statistics that cover complete populations. The psychiatric register is virtually defunct these days because it is expensive to maintain, was not used as much as had been expected for research, and ran afoul of privacy laws. But even had registers thrived, record linkage has its own problems. If the updating of the two registers is not in synchrony, a case may be missed simply because the data entry has been delayed. There are always problems in matching names and identifiers due to misspellings or absence of a middle initial or birthdate errors. If strict matches are required, cases are missed and the proportion of suicides in the linked register is underestimated. If the criteria are loose, the linkage is overestimated. Nonetheless, the ability to link rosters greatly increases the potential for finding explanatory variables.

Overview of Death Record Studies

These studies utilizing death certificates have suggested a variety of causal factors in suicide, among them national attitudes, easy availability of highly lethal means, economic stress, age and sex roles, and physical illness. They have simultaneously raised questions as to whether apparent differences in rates are real or whether they are artifacts of ascertainment and reporting. Other methods linking individuals' histories to their suicidal behavior are necessary to make the causal arguments more convincing.

RETROSPECTIVE STUDIES OF COMPLETED SUICIDE

Retrospective studies of completed suicides are investigations in which the researcher collects data on events or circumstances prior to the suicide in hopes of identifying its causal antecedents. In clinical research seeking risk factors for an illness, the preferred design for restrospective studies is the case control design, in which those affected, along with control subjects similar to them in ways thought not to be causes of the disorder of interest, are either interviewed or investigated through records about the circumstances present during the time period before those affected became sick. The chief design issues in case control studies are getting representative samples of those affected, choosing the proper control subjects, and dating onset to be sure that the time frame of inquiry is appropriate. Retrospective studies of suicide have two advantages over studies of illness: representativeness of the cases is generally not an issue because a consecutive series or random sample of all suicides recorded in the local Department of Vital Statistics records within a specified time period can be studied; and the date of occurrence is certain. However, it is obviously impossible to interview affected persons, and it is so unclear who the relevant controls should be that most studies include none.

Lacking the opportunity to interview the proband, retrospective studies have utilized a variety of sources of information, principally relatives, physicians, employers, medical records, suicide notes, and coroners' reconstruction of events surrounding the suicide itself. When this technique has centered on reconstructing the events immediately surrounding the death, it has been called the "psychological autopsy" (Shneidman, 1981b). But the search for causes has also covered earlier histories, including earlier suicide attempts, histories of psychiatric treatment, and losses or threats of losses that might explain the suicide victim's hopelessness.

Reconstruction of Events Preceding the Suicide

The studies of Dorpat and Ripley (1960), Barraclough and colleagues (1974), and Robins (1981), all of which used retrospective reconstruction of events preceding the suicide, agree that almost all suicide victims were psychiatrically ill at the time of death. In all three studies, depression and alcoholism were the predominant diagnoses. Many of the suicide victims had been in touch with a physician shortly before the event and many had made prior unsuccessful suicide attempts (Robins, 1981). The agreement across studies about psychiatric status at the time of death shows that interviews with relatives of the suicide victim allow one to formulate retrospective diagnoses. Also, the fact that many suicide victims had been in psychiatric treatment shortly before the event shows that there is no exaggeration of the attendant psychiatric problems by relatives in an effort to understand reasons for the suicide.

Although none of these studies provided a control group for comparison, the rates of psychiatric disorder reported for the suicides were so high that no control group is necessary to convince us that suicide victims have higher rates of disorder than do members of the general population. What one would like to know, however, is how psychiatrically disordered persons who commit suicide differ from psychiatrically disordered persons who do not, so that preventive measures could be instituted with the appropriate patients. To learn this, one needs to compare patients who committed suicide with a control group of patients who did not. Farberow and Shneidman (1955) compared 32 male patients in a Veterans Administration mental hospital who committed suicide with three other groups of patients: those who attempted suicide, those who threatened suicide, and those who were nonsuicidal. The suicidal patients were distinguished from the nonsuicidal group by a diagnosis of depression or paranoid schizophrenia. A family history of mental hospitalization differentiated the completed suicides from the other three groups. Social and environmental factors revealed no differences among groups.

Researchers concerned with social factors that may predict suicide have also found a need for control subjects. Breed (1963) selected controls (matched by age, sex, and race to the suicides) from the neighborhoods where the suicides had lived. He found the suicides to have had more occupational problems, including downward mobility, lower income, and more unemployment.

Retrospective studies have also permitted contrasting diagnostic groups with respect to their apparent motives for suicide (Murphy and Robins, 1967) and the methods selected (Murphy, 1975). Alcoholics were particularly likely to have been left by their spouses or to have received a serious threat of such leaving shortly before the attempt.

Despite the remarkable amount of information available through retrospective studies, these studies cannot provide certain crucial information. What is missing is information as to how high the risks of suicide are in known high risk groups such as elderly white males, or unemployed men with alcohol problems, or depressed persons who have suffered certain types of loss, and how long the risk persists. Prospective studies have addressed some of these issues.

PROSPECTIVE STUDIES

The Problem of Rare Events

To be financially feasible, prospective studies of suicide generally require samples enriched by subjects known to be at high risk on the basis of clinical or socio-demographic characteristics, or of critical life events. But even high risk samples have seldom turned out to be large enough to yield sufficient suicides within a reasonable time span to distinguish the antecedents of the act. Cobb and Kasl (1972), for example, assuming that unemployment puts men at high risk for suicide, followed men working for a plant that was about to be closed in order to learn what the risk and predictive factors in suicide were, under conditions of high stress. However, they could not tell because they found only two suicides.

To be useful for prevention, the factors found to predict suicide must predict a reasonably high frequency of its occurrence. Yet MacKinnon and Farberow (1976) noted that even with the most conservative estimates of predictive error in a psychiatric inpatient population, certainly a population with an elevated risk, suicides are still too rare even among the highest risk segments to justify taking strenuous preventive action, because too many patients who did not need such action would be inconvenienced. A number of studies confirm their conclusion. Motto (1979) attempted to predict suicide in depressed and suicidal psychiatric inpatients on the basis of social and situational factors derived by discriminant analysis. He found statistically significant results, but results of limited practical utility for intervention. Pokorny (1983) followed a sample of 4,800 psychiatric inpatients to assess the number of completed suicides and parasuicides. A total of 67 suicides were identified and 179 unsuccessful suicide attempts. The predictors derived produced too many false positive cases to be useful in planning interventions.

One population that might be expected to yield a high enough rate of positives to be useful as a basis for planning interventions is that of suicide attempters, since retrospective studies found that many completed suicides had been preceded by unsuccessful attempts. Dorpat and Ripley (1967) summarized 15 studies of the rate of committed suicide following attempted suicide. The percentage who were found at follow-up to have committed suicide ranged from 0.03 percent to 22.0 percent, depending on the length of the follow-up. A rate of two percent was found by Schmidt and colleagues (1954), when attempters seen in an emergency room were followed for eight months. Tuchman and Youngman (1968) compared the suicide risk in 1,112 consecutive attempted suicides with the risk for the general population, and found a 139-fold increase (1.9 percent versus 0.01 percent), despite the fact that attempters tend to be female, young, and nonwhite, while suicides tend to be older white males. Attempters are at considerably higher risk for suicide, for example, than persons with terminal illnesses such as cancer, where the excess is only twofold (Marshall et al, 1983). But despite the fact that attempters have a more elevated risk than any other identified population, the risk does not appear high enough to warrant taking preventive action over a prolonged period, since 98 percent of the attempters do not require such intervention.

Even if prospective studies were to yield high enough rates of suicide to make our efforts to intervene practical, they would not tell us much about the causes closest in time to the event. Murphy (1984) points out that although a prospective study allows personal interviews with the prospective suicide victim, and thus provides more and better quality information about psychiatric symptoms and life events than that obtainable after death from an informant, it yields less data than do retrospective studies about circumstances immediately antecedent to the suicide act, since it is unlikely that the suicide will follow closely upon an interview. In addition, the ethical requirement to attempt to prevent a suicide if there is a clear and imminent danger compromises the scientific objectivity of prospective studies.

Suicide as One of Several Outcomes

The studies discussed thus far were designed specifically to study suicide. An alternative design is to follow a high risk population with respect to a variety of outcomes, of which suicide is one. The advantage of this design is that it allows for comparison of the frequency of suicide with that of other possible results. It also makes follow-up studies more attractive economically, since the study will yield some important results even if suicide rates turn out to be low. However, to include suicide as an outcome may lead to a longer follow-up interval than would be needed to study other outcomes. Since risk increases with age, it would be most informative to follow all cases to death, so that all the suicides that will ever occur will be discovered. No such study has yet been carried out.

A study of children seen in a child guidance clinic followed them into their mid-forties (Robins, 1966), and Terman and Oden's (1947) follow-up of children with very high IQs reported its last contact with them in their forties and fifties. These studies discovered childhood predictors of many adult outcomes, but they fell short of achieving this goal for suicide. The child guidance clinic study found a slightly higher rate of suicide (two percent) in those who received a consensus diagnosis of antisocial personality than in those with other adult disorders or in a control group of nonpatients. However, the numbers were too small to conclude that antisocial personality is a risk factor for suicide. But even had differences been statistically significant, the fact that follow-up ended when the subjects were in their mid-forties meant that the results might only indicate that antisocial personality is associated with earlier suicide, not more suicides. The follow-up of children with high IQs was reanalyzed (Shneidman, 1981a) to seek childhood antecedents and intercurrent events differentiating five who shot themselves from a control group who died a natural death. Despite the special sample and small number, the familiar variables of alcoholism and occupational instability were noted.

TESTING ECOLOGIC HYPOTHESES IN POPULATION SURVEYS

The studies we have just reviewed sought predictors of suicide either by comparing aggregate data across time and place or by comparing individual cases of suicides with nonsuicides. These studies have produced a host of correlates from demographic, psychiatric, and life event domains. What has not yet happened is some bridging of the aggregate and individual approaches so that differences between aggregate rates in deomgraphically defined populations can be explained. Accomplishing this is difficult for the reasons outlined above—suicides are rare and the victims cannot be interviewed.

There have been two attempts to circumvent these problems by approaching the problem obliquely. The argument goes as follows: If suicide is more common in certan populations than in others, and if suicidal individuals have character-isitics that distinguish them from nonsuicidal persons, then those distinguishing characteristics should be particularly common in the populations that provide the highest suicide rates. This approach has been applied by Hendin (1964) in an attempt to explain the fact that suicide rates are high in Denmark and low in Norway, and by Robins and colleagues (1977) in an attempt to explain why, in America, older white men have much higher suicide rates than older black men. Both studies began with interviews comparing suicidal patients with other patients, and then tested their results by interviewing members of the general populations that produce high and low suicide rates. Those characteristics that distinguished both suicidal from nonsuicidal patients, and general populations at high risk for suicide from general populations at low risk, were likely to help explain the population differences in suicide rates. In the study seeking to explain the high suicide rates in older white men (Robins et al, 1977), six findings from the clinical study of suicidal patients were confirmed as relatively more common in the general population of older white than black men: depression, alcohol abuse, low religiosity, family members or friends who had committed suicide, not living with a spouse, and expecting old age to be unrewarding.

PROPOSALS FOR VALIDATING CAUSAL HYPOTHESES

This indirect approach joining clinical and population studies is only one necessary step in producing a unified body of theory of suicide causation that can accommodate findings at both the aggregate and individual levels. Although it allows weeding out hypotheses that are not promising on the aggregate level, it fails to prove the correctness of the hypotheses that are sustained. A next step should be a prospective study of members of high risk populations with and without the postulated risk characteristics. In the United States, such a sample would be white men over 65 who are allocated to high and low risk groups on the basis of their history of alcohol problems and depression, their family histories of suicide, their religiosity, their marital status, and their attitudes toward aging. If our hypotheses are correct, the suicide rate in the population with all these predictors will be so high that it will be possible to validate the potency of these predictors even for an event as rare in the general population as suicide within a reasonable study period—perhaps 10 years—and in a sample of only moderate size. The most exciting finding that such a study could yield would be that older white men *without* any of these personal risk factors had suicide rates no higher than those found in low risk demographic categories (women, blacks, and young white men). With such results, we would be encouraged to believe that if older white men could be protected from these risk factors, their rates might decline to the levels experienced by the rest of the population. The next step would then be experimental epidemiology: an effort to change the experience of older white men in a few communities to see whether the rate can in fact be reduced. If this step were to succeed, we would be ready for a national trial, and some expectation that the promise of what epidemiological and clinical studies of suicide can offer will be fulfilled—a successful program of prevention.

REFERENCES

Barraclough BM: Differences between national suicide rates. Br J Psychiatry 1973; 122:95-96

Barraclough B, Bunch J, Nelson B, et al: A hundred cases of suicide: clinical aspects. Br J Psychiatry 1974; 125:355-373

Boyd JH: The increasing rate of suicide by firearms. N Engl J Med 1983; 308:872-874

Breed W: Occupational mobility and suicide among white males. American Sociological Review 1963; 28:179-188

Brenner MH: Mortality and the national economy: a review, and the experiences of England and Wales, 1936-1976. Lancet 1979; 2:568-573

Brown JH: Suicide in Britain: more attempts, fewer deaths, lessons for public policy. Arch Gen Psychiatry 1979; 36:1119-1124

Centers for Disease Control: Suicide Surveillance, 1970-1980. Atlanta, GA, United States Department of Health and Human Services, Public Health Service, 1985

Cobb S, Kasl SV: Some medical aspects of unemployment. Industrial Gerontology 1972; 8:8-15

Diekstra RFW: Suicide and suicide attempts in the European Economic Community: an analysis of trends, with special emphasis upon trends among the young. Suicide and Life-threatening Behavior 1985;15:27-42

Dorpat TL, Ripley HS: A study of suicide in the Seattle area. Compr Psychiatry 1960; 1:349-359

Dorpat TL, Ripley HS: The relationship between attempted suicide and committed suicide. Compr Psychiatry 1967; 8:74-79

Durkheim E: Suicide. New York, Free Press, 1951

Farberow NL, Shneidman ES: Attempted, threatened, and completed suicide. Journal of Abnormal and Social Psychology 1955; 50:230

Farmer R, Rohde J: Effect of availability and acceptability of lethal instruments on suicide mortality: an analysis of some international data. Acta Psychiatr Scand 1980; 62:436-446

Hendin H: Suicide and Scandinavia. New York, Grune & Stratton, 1964

Henry AF, Short JF: Suicide and Homicide. London, The Free Press of Glencoe, 1954

Holinger PC, Klemen E: Violent deaths in the United States, 1900-1975. Relationships between suicide, homicide, and accidental deaths. Soc Sci Med 1982; 16:1929-1938

Kleinbaum DG, Kupper LL, Morgenstern H: Epidemiologic Research: Principles and Quantitative Methods. Belmont, CA, Lifetime Learning Publications, 1982

Kraft DP, Babigian HM: Suicide by persons with and without psychiatric contacts. Arch Gen Psychiatry 1976; 33:209-215

Kreitman N: The coal gas story: United Kingdom suicide rates, 1960-1971. British Journal of Preventive and Social Medicine 1976; 30:86-93

Lester D: Letter. Med J Aust 1972; 1:941

Lester D, Murrell ME: The influence of gun control laws on suicidal behavior. Am J Psychiatry 1980; 137:121-122

MacKinnon DR, Farberow NL: An assessment of the utility of suicide prediction. Suicide and Life-threatening Behavior 1976; 6:86-91

MacMahon K: Short-term temporal cycles in the frequency of suicide, United States, 1972-1978. Am J Epidemiol 1983; 117:744-750

Malla A, Hoenig J: Differences in suicide rates: an examination of under-reporting. Can J Psychiatry 1983; 28:291-293

Markush RE, Bartolucci AE: Firearms and suicide in the United States. Am J Public Health 1984; 74:123-127

Marshall JP, Burnett W, Brasure J: On precipitating factors: cancer as a cause of suicide. Suicide and Life-threatening Behavior 1983; 13:15-27

Miller HL, Coombs DW, Leeper JD, et al: An analysis of the effects of suicide prevention facilities on suicide rates in the United States. Am J Public Health 1984; 74:340-343

Motto JA: The psychopathology of suicide: a clinical model approach. Am J Psychiatry 1979; 136:516-520

Murphy GE: The physician's responsibility for suicide, I: an error of commission. Ann Intern Med 1975; 82:301-304

Murphy GE: The prediction of suicide: why is it so difficult? Am J Psychotherapy 1984; 38:341-349

Murphy GE, Robins E: Social factors in suicide. JAMA 1967; 199:303-308

Murphy GE, Gantner GE, Wetzel RD, et al: On the improvement of suicide determination. J Forensic Sci 1984; 19:276-283

National Center for Health Statistics: Health, United States, DHHS Publication No. (PHS) 85–1232. Public Health Service. Washington, DC, U.S. Government Printing Office, 1984

Nelson FL, Farberow NL, MacKinnon DR: The certification of suicide in eleven western states: an inquiry into the validity of reported suicide rates. Suicide and Life-threatening Behavior 1978; 8:75-88

Oliver RG, Hetzel BS: An analysis of recent trends in suicide rates in Australia. Int J Epidemiol 1973; 2:91-101

Platt S: Unemployment and suicidal behavior: a review of the literature. Soc Sci Med 1984; 19:93-115

Platt S, Kreitman N: Parasuicide and unemployment among men in Edinburgh 1968-1982. Psychol Med 1985; 15:113-123

Pokorny AD: Prediction of suicide in psychiatric patients: report of a prospective study. Arch Gen Psychiatry 1983; 40:249-257

Robins E: The Final Months. New York, Oxford University Press, 1981

Robins LN: Deviant Children Grown Up. Baltimore, Williams & Wilkins, 1966

Robins LN, West PW, Murphy GE: The high rate of suicide in older white men: a study testing ten hypotheses. Social Psychiatry 1977; 12:1-20

Sainsbury P: Validity and reliability of trends in suicide statistics. World Health Statistics Quarterly 1983; 36:339-345

Sainsbury P, Barraclough BM: Differences between suicide rates. Nature 1968; 220:1252

Sainsbury P, Jenkins JS: The accuracy of officially reported suicide statistics for purposes of epidemiological research. J Community Health 1982; 36:43-48

Schmidt EH, O'Neal P, Robins E: Evaluation of suicide attempts as a guide to therapy: clinical and follow-up study of 109 patients. JAMA 1954; 155:549-555

Selkin J: The Legacy of Emile Durkheim. Suicide and Life-threatening Behavior 1983; 13:3-13

Shneidman ES: Suicide among the gifted. Suicide and Life-threatening Behavior 1981a; 11:254-281

Shneidman ES: The psychological autopsy. Suicide and Life-threatening Behavior 1981b; 11:325-340

Terman LM, Oden MH: The Gifted Child Grows Up, vol. IV. Genetic Studies of Genius. Stanford, CA, Stanford University Press, 1947

Tuckman J, Youngman WF: Assessment of suicide risk in attempted suicides, in Suicide Behaviors. Edited by Resnik HLP. Boston, Little, Brown, 1968

Wasserman IM: The influence of economic business cycles on United States suicide rates. Suicide and Life-threatening Behavior 1984; 14:143-156

World Health Organization Regional Office for Europe: Changing patterns in suicide behaviour: report on WHO working group. Copenhagen, EURO Reports and Studies 74, 1982

Chapter 14

Risk Factors for Suicide

by Robert M.A. Hirschfeld, M.D., and Lucy Davidson, M.D., Ed.S.

Suicide and suicide attempts represent a serious public health problem in the United States. Each year more than 29,000 persons commit suicide, making this the eighth leading cause of death in the United States. The suicide rate for all ages combined remains approximately 12 per 100,000 population, although in recent years suicide rates have decreased for older persons and increased for youth (National Center for Health Statistics, 1986). A moderate estimate of the number of suicide attempts at 10 times the reported number of suicides means that nearly 300,000 persons attempted suicide last year—approximately one person every two minutes (Davidson, 1986).

Identifying characteristics of persons at high risk for attempting or committing suicide expands the psychiatrist's reference base in assessing suicidal potential. The patient who shares characteristics typical of most persons who commit suicide heightens one's estimate of the danger of suicide. On the other hand, one cannot dismiss the possibility of suicide in, say, a thirty-year-old, married black woman simply because she doesn't fit the epidemiologic profile of a high risk patient. Familiarity with risk factors for suicidal behavior helps the physician register the import of the data from the psychiatric interview and make a more cogent appraisal of the possibility of suicide.

This chapter presents current knowledge on major risk factors for suicide and suicide attempts, predominantly in psychiatric patients. Risk factors in general population samples are to be found in Chapter 13. After a section on definitions and data sources, risk factors for suicide in psychiatric patients are described. Following this is a section on risk factors for alcoholic and substance abuse patients. Finally there is a section on suicide attempts, which compares risk factors for completed suicide and attempted suicide.

DEFINITIONS AND DATA SOURCES

Suicide is defined as a self-inflicted, intentional death. A suicide attempt is a nonlethal, self-inflicted act that has death as its intended purpose, or the appearance of willingness to die. The term suicide gesture usually refers to a suicide attempt of low lethality, implemented manipulatively. Suicidal ideation refers to a range of thoughts, from the idea that death would be welcome, to the immediate intent to kill oneself. Ideation shades over into suicidal plans as the person's wish to die assumes a concrete, logistical form.

Data on suicides are ultimately dependent on the official certification of the manner of death as suicide. Each death certificate must have the manner of death specified as either natural, accident, suicide, homicide, or undetermined. The coroner or medical examiner's determination of suicide requires establishing that the death was both self-inflicted and intentional. Intentionality is the more problematic criterion to establish. The certifier's suspicion of suicide may be blunted by reluctance to stigmatize the deceased's family. An unambiguous suicide note may be required by the certifier, although only about one-third of those who commit suicide leave a note (Litman et al, 1963). Uniform criteria for the classification of suicide have not been implemented by coroners and medical examiners.

The reluctance to classify deaths as suicide and the nonuniformity of the certification guidelines contribute to a major underreporting of suicides. Death certificates that do list suicide as the official manner of death are presumed valid, since the impetus in certifying the manner of death is against suicide, favoring the designations "accidental" or "otherwise." The reporting errors that occur in cases of suicide do not appear to have changed much over time (Brugha and Walsh, 1978).

The majority of data forming the basis of this chapter are derived from studies using three methodological approaches. The first of these is surveillance. The United States suicide statistics compiled annually by the National Center for Health Statistics (NCHS) are the primary source for information about suicide. These data are abstracted from death certificates and are descriptive in nature. Information is available to calculate suicide rates by sex, age, race, marital status, method of suicide, and geographic region. Information is not available for socioeconomic status, educational level, motive, or most psychiatric diagnoses. Although death certificate data are limited, NCHS is the only source of information on all reported suicides in the United States. Analysis of these rates over time illuminates trends in suicidal behavior. No such national reporting system exists for suicide attempts. Thus, data from studies of suicide attempts are much less representative and generalizable.

Retrospective empiric investigations are a second methodological approach. Researchers have used the "psychological autopsy" method to gather information about the decedent's life circumstances, emotional state, and activities. Generally, a consecutive series of suicides is identified from death records and persons close to the decedents are interviewed. Hospital, school, and employment records can provide additional data. The suicide group may be compared with a nonsuicide control group or the general population on some variable of interest. Similar retrospective investigations have been conducted with suicide attempters, although, of course, the subjects can be interviewed directly.

Prospective empirical investigations are the third methodological approach. Most of these studies are based on samples of psychiatric patients who are followed for a specified period of time. Those who subsequently attempt or commit suicide are compared with those who have not on a variety of characteristics, usually clinical. The length of follow-up varies in these studies and is generally short in comparison to a lifetime. Thus, they provide information about the characteristics of persons who attempt or commit suicide relatively soon after their clinical experience.

Both the types and quality of information about risk factors for suicide are limited. The available data sources may be thought of as pieces of a mosaic, which have been collected over time and assembled. They reflect various methodologies, sample populations, and aspects of suicidality. Although the mosaic has quite a few missing pieces, one can describe its salient features, as follows in this chapter.

SUICIDE COMPLETIONS AMONG PSYCHIATRIC PATIENTS

This section describes 11 recent studies on suicide completions among psychiatric patients. The studies range in type from a long-term prospective study of an epidemiologic sample to retrospective reviews of hospital charts (see Table 1). Each of the studies will be briefly described and major findings summarized.

Essen-Moeller and three psychiatric colleagues (1956) conducted psychiatric diagnostic interviews on nearly all the inhabitants in a small community in Sweden in 1947. Reexaminations were done 15 and 25 years later, and Hagnell (Hagnell and Rorsman, 1978) has reported on the suicides. All deaths in the area were registered and causes of death confirmed in parish registers. He found that among the 3,563 persons (1,823 men and 1,730 women), 23 men and 5 women had committed suicide.

The overall rate of suicide among men was 51 per 100,000 person-years (see Table 2). Among those without psychiatric history the rate was 8.3, and among those with a psychiatric disorder other than depression the rate was 10 times that, or 83. Among men with a history of depression, the rate was 650, nearly 80 times that among men without psychiatric history. When the depressions were categorized according to mild, medium, and severe impairment, the rates went from 0 to 220 to 3,900, respectively. For the nondepressed mental disorder group, the respective figures were 0, 110, and 290. Thus the rate of suicide among men who had suffered a severe impairment associated with depression were nearly 500 times more likely to commit suicide than men without psychiatric diagnosis. Hagnell found that the suicides were preceded by undesirable events such as a blow to self-esteem, object loss, personal sickness, and moving. Humiliating events, particularly in the areas of work and legal problems, were especially ominous. In his overall sample he found that acute psychiatric illness preceded 26 of the 28 suicides.

Alec Roy (1982) identified 90 patients (53 men and 37 women) from the Clarke Institute in Toronto who had committed suicide in the decade beginning in 1968. Each of these patients were individually matched for sex and age with the next psychiatric patient to be admitted.

Many differences were identified between the suicide group and the control group. The average age of the men was 30 at the time of suicide, compared with 38 for the women. Depression and schizophrenia made up nearly 80 percent of the diagnoses of the patients who committed suicide. The social factors that distinguished the suicide from the control group were being unmarried, living alone, and being unemployed. The patients who committed suicide were much more likely to have had previous psychiatric episodes. Among the 15 inpatients who committed suicide, 3 killed themselves while in the hospital. Among the outpatients, over 80 percent committed suicide shortly after changing from inpatient to outpatient status. Forty-seven percent had a history of suicide attempts.

Borg and Stahl (1982) identified 34 psychiatric patients whom they had prospectively followed until their deaths, and matched them on age, sex, diagnosis, and patient status with 34 nonsuicidal psychiatric patients. The suicide group had a significantly higher percentage of nonmarrieds, of those who more often lived alone, and of those who had more often lost a key person by death (but not by divorce or separation).

Table 1. Studies of Suicide among Psychiatric Patients

Principal Investigator	Type of Study	Sample	Follow-up Length	Suicide Rate (per 100,000 person-years)
Hagnell	epidemiologic prospective follow-up	3,563 persons, the entire population of "Lundby" in Sweden	15 and 25 years	nondepressive psychiatric condition (men): 83 depression (men): 650 nonpsychiatric (men): 8.3
Roy	retrospective chart review	90 suicides among psychiatric in- and outpatients, and matched controls	not applicable	not applicable
Evenson	registry	207 patients of Missouri state mental health system	not applicable	148 for men 73 for women
Borg and Stahl	prospective follow-up	34 patients who committed suicide and a matched control group	2 years	not applicable
Pokorny	prospective follow-up	4,800 Veterans Hospital psychiatric inpatients	5 years	279
Beck	prospective follow-up	207 psychiatric inpatients admitted for suicidal ideation, but *not* recent attempts	5 to 10 years	1,000 (estimate)

Table 1. Studies of Suicide among Psychiatric Patients *(continued)*

Principal Investigator	Type of Study	Sample	Follow-up Length	Suicide Rate (per 100,000 person-years)
Black	registry and chart review	5,412 psychiatric inpatients	4 years	314 (estimate)
Egeland	retrospective record review	all suicides ascertained among the Old Order Amish	100 years (1880–1980)	4.3 for men and 3.7 for women
Motto	prospective follow-up	2,753 psychiatric inpatients from a variety of hospitals	2 years	2,500 (estimate)
Barner-Rasmussen	registry	All suicides in Denmark within one year of discharge from a psychiatric hospital between 1971 and 1981	1 year	1,800 (men) 1,400 (women)
Fawcett	prospective follow-up	929 in- and outpatients with affective disorder	4 years	

Table 2. Findings of Studies of Suicide of Psychiatric Patients

Principal Investigator	Diagnosis (%)			Other Findings
	Schizophrenia	Depression	Substance Abuse	
Hagnell				rates among men with severe depression were 3,900 per 100,000 person-years, nearly 80 times the overall rate for men; suicides were nearly 5 times higher in men than women; undesirable life events, especially humiliating experiences
Roy	33	66	?	highest among those with previous suicide attempts, young, unemployed, living alone, and unmarried
Evenson				suicide rates are highest (180 to 220 per 100,000) among young men who are inpatients, depressed, or schizophrenic); male:female ratio lower than among general population
Borg and Stahl				higher in nonmarried and those with loss of a key person
Pokorny	28	27	32	peaks in young (20–29) and middle aged (40–59); 58% within six months of discharge; lower in blacks; least among married
Beck	35	57	?	best predictor was hopelessness score; lower in blacks
Black				first six months postdischarge very high risk for women; low among elderly, highest among middle aged; add diagnosis

Table 2. Findings of Studies of Suicide of Psychiatric Patients *(continued)*

Principal Investigator	Diagnosis (%)			Other Findings
	Schizophrenia	Depression	Substance Abuse	
Egeland	0	92	0	suicide was highly familial and highly associated with affective disorder
Motto				high risk factors include older age, "special" stress, suicidal impulses, history of previous lethal attempts
Barner-Rasmussen				risk factors include history of psychosis, manic-depressive disease, male sex, middle age; did not find increase among young in Denmark
Fawcett				hopelessness, loss of pleasure, fewer prior episodes, delusions of thought insertion, and cycling were predictive; age, affective subtype, and history of suicide attempts were not. Over one-half occurred within one year of discharge

Evenson and colleagues (1982) identified 220 people who had committed suicide between 1972 and 1974 who had received psychiatric treatment according to the Missouri Department of Public Health, which gathered this information by using death certificates and a computerized patient registry. They investigated suicides only among Caucasians because there were too few among nonwhites to permit adequate statistical analysis. Suicide rates were highest among middle aged (30–49) men. The age-adjusted suicide rate for inpatient men was six times higher than that for the male general population, and for women the figure was 11 times higher. In general, the sex ratio for suicides was higher among the general population (ranging from 2:3 for males:females) than among psychiatric patients (1:2 for males:females), except among the 30–39-year-old age group, in which male patients were nearly 7 times more likely than women to commit suicide. Male inpatients were found to commit suicide at a rate 5.7 times more often than men in the general population, and women about 10 times more often than women in the general population.

Evenson reports that patients with major affective disorder were twice as likely as any other diagnostic group to commit suicide. Other high risk patient diagnostic groups include schizophrenia, depressive neuroses, and substance abuse.

An analysis of variance was performed to determine the most important variables. Diagnostic category accounted for more than 57 percent of the variance, followed by sex (14.6 percent), with age surprisingly adding very little.

Pokorny prospectively followed 4,800 inpatients for an average of 5 years at the Houston Veterans Administration Hospital (Pokorny, 1983). There were 67 suicides among this almost exclusively male group, resulting in a suicide rate of 279 per 100,000 per year. This is more than 10 times higher than the age- and sex- adjusted suicide rate for veterans, which is 23 per 100,000 per year.

Pokorny found two peaks in suicide—38 percent between the ages of 20 and 29, and 44 percent between the ages of 40 and 59. The rate was substantially lower in black men. The suicides were almost evenly split among affective disorders, schizophrenia, and substance abuse. Five of the suicides occurred while in the hospital, and nearly 60 percent of the rest occurred within six months of discharge. Less than one-fourth of the patients had made a previous suicide attempt.

Using a number of sophisticated multivariate statistical techniques, Pokorny was not highly successful in identifying those who would commit suicide with sufficient sensitivity and specificity to be useful. He concluded that identification of individuals who would go on to commit suicide was not currently feasible.

Beck and his colleagues (1982) studied 207 patients who had been hospitalized with suicidal ideation but who had not made recent suicide attempts. In the subsequent 5 to 10 years, 14 patients committed suicide. There was a low percentage of blacks among those who committed suicide. Fifty-seven percent had a diagnosis of depression, while 35 percent had a diagnosis of schizophrenia. Beck reported that the best predictor of subsequent suicide was an increase in hopelessness on a self-report scale. Overall severity of depression and amount of suicidal ideation did not predict suicide. In addition, alcohol and drug abuse, and family history of suicide were not good predictors.

Black and colleagues (1985a) cross-referenced all psychiatric inpatients at the University of Iowa Hospital admitted for the decade beginning 1972 with the register of Iowa state death certificates. Of the 5,412 patients, 68 had committed suicide during the four-year follow-up period. Using a standardized mortality ratio (SMR), defined as the ratio of observed deaths to expected deaths in a particular group, Black found the highest SMRs among women between the ages of 30 and 49, even though overall sex ratio was 37:31 (male:female). The reason for this finding is the much lower expected suicide rate in women compared with men in all age categories (the male:female ratio ranged from 4:10).

Over one-half of the women killed themselves within six months of discharge from the hospital, compared with less than 25 percent of the men during the same period. Affective disorders accounted for approximately one-third of the suicides, schizophrenia for 21 percent, personality disorders for 10 percent, alcohol and drug abuse for 8.8 percent, and acute schizophrenia and depressive neuroses, each, for 7.4 percent.

In a particularly fascinating study, Egeland and Sussex (1985) examined all suicides ascertained among a group of Old Order Amish in Pennsylvania over the course of a century. This group is highly insulated from the outside world, has no alcohol or substance abuse, and regards suicide as an "abominable sin." Twenty-six cases of suicide (21 males and 5 females) were identified by record review.

The most striking finding was the clustering of the suicides and the affective disorders among four primary pedigrees, indicating a strong genetic component. Twenty-four of the 26 suicides met Research Diagnostic Criteria (RDC) for major affective disorder, including 12 who met the criteria for bipolar disorder. Although the suicide victims appeared to have a high rate of affective disorder, there were many families with clustering of affective disorders where suicide was absent. So it is possible that affective disorders may be genetically determined independently of suicide risk.

Motto (1980) prospectively followed 2,753 inpatients who had been admitted for a "depressive or suicidal state" to any of nine mental health facilities around the San Francisco area. Their purpose was to develop a clinical instrument to estimate suicide risk. One hundred and thirty-six subjects (five percent) committed suicide within the two-year follow-up period. Among the best predictors were older age, experiencing a special stress (which was defined as situations "too varied to classify individually—for example, an anticipated amputation or the full realization that a life-long goal must be relinquished"), high suicidal impulses, and highly lethal intent of present suicide attempt.

Other variables that tended to be predictive were having increased financial resources, having a bisexual, gay, or inactive sexual orientation, a history of previous psychiatric hospitalizations, and negative results of previous efforts to obtain help.

All persons who completed suicide and who had a psychiatric history in Denmark between the years 1970 and 1980 were studied by Barner-Rasmussen and colleagues (Barner-Rasmussen, 1986; Barner-Rasmussen et al, 1986). Nearly 3,998 inpatients committed suicide either during hospitalization or up to one year following discharge. Amazingly, more than one in five of these patients committed suicide *during* the hospitalization.

The yearly rates per 100,000 were 1,800 for the men 1,400 for the women. In contrast to the United States, there was no increase for individuals aged 15 to 25 committing suicide. In fact, the total number of suicides among people under 25 years of age actually decreased from 6.5 in the first half of that decade to 5.3

in the second half. The overwhelming majority of suicides were among people in their middle years. There was a sharp rise in the proportion of suicides among the rural population throughout the decade, although the rate was still approximately one-third that of the larger cities in Denmark.

Depressive diagnoses were the most frequent, with 31 percent of the men and 43 percent of the women carrying such a diagnosis. Nearly one-half of both sexes who committed suicide carried a diagnosis of an affective or schizophrenic psychosis. Substance abuse accounted for 19 percent of the men and 8 percent of the women.

In results similar to those found in other studies, suicide occurred close to the time of hospitalization. Among the suicides who had left the hospital, nearly 50 percent had killed themselves within six months.

The highest suicide rates were found among men over the age of 65 with reactive psychoses, and among men between the ages of 45 and 64 suffering from manic depressive or reactive psychoses. These rates were twice as high as the highest among any age–diagnosis specific rate among women. Fawcett and his colleagues in the Clinical Studies of the NIMH Collaborative Study on the Psychobiology of Depression (1987) followed 929 in- and outpatients with moderate to severe affective disorders every six months for a mean of 4 years. Twenty-five patients (14 men and 11 women) had committed suicide. As in other studies, suicide tended to occur early in the follow-up period—32 percent in the first six months, and 52 percent by one year. The mean age of the male suicide completers was 35.5 years, and the women, somewhat older, at 44.6 years. However, their ages were not significantly different from those of the survivors.

The most powerful clinical predictors of suicide, as compared with the survivors, included hopelessness, loss of pleasure or interest, fewer previous episodes of depression (perhaps suicide occurs earlier in the life course of the disorder), loss of reactivity, mood cycling within an episode, and several psychotic delusions. Surprisingly, affective subtype (including bipolar, unipolar, psychotic, endogenous, and primary), history of suicide attempt (although there was a trend), and life stress at entry did not discriminate between the two groups.

ALCOHOL AND SUICIDAL BEHAVIOR

Persons who abuse or are dependent upon alcohol have long been recognized as being at high risk for suicidal behavior (Dahlgren, 1951). Alcohol and suicide can relate in two ways. First, alcohol can be involved in the suicidal act itself, usually as a precipitant. Second, alcoholism itself can be considered a risk factor. Both of these will be discussed. Findings are summarized in Tables 3 and 4.

Alcohol Use Prior to the Act

Alcohol is often consumed just prior to suicide, although various studies reporting the prevalence of consumption have ranged from 21 to 89 percent. Approximately one in five were legally intoxicated (blood alcohol content [BAC] of 0.1g percent or greater) (Centers for Disease Control, 1984; Haberman and Baden, 1978; Crompton, 1985; Dorpat and Ripley, 1960). Part of the large variance in these ranges is attributable to differences among the populations studied: for example, single vehicle fatalities, alcoholics, or self-poisoning patients. Some

Table 3. Descriptive Studies of Alcohol Involvement in Self-Directed Violence

Reference	Data Source	Dimension of Alcohol Use	Population Studied	Results/Findings
Beck et al, 1982	Scale for Suicidal Ideation, Beck Depression Inventory, and Hopelessness Scale	alcoholism, not defined	105 consecutive admissions to the alcoholism program of a large metropolitan community mental health center	—26.7% had made previous suicide attempts —12% had current suicidal ideation
Berglund, 1984	psychiatrists' discharge ratings and death registers	chronic alcohol intoxication indicating a chronic habit of drinking until intoxication and not necessarily social or occupational impairment	all (1,312) first admissions with chronic alcohol intoxication to University Hospital, Lund, Sweden, 1949–1969; followed through 1980	—7% risk of suicide overall —9% if depression or dysphoria also present at admission —18% if had history of peptic ulcer
Centers for Disease Control, 1984	medical examiner's records	BAC intoxicated = 0.1 g% BAC or higher at time of death	persons 15 years or older who died within 8 hours of injury during 1973–1983 in Erie County, New York	—22% of the 655 suicide victims were intoxicated at time of death

BAC = blood alcohol content

Table 3. Descriptive Studies of Alcohol Involvement in Self-Directed Violence *(continued)*

Reference	Data Source	Dimension of Alcohol Use	Population Studied	Results/Findings
Berkelman et al, 1985	medical examiner records	BAC legally intoxicated = 0.1 g% BAC or greater at time of death	368 homicides, suicides, or victims of unintentional fatal injuries who died within 6 hours of injury in 1982	—18% of the suicides were legally intoxicated at the time of death —another 38% of the suicides had consumed alcohol
Cheynoweth et al, 1980	interviews, medical records and coroner's reports	drug dependent group = "evidence of impairment of physical, mental or social functioning as a direct result of the use of sedatives or alcohol"	135 consecutive suicides in Brisbane, Australia from 3–1–73 to 2–28–74	—22% of suicides had principal diagnosis of alcohol dependence —34% had principal or secondary diagnosis of drug dependency
Crompton, 1985	coroners' records	BAC	406 cases of violent accidental death or suicide (228) of persons over 15 years old in London from 1-1-70 to 1-1-81	—21.1% of suicides had positive BAC

BAC = blood alcohol content

Table 3. Descriptive Studies of Alcohol Involvement in Self-Directed Violence (*continued*)

Reference	Data Source	Dimension of Alcohol Use	Population Studied	Results/Findings
Makela, 1983	hospital records	alcoholism and problem drinking, not defined; history of consumption	self-poisoning patients admitted to the ICU or seen in the ER of University Central Hospital of Tampere, Finland in 1970–1971 and 1974–1979	—33% of the male and 7% of the female patients were diagnosed as alcoholic —54% of the male and 32% of the female patients were problem drinkers —54% of the emergency room and 25%–53% of the ICU patients had consumed alcohol
National Institute on Drug Abuse, 1984	emergency room and medical examiner's records	history or BAC	42,294 suicide attempts and 1,097 suicides by the nonmedical use of drugs in 1983	—19.7% of the suicide attempters had consumed alcohol —21% of the suicides had consumed alcohol
Norvig and Nielsen, 1956	patient interviews and death records	chronic alcoholism if patient had psychic or somatic changes secondary to alcohol or abusers spertuosorum otherwise	221 alcohol addicts treated at Sanct. Hans Hospital, Denmark between 7-1-48 and 12-31-50 and followed until 10–53	—6.8% of alcohol addict patients committed suicide during follow-up period

BAC = blood alcohol content

Table 3. Descriptive Studies of Alcohol Involvement in Self-Directed Violence *(continued)*

Reference	Data Source	Dimension of Alcohol Use	Population Studied	Results/Findings
Ojesjo, 1981	personal interviews, agency records, clinic records, and temperance board records	abusers = high quantity/high frequency drinking plus repeated acute medical and social disabilities; addicts = drinkers with generalized dependence and medical sequelae	96 alcoholic men identified from a population survey in Lundby, Sweden 7-1-47 and followed until 7-1-72	—12% of the decedents were suicides —3.1% committed suicide during follow-up period
Ulmanen, 1983	hospital records	alcohol abuse, not defined	299 self-poisoning patients admitted to the ICU of University Central Hospital of Tampere, Finland during 1976–1977	—31.8% of the self-poisoning attempters were alcohol abusers

BAC = blood alcohol content

Table 4. Studies of Alcohol Involvement in Self-Directed Violence Using Comparison Groups

Reference	Data Source	Dimension of Alcohol Use	Population Studied	Results/Findings
Black et al, 1985b	hospital records and Iowa death certificates	alcohol and other drug abuse (ICD–9, 303–305)	5,412 psychiatric patients admitted between 1–1–72 and 12–31–81 compared to Iowa vital statistics mortality tables	—8.8% of suicides in study group had been treated for alcohol —ratio of observed to expected deaths among the alcohol or drug abuse suicides was 11.11 for males ($p < .05$) and 60.00 for females ($p < .01$)
Combs-Orme et al, 1983	death certificates	alcoholism—excessive drinking within 6 months prior to admission and at least 2 problems or symptoms, e.g., tremors, marital difficulties, delirium tremens, job problems	1,289 alcoholics followed 6–9 years after admission in St. Louis compared to St. Louis vital statistics mortality tables	—3.5% of those dying committed suicide —rate ratios for alcoholic suicides were 6.5 overall, 7.5 for whites, 4.6 for blacks, 13.5 for women —0.7% committed suicide during follow-up period

Table 4. Studies of Alcohol Involvement in Self-Directed Violence Using Comparison Groups *(continued)*

Reference	Data Source	Dimension of Alcohol Use	Population Studied	Results/Findings
Goldney, 1981	interviews, hospital records, coroner's records	history, BAC	110 women 18–30 years old admitted after drug overdose and 32 female suicides with BAC determination from the Adelaide, Australia, coroner's office compared with 21 female controls attending a community health center	—28% of the suicides had positive BACs —31.8% of the attempters reported alcohol consumption immediately before their attempted suicide —the proportion consuming alcohol before suicide (28%) was greater than the high-lethality attempters (15%) but less than intermediate (34%) or low-lethality groups (48%), N = 7.224, $p < 0.05$

Table 4. Studies of Alcohol Involvement in Self-Directed Violence Using Comparison Groups *(continued)*

Reference	Data Source	Dimension of Alcohol Use	Population Studied	Results/Findings
Motto, 1980	clinical interview	alcohol abuse—"the subject was drinking and did not have control over the amount of alcohol ingested"	978 persons admitted to a hospital for depression or suicidality who abused alcohol, divided into an index group (N = 731; 42 suicides) and a cross-validation group (N = 247; 11 suicides)	high risk categories for suicide were identified: —more than 2 prior suicide attempts —serious present attempt or intent —high intelligence —physical health with minor impairment or getting worse in past year —job change in past 2 years —other than good present health

differences in alcohol consuption rates may also reflect different background rates of consumption in the geographic regions studied.

Alcohol effect can be disinhibiting, allowing an individual to overcome fears or other constraints on committing suicide (Patel et al., 1972). Its effects on higher cortical functions may usurp self-regulatory prohibitions against violence. Whether alcohol releases covert aggressive feelings or whether the consumption of alcohol is an expression of such aggression is controversial (Whitlock and Broadhurst, 1969). Alcohol may also be used as a self-medication that may have the opposite effect, that of mitigating suicidal intent (Goldney, 1985).

It is paradoxical that alcohol consumption preceding suicidal behavior may actually contribute to an underreporting of suicides and attempts. When the BAC exceeds some levels of intoxication, coroners may, as a matter of policy, classify the death as accidental rather than as suicide (Crompton, 1985). The coroner reasons that mental faculties would be impaired to the point that the victim could not appreciate the potentially fatal consequences of the act. Thus, our information regarding alcohol ingestion prior to suicidal behavior is skewed toward lower ranges of BAC.

Alcohol Abuse and Alcoholism

Although the risk of suicide among alcoholics has often been placed at 15 percent, research studies show a range of 0.2 to 11 percent (Choi, 1975; Lemere, 1953). This wide range is mostly due to the varying lengths of follow-up in studies from three years to death. In general, the estimate of suicide risk increases with increasing length of follow-up. Since suicide among alcoholics appears to be a late sequela of the disease, studies with short follow-up periods after admission, especially first admissions, underestimate the risk of suicide. Suicides comprise between 4.8 and 12 percent of deaths during follow-up of alcoholics (Tashiro and Lipscomb, 1963; Ojesjo, 1981).

Alcoholics are at greater risk for suicide than the general population. The ratios of observed deaths among alcoholic samples to expected suicides among age-matched mortality records range from 3.2:1 to 86:1 (Dahlgren, 1951; Kessel and Grossman, 1961).

Alcoholism is often included among variables assessed in many studies of suicide. The percentage diagnosed as alcoholic in studies of consecutive suicide ranges from 15 to 31 percent (Dorpat and Ripley, 1960; Barraclough et al, 1974).

Barraclough and colleagues (1974) compared the alcoholic suicides in their series to a previous survey of living alcoholics in Cambridgeshire, England, highlighting factors which increase the alcoholics' susceptibility to suicide. More of the alcoholic suicides were divorced or widowed. A history of previous suicide attempts was obtained for 67 percent of the alcoholic suicides versus 10 percent of the living Cambridgeshire alcoholics. The alcoholic suicides comprised an older population than their controls. When compared to nonalcoholic suicides in the series, more alcoholic suicides had made an overt suicide threat and more had seen a doctor/psychiatrist in the week before death.

Robins' study underscores the long duration of alcoholic illness before suicide and the very high percentage (77 percent) of alcoholic suicides who had communicated their suicidal intent. In their series, only 40 percent of the alcoholics had received medical or psychiatric care in the year preceding their suicide (Robins, 1981; Robins et al, 1959).

Risk factors for suicide among alcoholics include a history of more than two prior attempts, a recent history of a serious attempt, and poor or failing health (Motto, 1980; Berglund, 1984). Job changes within the past two years and higher intelligence also were shown to increase risk (Motto, 1980).

Disruption of a close interpersonal relationship is a common precipitant of suicide among alcoholics (Murphy et al, 1979). Having a concurrent affective disorder or history of dysphoria also increases the risk of suicide (Murphy et al, 1979; Berglund, 1984). Suicide is more common as a late sequela of alcoholism (Robins et al, 1959).

SUICIDE AMONG MEDICAL AND SURGICAL PATIENTS

Suicide among medical and surgical patients in the general hospital would seem to be especially preventable, since the patient has the opportunity for frequent contact with medical professionals. Studies of self-destructive behavior among hospitalized medical and surgical patients highlight characteristics of those at higher risk and situations likely to be hazardous.

Several diagnostic groups have been associated with higher rates of suicide and suicide attempts. Cancer patients were traced through the Finnish Cancer Registry (Louhivouri and Hakama, 1979). The risk of suicide for male cancer patients was 1.3 and for females 1.9 times that of the general population. Higher relative risk was associated with having a nonlocalized cancer or a gastrointestinal cancer. Patients treated by surgery or radiation therapy were not at increased risk, while those receiving no treatment or other treatment (including chemotherapy) were at significantly higher risk. A design limitation of the study is that the "no treatment" group included those whose cancers were so far advanced that only palliative treatment was offered as well as those who committed suicide before any treatment could be initiated. Thus, one cannot make conclusions regarding suicide and the prognosis of the patient's cancer.

Terminal illnesses raise the spectre of pain, loss of function, alienation, and possible disfigurement. Any of these may precipitate suicide in the vulnerable patient. It may seem natural and inevitable for the terminally ill patient to be depressed. The physician may then miss the opportunity to treat major depression and thereby prevent an untimely death.

Brown and colleagues (1986) have investigated the prevalence of wishes for death among the terminally ill. They studied terminally ill patients on a palliative care service who were aware of their illness and its prognosis and had either pain, severe disfigurement, or severe disability. Of the 44 patients eligible for study, 34 had never been suicidal nor had wished for death. All of the patients desiring death had severe depressive illness either by *Diagnostic and Statistical Manual of Mental Disorders, Third Edition (DSM-III)* (American Psychiatric Association, 1980) criteria or by the criteria of the Beck Depression Inventory (short version). None of the patients without clinical depression had suicidal ideation or wishes for premature death. Although generalizability is limited by the small sample size available, results indicate that clinical depression is not an inevitable feature of terminal illness and that suicidal thoughts in the terminally ill are present only when there is a concurrent depression.

Patients with severe respiratory diseases have been overrepresented among hopsital suicides (Baker, 1984). In this study of the Veterans Administration medical system, respiratory diseases accounted for 23 percent of the primary diagnoses among suicides in their general medical/surgical population; while that diagnostic group represented only 8 percent of the hospital population. Shapiro and Waltzer (1980) reported a similar overrepresentation of respiratory diseases among suicides and suicide attempters in the general hospital setting. Acute episodes of respiratory insufficiency frequently preceded the suicide attempts and raise the question of how cerebral anoxia may contribute to suicide risk. The authors were concerned with the failure of medical staff to request psychiatric consultation for agitated, medically ill patients, even when body restraints had been necessary.

Hemodialysis patients have characteristics that contribute to their extraordinarily high suicide rates. Whether by ordinary means or through discontinuation of dialysis or intentionally fatal breaches of the treatment regimen, approximately five percent of dialysis patients commit suicide. Suicide is up to 400 times more frequent among dialysis patients than it is in the general population (Abram et al, 1971; Haevel et al, 1980). Suicide and suicide attempts are less common among home dialysis than among center dialysis patients. This may reflect greater family support or the patients feeling more in control of the treatment.

The dialysis patient combines impaired quality of life, the ever present possibility of unintended death, and ready access to lethal methods of suicide. The choice of a method intrinsic to one's illness comprises a statement about its intolerability. The patient can readily disconnect a shunt, binge-induce hyperkalemia, or sever the arteriovenous fistula.

Initiating dialysis occasions many losses—social, occupational, and interpersonal. An even more painful sense of loss may accompany transplant failure when the patient has been sustained by the hope of being "normal" again through transplantation. Psychological problems are nearly universal among dialysis patients, and so, effective suicide prevention requires ongoing psychiatric support instead of treatment initiated at crisis points (Haevel et al, 1980).

Patients in delirium tremens comprise another group of medical/surgical patients at high risk for suicide (Glickman, 1980; Keller et al, 1985). In Glickman's series, suicides were most often enacted within 24 hours of the onset of the delirium tremens and occurred among patients inadequately sedated. Difficulties in eliciting a history of alcohol consumption from emergency patients may contribute to their likelihood of having withdrawal symptoms unanticipated by the physician.

Recent studies summarizing suicides among medical and surgical patients have used the Veterans Administration hospital system; so conclusions are less likely to be generalizable to women patients (Baker, 1984; Farberow and Williams, 1982). However, medical/surgical patients who committed suicide were older than neuropsychiatric patients who did so. Few (3 percent) made nonfatal suicide attempts during the hospitalization, but 16 percent had made prior attempts and 6 percent were admitted as the result of an attempt. Nearly 20 percent were assaultive during their admissions. Respiratory system diseases were common. Most suicides were carried out by cutting, piercing, or jumping (Farberow and Williams, 1982).

RISK FACTORS FOR SUICIDE ATTEMPTS

Despite overlap between two groups, suicide completers and attempters represent distinct populations. Suicide attempts occur much more frequently in the
general population than do completed suicides. Conservative estimates place
the ratio of attempters to completers at 8:1. (Cross and Hirschfeld, 1985).

Even though only 10 to 20 percent of attempters go on to complete suicide,
a history of suicide attempts significantly increases the likelihood of subsequent
suicide.

Risk factors for suicide attempts differ from those for suicide completion in
some areas, and are quite similar in others (see Table 5). They differ considerably
for age and sex. An average of three men commit suicide for every woman. The
ratio is reversed for suicide attempts—60 to 70 percent of attempts are made by
women (Cross and Hirschfeld, 1985). Similarly, although suicide rates are highest in those over 50 years of age, suicide attempts are much more likely to occur
in the young, with approximately 50 percent occurring in those under 30 years
of age. The peak period for attempts is between ages 20 and 24 (Cross and
Hirschfeld, 1985).

A recent Danish study has reported findings somewhat at variance with the
traditional literature (Bille-Brahe et al, 1985; Wang et al, 1985). Ninety-nine
psychiatric patients who had attempted suicide were randomly selected from
those admitted to the department of psychiatry at a Danish university hospital.
Slightly more than one-half of the attempters were men (the male:female ratio
was 51:48). The men were typically fairly young (more than three-fourths were
under 40, and more than 40 percent were under 30). The women were somewhat
older. Nearly three-fourths were aged 30 or older.

Risk factors for completers and attempters are very similar for marital status,
employment status, and psychiatric diagnosis. Both are much more frequent
among the unmarried (particularly among those who are divorced and living
alone), the unemployed, those without a confidant, and those with depression.

The presence of alcoholism in patients with other psychiatric disorders may
substantially increase the likelihood of suicidal behavior. For example, in one
study 80 percent of alcoholic patients with manic-depressive illness had attempted
suicide, versus only 13 percent of the nonalcoholic manic-depressives (Johnson
and Hunt, 1979).

Table 5. Risk Factors for Suicide Completers versus Attempters
among Psychiatric Patients

Risk Factor	Suicide Completion	Suicide Attempt
Sex	Males	Females
Age	30s and 40s	Under 30
Marital status	Unmarried	Unmarried
Employment status	Unemployed	Unemployed
Psychiatric diagnosis	Depression and Schizophrenia	Depression

One reason for this striking increase is that alcohol intoxication can increase impulsivity and decrease inhibitions. Conn and colleagues (1984) found this to be true in their study of near-lethal suicide attempts by gunshot wound. They found that the attempts occurred when the subject was depressed or perceived threats to a dependent relationship, suggesting that alcohol consumption alone is usually insufficient to precipitate a suicide attempt.

Adverse life events have been associated with both suicide completions and attempts in a number of studies. Paykel's classic 1975 study compared 53 predominantly young female attempters with matched nonsuicidal psychiatric patients and matched normals (Paykel et al, 1975). He found that the attempters had four times as many life events as the normals, and had 1½ times as many as the depressed group, in the six months before the attempt, with a marked peak in the month prior to the attempt. The attempters' events were characterized as undesirable interpersonal, health, and legal problems.

The literature on the relationship between early loss and suicide attempts is somewhat inconsistent, and riddled with methodologic problems. Overall, however, it suggests that individuals who experience loss of a parent through death or divorce are more likely to exhibit suicidal behavior in adulthood (Cross and Hirschfeld, 1986).

Personality features of patients who have attempted suicide have been the subject of several studies. Unfortunately, all of the assessments were made shortly after the attempt, when the patients were in crisis and psychiatrically ill. As Hirshfeld and colleagues have shown, even slight levels of depression greatly affect personality assessment (Hirschfeld et al, 1983), a finding which is very relevant to these investigations. In general, attempters have been characterized by increased locus of control and greater introversion when compared with controls (Cross and Hirschfeld, 1985).

Although only a minority of suicide attempters go on to commit suicide, they represent a significant risk group. An excellent example of this is contained in a recent 10-year follow-up of 262 suicide attempters by Katschnig in Vienna (Katschnig and Fuchs-Robetin, 1985). Fourteen patients (five percent) committed suicide within the follow-up period. Two clusters were identified in which the suicide risk was considerably increased. The first was the "failed suicide" cluster, which was characterized by advanced age, retired employment status, and first admission. The second was the "chronic" cluster, which was characterized by younger age and multiple admissions.

The combination of alcohol abuse and a history of suicide attempts increases the risk for suicide. In the Cambridgeshire study Barraclough and colleagues (1974) reported that a history of previous suicide attempts was obtained for 67 percent of the alcoholic suicides versus 10 percent of the living Cambridgeshire alcoholics.

SUMMARY OF RISK FACTORS FOR SUICIDE IN PSYCHIATRIC PATIENTS

Table 6 summarizes the major risk factors for suicide in psychiatric patients. The most important factor is simply being a psychiatric patient. Rates of suicide in psychiatric patients, particularly inpatients, ranges from 5 to 6 times to nearly

Table 6. Summary of Risk Factors for Suicide in Psychiatric Patients

- Being a psychiatric patient
- Being male: although the gender distinction is less important than among the general population
- Age: middle years, in contrast to the general population
- Race: whites are at much higher risk than blacks
- Diagnosis: depression and schizophrenia
- History of suicide attempts, except among psychotic patients
- Undesirable life events, especially humiliating ones or loss of a key person
- Timing: during hospitalization and in the 6–12 months postdischarge

40 times the comparable rate in the general population. Therefore, simply being a psychiatric patient puts one at a substantially increased risk for suicide.

Men are at higher risk for suicide in psychiatric populations, although the sex ratio is substantially lower among psychiatric patients than it is in the general population. The male:female ratio in all but one of these studies (excluding the VA study) reported a sex ratio below 1.5:1.

Among the general population the sex ratio for suicide in the United States was 2.5:1 (ranging from approximately 2 to 10 for various age groups). Therefore, being a psychiatric patient tends to increase the risk of suicide in women much more so than it does in men.

In the general population, suicide is very much a phenomenon of older white men. This is not nearly as true among psychiatric patients, whose peak suicide rate tends to be in the middle years. Male psychiatric patients tend to commit suicide at a somewhat younger age, perhaps around the ages of 25 to 40, whereas the peak in female patients tends to be between the ages of 35 and 50.

In psychiatric populations, Caucasians kill themselves at a much higher rate than do blacks and other nonwhite groups. Depression, schizophrenia, and substance abuse are also associated with a substantially increased risk of suicide. However, depression, especially psychotic depression or severely incapacitating depression, causes the risk of suicide to soar. Given the high prevalence of depression, its importance as a risk factor puts it at the top of the list. In contrast to most other psychiatric disorders, suicide among alcoholics is often a late sequela of the disease. Therefore, short-term follow-up studies, especially those of first admissions, may vastly underestimate suicidal risk among alcoholics.

A psychiatric history increases one's risk of suicide, and a history of prior suicide attempts substantially increases suicide risk. However, the predictive value of suicide attempts does not hold up among psychotic patients, who are much more likely to kill themselves without any warning.

Finally, the timing during the course of treatment for the disorder is extremely important. Even though patients are being actively administered to and are being observed for suicidal tendencies while in the hospital, a substantial proportion of them nonetheless kill themselves while they are in the hospital. In addition, the period of 6 to 12 months immediately following discharge is one of very high risk. This is particularly true among women in the first six months following hospitalization.

Alcohol is an important consideration in the study of suicide. It may have a disinhibiting effect, breaking down normal constraints on self-destructive behavior. In fact alcohol is often consumed prior to suicides, and one in five suicide victims are intoxicated at the time of death.

Risk factors for suicide among alcoholics are similar to those among other psychiatric patients. In contrast to other patients, however, alcoholics are more likely to kill themselves late in the course of their disease. Alcoholics are especially likely to communicate suicidal wishes prior to suicide. The risk substantially increases if there is a concurrent depression.

Certain medical and surgical patients present special suicidal risks, and bear more intensive psychiatric attention. Patients with respiratory diseases are three times more likely to commit suicide than are other medical patients. Similarly, patients on hemodialysis are a high risk group. Patients with cancer are slightly more likely to kill themselves than the general population, but, if untreated, they may be at very high risk. In this group it is unclear how many of the suicides occurred prior to treatment; so generalizations must be tentative.

Most medical patients who commit suicide, even those with terminal illnesses, have concurrent treatable major depressions. So careful assessment of psychiatric status in these patients can literally be lifesaving, or at least substantially increase the quality of remaining life.

CONCLUSION

All of this information on risk factors might lead some to the conclusion that prediction of suicide should be a fairly straightforward and easy matter at this time. Unfortunately, this is far from the truth, as Pokorny reported in his large follow-up study. He found that any technique that is sufficiently sensitive to identify individuals who will go on to commit suicide will also select an extremely large number of "false positives"; that is, individuals who will not go on to commit suicide. Therefore, we must be conservative and humble in our claims about identification of individuals at risk, and not overestimate our abilities in such matters.

REFERENCES

Abram HA, Moore GL, Westervelt FB: Suicidal behavior in chronic dialysis patients. Am J Psychiatry 1971; 127:199-200

American Psychiatric Association: Diagnostic and Statistical Manual of Mental Disorders, Third Edition (DSM-III). Washington, DC, American Psychiatric Association, 1980

Baker JE: Monitoring of suicidal behavior among patients in the VA health care system. Psychiatric Annals 1984; 14:272-275

Barner-Rasmussen P: Suicide in psychiatric patients in Denmark, 1971-1981. Acta Psychiatr Scand 1986; 73:449-455

Barner-Rasmussen P, Dupont A, Bille H: Suicide in psychiatric patients in Denmark, 1971-81. Acta Psychiatr Scand 1986; 73:441-448

Barraclough B, Bunch J, Nelson B, et al: A hundred cases of suicide: clinical aspects. Br J Psychiatry 1974; 125:355-373

Beck AT, Steer RA, McElroy MG: Relationships of hopelessness, depression, and previous suicide attempts to suicidal ideation in alcoholics. J Stud Alcohol 1982; 43:1042-1046

Berglund M: Suicide in alcoholism. Arch Gen Psychiatry 1984; 41:888-891

Berkelman RL, Herndon JL, Calloway JL, et al: Fatal injuries and alcohol. American Journal of Preventive Medicine 1985; 1:21-28

Bille-Brahe U, Hansen W, Kolmos L, et al: Attempted suicide in Denmark, I: some basic social characteristics. Acta Psychiatr Scand 1985; 71:217-226

Black DW, Warrack G, Winokur G: The Iowa record-linkage study, I: suicides and accidental deaths among psychiatric patients. Arch Gen Psychiatry 1985a; 42:71-75

Black DW, Warrack G, Winokur G: The Iowa record-linkage study, II: excess mortality among patients with organic mental disorders. Arch Gen Psychiatry 1985b; 42:78-81

Borg ES, Stahl M: A prospective study of suicides and controls among psychiatric patients. Acta Psychiatr Scand 1982; 65:221-232

Brown JH, Henteleff P, Barakat S, et al: Is it normal for terminally ill patients to desire death? Am J Psychiatry 1986; 143:208-211

Brugha T, Walsh D: Suicide past and present—the temporal constancy of under-reporting. Br J Psychiatry 1978; 132:177-179

Centers for Disease Control: Alcohol and violent death—Erie County, New York, 1973–1983. Morbidity and Mortality Weekly Report 1984; 33:226-227

Cheynoweth R, Tonge JI, Armstrong J: Suicide in Brisbane: a retrospective psychosocial study. Aust NZ J Psychiatry 1980; 14:37-45

Choi SY: Death in young alcoholics. J Stud Alcohol 1975; 36:1224-1229

Combs-Orme T, Taylor JR, Scott EB, et al: Violent death among alcoholics. J Stud Alcohol 1983; 44:938-949

Conn LM, Rudnick BF, Lion JR: Psychiatric care for patients with self-inflicted gunshot wounds. Am J Psychiatry 1984; 141:261-263

Crompton MR: Alcohol and violent accidental and suicidal death. Med Sci Law 1985; 25:59-62

Cross CK, Hirschfeld RMA: Epidemiology of disorders in adulthood: suicide, in Psychiatry; a Multi-Volume Textbook, vol. 6. Edited by Cavenar JO, Michels R. Philadelphia, JB Lippincott, 1985

Cross CK, Hirschfeld RMA: Psychosocial factors and suicidal behavior, in Psychosocial Factors and Suicidal Behavior. Edited by Mann J, Stanley M. New York, The New York Academy of Sciences, 1986

Dahlgren KG: On death-rates and causes of death in alcohol addicts. Acta Psychiatr Scand 1951; 26:297-311

Davidson LE: Study of suicide attempts during a cluster of suicides. Paper presented at the Epidemic Intelligence Service Conference, Atlanta, April 1986

Dorpat TL, Ripley HS: A study of suicide in the Seattle area. Compr Psychiatry 1960; 1:349-359

Egeland JA, Sussex JN: Suicide and family loading for affective disorders. JAMA 1985; 254:915-918

Essen-Moller E, Larsson H, Uddenberg CE, et al: Individual traits and morbidity in a Swedish rural population. Acta Psychiatrica Neurologica Scandinavica 1956; Suppl 100

Evenson RC, Wood JB, Nuttall EA, et al: Suicide rates among public mental health patients. Acta Psychiatr Scand 1982; 66:254-264

Farberow NL, Williams JL: Status of suicide in Veterans Administration hospital. Report VI, Central Research Unit, VA Wadsworth Medical Center, Los Angeles, CA, 1982

Fawcett J, Scheftner W, Clark D, et al.: Clinical predictors of suicide in patients with major affective disorders: a controlled prospective study. Am J Psychiatry 1987; 144:1, 35-40

Glickman LS: Psychiatric consultation in the general hospital. New York, Marcel Dekker, 1980

Goldney RD: Attempted suicide in young women: correlates of lethality. Br J Psychiatry 1981; 139:382-390

Goldney RD: Parental representation in young women who attempt suicide. Acta Psychiatr Scand 1985; 72: 230-232

Haberman PW, Baden MM: Alcohol, other drugs and violent death. New York, Oxford University Press, 1978

Haevel T, Brunner F, Battegay R: Renal dialysis and suicide: occurrence in Switzerland and in Europe. Compr Psychiatry 1980; 21:140-145

Hagnell O, Rorsman B: Suicide and endogenous depression with somatic symptoms in the Lundby study. Neuropsychobiology 1978; 4:180-187

Hagnell O, Lanke J, Rorsman B: Suicide and depression in the male part of the Lundy study. Neuropsychobiology 1982; 8:182-187

Hirschfeld RMA, Klerman GL, Clayton PJ, et al: Assessing personality: effects of depressive state on trait measurement. Am J Psychiatry 1983; 140:695-699

Johnson GF, Hunt G: Suicidal behavior in bipolar manic-depressive patients and their families. Compr Psychiatry 1979; 20:159-164

Katschnig H, Fuchs-Robetin G: A typology of attempted suicide, in Psychiatry: The State of the Art. Edited by Pichot P, Berner P, Wolf R, et al. New York, Plenum Press, 1985

Keller CH, Best CL, Roberts JM, et al: Self-destructive behavior in hospitalized medical and surgical patients. Psychiatr Clin North Am 1985; 8:279-289

Kessel N, Grossman G: Suicide in alcoholics. Br Med J 1961; 2:1671-1672

Lemere F: What happens to alcoholics? Am J Psychiatry 1953; 109:674-676

Litman RE, Curphey TJ, Schneidman ES, et al: Investigations of equivocal suicides. JAMA 1963; 184:924-929

Louhivouri KA, Hakama M: Risk of suicide among cancer patients. Am J Epidemiol 1979; 109:59-65

Makela R: Alcohol and self-poisonings. Psychiatria Fennica 1983; Suppl: 85-92

Motto JA: Suicide risk factors in alcohol abuse. Suicide and Life-Threatening Behavior 1980; 10:230-238

Murphy GE, Wetzel RD: Suicide risk by birth cohort in the United States, 1949 to 1974. Arch Gen Psychiatry 1980; 37:519-523

Murphy GE, Armstrong JW Jr, Hermele SL, et al: Suicide and alcoholism: interpersonal loss confirmed as a predictor. Arch Gen Psychiatry 1979; 36:65-69

National Center for Health Statistics: Monthly Vital Statistics Report, Annual Summary of Births, Marriages, Divorces, and Deaths: United States, 1985. DHHS publication no. (PHS) 86-1120. Hyattsville, MD, NCHS, vol. 34, no. 13, September 19, 1986

National Institute on Drug Abuse: Annual Data 1983. DHHS publication no. (ADM)84-1353. Rockville, MD, NIDA, 1984

Norvig J, Nielsen B: A follow-up study of 221 alcohol addicts in Denmark. J Stud Alcohol 1956; 17:633-642

Ojesjo L: Long-term outcome in alcohol abuse and alcoholism among males in the Lundby general population, Sweden. British Journal of Addiction 1981; 76:391-400

Patel AR, Roy M, Wilson GM: Self-poisoning and alcohol. Lancet 1972; 2:1099-1103

Paykel E, Prusoff BA, et al: Suicide attempts and recent life events: a controlled comparison. Arch Gen Psychiatry 1975; 32:327-333

Pokorny AD: Prediction of suicide in psychiatric patients. Arch Gen Psychiatry 1983; 40:249-257

Robins E: The Final Months. New York, Oxford University Press, 1981

Robins E, Murphy GE, Wilkinson RB, et al: Some clinical considerations in the prevention of suicide based on a study of 134 successful suicides. Am J Public Health 1959; 49:888-889

Roy A: Risk factors for suicide in psychiatric patients. Arch Gen Psychiatry 1982; 39:1089-1095

Shapiro S, Waltzer H: Successful suicides and serious attempts in a general hospital over a 15-year period. Gen Hosp Psychiatry 1980; 2:118-126

Tashiro M, Lipscomb WR: Mortality experience of alcoholics. Quarterly Journal for the Study of Alcoholism 1963; 24:203-212

Ulmanen I: Self-poisoning patients with several suicide attempts. Psychiatria Fennica; 1983 Suppl: 115-118

Wang AG, Nielsen B, Billie-Brahe U, et al: Attempted suicide in Denmark, III: assessment of repeated suicidal behavior. Acta Psychiatr Scand 1985; 72:389-394

Whitlock FA, Broadhurst AD: Attempted suicide and the experience of violence. J Biosoc Sci 1969; 1:353-368

Chapter 15

Biological Factors Associated with Suicide

by Michael Stanley, Ph.D., and J. John Mann, M.D.

Until recently suicide research has been limited to determining psychosocial and epidemiological factors associated with this behavior (Monk, 1975; Perlin and Schmitt, 1975; Goldney, 1982). In addition, most suicide research has been conducted within the context of studies of affective illness (McHugh and Goodell, 1971; Pallis and Sainsbury, 1976). This work has identified several variables that significantly correlate with suicide (Sainsbury, 1973; Platts, 1984). However, the correlations between these variables and suicide are too weak to be of practical clinical utility (Cohen, 1986). Furthermore, these indicators tend to overpredict suicide potential and thus, many individuals are falsely identified as suicide risks (Lettieri, 1974; Pokorny, 1983).

Because behavioral factors alone have been of limited clinical utility, more recent studies have tried to determine whether there might be biochemical changes associated with suicide and attempted suicide.

Biochemical studies of suicide were initially undertaken in the 1960s with postmortem examination of biogenic amines and their metabolites in the brains of suicide victims compared with controls. Subsequently, in the early 1970s, clinical studies that examined biogenic amine metabolites in the cerebrospinal fluid (CSF) began to observe a relationship between the serotonin metabolite 5-hydroxyindoleacetic acid (5-HIAA) and suicidal behavior. As previously noted, this early suicide research was conducted in those suffering from an affective illness. In the 1980s two important factors have had a significant impact on studies of suicide. The first was the development and application of receptor binding technology to the field of suicide research (Stanley et al, 1982; Stanley and Mann, 1983; Kaufman et al, 1984). The second was the change in the conceptual approach investigators had begun to use in the study of suicide. Recent investigations into suicide have focused on the act of suicide or attempted suicide as a behavior that is characteristic of multiple diagnostic categories and as a result of these investigations, depressive disorders are no longer regarded as the sole source of research material for the study of suicide (Meyendorff et al, 1986).

This chapter will describe: 1) postmortem studies of biogenic amines and their metabolites in suicide victims and controls; 2) postmortem studies that have applied receptor binding methods; 3) CSF studies that have been conducted in various diagnostic groups of suicide attempters; and 4) neuroendocrine studies in suicide and suicidal behavior.

This work was supported in part by grants from The NIMH (MH41847), Lowenstein Foundation, and the Scottish Rite to Dr. Stanley, and by an NIMH grant (MH40201) and an Irma T. Hirschl Trust Research Scientist Award to Dr. Mann.

POSTMORTEM FINDINGS IN SUICIDE VICTIMS

Biogenic Amines and Metabolites

The advances in analytic methods in neurochemistry in the 1960s and 1970s made postmortem studies of the brains of suicide victims feasible. The first series of studies on suicide victims had as their focus the determination of levels of the biogenic amines serotonin (5-HT), norepinephrine (NE), and dopamine (DA), and their respective metabolites 5-hydroxyindoleacetic acid (5-HIAA), 3-methoxy, 4-hydroxyphenylglycol (MHPG), and homovanillic acid (HVA). The concentrations of these compounds in suicide victims were compared with those in nonsuicide controls. Thus far, a total of 11 postmortem studies of suicide victims have been published.

A review of the neurochemical measures reported in these studies indicates that differences in the concentration of either 5-HT and/or 5-HIAA are the most consistently reported findings. In general, decreases were noted in the area of the brain stem (raphe nuclei) and in other subcortical nuclei (for example, hypothalamus). Lloyd and colleagues (1974) measured 5-HT and 5-HIAA in raphe nuclei of five suicide victims and five controls. Three of the five suicide victims had died by drug overdose. They found no significant difference in 5-HIAA levels between the two groups. There was, however, a significant reduction in 5-HT levels for the suicide group. Pare and associates (1969) determined norepinephrine, dopamine, 5-HT, and 5-HIAA levels in suicide victims who died by carbon monoxide poisoning. They found no significant difference between the two groups for norepinephrine, dopamine, and 5-HIAA. They did report a significant reduction in brainstem levels of 5-HT for the suicide group. Shaw and co-workers (1967) found lower brainstem levels of 5-HT in suicide victims compared with controls, a statistically significant difference. However, it should be noted that approximately one-half of the suicide group died of barbiturate overdose and the other half died of carbon monoxide poisoning.

More recently, Korpi and colleagues (1983) reported significant decreases in the hypothalamic concentration of 5-HT of suicide victims compared with nonsuicide controls. Similar findings were reported by Kleinman (1985), who noted that 5-HT levels were significantly lower in the hypothalamus of suicide victims compared with controls.

Three studies have reported significant reductions in the levels of 5-HIAA in suicide victims. Bourne and associates (1968) measured NE, 5-HT, and 5-HIAA in the hindbrain and found significantly lower levels for only 5-HIAA. Beskow and co-workers (1976) measured DA, NE, 5-HT, and 5-HIAA in brainstem areas of suicide victims and controls. They noted significant reductions in 5-HIAA levels for the suicide group. Changes in DA, NE, or their metabolites were either negative or inconsistent (Table 1).

Monoamine Oxidase

One important area of postmortem research on suicide related to the 5-HT findings is the assessment of monoamine oxidase (MAO) in the brains of suicide victims. The rationale for such studies arises from the fact that 5-HT is a substrate for MAO, and that the decreased levels of 5-HT and 5-HIAA reported in studies of suicide victims previously described might be reflected by alterations in MAO activity in this population.

Table 1. Postmortem Neurotransmitter and Metabolite Studies
of Suicide Victims

Study		Patient Group	Findings
Shaw et al	(1967)	Completed suicides	↓ Brainstem 5-HT
Beskow et al	(1976)	Completed suicides	↓ Brainstem 5-HIAA
Bourne et al	(1968)	Completed suicides	↓ Brainstem 5-HIAA
Pare et al	(1969)	Completed suicides	↓ Brainstem 5-HT
Lloyd et al	(1974)	Completed suicides	↓ Brainstem 5-HT
Korpi et al	(1983)	Completed suicides	↓ Hypothalamus 5-HT ↓ Nucleus accumbens 5-HIAA
Cochran et al	(1976)	Completed suicides	No change in brain 5-HT
Stanley et al	(1983)	Completed suicides	No change in 5-HIAA or 5-HT levels in frontal cortex
Crow et al	(1984)	Completed suicides	No change in 5-HIAA or 5-HT levels in frontal cortex
Owens et al	(1983)	Completed suicides	No change in 5-HIAA levels in frontal cortex

↓ = decrease

There have been three studies which have examined postmortem MAO activity in suicide victims (Grote et al, 1974; Gottfries et al, 1975; Mann and Stanley, 1984). One study reported no differences in MAO activity compared with controls (Grote et al, 1974). A second study found reduced MAO activity in patients where the suicide was associated with alcoholism but not in depressives without a history of alcoholism (Gottfries et al, 1975). These studies, however, include a significant proportion of patients who had died by carbon monoxide poisoning or drug overdose, which may have altered this enzyme's activity. They also employed a single substrate concentration, a method that is less informative and less sensitive than enzyme kinetic studies.

Mann and Stanley (1984) assayed MAO-A and -B in the frontal cortex of suicide victims and controls using labeled 5-HT and phenylethylamine (PEA) as substrates for MAO-A and -B, respectively. Suicide methods in this study were generally by violent means, with the exception of one overdose. There were no significant differences between the suicide and control group with respect to factors such as age, sex, and postmortem interval. The results of this kinetic study show no significant difference between the groups for either substrate (5-HT or PEA) with respect to MAO V_{max} or Km. There was significant positive correlation between age and MAO-B V_{max} for both groups. The suicide victims in this study could be distinguished from those in other studies of brain MAO in suicide largely because those who died by overdose were excluded, thereby avoiding the potential problem of drug effects contaminating the findings. These data further suggest that the reported lower brain MAO activity in alcoholic suicides (Gottfries et al, 1975), if confirmed, may be related primarily to alcoholism rather than to suicidal behavior.

Platelet Monoamine Oxidase Activity

With regard to the activity of MAO in platelets, the experimental evidence is less clear. However, platelet MAO activity was reported to be low in normal volunteers with a family history of suicide or suicide attempts (Buchsbaum et al, 1979; Gottfries et al, 1980). Two subsequent studies failed to find lower platelet MAO activity in patients who had attempted suicide (Oreland et al, 1981; Meltzer and Arora, 1986).

Thus, although low platelet MAO may predict a family history of suicidal behavior, it does not appear to predict suicide risk in the proband.

METHODOLOGICAL CONSIDERATIONS

In many of the postmortem studies, which have measured 5-hydroxyindole-acetic acid (5-HIAA), it is important to note that some diagnostic information was available for the suicide victims. These data indicate that approximately 50 percent of the suicide victims were diagnosed as endogenously depressed; the remaining cases carried a variety of diagnoses including schizophrenia, personality disorders, alcoholism, and reactive depression. These diagnostic groupings are consistent with a number of studies that have made a retrospective diagnostic analysis of individuals who have committed suicide (Dorpat and Ripley, 1960; Barraclough et al, 1974; Robins et al, 1959). In general, these studies found that in addition to the diagnosis of depression, individuals classified as schizophrenic, alcoholic, and having personality disorders were also represented. Thus it is of both theoretical and practical importance to note that suicide victims typically represent a diagnostically heterogeneous group of individuals. With regard to biochemical findings within this population, the diagnostic heterogeneity suggests that differences in neurochemistry may be related more to suicidal behavior than to depression per se.

While the biochemical findings reported above provided useful information regarding the role of 5-HT in this behavior, a note of caution should be added. In many of the foregoing studies, factors such as death by overdose or carbon monoxide poisoning, extensive postmortem delay, and lack of age-matched control groups figure significantly in the interpretation of these findings. These variables may also account, in part, for the lack of uniformity of findings among the postmortem studies. In addition to these potential sources of error, the levels of monoamines and their metabolites are known to be influenced by factors such as diet (Muscettola et al, 1977), acute drug use (Banki et al, 1983), alcohol (McEntee and Mair, 1978), and other factors. While it is possible to control for the acute influence of these factors in CSF studies, for obvious reasons this is not always the case in postmortem assessments.

CSF STUDIES OF SUICIDE ATTEMPTERS

Theoretical Background and Methodological Issues

The biogenic amine hypothesis of affective illness has postulated that manic symptoms may arise from an excess of available neurotransmitter and, conversely, depressive symptoms might be a consequence of too little available transmitter (Schildkraut, 1965; Lapin and Oxenkrug, 1969). While this hypothesis was very effective in stimulating inquiries into the biochemical basis of affective illness, the results obtained have been, nevertheless, equivocal (Koslow et al, 1983).

Many of the investigations into the role of biogenic amines in affective disorders involved measures of metabolites in CSF. One issue that is frequently raised concerning measures derived from CSF relates to the validity of these values as indicators of central turnover of the parent aminergic system. For example, it has been argued that CSF levels of 5-HIAA may be more indicative of local 5-HT turnover in spinal cord rather than 5-HT turnover in brain (Ashby et al, 1976). There have been a number of studies that have addressed this question using a variety of indirect measures, which have yielded equivocal findings (Curzon et al, 1971; Post et al, 1973). In an attempt to directly assess the degree to which 5-HIAA in the CSF reflects brain levels of 5-HIAA, Stanley and colleagues (1985) measured 5-HIAA in the brain and CSF of the same individual in samples obtained at autopsy. They found that there was a significant positive correlation (n = .78) between CSF and brain 5-HIAA levels. These findings provide the best proof that CSF metabolites do, in fact, reflect biogenic amine metabolism in the brain.

Historical Introduction

In the course of one of their studies of affective illness, Asberg and colleagues (1976) observed a bimodal distribution of 5-HIAA in the CSF of a group of depressed individuals. Within the group that had the lowest levels of CSF 5-HIAA, they found a significant proportion of individuals who had either committed or attempted suicide by violent means. Since this initial observation there have been numerous separate studies that have examined the relationship between CSF levels of 5-HIAA and suicidal behavior (contact J. Mann and M. Stanley for additional references).

CSF Serotonergic Studies and Suicidal Behavior

DEPRESSIVE DISORDERS. Following the report of Asberg and colleagues (1976), Agren was among the first to confirm that suicidal depressed patients had lower CSF levels of 5-HIAA than did nonsuicidal depressed patients (Agren, 1980). Other confirmatory studies in depression include those by Van Praag (1982), Montgomery and Montgomery (1982), Palanappian and associates (1983), Banki and colleagues (1984), and Perez De Los Cobos and co-workers (1984).

It should be noted that not all studies that have examined CSF levels of 5-HIAA in suicidal patients with affective illness have reported significant decreases in this measure. It is interesting that, for the most part, the absence of finding for decreased levels of CSF 5-HIAA can be attributed to those studies in which the diagnosis of bipolar disorder predominates (Roy-Byrne et al, 1983; Berrettini et al, 1986). Although it is well known that manic-depressive illness carries a particularly high risk of suicide (Jamison, 1986), it has been suggested that a significant degree of serotonergic dysfunction may be directly related to the illness itself and therefore obscure any potential suicide–serotonin relationship (Goodwin, 1986).

NONAFFECTIVE DISORDERS. In addition to depression and affective illness, decreased levels of CSF 5-HIAA have also been reported for suicidal patients with personality disorder. Brown and colleagues (1979, 1982) reported that in two groups of personality disorders (antisocial and borderline) it was possible to identify those who had a history of suicidal behavior on a group basis, by the presence of lower concentration of 5-HIAA in the suicide group. Traskman and associates (1981) obtained similar results in a group of patients with personality disorders compared to normal controls. Linnoila and colleagues (1983) found lower levels of 5-HIAA in the CSF of a group of violent prisoners who had attempted suicide.

CSF SEROTONERGIC STUDIES AND VIOLENCE. In conjunction with the 5-HIAA/suicide findings for this patient group, it is interesting to note that in the study by Brown and colleagues (1982) a significant inverse correlation was observed between 5-HIAA and a history of aggressive behavior. In the Linnoila study it was observed that those individuals who had committed their violent crimes impulsively had the lowest level of CSF 5-HIAA (Linnoila et al, 1983). These findings provide some support for the contention that aggressive/impulsive behaviors may be related to changes in serotonergic function, and that these may in turn exert an additional influence on individuals at risk for suicide.

Schizophrenic patients are a patient group that has been identified as being at high risk for suicide (Miles, 1977; Tsuang, 1978; Roy, 1982). In 1983, Van Praag reported that 5-HIAA levels were significantly lower in schizophrenic patients who had attempted suicide in comparison to those who had never attempted suicide. These findings have subsequently been replicated by two separate research groups (Ninan et al, 1984; Stanley et al, 1986). However, two other groups have failed to observe a difference in CSF levels of 5-HIAA between schizophrenic suicide attempters and nonattempters (Roy et al, 1985; Pickar et al, 1986).

Suicide and attempted suicide in alcoholic patients occurs at a high rate (270 per 100,000 per year) (Miles, 1977). In those alcoholic patients who commit suicide, more than one-third had made a previous attempt (Roy, 1985). Despite the clear vulnerability of these individuals for suicidal behavior, they represent a particularly difficult group in whom to conduct biochemical studies, since alcohol is known to affect the turnover of biogenic amines (Tabakoff and Ritzmann, 1975; Ellingboe, 1978; Herrero, 1980).

It has been suggested that alcoholic patients have a lower level of 5-HT turnover in the central nervous system (CNS) (Ballenger et al, 1979) and that acute ethanol consumption promotes an increase in 5-HT release and turnover. The experimental data in support of this theory indicate that CSF 5-HIAA levels in acutely abstinent (48 hours) alcoholics are significantly higher than those values obtained after four weeks of continued abstince (Ballenger et al, 1979). Similar findings were reported by Banki (1981), who noted a significant inverse correlation between 5-HIAA levels in CSF and the number of days abstinent. Banki further noted that alcoholics who had made a suicide attempt had lower CSF levels of 5-HIAA than did alcoholics who had not attempted suicide (Banki et al, 1986). However, these findings must be viewed in this context: that the effects of ethanol consumption on biogenic amine metabolism in man are poorly understood and have not been studied extensively in alcoholic suicide attempters.

The CSF finding of decreased levels of the serotonin metabolite 5-HIAA is consistent with postmortem studies which have reported decreased levels in either 5-HIAA or serotonin itself. These observations suggest that suicide and suicidal behavior are largely independent of diagnostic boundaries, as is their correlation with serotonergic measures. Thus, we find numerous reports of decreased levels of 5-HIAA in the CSF of suicidal patients, not only those who have a diagnosis of a depressive illness, but also in those patients who have personality disorders, schizophrenia, and alcoholism (Table 2).

POSTMORTEM RECEPTOR BINDING STUDIES

In reviewing the postmortem studies of suicide victims that had measured the concentration of biogenic amines and their metabolites in various brain regions, it can be observed that intervening variables such as the cause of death (carbon monoxide poisoning, drugs, and so on), postmortem interval, age, gender, and

Table 2. CSF Studies of Suicide Attempters

Study		Patient Group	Findings
Asberg et al	(1976)	Depression	↓ CSF 5-HIAA
Brown et al	(1979)	Personality disorders	↓ CSF 5-HIAA
Agren	(1980)	Depression	↓ CSF 5-HIAA
Banki et al	(1981)	Depression	↓ CSF 5-HIAA
Traskman et al	(1980)	Depression and personality disorders	↓ CSF 5-HIAA
Ninan et al	(1984)	Schizophrenia	↓ CSF 5-HIAA
Banki et al	(1984)	Alcoholism	↓ CSF 5-HIAA
Stanley et al	(1986)	Schizophrenia	↓ CSF 5-HIAA
Banki et al	(1983)	Schizophrenia	↓ CSF 5-HIAA
Roy et al	(1985)	Schizophrenia	no significant difference in CSF 5-HIAA
Berrettini et al	(1985)	Bipolar patients	no significant difference in CSF 5-HIAA
Secunda et al	(1986)	Depression	no significant difference in CSF 5-HIAA

↓ = decreased levels

the control group may have influenced the results. Similarly, acute drug and alcohol use may exert an effect on the same measures. In an effort to minimize the impact of the aforementioned variables, several investigators decided to examine receptor binding, which has been shown to be be generally nonresponsive to acute influences (Peroutka and Snyder, 1980).

Binding studies have shown that changes in the number of sites (or their density) can be induced by either a sustained increase in transmitter following chronic exposure to a chemical agent—for example, antidepressants (Peroutka and Snyder, 1980)—or by a sustained reduction in the level of a particular amine—for example, by lesioning neurons (Brunello et al, 1982). Recently, assays of receptors that appear to be associated with pre- and postsynaptic 5-HT neurons have been developed (Langer et al., 1980; Brunello et al., 1982). Imipramine binding sites, associated with presynaptic binding sites, have been characterized in platelets and various regions of the brain (Langer et al, 1980; Rehavi et al, 1982).

The idea of studying imipramine binding in suicide victims was derived in part from the clinical findings of Langer and associates, who had reported significantly reduce B_{max} values in platelets of depressed patients compared to controls (Raisman et al, 1981). The combined association of imipramine binding with 5-HT function, as well as the significant reduction in binding density in depressives, suggested the possibility that alterations in imipramine binding might be present in suicide victims. To test this hypothesis, Stanley and colleagues (1982) determined imipramine binding in the brains of suicide victims and controls. Because of the problems previous research groups had encountered conducting postmortem studies, particular care was taken in selecting cases matched for age, gender, and postmortem delay for this study. The suicide victims died in a determined manner (for example, gunshot wound, hanging, jumped from height) and the control group was similarly chosen to match for sudden and violent deaths. The findings indicated a significant reduction in the number of imipramine binding sites in frontal cortex with no difference in binding affinity (K_d). The results of this experiment are consistent with the accumulating evidence suggesting the involvement of 5-HT in suicide. Specifically, reduced imipramine binding (associated with presynaptic terminals) may indicate fewer functional serotonergic terminals, which may result in reduced 5-HT release and be in agreement with reports of reduced postmortem levels of 5-HT and 5-HIAA in suicides, as well as lower levels of 5-HIAA in the CSF of suicide attempters.

Since the completion of this study, there have been four studies that have measured imipramine binding either in suicide victims or in depressive persons who died from natural causes.

Paul and co-workers (1984) measured imipramine binding in hypothalamic membranes from suicides and controls. Both groups were matched for age, gender, and postmortem interval. Imipramine binding was significantly lower in the brains of the suicide victims compared with controls. This group also measured desipramine binding in the same samples and noted no significant difference between the suicide and control group. The selective reduction in imipramine binding argued against the possibility that this finding could be attributed to a drug-induced effect. Perry and colleagues (1983) measured imipramine binding in the occipital cortex and hippocampus of depressed individuals dying from nonsuicidal causes. They reported a significant reduction in imipramine binding in the depressive group relative to a nondepressed control group that had been matched for age, sex, and postmortem interval. Crow and co-workers (1984) also reported a significant decrease in imipramine binding in the cortex of suicide victims compared with controls. In contrast to the findings cited above, one study found an increase in imipramine binding in the brains of suicides compared with controls (Meyerson et al, 1982). Possible explanations offered to address this discrepant finding include use of single concentration analysis instead of saturation isotherms, and an inadequate matching of factors such as age, gender, and postmortem interval.

In summary, five published postmortem studies have measured imipramine binding. Thus far, four of the five studies reported a decrease in imipramine binding and one study found an increase.

In addition to assessing postmortem presynaptic function of the 5-HT system in suicide, it is possible to measure postsynaptic 5-HT binding sites using ligands such as ^{3}H-spiroperidol or ^{3}H-ketanserin. 5-HT_2 binding in animals has been shown to be down-regulated or reduced in response to chronic antidepressant treatment, and lesioning of 5-HT nuclei produces up-regulated or increased 5-HT_2 receptor binding (Peroutka and Snyder, 1980; Brunello et al, 1982).

Stanley and Mann (1983) measured 5-HT_2 binding kinetics in the frontal cortex of suicide victims compared with controls and both groups were matched for age, sex, postmortem interval, and suddenness of death. Also, care was taken to select individuals who had died by nonpharmacologic means.

The study found significant increase in the number of 5-HT_2 binding sites in the frontal cortex of suicide victims with no change in binding affinity.

Because many of the brains had also been used in the previous report on imipramine binding by Stanley and colleagues (1982) it was possible to assess the degree to which these measures of receptor function correlated. The number of binding sites (B_{max}) for 5-HT_2 and imipramine showed a trend for a negative correlation ($r = -.42, p > .1$). Such a relationship supports the suggestion that the increase in 5-HT_2 binding might reflect a compensatory increase in post-synaptic binding sites secondary to a reduction in presynaptic input. It may be that despite the compensatory postsynaptic changes there is still an overall hypofunction of the serotonergic system. Thus, reduced levels of 5-HIAA in the CSF of suicide attempters as well as reduced levels of 5-HT and 5-HIAA in the brains of suicide victims are consistent with a hypofunctioning serotonergic system.

Subsequent to the study done by Stanley and Mann (1983), there have been four additional reports of 5-HT_2 binding in suicides. Owens and colleagues (1983) reported an increase in 5-HT_2 binding in nonmedicated suicide victims. Crow and colleagues (1984) found no change in 5-HT_2 binding between suicides and controls. In a larger series of suicide victims and controls, Mann and associates (1986) found a significant increase in suicide victims in 5-HT_2. Finally, Meltzer and co-workers (1987) also reported a significant increase in 5-HT_2 binding in frontal cortex.

In addition to serotonergic binding sites, several groups have measured muscarinic and beta-adrenergic binding sites in the brains of suicide victims. There have been three studies that have examined muscarinic binding sites in the frontal cortices and other regions of the brains of suicide victims (Stanley, 1984; Kaufman et al, 1984; Meyerson et al, 1982). The rationale for these studies was suggested by the cholinergic-adrenergic imbalance theory postulated by Janowsky and colleagues (1972) and by the known high proportion of suicide victims who are diagnosed as suffering from an affective disorder.

In a study comparing a large group of suicide victims and nonsuicide controls Stanley (1984) found no difference between the number of binding sites in the frontal cortex for the two groups. Similarly, no changes in binding affinity were observed between the two groups. Further analysis revealed that no significant differences existed for factors such as age, gender, and postmortem interval between the two groups. This finding was replicated by Kaufman and associates (1984) who determined QNB binding in three brain regions (including the frontal cortex) in suicide victims. They found no differences in binding parameters for either group in any of the brain regions studied.

In contrast to the findings observed in the two previously described studies, Meyerson and co-workers (1982) reported a significant increase in QNB binding sites in a small group of suicide victims compared with a control group that was not matched for age, gender, and postmortem interval.

In an attempt to better understand the functional status of central noradrenergic neurons in suicidal behavior, Mann and colleagues (1986) measured beta-adrenergic receptors in suicide victims. It has been suggested that alterations in beta-adrenergic receptors might be linked to the therapeutic actions of antidepressant drugs (Sulser and Robinson, 1978). Mann and colleagues (1986) noted a significant increase in specific beta-adrenergic binding in suicide victims compared with controls.

In addition to this study, Zanko and Biegon (1983) reported an increase in the number of binding sites (B_{max}) with no change in K_d in a small series of six suicide victims and matched controls. In contrast with the above studies, Meyerson and associates (1982) reported no alteration in DHA binding in suicide victims. Thus, two of three studies measuring beta-adrenergic receptors have reported an increase in binding in suicide victims. It should be noted that antemortem use of antidepressants would not explain the receptor alterations observed by Mann and colleagues (1986) and Zanko and Biegon (1983). Data from animal studies indicate that chronic antidepressant treatment causes a down-regulation of beta-adrenergic receptors (Sulser and Robinson, 1978).

It is interesting to note that the combination of 5-HT$_2$ binding data, together with the results obtained for beta-adrenergic binding, may provide additional sensitivity and specificity in the identification of suicide victims. For example, in the study of Mann and colleagues (1986), victims were found to have increases in both 5-HT$_2$ and beta-adrenergic binding. Conversely, no suicide victims had low levels of both receptor types. These findings may have potential therapeutic and forensic applications (Table 3).

In addition to those studies that have measured receptor sites for the biogenic amines in suicide victims, a recent study measured binding sites for corticotropin releasing factor (CRF). In studies in depression, the levels of CRF in CSF have been reported to be significantly elevated relative to normal controls (Nemeroff et al, 1984) and to those of schizophrenic patients (Banki et al, in press). CFR binding sites in the frontal cortex of suicide victims were found to be lower than in nonsuicidal controls (Nemeroff, submitted for publication). The findings of the above studies suggest that the increased levels of CRF observed in depression may subsequently result in a down-regulation of CRF receptors in suicide

Table 3. Postmortem Receptor Studies of Suicide Victims

Imipramine Binding

Stanley et al	(1982)	Completed suicides	↓ ^{3}H-imipramine binding in cortex
Paul et al	(1984)	Completed suicides	↓ ^{3}H-imipramine binding in brain
Perry et al	(1983)	Depressed dying of natural causes	↓ ^{3}H-imipramine binding in cortex
Crow et al	(1984)	Completed suicides	↓ ^{3}H-imipramine binding in cortex
Meyerson et al	(1982)	Completed suicides	↑ ^{3}H-imipramine binding in cortex

5-HT$_2$ Binding

Stanley and Mann	(1983)	Completed suicides	↑ 5-HT$_2$ binding in cortex
Mann et al	(1986)	Completed suicides	↑ 5-HT$_2$ binding in cortex
Meltzer et al	(1987)	Completed suicides	↑ 5-HT$_2$ binding in cortex
Owens et al	(1983)	Completed suicides	Increase but not significantly
Cheetam et al	(1987)	Completed suicides	↓ 5-HT binding in cortex

Muscarinic Binding

Stanley	(1984)	Completed suicides	No change in muscarinic cholinergic receptor binding in cortex
Kaufman et al	(1984)	Completed suicides	No change in muscarinic cholinergic receptor binding
Meyerson et al	(1982)	Completed suicides	↑ in muscarinic cholinergic receptor binding

Beta-adrenergic Binding

Zanko and Biegon	(1983)	Completed suicides	↑ in beta receptor binding
Mann et al	(1986)	Completed suicides	↑ in beta receptor binding
Biegon	(1987)	Completed suicides	↑ in beta receptor binding
Meyerson et al	(1982)	Completed suicides	No change in beta receptor binding

↑ = increase
↓ = decrease

victims, many of whom would be diagnosed as depressed. However, a separate study which measured CSF levels of CRF in depressed patients who were either suicidal or nonsuicidal found no difference between the groups (Arato et al, 1986). Both groups of depressives did, however, have significantly higher levels of CRF compared to nondepressed controls. The results of that study suggest that CRF changes are associated with a depressive disorder rather than suicidal behavior.

HYPOTHALAMIC–PITUITARY–ADRENAL AXIS FUNCTION AND SUICIDAL BEHAVIOR

Two indices of hypothalamic-pituitary-adrenal (HPA) axis function, namely cortisol levels and dexamethasone suppression of cortisol levels, have been studied extensively in psychiatric patients. An association between hypercortisolemia and resistance to dexamethasone suppression of cortisol levels has been reported for patients with endogenous depression or melancholia (Carroll et al, 1981a, or 1981b).

What has proven more difficult is to distinguish alterations in HPA axis function associated with a depressive illness from those alterations associated specifically with suicidal behavior. Most studies reporting correlations of HPA indices with suicidal behavior have failed to control for the effects of a concurrent depressive illness. We will present data that suggest there is no specific correlation with suicide.

Several studies have reported increased levels of 24-hour urinary 17-hydroxy-corticosteroids or urinary free cortisol in suicidal patients, or in patients who subsequently committed suicide (Bunney and Fawcett, 1965, 1969; Ostroff et al, 1982). However, other studies reported normal or low levels of urinary cortisol in patients who have attempted or completed suicide (Krieger, 1970; Levy and Hansen, 1969).

Two studies reported the absence of a significant correlation between suicide attempts and hypercortisolemia, and these findings have been summarized by Kocsis and colleagues (1986). No significant association appears to exist between suicidal behavior and cerebrospinal fluid (CSF) levels of cortisol, adrenocorticotropin hormone (ACTH) and CRF (Asberg and Traskman, 1981; Arato et al, 1986). Measurement of ACTH and cortisol in CSF obtained from suicide victims and controls at autopsy has revealed no significant differences (Arato et al, 1986).

There is no clear agreement regarding the question of an association between suicidal behavior and resistance to dexamethasone. Four studies reported such an association (Carroll et al, 1981b; Coryell and Schlesser, 1981; Targum et al, 1983; Banki and Arato, 1983) and three studies failed to find an association (Van Waltere et al, 1983; Kocsis et al, 1986). Thus, although HPA abnormalities appear to be associated with depressive illness, a specific association has not been established with suicidal behavior.

NEUROENDOCRINE STUDIES OF THE SEROTONERGIC SYSTEM AND SUICIDAL BEHAVIOR

Administration of drugs that activate the serotonergic system in the brain permit assessments of serotonin function in vivo and the study of potential correlations with current symptomatology and diagnosis. Meltzer and colleagues (1984) reported an enhanced cortisol response to 5-hydroxytryptophan, a precurser of serotonin, in depressed patients who made a suicide attempt compared to patients who had not. They explained this finding as evidence of postsynaptic serotonin receptor supersensitivity in the brains of suicide attempters. Recently, Meltzer (1987) reported a similar result using the serotonin agonist MK212, which acts directly on serotonin receptors. These data are consistent with reports by Stanley and Mann (1983) and Stanley and colleagues (1986) on an increased number of 5-HT_2 binding sites in the brains of suicide victims.

Although there is evidence of postsynaptic serotonin receptor supersensitivity in suicidal patients, overall net serotonergic activity is reduced. Support for this conclusion comes from the work of Cocarro and colleagues (1987), who have reported a negative correlation among severity of suicidal behavior, impulsivity and aggressivity, and prolactin response induced by fenfluramine. Fenfluramine is an indirect-acting serotonin agonist that releases endogenous stores of serotonin and inhibits its reuptake. Therefore, prolactin release by this drug is the result of net serotonin release and receptor sensitivity. Since prolactin release is lower in suicidal patients, it may be inferred that despite the increase in serotonin receptors, net transmission is still lower.

In summary, neuroendocrine studies of the serotonin system are consistent with the postmortem receptor findings and support the hypothesis that suicidal behavior may be correlated with lower serotonergic activity.

POTENTIAL OF BIOLOGICAL MEASURES AS PREDICTORS OF RISK FOR SUICIDE

As biological factors associated with suicide and attempted suicide are identified, it is appropriate to ask whether there may be a practical application of these findings. While it may still be premature to seek direct application, there have been some investigators who have begun to explore this possibility. The high prevalence of decreased CSF levels of 5-HIAA in suicide attempters raises the intriguing possibility that this measure may be of some clinical utility in determining the risk of sucide.

Asberg and colleagues have reported that individuals who attempt suicide and have low levels of 5-HIAA in their CSF are at 10 times greater risk for committing suicide than those with higher 5-HIAA levels (Asberg et al, 1986). These findings are also supported by the findings of Roy and associates (personal communication) who observed a similar increase in suicide mortality. Thus it would appear that biochemical findings may prove to have practical clinical value, and perhaps when combined with other known risk factors (gender, history of previous suicide attempt, marital status, and so on), contribute significantly to the more precise identification of the high-risk patient.

TREATMENT IMPLICATIONS

One issue related to the biochemical findings described in this chapter pertains to the issue of treatment. Two considerations seem important in regard to treatment: 1) the psychiatric syndrome a given individual who attempts suicide suffers from and 2) the presumed abnormality in serotonergic function that predisposes or renders vulnerable an individual for attempted suicide.

In the first instance it is clear that psychiatric illness itself represents a significant risk factor for suicide. Furthermore, it is known that suicide and attempted suicide occur in many psychiatric disorders. These observations suggest that adequate control of psychiatric symptoms may be an important consideration in the management of suicidal behavior (for example, affective or psychotic symptoms). If the second consideration (that is, abnormal serotonergic function) becomes firmly established, this may suggest that suicidal behavior may be controlled through pharmacological alterations of central 5-HT function. Thus it may develop that the treatment of a specific psychiatric illness in the individual who attempts suicide may be necessary but not sufficient to achieving adequate control of suicidal behavior. What might be required is some form of additional pharmacologic treatment that would more specifically target the presumed underlying biochemical abnormality in the serotonergic system of these individuals.

A recent example of a pharmacologic trial utilizing this strategy was conducted by a research group using the serotonergic depleting drug fenfluramine (Meyendorff, 1986).

REFERENCES

Agren H: Symptom patterns in unipolar and bipolar depression correlating with monomine metabolites in the cerebrospinal fluid, II: suicide. Psychiatry Res 1980; 3:225-236

Arato M, Banki CM, Nemeroff CB, et al: Hypothalamic-pituitary-adrenal axis and suicide, in Psychobiology of Suicide Behavior. Edited by Mann JJ, Stanley M, New York, New York Academy of Sciences, 1986

Asberg M, Thoren P, Traskman L, et al: Serotonin depression: a biochemical subgroup within the affective disorders? Science 1976; 191:478-480

Asberg M, Traskman L: Studies of CSF 5-HIAA in depression and suicidal behavior. Exp Med Biol 1981; 133:739-752

Asberg M, Nordstrom P, Traskman-Bendz L: Cerebrospinal fluid studies in suicide: an overview, in Psychobiology of Suicidal Behavior. Edited by Mann JJ, Stanley M, New York, New York Academy of Sciences, 1986

Ashby P, Verrier M, Warsh JJ, et al: J Neurol Neurosurg Psychiatry 1976; 39:1191

Ballenger JC, Goodwin FK, Major LF, et al: Alcohol and central serotonin metabolism in man. Arch Gen Psychiatry 1979; 36:224-227

Banki C: Factors influencing monoamine metabolites and tryptophan in patients with alcohol dependence. J Neural Transm 1981; 50:98-101

Banki CM, Arato M: Amine metabolites and neuroendocrine responses related to depression and suicide. J Affective Disord 1983; 5:223-232

Banki CM, Arato M, Papp Z, et al: The influence of dexamethasone on cerebrospinal fluid monoamine metabolites and cortisol in psychiatric patients. Pharmacopsychiatria 1983; 16:77-81

Banki CM, Arato M, Papp Z, et al: Biochemical markers in suicidal patients: investigations with cerebrospinal fluid amine metabolites and neuroendocrine tests. J Affective Disord 1984; 6:341-350

Banki C, Arato M, Kilts C: Aminergic studies and cerebrospinal fluid cautions in suicide, in Psychobiology of Suicidal Behavior. Edited by Mann JJ, Stanley M. New York, New York Academy of Sciences, 1986

Banki CM, Bissett G, Arato M, et al: CSF corticotropin-like immunoreactivity in depression and schizophrenia. Am J Psychiatry (in press)

Barraclough B, Bunch J, Nelson B, et al: A hundred cases of suicide: clinical aspects. Br J Psychiatry 1974; 125:355-373

Berrettini W, Nurenberger J, Narrow W, et al: Cerebrospinal fluid studies of bipolar patients with and without a history of suicide attempts, in Psychobiology of Suicidal Behavior. Edited by Mann JJ, Stanley M. New York, New York Academy of Sciences, 1986

Beskow J, Gottfries CG, Roos BE, et al: Determination of monoamine and monoamine metabolites in the human brain: post mortem studies in a group of suicides and in a control group. Acta Psychiatr Scand 1976; 53:7-20

Bourne HR, Bunney WE Jr, Colburn RW, et al: Noradrenaline, 5-hydroxytryptamine, and 5-hydroxyindoleacetic acid in the hindbrains of suicidal patients. Lancet 1968; 2:805-808

Brown GL, Goodwin FK, Ballenger JC, et al: Aggression in humans correlates with cerebrospinal fluid amine metabolites. Psychiatry Res 1979; 1:131-139

Brown GL, Ebert MH, Goyer PF, et al: Aggression, suicide, and serotonin: relationships to CSF amine metabolites. Am J Psychiatry 1982; 139:741-746

Brunello N, Chuang DM, Costa E: Different synaptic location of mianserin and imipramine binding sites. Science 1982; 215:1112-1115

Buchsbaum MS, Hairr RJ, Murphy DL: Suicide attempts, platelet monoamine oxidase and the average evoked response. Acta Psychiatr Scand 1979; 56:69-77

Bunny WE Jr, Fawcett JA: Possibility of a biochemical test for suicidal potential. Arch Gen Psychiatry 1965; 13:232-239

Bunney WE Jr, Fawcett JA, Davis JM, et al: Further evaluation of urinary 17-hydroxycorticosteroids in suicidal patients. Arch Gen Psychiatry 1969; 21:138-150

Carroll BJ, Feinberg M, Greden JF, et al: A specific laboratory test for the diagnosis of melancholia: standardization, validation and clinical utility. Arch Gen Psychiatry 1981a; 38:15-22

Carroll BJ, Greden JF, Feinberg M: Suicide, neuroendocrine dysfunction and CSF 5-HIAA concentrations in depression, in Recent Advances in Neuropsychopharmacology. Edited by Angrist B. Oxford, Pergamon Press, 1981b

Cocarro EF, Siever LJ, Klar H, et al: 5-HT Function and History of Suicidal Behavior: New Research Abstracts NR158 105. Washington, DC, American Psychiatric Association, 1987

Cochran E, Robins E, Grate S: Regional serotonin levels in the brain: a comparison of depressive suicides and alcoholic suicides with controls. Biol Psychiatry 1976; 11:283-294

Cohen J: Statistical approaches to suicidal risk factor analysis, in Psychobiology of Suicidal Behavior. Edited by Mann JJ, Stanley M. New York, New York Academy of Sciences, 1986

Coryell W, Schlesser MA: Suicide and the dexamethasone suppression test in unipolar depression. Am J Psychiatry 1981; 138:1120-1121

Crow TJ, Cross AJ, Cooper SJ, et al: Neurotransmitter receptors and monoamine metabolites in the patients with Alzheimer-type dementia and depression and suicides. Neuropharmacology 1984; 23:1561-1569

Curzon G, Gumpert EJ, Sharpe DM: Amine metabolites in the lumbar cerebrospinal fluid of humans with restricted flow of cerebrospinal fluid. Nature 1971; 231:189

Dorpat TL, Ripley HS: A study of suicide in the Seattle area. Compr Psychiatry 1960; 6:349-359

Ellingboe J: Effect of alcohol on neurochemical process, in Psychopharmacology: A Generation of Progress. Edited by Lipton M, DiMascio A, Killman K. New York, Raven Press, 1978

Goldney R: Loss of control in young women who have attempted suicide. J Nerv Ment Dis 1982; 4:198-201

Goodwin FK: Suicide, aggression and depression: a theoretical framework for future research, in Psychobiology and Suicidal Behavior. Edited by Mann JJ, Stanley M. New York, New York Academy of Sciences, 1986

Gottfries CG, Oreland L, Wiberg A, et al: Lowered monoamine oxidase activity in brains from alcoholic suicides. J Neurochem 1975; 25:667-673

Grottfries CG, Knorring LV, Oreland L: Platelet monamine oxidase activity in mental disorders. Neuropsychopharmacology 1980; 4:185-192

Grote SS, Moses SG, Robins E, et al: A study of selected catecholamine metabolizing enzymes: a comparison of depressive suicides and alcoholic suicides with controls. J Neurochem 1974; 23:791-802

Herrero E: Monoamine metabolism in rat brain regions following long-term alcohol treatment. J Neural Transm 1980; 47:227-236

Jamison KR: Suicide and bipolar disorders, in Psychobiology of Suicidal Behavior. Edited by Mann JJ, Stanley M. New York, New York Academy of Sciences, 1986

Janowsky DS, El-Yousef MK, David JM, et al: A cholinergic-adrenergic hypothesis of mania and depression. Lancet 1972; 1:632

Kaufman CA, Gillin JC, Hill B, et al: Muscarinic binding in suicides. Psychiatry Res 1984; 12:47-55

Kleinman J: Muscarinic receptor density in skin fibroblasts and autopsied brain tissue in affective disorder. Paper presented at Psychobiology of Suicide Behavior. New York, New York Academy of Sciences, September 1985

Kocsis JH, Kennedy S, Brown RP, et al: Neuroendrocrine studies in depression: relationship to suicidal behavior, in Psychobiology of Suicidal Behavior. Edited by Mann JJ, Stanley M. New York, New York Academy of Sciences, 1986

Korpi ER, Kleinman JE, Goodman SI, et al: Serotonin and 5-hydroxyindoleacetic acid concentrations in different brain regions of suicide victims: comparison in chronic schizophrenic patients with suicide as cause of death. Presented at the International Society for Neurochemistry, Vancouver, Canada, 1983

Koslow SH, Mass JW, Bowden CL, et al: CSF and urinary biogenic amines and metabolites in depression and mania: a controlled, univariate analysis. Arch Gen Psychiatry 1983; 40:999-1010

Krieger G: Biochemical predictors of suicide. Diseases of the Nervous System 1970; 31:478-482

Langer SZ, Moret C, Raisman R, et al: High-affinity [^{3}H] imipramine binding in rat hypothalamus: association with uptake of serotonin but not of norepinephrine. Science 1980; 210:1133-1135

Lapin IP, Oxenkrug GF: Intensification of the central serotonergic process as a possible determinant of the thymoleptic effect. Lancet 1969; 1:132-136

Lettieri D: Suicidal death prediction scales, in The Prediction of Suicide. Edited by Beck A, Resnik H, Lettieri D. Bowie, MD, Charles Press, 1974

Levy B, Hensen E: Failure of the urinary test for suicidal potential. Arch Gen Psychiatry 1969; 20:415-418

Linnoila M, Virkkunen M, Scheinin M, et al: Low cerebrospinal fluid 5-hydroxyindoleacetic acid concentrations differentiates impulsive from nonimpulsive violent behavior. Life Sci 1983; 33:2609-2614

Lloyd KG, Farley IJ, Deck JHN, et al: Serotonin and 5-hydroxyindoleacetic acid in discrete areas of the brainstem of suicide victims and control patients. Advances in Biochemical Psychopharmacology, vol. II. New York, Raven Press, 1974

Mann JJ, Stanley M: Postmortem monoamine oxidase enzyme kinetics in the frontal cortex of suicide victims and controls. Acta Psychiatr Scand 1984; 69:135-139

Mann JJ, Stanley M, McBride AP, et al: Increased serotonin and beta-adrenergic receptor binding in the frontal cortices of suicide victims. Arch Gen Psychiatry 1986; 43:954-959

McEntee WJ, Mair RG: Memory impairment in Korsakoff's psychosis: a correlation with brain noradrenergic activity. Science 1978; 202:905-907

McHugh PR, Goodell H: Suicidal behavior: a distinction of patients with sedative poisoning seen in a general hospital. Arch Gen Psychiatry 1971; 25:456-464

Meltzer HY, Arora RC: Platelet markers of suicidality, in Psychobiology of Suicidal Behavior. Edited by Mann JJ, Stanley M. New York, New York Academy of Sciences, 1986

Meltzer HY, Perline R, Tricou BJ, et al: Effect of 5-hydryoxytryptophan or serum cortisol levels in major affective disorders, II: relation to suicide, psychosis and depressive symptoms. Arch Gen Psychiatry 1984; 41:379-387

Meltzer HY, Nash JF, Ohmori T, et al: Neuroendocrine and Biochemical Studies of Serotonin and Dopamine in Depression and Suicide. International Conference on New Directions in Affective Disorders. Book of Abstracts (S60), 1987

Meyendorff E, Jain A, Traskman-Bendz L, et al: The effects of fenfluramine on suicidal behavior. Psychopharmacol Bull 1986; 22:155-159

Meyerson LR, Wennogle LP, Abel MS, et al: Human brain receptor receptor alterations in suicide victims. Pharmacol Biochem Behav 1982; 17:159-163

Miles C: Conditions predisposing to suicide. J Nerv Ment Dis 1977; 164:231-246

Monk M: Epidemiology, in A Handbook for the Study of Suicide. Edited by Perlin S. New York, Oxford University Press, 1975

Montgomery SA, Montgomery D: Pharmacological prevention of suicidal behavior. J Affective Disord 1982; 4:291-298

Muscettola G, Wehr T, Goodwin PK: Effect of diet on urinary MHPG excretion in depressed patients and normal control subjects. Am J Psychiatry 1977; 134:914-916

Nemeroff CB, Widerlow E, Bissett G, et al: Elevated concentrations of CSF corticotropin-releasing factor-like immunoreactivity in depressed patients. Science 1984; 226:1342-1344

Ninan PT, Van Kammen DP, Scheinin M, et al: CSF 5-hydroxyindoleacetic acid in suicidal schizophrenic patients. Am J Psychiatry 1984; 141:566-569

Oreland L, Wiberg A, Asberg M, et al: Platelet MAO activity and monoamine metabolites in cerebrospinal fluid in depressed and suicidal patients and in healthy controls. Psychiatry Res 1981; 4:21-29

Ostroff R, Giller E, Bonese K, et al: Neuroendocrine risk factors of suicide. Am J Psychiatry 1982; 139:1323-1325

Owens F, Cross AJ, Crow TJ, et al: Brain 5-HT$_2$ receptors and suicide. Lancet 1983; 2:1256

Palanappian V, Ramachandran V, Somasundaram O: Suicidal ideation and biogenic amines in depression. Indian J Psychiatry 1983; 25:268-292

Pallis DJ, Sainsbury P: The value of assessing intent in attempted suicide. Psychol Med 1976; 6:487-492

Pare CMB, Yeung DPH, Price K, et al: 5-hydroxytryptamine, noradrenaline, and dopamine in brainstem, hypothalamus, and caudate nucleus of controls of patients committing suicide by coal-gas poisoning. Lancet 1969; 1:131-135

Paul SM, Rehavi M, Skolnick P, et al: High affinity binding of antidepressants to a biogenic amine transport site in human brain and platelet: studies in depression, in Neurobiology and Mood Disorders. Edited by Post RM, Ballenger JC. Baltimore, Williams & Wilkins, 1984

Perez de los Cobos JZ, Lopez-Ibor Alino JJ, Saiz Ruiz J: Correlatos biologicos del suicido y la agresividad en depressiones mayores (con melancolia): 5-HIAA en LCR, DST, y respuesta terapeutica a 5-HTp. Presented to the First Congress of the Spanish Society for Biological Psychiatry, Barcelona, 1984

Perlin S, Schmitt S: Psychiatry, in A Handbook for the Study of Suicide. Edited by Perlin S. New York, Oxford University Press, 1975

Peroutka SJ, Snyder SH: Multiple serotonin receptors: differential binding of ^{3}H-5 hydroxytryptamine, ^{3}H-lysergic acid diethylamide and ^{3}H-spiroperdol. Mol Pharmacol 1979; 16:687-699

Peroutka SJ, Snyder SH: Regulation of serotonin (5-HT$_2$) receptors labeled with [^{3}H] spiroperidol by chronic treatment with antidepressant amitriptyline. Pharmacol Exp Ther 1980; 215:582-587

Perry EK, Marshall EF, Blessed G, et al: Decreased imipramine binding in the brains of patients with depressive illness. Br J Psychiatry 1983; 142:188-192

Pickar D, Roy A, Breier A, et al: Suicide and aggression in schizophrenia: neurobiologic correlates, in Psychobiology of Suicidal Behavior. Edited by Mann JJ, Stanley M. New York, New York Academy of Sciences, 1986

Platts S: Unemployment and suicidal behavior: a review of the literature. Soc Sci Med 1984; 19:93-115

Pokorny AD: Prediction in suicide in psychiatric patients. Arch Gen Psychiatry 1983; 40:249-257

Post RM, Goodwin FK, Gordon E, et al: Amine metabolites in human cerebrospinal fluid: effects of cord transection and spinal fluid block. Science 1973; 179:897

Raisman R, Sechter D, Briley MS, et al: High affinity ^{3}H-imipramine binding in platelets from untreated and treated depressed patients compared to healthy volunteers. Psychopharmacology 1981; 75:368-371

Rehavi M, Skolnick P, Paul SM: Solubilization and partial purification of the high affinity [3H] imipramine binding site from human platelets. Federation of European Biochemical Societies Letters 1982; 150:514-518

Robins E, Murphy GE, Wilkinson RH Jr, et al: Some clinical considerations in the prevention of suicide based on a study of 134 successful suicides. Am J Public Health 1959; 49:889

Roy A: Suicide in chronic schizophrenia. Br J Psychiatry 1982; 141:171-177

Roy A: Suicide and psychiatric patients. Psychiatr Clin North Am 1985; 8:227-241

Roy A, Ninan P, Mazonson A, et al: CSF monoamine metabolites in chronic schizophrenic patients who attempt suicide. Psychol Med 1985; 15:335-340

Roy-Byrne P, Post RM, Rubinow DR, et al: CSF 5-HIAA and personal and family history of suicide in affectively ill patients: a negative study. Psychiatry Res 1983; 10:263-274

Sainsbury P: Suicide: opinions and facts. Proceedings of the Royal Society of Medicine 1973; 66:579

Schildkraut JJ: The catecholamine hypothesis of affective disorders: a review of supporting evidence. Am J Psychiatry 1965; 122:509-522

Secunda SK, Cross CK, Koslow S, et al: Biochemistry and suicidal behavior in depressed patients. Biol Psychiatry 1986; 21:756-767

Shaw DM, Camps FE, Eccleston EG: 5-hydroxytryptamine in the hind-brain of depressive suicides. Br J Psychiatry 1967; 113:1407-1411

Stanley M: Cholinergic receptor binding in the frontal cortex of suicide victims. Am J Psychiatry 1984; 141:1432-1436

Stanley M, Mann JJ: Increased serotonin-2 binding sites in frontal cortex of suicide victims. Lancet 1983; 2:214-216

Stanley M, Virgilio J, Gershon S: Triated imipramine binding sites are decreased in the frontal cortex of suicides. Science 1982; 216:1337-1339

Stanley M, Traskman-Bendz L, Dorovini-Zis K: Correlations between aminergic metabolites simultaneously obtained from human CSF and brain. Life Sci 1985; 37:1279-1286

Stanley M, Stanley B, Traskman-Bendz L, et al: Depressive symptoms and CSF levels of 5-HIAA in schizophrenic patients who have attempted suicide. American College of Neuropsychopharmacology, 1986

Sulser F, Robinson SE: Clinical implications of pharmacological differences among antipsychotic drugs, in Psychopharmacology: A Generation of Progress. Edited by Lipton MA, DiMascio A, Killam KF. New York, Raven Press, 1978

Tabakoff B, Ritzmann R: Inhibition of the transport of 5-hydroxyindoleacetic acid from brain by ethanol. J Neurochem 1975; 24:1043-1051

Targum SD, Rosen L, Capodanno AE: The dexamethasone suppression test in suicidal patients with unipolar depression. Am J Psychiatry 1983; 140:877-879

Traskman L, Asberg M, Bertilsson K, et al: Monoamine metabolites in CSF and suicidal behavior. Arch Gen Psychiatry 1981; 38:631-636

Tsuang MT: Suicide in schizophrenics, manics, depressives, and surgical controls. Arch Gen Psychiatry 1978; 35:153-155

Van Praag HM: Depression, suicide and the metabolism of serotonin in the brain. J Affective Disord 1982; 4:275-290

Van Praag HM: CSF 5-HIAA and suicide in nondepressed schizophrenics. Lancet 1983; 2:977-978

Van Waltere JP, Charles G, Wilmotte J: Test de function a la dexamethasone et suicide. Acta Psychiatry Scand 1983; 83:569-578

Zanko MT, Biegon A: Increased B-adrenergic receptor binding in human frontal cortex of suicide victims. Abstract of the Annual Meeting, Society of Neuroscience, Boston, MA 1983

Chapter 16

The Assessment and Treatment of Patients at Risk for Suicide

by David A. Brent, M.D., David J. Kupfer, M.D.,
Evelyn J. Bromet, Ph.D., and Mary Amanda Dew, Ph.D.

Suicide remains among the most dreaded outcomes of psychiatric disorder. Regrettably, it is also one of the most common (Bromet et al, 1985). The risk of suicide among psychiatric patients is at least 10 times that among the general population (Guze and Robins, 1970; Hillard et al, 1983; Morrison, 1982, Pokorny, 1983). Moreover, 10 to 15 percent of patients with major psychiatric disorders such as substance use disorder, affective disorder, and schizophrenia will die by suicide (Miles, 1977). Therefore, the assessment and diminution of suicidal potential among psychiatric patients should be a task of the highest priority for the practicing psychiatrist.

In this chapter, we examine salient issues of assessment of suicidality and suicidal risk in psychiatric patients. This will include the assessment of suicidal potential in the patient who has already engaged in a suicide attempt, as well as a delineation of the contribution of psychosocial stressors, personality and cognitive style, intercurrent medical illness, and specific psychiatric syndromes to suicidal risk in psychiatric patients. In the second half of this chapter, we apply our current knowledge about risk factors for suicide in psychiatric patients to prevention of suicidality through rational, empirically based psychiatric treatment of patients at high risk for suicide. In this latter section, we also discuss the indications for psychiatric inpatient treatment. Finally, both somatic and psychosocial treatments for patients who attempt suicide and/or who have major psychiatric disorders are examined with respect to their potential effectiveness in diminishing the risk for subsequent suicide and suicidal behavior.

ASSESSMENT

Assessment of Suicidal Patients

SUICIDALITY.   An assessment of the presence and extent of suicidality is an essential part of the psychiatric examination. Suicidality exists as a spectrum from nonspecific suicidal ideation, such as thoughts of death, to thoughts of one's own death, and finally to suicidal thoughts with a plan and intent to die. Individuals with more severe forms of suicidal ideation are also likely to have less severe manifestations of this clinical phenomenon as well (Paykel et al, 1974b; Brent et al, 1986a). For example, a patient who has suicidal ideation with

Preparation of this chapter was supported in part by NIMH Grants #1 KO8 MH00581–01 and MH15169–09. Portions of this chapter were based upon a report prepared under NIMH Contract #85M05914601S (Bromet, Dew, and Brent, 1985).

a plan is likely to have had nonspecific thoughts of death or dying as well. Therefore, one should screen for the presence of suicidality by asking about nonspecific suicidality, then proceed to more specific forms of suicidal ideation if the initial screening questions are positive.

The severity of suicidal ideation appears to be correlated with the intensity of depression and hopelessness in children, adolescents, and adults (Beck et al, 1979b; Brent et al, 1986a; Carlson and Cantwell, 1982; Paykel et al, 1974b; Pfeffer et al, 1979, 1980; Pfeffer, 1981). Therefore, within the subgroup of patients who are suicidal, those with the greatest severity of suicidal ideation are likely to be at the highest risk.

However, those patients who demonstrate *any* degree of suicidality—ideation, threat, or even actual suicidal behavior—are all at much higher risk for completed suicide than are nonsuicide psychiatric patients. A similarity among persons with suicidal ideation and those who actually attempt suicide has been substantiated in cross-sectional studies of children and adolescent outpatients (Brent et al, 1986a; Pfeffer et al, 1979, 1980), affectively disordered adults attending a medication clinic (Stallone et al, 1982), and community samples (Goldberg, 1981; Vandivort and Locke, 1979). Pokorny (1966) has shown that the suicide rates for psychiatric patients admitted for suicidal ideation, threats, and attempts are 30, 35, and 40 times higher than nonsuicidal psychiatric controls, respectively, suggesting that distinctions among subtypes of suicidality are less important in the prediction of risk for suicide than the presence of *any* suicidal indicators. Similarly, persons who call suicide crisis centers, although not "patients" in the strictest sense, are on the average 25 times more likely to commit suicide than are members of the general population (Dew et al, 1987). Therefore, suicidality in any form should not elude the clinician, as the outcome may prove to be fatal.

In this section, we will focus on descriptors of actual suicidal behavior. Four parameters will be discussed: 1) precipitant; 2) motivation; 3) suicidal intent; and 4) medical lethality of the attempt.

PRECIPITANT. We define precipitants for suicidal behavior as stressful events that occur within six weeks prior to the attempt (see Murphy et al, 1979; Paykel, 1986), and which appear to have provided some motivation for the episode of self-destructive behavior. Examples of such stressors include interpersonal loss, interpersonal discord, an impending disciplinary crisis or incarceration, or loss of a job. These are events that are generally acknowledged to be stressful for the general population, although it is probably only in the context of other vulnerability characteristics (for example, alcoholism; see Murphy et al, 1979) that such events may engender suicidal behavior. Paykel (1986) has noted that suicide attempters, compared to matched nonsuicidal depressed controls, were likely to have experienced a greater number of stressful life events within the week and month prior to the attempt. Cohen-Sandler and colleagues (1982) found a similar accumulation of stressors in the 12 months preceding admission to a child psychiatric inpatient unit for suicidal ideation or behavior, which suggests that the effects of stress may be cumulative over a longer period of time than six weeks. The most common precipitants of suicidal behavior are interpersonal discord with a significant other, and the threatened or actual loss of an important relationship, such as a conjugal partner or parent (Cohen-Sandler et al, 1982; Paykel et al, 1975; Paykel, 1986). Alcoholics who commit suicide are especially likely to have experienced an interpersonal loss within six weeks prior to their death (Murphy et al, 1979). Other frequent precipitants for suicidal behavior include threat of incarceration, other disciplinary crisis, and specifically in older patients, onset of terminal illness such as cancer (Cohen-Sandler et al, 1982; Fox et al, 1982; Murphy et al, 1979; Paykel et al, 1975; Paykel, 1986; Shaffer, 1974).

The identification of precipitants of suicidal behavior is important for three reasons. First, in concert with other risk factors, knowledge of the occurrence of specific stressors can be used to identify those patients at highest risk for suicide (for example, divorce in an alcoholic male). Second, the nature of the individual's immediate reactions to the precipitant gives some clues as to how the patient solves problems and perceives his or her own life situation. For example, a patient who wants to commit suicide after a break-up in a relationship may have thoughts such as, "Without him/her, I am nothing." The modification of such dysfunctional cognitions might well be one of the first tasks in the amelioration of suicidality in such a patient. Similarly, a person who become suicidal after an angry interpersonal encounter may need to learn to manage negative affect more effectively, thereby obviating the desire or perceived need to resort to suicidal behavior. Finally, if interpersonal conflict is a precipitant of suicidal behavior, then the social environment of the suicidal patient requires investigation. For example, if marital discord precipitates a suicide attempt, then therapeutic efforts should target both a reduction in marital conflict concurrent with a diminution in the strength of the patient's reaction to criticism.

MOTIVATION. Motivations for engaging in suicidal behavior can be quite diverse, and different motivations have different implications for treatment and disposition. Patients can have multiple and even contradictory motivations for exhibiting suicidal behavior. For example, it has been demonstrated that suicidal individuals can simultaneously hold strong desires to live *and* die (Kovacs and Beck, 1977). Therefore, it is important to assess a wide range of possible motivations, since the presence of a motivation with a future orientation (for example, trying to get a conjugal partner back) does *not* necessarily rule out a strong desire to die.

Nevertheless, most suicide attempters evidence motivations other than a wish to die. The most frequent motivations reported in both adolescent and young adult suicide attempters are: desire to influence another person's behavior (for example, to gain attention, to make someone feel guilty), to express anger, and to escape (Hawton et al, 1982a; Hawton and Catalon, 1982). Younger children who have lost a parent or close relative to death sometimes express a desire to join that relative through suicide (Pfeffer, 1980). The nature of the motivation for suicidal behavior has important implications for treatment planning. For example, the person who is depressed, hopeless, and truly wants to die may need inpatient hospitalization, pharmacotherapy, and/or cognitive therapy that targets hopelessness and related cognitive distortions. On the other hand, a person who uses suicidal behavior as a method for influencing other people may benefit from the acquisition of such social skills as direct communication of feelings, assertiveness, and skills in interpersonal problem solving (Clum et al, 1979; Schotte and Clum, 1987).

SUICIDAL INTENT. The motivation for suicidal behavior that should cause greatest concern is the wish to die, otherwise known as suicidal intent. This construct has been carefully studied and refined by Beck and colleagues, and their work has resulted in a 15-item Suicidal Intent Scale (Beck et al, 1974a). This measure taps the patient's thoughts and behaviors just prior to the suicidal act in order to determine to what extent the patient desired a lethal outcome. In general, patients who leave notes, make wills, express suicidal intent before their act, and take precautions not to be discovered are judged to have the highest suicidal intent. High suicidal intent has been found to predict reattempts among adolescent and adult suicidal attempters (Beck et al, 1974a; Hawton et al, 1982b) as well as to predict suicide completion among adults (Beck et al, 1974a; Pierce, 1981). Intent is also highly correlated with the severity of depression, and even more closely related to hopelessness (Beck et al, 1974b; Dyer and Kreitman, 1984; Wetzel, 1976). Most often, youthful suicide attempters do *not* show high suicidal intent (Brent, 1987; Hawton et al, 1982b) but when high suicidal intent *is* present, it is an indication for psychiatric hospitalization.

LETHALITY. While it is clear that the medical dangerousness of a suicide attempt is the final arbiter of its lethality, the relationship between lethality and intent is only modestly positive at best (Beck et al, 1979a; Brent, 1987). Therefore, it is a mistake to judge the risk for suicide based *solely* on the medical seriousness of a suicide attempt. For example, an attempt of low intent can result in a fatality if the person who is supposed to discover the victim fails to appear. Similarly, particularly in young children and adolescents, the lack of knoweldge of lethality of various methods interferes with the ability to plan and execute a lethal attempt (Shaffer, 1974; Shaffer and Fisher, 1981). In fact, Beck and colleagues (1979b) have shown that the relationship between lethality and intent is negligible *except* in those suicide attempters whose knowledge of the lethality of the method employed was adequate.

However, there is some evidence that use of violent methods is predictive of future suicide both in adolescents and adults who attempt suicide (Otto, 1972; Tuckman and Youngman, 1968). This is convergent with biochemical investigations of suicide attempters—those who make violent attempts are most likely to have low cerebrospinal fluid (CSF) 5-hydroxyindoleacetic acid (5-HIAA), and in turn are most likely to die by suicide (Asberg et al, 1976; Asberg, 1986). Therefore, use of a violent method, or use of a less-than-lethal method that one mistakenly thought would result in death, are both signs of a serious suicide attempt.

A related issue concerns the relationship of the availability of lethal agents to the risk for suicide. There is now convergent ecologic evidence linking the availability of firearms and the suicide rate by this method in adults (Boyd, 1983; Boyd and Moscicki, 1986; Kellerman and Reay, 1986; Lester and Murell, 1980, 1982; Markush and Bortolucci, 1984) and adolescents (Brent et al, 1986b). In addition, the suicide rate has dropped following the detoxicification of domestic gas in Great Britain (Kreitman, 1976) and the restriction of the quantity of prescriptions for hypnotics in Australia (Goldney and Katsikitas, 1983). This lends further support to a relationship between the availability of lethal agents and the suicide rate.

ASSESSMENT OF PATIENTS WITH PSYCHIATRIC DISORDER

The risk for suicide and suicidal behavior is increased in virtually every major psychiatric syndrome (Miles, 1977; Pokorny, 1983; Morrison, 1982). All of the psychological autopsy studies of adult (Barraclough et al, 1974; Dorpat and Ripley, 1960; Robins et al, 1959) and adolescent suicide victims (Shaffer et al, 1985; Shafii et al, 1985; Shafii, 1986) indicate that nearly all had a major current psychiatric disorder at the time of death, although only a minority were engaged in active psychiatric treatment (Brent et al, 1986b; Robins et al, 1959; Shafii et al, 1985). These studies indicate that suicide victims most frequently have a diagnosis of affective disorder, for which suicidality is actually a serious *symptom*, and for which remission of the disorder should be accompanied by remission of the suicidality. In addition, a substantial minority of suicide victims shows other psychiatric disorders such as alcohol or drug abuse, personality disorder, and schizophrenia. For patients with any of these disorders, proper evaluation, treatment, and follow-up is key to the prevention of suicide within this population. However, before discussing the aspects of each specific psychiatric syndrome that constitute risk factors for suicide, we will address some general factors that contribute to suicidal risk. These contributory factors appear to operate *across* psychiatric syndromes and include: previous suicidal behavior, exposure (both intra- and extrafamiliarly) to suicidal behavior, other family/environmental stressors, personality variables, and medical illness.

Previous Suicidal Behavior

Patients who have been suicidal previously are at higher risk to complete suicide, regardless of psychiatric diagnosis. The suicide rate among those who attempt suicide varies with demographic and psychiatric characteristics, but has been reported to be as high as one to two percent per year of follow-up in male psychiatric patients (Motto, 1965; Otto, 1972; Pokorny, 1983). Other follow-up studies of psychiatric patients indicate that those who have made multiple suicide attempts are at especially high risk for suicide (Tuckman and Youngman, 1968). Patients who have suicidal ideation with a plan, or who threaten suicide, appear to have a risk for suicide almost as high as those who actually attempt suicide (Pokorny, 1966). Similarly, clients of suicide prevention centers show a risk for suicide that is markedly above the general population rate (Dew et al, 1987). Moreover, the presence of suicidality in psychiatric patients may be a sensitive and specific predictor of future suicide. In a 40-year follow-up of 225 recurrent unipolar depressed patients, 15 completed suicide, all of whom had previously threatened suicide (Fowler et al, 1979). Moreover, this indicator was *specific*, as none of those unipolar patients who did *not* complete suicide had *ever* threatened suicide during the follow-up period.

Familial and Extrafamilial Exposure to Suicidal Behavior

A family history of suicide should be inquired after, as such a history in adopted–away persons conveys a sixfold risk for suicide among their first-degree biological relatives (Schulsinger et al, 1979). Tsuang (1983) found a fourfold increase of suicide in the first-degree relatives of psychiatric patients who committed suicide, and Egeland and Sussex (1985) reported familial aggregation of suicide in Amish pedigrees. While these and related studies (Wender et al, 1986) suggest a genetic etiology, the clustering of suicides in families could also be mediated by family stress or contagion (Keller et al, 1986; Pfeffer, 1986).

For example, there is some evidence that extrafamilial exposure (such as through friends or through media publicity) may render individuals, particularly adolescents, more vulnerable to suicide (Gould and Shaffer, 1986; Kreitman et al, 1970; Phillips and Carstensen, 1986; Robbins and Conroy, 1983; Shafii et al, 1985). Treatment of patients who are exposed to these influences should aim to diminish the appeal of such models, and therefore should decrease the likelihood of imitation.

Other Family/Environment Factors

Family history of psychiatric disorder, particularly affective disorder, renders patients much more vulnerable to suicide and suicidal behavior (Linkowski et al, 1985; Roy, 1982a, 1983; Tsuang, 1983; Wender et al, 1986). Such a family history is particularly important to ascertain in younger patients for two reasons: first, younger patients still dependent on their parents may be particularly vulnerable to the effects of living with a psychiatrically ill parent (Beardslee et al, 1983; Keller et al, 1986; Rutter and Quinton, 1984); and second, the early psychiatric manifestations of an adolescent's genetic and familial endowment may be subtle enough to elude detection (Akiskal et al, 1985).

Social support is a key parameter to assess in the evaluation of the potentially suicidal patient. Although there are only a few reports to link the lack of social support with suicide or suicidal behavior in adults and adolescents (Murphy et al, 1979; Topol and Reznikoff, 1982), it is well known that such supports play an important role in the etiology of psychological distress (Brown and Harris, 1978), treatment seeking and compliance with treatment (Frank et al, 1985; Haas et al, 1986; Miklowitz et al, 1986), and response to both psychosocial and pharmacologic treatments (Downing and Rickels, 1973; Hogarty et al, 1986; Steinmetz et al, 1983). Among the important aspects of social support to evaluate are: 1) the presence of a confiding relationship (Brown and Harris, 1978); 2) the ability of a significant other to monitor the behavior of the patient in question (Frank et al, 1985; Haas et al, 1986; Miklowitz et al, 1986); and 3) the extent to which the quality of significant relationships protect and/or contribute to suicidal potential. For example, a spousal relationship that is fraught with tension and discord may be more of a stressor than a support.

Personality and Cognitive Style

There is growing evidence that personality and cognitive traits play a role in suicidal behavior and completed suicide. For example, hostility, aggression, interpersonal maladjustment, and sensation seeking have been noted to be more common among patients who attempt suicide than among matched psychiatric controls (Steiner et al, 1972; Weissman et al, 1973). Moreover, various deficits in interpersonal problem solving may put psychiatric patients at higher risk for engaging in suicidal behavior (Clum et al, 1979; Schotte and Clum, 1987). As already noted, dysfunctional cognitions such as hopelessness are associated with suicidal intent (Beck et al, 1974b; Beck et al, 1975) and suicide completion (Beck et al, 1985). Rapidity to habituate to stimuli in physiologic studies, which may be a correlate of an impulsive cognitive style, has also been reported to predict suicide in psychiatric patients (Edman et al, 1986). An exploration of the association between categorical classifications of personality disorder and suicide has tended to confirm that patients with various personality disorders, including Briquet's syndrome and antisocial personality disorder, have an elevated risk of suicide (Martin et al, 1985; Morrison, 1982). The common denominator in many of these predisposing characteristics may be a tendency toward impulsive violence, one which may be both mediated through low CSF 5-HIAA and closely associated with risk for suicide (Asberg et al, 1976; Asberg, 1986; Brown et al, 1979, 1982a; Linnoila et al, 1983). Blumenthal and Kupfer (1986b) have suggested that those patients who show comorbidity—that is, who have *both* a major psychiatric syndrome *and* some predisposing personality and cognitive variables—may be at highest risk for suicide. In any case, it is clear that patients with comorbidity of affective disorder *and* personality disorder are more difficult to treat than those patients with "pure" affective disorder (Weissman et al, 1978; Zuckerman et al, 1980), which may make this subgroup at higher risk for suicide. However, conclusive studies on the relationship between personality disorder and suicide have been problematic until recently, when some promising assessment measures for personality disorder have been developed (Loranger et al, 1984; Pfohl et al, 1983; Spitzer et al, 1986). None of these has yet been applied to area of suicide.

Medical Disorders

An integral part of the psychiatric evaluation of the potentially suicidal patient is a history, physical examination, and appropriate laboratory tests. Among those disorders that have been associated with suicide are cancer, peptic ulcer disease, Huntington's chorea, and epilepsy (Mackenzie and Popkin, 1987). Furthermore, several other medical conditions, while not specifically linked to suicide, have been associated with depression, including endocrinopathies, collagen vascular disorders, myasthenia gravis, and multiple sclerosis (Kupfer and Spiker, 1981). Finally, certain medical therapeutics such as antihypertensives, antiepileptic medication, and steroids may be associated with psychiatric manifestations.

Cancer has been associated with suicide in a number of studies (Campbell, 1966; Dorpat et al, 1968; Farberow and Schneidman, 1963; Fox et al, 1982; Louhivuori and Hakama, 1979). There is some evidence to suggest that the risk of suicide is greatest soon after diagnosis (Fox et al, 1982), and that the risk of suicide is highest in those with nonfocalized disease and in those who receive chemotherapy (Louhivouri and Hakama, 1979). However, while these studies suggest that the suicide is a response to the news of a potentially terminal and debilitating illness, alternative hypotheses should be considered. For example, the association between malignancy and cancer may be strongest for digestive organ cancers (Louhivuori and Hakama, 1979), which in turn are often associated with alcohol abuse (Morson and Lyon, 1975). Therefore, it is possible that the association between cancer and suicide is confounded by alcohol abuse. Moreover, it has been shown that patients with certain types of cancer (for example, pancreatic cancer) may show depressive symptoms which *antedate* their diagnosis (Fras et al, 1967). Furthermore, Kerr and colleagues (1969) showed that a cohort of patients hospitalized for affective disorders had a higher rate of subsequent malignancies than would be expected. Therefore, it is possible that the association between suicide and malignancy may be confounded by either depression predisposing to malignancy or occult malignancy predisposing to depression.

Peptic ulcer disease has been found to be overrepresented in victims of completed suicide (Dorpat et al, 1968). In addition, follow-up studies of adult medical/surgical patients with peptic ulcer disease have yielded higher-than-expected rates of suicide (Knop and Fisher, 1981; Viskun, 1975). It is possible that the overrepresentation of peptic ulcer patients among suicide victims may be related to the prevalence of alcoholism among patients with this medical illness (Knop and Fisher, 1981; Mackenzie and Popkin, 1987). However, peptic ulcer disease was found to be associated with suicide even among alcoholics (Knop and Fisher, 1981).

Huntington's chorea has been associated with approximately a sixfold increase in the rate of suicide compared to population norms (Chandler et al, 1960). Furthermore, family relations of index cases who may not as yet have manifested the disorder also may have a higher rate of suicide (Dewhurst et al, 1970). It is unclear whether the latter finding is due to depression mediated by clinically latent, but biochemically active, aspects of this inherited disorder, or whether suicide is motivated by the desire to avoid this frightening and debilitating neurologic illness.

The suicide rate among patients with epilepsy is approximately four times that of normal controls (Matthews and Barabas, 1981). While there are various theoretical reasons to link disturbances of mood and epilepsy (Corbett and Trimble, 1983), it is possible that treatment with phenobarbital may predispose to suicidal ideation and behavior both in children and adults with epilepsy (Brent et al, in press; Brent, 1986; Hawton et al, 1980; Mackay, 1979). Therefore, any epileptic patient who is seen for a psychiatric evaluation of mood disturbance and is receiving a barbiturate anticonvulsant should be switched to an alternative anticonvulsant if this is clinically feasible. Preliminary evidence suggests, at least in younger patients, that those with a family history of an affective disorder are most vulnerable to the affective side effects of phenobarbital (Brent et al, in press). Other pharmacologic factors associated with psychiatric disburbance in this population include polytherapy and decreased serum folate secondary to anticonvulsant treatment (Corbett and Trimble, 1983). Moreover, other factors, such as the neurophysiological alterations associated with epilepsy, and occupational and social discrimination experienced by epileptic patients, may also account for the high suicide rate in this particular chronic illness (Barraclough, 1981; Corbett and Trimble, 1983; Matthews and Barabas, 1981).

Endocrine disorders have long been associated with mood disturbance, particularly hypo- and hyperthyroidism, Cushing's disease, and hyperparathyroidism (Lishman, 1978), although no endocrinopathies have specifically been linked to suicide. Laboratory screens for all psychiatric patients should include thyroid function tests, calcium, and phosphorus. A fundoscopic and general physical examination should enable one to diagnose Cushing's disease, which has often been associated with depression (Starkman et al, 1981). Not only can hypothyroidism present as an affective disorder, but subclinical hypothyroidism can render unipolar and bipolar patients refractory to standard pharmacologic management (Cowdrey et al, 1983; Targum, 1983). Other intercurrent medical illnesses appear to render depressed patients more refractory to pharmacotherapy as well (as reviewed in Thase and Kupfer, 1987; Griest and Griest, 1979; Klerman and Hirschfeld, 1979).

The use of antihypertensives, such as propranolol, is associated with depression (Paykel et al, 1982), particularly in the presence of a family history of affective disorder (Griffin and Friedman, 1986). Patients with antihypertensive agents that affect mood should be closely monitored for depression. If depressive symptomatology develops, a change in antihypertensive regimen to a calcium channel blocker or beta-blocker without central effects should be considered. However, there is no conclusive evidence that the suicide rate is higher in patients with hypertension (Mackenzie and Popkin, 1987).

Steroids are another type of widely used medication associated with both mania and depression, although again, there is no conclusive evidence linking their use to suicide. While the effects have not been systematically studied, there is no question that these agents are associated with behavioral and sleep disturbance, mood lability, and even psychosis (Harris et al, 1986; Lerner et al, 1986; Ling, 1981). In one study, patients treated with methylprednisdone seemed to be protected from this effect, in contrast to the pronounced adverse effects associated with the other types of steroid agents (Lerner et al, 1986). While some investigators argue that psychiatric manifestations of some disorders, such as central nervous sytem (CNS) lupus, can be suppressed by large doses of steroids (Bennett et al, 1972), others feel that the psychiatric and medical iatrogenic effects of high dose steroids outweigh the benefits (Sergent et al, 1975). Psychiatric morbidity of patients treated with steroids can be minimized by use of the dosage with minimal psychiatric side effects that is still medically beneficial.

In conclusion, it is important to be aware of the psychiatric manifestations of medical disease and medical therapeutics. While this discussion highlights some of the more important contributions to the risk for suicide, it is by no means exhaustive. For more detailed discussion of this complex issue, the clinician is referred to appropriate texts and reviews (Griest and Griest, 1979; Klerman and Hirshfeld, 1979; Lishman, 1978; Mackenzie and Popkin, 1987).

Affective Disorders

The assessment of depressive symptomatology is an integral part of the evaluation of the suicidal patient. Psychological autopsy studies (Barraclough et al, 1974; Dorpat and Ripley, 1960; Robins et al, 1959) show that between 40 and 70 percent of all suicide victims have an affective disorder. Follow-up studies (reviewed in Miles, 1977) indicate that 10 to 15 percent of patients with a major affective disorder commit suicide. Of particular note is that suicide appears to occur relatively *early* in the course of affective illness (Guze and Robins, 1970; Miles, 1977). This has been attributed to the inability of hopeless, depressed individuals who have never experienced a remission to believe that their illness will, in fact, remit. Therefore, in the ongoing care of depressed patients, providing hope and education about the expected course of affective disorders is likely to help in preventing suicide in this high-risk sample.

One very controversial question centers around the relationship of nonlethal suicidal behavior to affective disorders. There is no question that the prevalence of suicidal behavior among affectively disturbed patients is high (for example, 20 to 40 percent) (Johnson and Hunt, 1979; Linkowski et al, 1985; Stallone et al, 1982), but some argue that the *majority* of adolescent (Carlson and Cantwell,

1982) and adult (Flood and Seager, 1968; Murphy and Wetzel, 1982) suicide attempters do *not* have an affective disorder. Recently, van Praag and colleagues (1985) have challenged this assumption by demonstrating that suicidal behavior appears to have a *cathartic* effect on psychiatric patients, and that retrospective assessment of their mood and associated symptoms *prior* to the suicidal episode indicates that the majority of attempters *were* in a depressive episode. It is unclear whether this "cathartic" effect is long-lasting, or whether, in fact, the depressive picture returns and requires specific psychosocial or pharmacologic intervention. Nevertheless, this underscores the importance of assessing the patient's symptomatology *prior* to the suicide attempt and not being overly influenced by the patient's appearance during the interview.

The specific type of affective disorder is important to determine because of the differential effect on prognosis and treatment. A history of hypomania or mania should be carefully sought, as there is some evidence that younger patients with bipolar disorder are at particularly high risk for suicide (Brent et al, 1986b; Welner et al, 1979) and suicidal behavior (Johnson and Hunt, 1979; Stallone et al, 1982). Prospective studies indicate that adult patients with mixed states and those undergoing a switch in polarity are particularly vulnerable to suicide (Fawcett et al, 1987). The old adage that depressed patients who commit suicide often become calm or euphoric just prior to suicide (Keith-Spiegel and Spiegel, 1967) must be reinterpreted in view of these findings, as some of these depressed patients may actually be bipolar patients who are experiencing a change in polarity. The association between bipolarity and suicide may, in part, account for the seasonal fluctuation in the suicide rate (Lester, 1971; Nayha, 1983), which happens to correspond to the seasonal pattern for recrudescences of bipolar disorder (Parker and Walter, 1982).

Seasonal affective disorder is gaining recognition as a *bona fide* subtype of affective disorder (Rosenthal et al, 1984). The diagnosis rests on the association of a hypersomnic, hyperphagic depressive syndrome with the winter months. While the relationship of seasonal affective disorder to suicide is not well delineated, suicide does have seasonal fluctuations, as noted above (Lester, 1971; Nayha, 1983; Zung and Green, 1974). Given the response of these patients to phototherapy (Rosenthal et al, 1984), it is important to attempt to elicit a seasonal component in patients with affective disturbance.

Premenstrual or perimenstrual exacerbation of affective disorders can occur in patients with an underlying affective disorder or with premenstrual syndrome (Abramowitz et al, 1982; Bancroft and Baskstrom, 1985; Halbreich and Endicott, 1983). There is evidence that suicidal behavior among women is more common perimenstrually (Fourestie et al, 1986). In addition, preliminary evidence from a series of psychological autopsies in adolescents indicates that two out of six girls who committed suicide suffered from severe premenstrual syndrome and were in fact premenstrual when they committed suicide (Brent et al, 1986).

Double depression, or depression on top of an underlying dysthymia, appears to be related to suicidal behavior in adolescents (Ryan et al, in press), although this relationship has not been established in adult patient populations. Studies of adults with double depression do indicate that these patients are less likely to achieve a full remission and are more likely to relapse than are patients with a more acute onset to their depressive syndrome (Keller et al, 1982a; 1982b, 1983). Akiskal (1982) emphasizes that a thorough medical work-up is particularly important in these patients, since underlying medical conditions may present as chronic depression.

There is evidence that patients with psychotic depression (delusional depression) are at higher risk for completed suicide than nonpsychotic depressed patients. Roose and colleagues (1983), reporting on the experience at Columbia, estimate that the risk for suicide among patients with delusional depression is 5.3 times that of patients with nondelusional depression. Delusional depression may be related to bipolar illness in adults (Weissman et al, 1984) and may be a harbinger of bipolar illness in younger patients (Strober and Carlson, 1982). In any case, psychotic features should always be elicited, as they have important implications for the assessment of suicidal risk as well as for treatment.

There is evidence that patients with affective disorder and comorbidity with *any* other psychiatric disorder are at particularly high risk for completed suicide. Shafii (1986) reports high rates of co-occurrence of affective and substance abuse disorders in youthful suicide victims, a finding confirmed by others (Brent et al, 1986b; Rich et al, 1986). Moreover, it is well known that patients with co-morbidity are more difficult to treat and are more likely to relapse (Akiskal, 1982; Clayton and Lewis, 1981; Weissman et al, 1978; Zuckerman et al, 1980). Finally, it is documented that alcohol and drug use and abuse can adversely affect the course of bipolar and unipolar depression (Akiskal, 1982; Clayton and Lewis, 1981; Himmelhoch and Garfinkel, 1986). Therefore, the presence of other diagnostic entities should always be carefully ascertained when evaluating suicidal risk patients with affective disorders.

Bereavement

The symptoms of grief and depression overlap considerably (Clayton et al, 1968, 1974). There is evidence that both short- and long-term consequences of interpersonal loss include suicide and suicidal behavior (Adams et al, 1980; Greer, 1974; Murphy et al, 1979). Therefore, psychiatrically vulnerable patients who experience bereavement may be particularly at risk for suicide, as has been noted by Murphy and associates (1979) in the case of alcoholic suicide victims. An important clinical issue is the differentiation between normal bereavement and depression. Symptoms that occur in both conditions include mood disturbance and neurovegetative signs, although in bereavement these frequently abate by two months after the loss. On the other hand, symptoms found in depression but *not* commonly in normal bereavement are functional impairment, suicidal ideation, feelings of worthlessness, and psychotic features (Clayton et al, 1974). Therefore, any patient who is bereaved but presenting with suicidal ideation, worthlessness, and functional impairment should be considered to be "pathologically" bereaved, and may merit pharmacotherapy and/or psychosocial intervention.

Alcohol and Chemical Dependency

Alcohol and substance abuse are also significant risk factors for completed suicide. A substantial minority of adult (Ford et al, 1979; James, 1966) and adolescent (Brent et al, 1987; Friedman, 1985) suicide completers are intoxicated at the time of death. Furthermore, alcohol intoxication may be related to suicide by firearms in youth (Brent et al, 1987).

In the case of alcohol dependence, suicide usually occurs late in the course of the disease, coinciding with the onset of medical complications such as cirrhosis (Barraclough et al, 1974; Miles, 1977; Robins et al, 1959). Therefore, the investigation of alcohol and substance abuse in the psychiatric patient should include physical and laboratory stigmata associated with these disorders, as well as historical information. Alcohol and drug abuse can also be a complication of other psychiatric disorders, such as affective disorder (Schuckit, 1979), anxiety disorder (Bibb and Chamblis, 1986; Quitkin et al, 1972), schizophrenia (Alterman et al, 1980, 1984), and antisocial personality disorder (Cadoret et al, 1986; Rounsaville et al, 1986). In addition, alcohol and drug abuse probably aggravate the course of these other attendant psychiatric disorders (Himmelhoch and Garfinkel, 1986; Klein, 1980; Negrete et al, 1986; Schuckit, 1979). Furthermore, alcoholism may predispose to depressive symptomatology (Behar et al, 1984; Pottenger et al, 1978).

Schizophrenia

The risk of suicide for patients with schizophrenia is comparable to that for patients with affective disorder (Miles, 1977). The archetypal schizophrenic suicide victim is a young, unemployed, white male with a chronic, relapsing illness who had been relatively functional and whose life ambitions had become incompatible with the perceived or apparent handicaps of schizophrenia (Drake et al, 1984, 1986; Roy, 1982b). The risk for suicide is highest among those schizophrenics who are hopeless, suicidal, fear mental disintegration, and have a negative attitude towards treatment (Drake et al, 1984; Drake and Cotton, 1986; Roy, 1982b; Virkkunen, 1976). Moreover, the risk is greatest early in hospitalization and just after discharge (Roy, 1982b). There have been anecdotal reports that the symptoms of akathisia may contribute to dysphoria, suicidal impulses, or even suicide (Drake and Erlich, 1985; Marder et al, 1984; Shear et al, 1983). In addition, although there have been no published studies, the co-occurrence of drug and alcohol abuse may make a significant contribution to risk for suicide in these patients. Some empirical support for this viewpoint comes from a study which correlates the severity of cannabis abuse with severity of psychiatric course in 137 schizophrenic patients in a six-month prospective study (Negrete et al, 1986).

It is of interest that hopelessness and fear of mental disintegration were more critical than psychotic symptoms in the prediction of suicide in these patients (Drake et al, 1984). Specifically, command hallucinations do *not* appear to be contributory to suicidal behavior (Hellerstein et al, 1987) or suicide (Drake et al, 1984). Therefore, assessment of the parameters of suicidal thoughts, feelings of worthlessness, hopelessness, dysphoria, drug and alcohol abuse, and akathisia in the schizophrenic patient are most likely to delineate suicidal risk.

TREATMENT

Overview

Pyschiatric treatment represents the opportunity to translate our knowledge, albeit incomplete, of risk factors for suicide into action. Therefore, psychiatric treatment of patients at high risk for suicide should ameliorate those risk factors that are most likely to result in suicide. It is difficult to study the relationship of treatment to suicide because suicide is a relatively rare outcome. In order to assess the relationship between psychiatric treatment and suicide, it is necessary to either study a very large cohort or to pool data across several studies. It is often necessary in practice to study outcome variables proximal to suicide, such as suicidal ideation and behavior, relapse of episode of psychiatric disorder, and functional impairment. There are several general principles that should guide the treatment of patients at high risk for suicide, and which apply across broad diagnostic categories. The most basic principle is that, since most suicide victims kill themselves in the midst of a psychiatric episode (Barraclough et al, 1974; Dorpat and Ripley, 1960; Robins et al, 1959; Shaffer, 1974; Shaffer et al, 1985; Shafii et al, 1985; Shafii, 1986), it is possible that proper diagnosis and treatment of the acute psychiatric disorder could dramatically alter the risk for suicide. Other general principles include family involvement for support and improved compliance; diagnosis and treatment of comorbid medical and psychiatric conditions; the provision of hope, particularly to new-onset patients; restriction of the availability of lethal agents; and indications for psychiatric hospitalization. These principles will now be examined.

Family Involvement and Compliance

There is evidence that adolescent and adult suicide victims are less likely to be or to *stay* in psychiatric treatment than surviving patients with comparable psychopathology (Brent et al, 1986b; Roy, 1982a). Therefore, efforts to maintain the patients' compliance once in treatment are likely to be important in the prevention of suicide as well. The importance of spouse and family involvement in maintaining compliance has been noted in bipolar, unipolar, and schizophrenic patients (Frank et al, 1985; Frank and Kupfer, 1986; Haas et al, 1986; Hogarty et al, 1986; Miklowitz et al, 1986). If family members can be sensitized to the signs and symptoms of decompensation, then the family can provide a safety net for the patient at risk. Therefore, the patient can be brought for treatment earlier and a potentially serious acute exacerbation can be averted. Conversely, family interactions that seem to provoke recrudescences can be attenuated through psychoeducation approaches (Frank et al 1985; Hogarty et al 1986; Miklowitz et al, 1986). Finally, family psychoeducation enables the family members to learn to live with a psychiatrically ill family member, which in turn facilitates a more supportive environment for the patient.

Comorbidity

In addition to the diagnosis and treatment of the disorder that has brought the patient for treatment, it is critical to scrutinize the patient closely for any attendant medical, personality, and other psychiatric disorders. As noted above, undiagnosed medical conditions, personality problems, or substance abuse disorders may render patients refractory to conventional psychiatric management. Therefore, the clinician should be alert to the presence of comorbidity, and should treat this problem aggressively.

Provision of Hope

In addition, it is important to remember that suicide is often an *early* complication of both affective and schizophrenic illness. A common thread in both illnesses may be the development of demoralization and hopelessness—hopelessness (the illness will *never* remit) and the belief that a return to premorbid functioning is completely out of the question. Therefore, providing hope is one of the most critical aspects of the treatment alliance between the psychiatrist and the newly diagnosed psychiatrically ill patient. Hope buys time for therapy and medication to take hold; hopelessness may propel the patient into a needless, lethal action from which there can be no return (Beck et al, 1985). Furthermore, a pervasive sense of hopelessness may not remit with pharmacologic treatment of depression or schizophrenia. Given the association between hopelessness and suicidal completion (Beck et al, 1985), it is important to attack this problem with psychosocial interventions if medication alone does not appear to be ameliorating this significant risk factor.

Availability of Lethal Agents

Another point regarding treatment is the importance of removal of firearms from the home of any patient felt to be at risk for suicide, since their availability may constitute a risk factor (Boyd, 1983; Boyd and Moscicki, 1986; Kellerman and Reay, 1986; Lester and Murrell, 1980, 1982; Markush and Bortolucci, 1984). Analogously, the prescription of tricyclic antidepressants or other psychotropic medication may constitute a risk factor for suicidal behavior (Avery and Winokur, 1978; Lonnqvist et al, 1974; Robin and Freeman-Browne, 1968). The size of these prescriptions should be limited (Goldney and Katsikitis, 1983). The clinician should be careful to prescribe antidepressants only for those patients for whom the medication is truly indicated, and at the proper dosage; in this way, the benefit/risk ratio with regard to the use of antidepressants can be maximized.

Psychiatric Hospitalization

The psychiatrist who is working with a potentially suicidal patient should make sure that the patient has access to a skilled clinician around the clock. The patient (and family) should be trained to look for warning signs of relapse and should have the telephone number of the treating clinician or back-up facility where emergency treatment can be obtained. It is clear that some patients cannot be maintained as outpatients, and these patients must be psychiatrically hospitalized.

Psychiatric hospitalization is indicated for patients who are judged to be in imminent danger of suicide unless monitored in a structured and protective environment. Patients who show preoccupation with death, evidence of a suicidal plan and the intent to carry it out, or who have made a suicide attempt with high intent or extreme medical dangerousness are best treated on an inpatient basis (Evenson et al, 1983; Kaplan et al, 1982). Furthermore, other indications for the hospitalization of suicidal patients include active substance abuse, psychosis, chronic medical illness, recent loss, hopelessness, and poor social support (Gerson and Bassuk, 1980; Patterson et al, 1983; Paykel et al, 1974a). Patients who resemble suicide completers most closely are at highest risk for completing suicide (Pallis et al, 1982, 1984), and therefore should be hospitalized. In general, suicide prediction will naturally result in large numbers of false positives. However, Murphy (1972) noted that the identification of persons who meet the risk profile for completed suicides is not wasted effort insofar as anyone meeting such a profile is likely to benefit from psychiatric intervention.

Psychiatric hospitalization may be opposed by the patient, in which case involuntary commitment should be sought. An exception to his is when both the patient and his or her family are opposed to hospitalization. In this case, hospitalization may antagonize both the patient and supportive others to psychiatric care, and the clinician may be better off trying to obtain an agreement from the family to seek outpatient care. However, whenever one refers a patient who has, for example, attempted suicide to outpatient treatment, it is important to recall that as many as one-half *never* show up for any therapy whatsoever (Paykel et al, 1974a). Also, if outpatient treatment is agreed upon, it is important to obtain a no-suicide contract from the patient and family; that is, an agreement that the patient will refrain from any suicidal behavior until the next appointment, and most important, that the patient will contact the therapist should he or she experience any overwhelming suicidal impulses (Drye et al, 1973; Strayhorn, 1982).

Hospitalization is, at best, a temporary respite from suicidality. Suicides frequently occur shortly after discharge from the hospital. Pokorny (1960) observed that 20 out of 37 suicides that occurred in ex-inpatients occurred within 20 days of discharge, and Roy (1982a), in a larger series, replicated these findings. Therefore, outpatient follow-up is key to the prevention of suicide in hospitalized patients, and particularly careful follow-up is required during the initial period postdischarge.

Unfortunately, despite the intense effort that professionals devote to hospitalized psychiatric patients, there is no evidence that inpatient hospitalization is a necessary or even helpful therapeutic intervention for acutely suicidal patients. Community standards and expert opinions continue to support this route for the high-risk patient, and ethical considerations may make a careful study of this problem impossible (Kirstein and Weissman, 1975; Paykel et al, 1974a).

Having discussed principles generic to the treatment of patients, we would like to discuss treatment interventions for more specific psychiatric problems: patients who attempt suicide, or who have unipolar and bipolar affective disorders, schizophrenia, and alcohol/substance abuse. In all of these topics, both psychotherapeutic and pharmacotherapeutic approaches are reviewed with respect to impact on remission, relapse, and, when data is available, relationship to suicidality.

Treatment of Suicide Attempters

The treatment of suicidality has two components—first, to treat the underlying psychiatric disorder that may have contributed to the suicide attempt; and second, to provide treatment designed to substitute more adaptive behavior for suicidal behavior in response to an interpersonal crisis.

Two early studies showed that suicide attempters who self-selected for treatment had a lower rate of recurrent suicide attempts than those who were not treated (Greer and Bagley, 1971; Kennedy, 1972). Although it is difficult to evaluate the results of treatment when one group was also noncompliant, this suggestion that treatment may be beneficial in the reduction of recidivism was important and had been followed by several more systematically designed studies.

Ettlinger (1975) compared the rates of suicide attempts and completions among suicide attempters treated between 1961 and 1964 with "traditional" outpatient approaches, as opposed to suicide attempters treated between 1964 and 1966 with a more aggressive outreach program. No difference in the rate of suicide attempts or completions was detected. However, as the author observed, a cohort effect of increased suicidal behavior among successively later birth cohorts might have masked the effectiveness of treatment. Motto (1976) conducted a four-year follow-up of depressed and suicidal psychiatric inpatients who dropped out of treatment and demonstrated a trend in favor of aggressive outreach over no follow-up, although the difference in the suicide rate was not statistically significant.

Several treatment studies of suicide attempters employed random assignment of patients to "traditional" outpatient treatment as opposed to a more flexible and intense modality (for example, telephone outreach, home visits, and so on). While some of these studies reported improvement in social functioning at follow-up (Chowdhury et al, 1973; Hawton et al, 1981; Welu, 1977), only Welu reported a lower rate of suicide attempts in the outreach group. However, the follow-up period of four months in Welu's study was especially brief and precludes forming a definitive conclusion about this particular treatment program. In this study, a diminished intake of alcohol was observed in the outreach group, but not in controls, suggesting that alcohol abuse may be a key variable affecting subsequent recidivism.

Other investigators used randomized clinical trials to study the efficacy of more focused psychotherapeutic interventions on the prevention of suicidal behavior. Gibbons and colleagues (1978) compared "task-centered" with traditional casework and found that, upon 12-month follow-up, the task-centered group showed greater improvement in social adjustment; however, no difference in the rate of suicidal behavior was found. In another study, 24 hospitalized suicide attempters who had made at least two prior attempts were randomly assigned to insight-oriented or behavioral therapy (Liberman and Eckman, 1981). At two-year follow-up, there was no difference between treatment groups in the suicide attempt rate, but the behavioral-treated group showed fewer suicidal plans, less depression, and better social adjustment. Obviously, suicidal behavior is a rare outcome, and the possibility of detecting meaningful treatment effects in a study of this size was small at best. However, the fact that the behavioral treatment preferentially ameliorated conditions which predispose to suicidal behavior (for example, suicidal ideation) holds future promise for this and related modalities in the treatment of recurrent suicidal behavior.

Three randomized clinical trials have examined the impact of pharmacotherapy on the prevention of suicide attempts among patients with recurrent suicidal behavior. In the first study, depot injectable neuroleptic was found to be more effective than placebo in reducing the attempted suicide rate on six-month follow-up in a high-risk group of 37 patients who had made at least four previous suicide attempts (Montgomery et al, 1979). While detailed diagnostic characteristics of these patients were not reported, their presentation (for example, multiple episodes of self-destructive behavior) and response to neuroleptics suggests that these patients may have had an underlying personality disorder, such as borderline personality disorder. These results are convergent with those of Soloff and colleagues (1986b), who demonstrated that patients with borderline personality disorder showed an improvement in symptomatology on low dose haloperidol. Therefore, low dose neuroleptic treatment may be of benefit in reducing suicidality in personality disordered patients with recurrent suicidal behavior.

Further studies are warranted to clarify the short- and long-term role of neuroleptics in the management of patients with recurrent suicidal behavior.

Antidepressants do not appear to have a useful role in the prevention of recurrent suicidal behavior in nonaffectively disordered patients. Two studies have compared the efficacy of second-generation heterocyclic antidepressants to placebo in the prevention of recidivism in nonaffectively disordered patients with recurrent suicidal behavior, and found that antidepressant treatment was ineffective (Hirsch et al, 1983; Montgomery et al, 1983). Moreover, at least in patients with borderline personality disorder, antidepressant treatment may be contraindicated. Soloff and colleagues (1986a) found a worsening of irritability and suicidality in borderline patients treated with amitryptiline, both compared to baseline and to patients treated with placebo and haloperidol. Therefore, amitryptiline (and perhaps other antidepressants) should be avoided in suicidal patients who demonstrate signs of borderline personality disorder and who show no evidence of an endogenomorphic depression. Given the association between low central serotonin and violent impulsive suicidal behavior (Asberg et al, 1976; Asberg et al, 1986), it is possible that serotonergic antidepressants (for example, trazodone, fluvoxamine) may hold future therapeutic promise for this group.

Unipolar Depression: The Role of Psychosocial Treatments

In the last decade, several clinical trials have been conducted comparing the efficacy of different types of somatic treatments as well as combinations of psychosocial therapies and medication in the treatment of unipolar depression. None of these studies specifically addresses the impact of therapy on the occurrence of suicidal behavior in depressed patients. However, there is some evidence of potential benefit of psychosocial treatment over pharmacotherapy alone in the management of suicidal, depressed patients.

First, the treatment drop-out rate has been found to be lower among patients who received behavioral (McLean and Hakistian, 1979), social skills (Bellack et al, 1981), or cognitive therapies (Blackburn et al, 1981; Rush et al, 1977) than among patients who received pharmacotherapy alone. Similarly, psychiatrically hospitalized depressed patients who were involved in psychoeducational family therapy were more compliant with outpatient follow-up treatment (Haas et al, 1986). These findings are important because suicidal patients have been shown to be difficult to sustain in treatment (Hawton, et al, 1982b; Paykel et al, 1974a) and some studies of suicidal patients suggest that aggressive follow-up treatment may have beneficial effects on suicidal outcomes (Welu, 1977; Motto, 1976).

Second, there is evidence, albeit equivocal, that short-term cognitive and interpersonal therapies, when compared to pharmacotherapy, may preferentially ameliorate hopelessness and suicidal ideation in unipolar depressed patients (DiMascio et al, 1979; Kovacs et al, 1981; Rush et al, 1977). Since these are symptoms closely associated with suicide (Beck et al, 1985; Fowler et al, 1979; Roy, 1982a), it follows that certain psychosocial approaches may be superior to pharmacotherapy alone in reducing the risk for suicide in this patient population. However, it should be noted that two studies found no evidence of such effects (Blackburn et al, 1981; Simons et al, 1984). Furthermore, Friedman (1975) found that amitryptiline was more strongly associated with amelioration of hopelessness and suicidal ideation than marital therapy. Moreover, the pharmacologic treatment in the studies that showed some superiority of psychosocial treatment might be considered inadequate by current standards (for example, dosage of 150 mg for a 16-week treatment, followed by complete discontinuation of medication). Studies of recurrent depression indicate that maintenance pharmacotherapy reduces the incidence of relapse (Prien and Kupfer, 1986) and that the optimal dose of imipramine for this patient population may be at least as high as 225 mg per day (Frank and Kupfer, 1986). Nevertheless, the ability to reduce these important correlates of suicide in depressed patients is potentially very important, and more research is needed to settle the issue of optimal treatment.

Third, there is evidence that the rate of relapse is lower in depressed patients treated with psychosocial treatment than in patients treated with pharmacotherapy. In fact, in all four studies that compare patients treated with either psychosocial treatment or pharmacotherapy at one-year follow-up all favor psychosocial therapy, insofar as the rate of relapses was lower in those patients who received psychosocial interventions (Kovacs et al, 1981; Rush et al, 1977; Simons et al, 1986; Weissman et al, 1981). Given that the prevention of suicidal behavior in high-risk individuals may require complex, long-term management, the results of short-term treatment trials may not be directly pertinent to the optimal treatment needs of suicidal patients.

Finally, there is some suggestion that *combinations* of psychosocial treatment and pharmacotherapy may result in outcomes that are superior to either treatment alone, suggesting a synergistic effect. This has been demonstrated across a wide variety of psychosocial interventions, including psychoeducational family therapies (Frank et al, 1985; Haas et al, 1986), interpersonal therapy (Weissman et al, 1979), and cognitive therapy (Blackburn et al, 1981). Psychoeducational family therapy appears to have a beneficial effect on compliance with medication (Frank et al, 1985; Haas et al, 1986) and, in addition, may improve response to pharmacotherapy through the relief of family and marital tensions (Thase and Kupfer, in press).

Unipolar Depression: Somatic Treatments

In reviewing the research on the effectiveness of different forms of therapy for the treatment of depressed patients, we located only one study that focused directly on the prevention of suicidal behavior in this group. Specifically, Avery and Winokur (1978) conducted an archival prospective study comparing the efficacy of electroconvulsive therapy (ECT) versus antidepressants over a one-year period. Limitations of this study include methods of data collection (chart review) and treatment assignment (naturalistic). Nevertheless, the study showed that the ECT-treated group had fewer suicide attempts than the antidepressant-treated group, despite the fact that patients who received ECT had a more severe depressive illness upon the initiation of treatment. These results were attributed to a greater efficacy of ECT compared to pharmacotherapy in the treatment of depression, results supported by the work of others (Janicak et al, 1985; Tsuang et al, 1979). These findings may also be due to the fact that the prescription of an antidepressant also provides an agent for a suicide attempt (Lonnqvist et al, 1974). Alternatively, the patients receiving antidepressants may not have received optimal pharmacologic management. At the very least, this study suggests a need to learn more about these patients who fail to respond to standard anti-depressant treatment (Thase and Kupfer, in press).

Pharmacologic Treatment

While it is accepted that tricyclic antidepressants are the standard treatments for adult depression, a significant minority of depressed patients appear to be refractory to this first-line pharmacologic intervention. There are several types of depressed patients who appear not to respond well to tricyclic antidepressants: 1) patients from nonsupportive environments (Downing and Rickels, 1973); 2) patients from lower socioeconomic classes (Deykin and Dimascio, 1972); 3) agitated, delusional patients, particularly over the age of 50 (Brown et al, 1982b; Kupfer and Spiker, 1981); 4) patients with atypical depression (Liebowitz et al, 1984); 5) bipolar, depressed patients (Himmelhoch et al, 1982); and 6) patients with comorbid medical, personality, or alcohol/drug disorders (Akiskal, 1982; Kupfer and Spiker, 1981). Several of these factors have been noted previously to be risk factors for completed suicide. This issue has been reviewed in detail by Thase and Kupfer (in press), who also observe that some cases of nonresponse may be due to noncompliance, inadequate or improper dose, or rapid metabolization of the antidepressant.

There are several therapeutic implications to be drawn from those clinical indicators of nonresponse. First, as noted above (Frank et al, 1985; Haas et al, 1986; Miklowitz et al, 1986), marital or psychoeducational family therapy may serve as a powerful adjunct to pharmacotherapy, particularly in cases in which marital discord is prominent. Psychosocial interventions may also improve compliance with pharmacotherapy. Additional psychopharmacologic interventions may also aid in the management of the antidepressant-resistant depressed patients. Patients who do not respond to a standard dosage of antidepressant should have a blood level determination, as they may be either noncompliant or rapid metabolizers. In the latter case, a higher dose may improve the clinical response. Agitated, delusional patients may respond better with the addition of a neuroleptic or with ECT. In addition, some depressed patients who are nonresponsive or only partially responsive to tricyclic antidepressants (TCAs) or monoamine oxidase inhibitors (MAOIs) may benefit from lithium augmentation (deMontigny et al, 1983; Himmelhoch et al, 1972; Heninger at al, 1983; Nelson and Mazure, 1986). We have discussed issues of comorbidity elsewhere; however, it is important to underscore the importance of detecting covert endocrinopathies, other forms of medical illness, and drug and alcohol abuse (Thase and Kupfer, in press).

Those patients with atypical depression deserve more detailed comment. Atypical depression refers to a pattern of mood lability, rejection sensitivity, hyperphagia, hypersomnia, and reversed diurnal mood variation (Quitkin et al, 1982). There is evidence that these patients, as well as patients with mixed features of both anxiety and depression, respond preferentially to MAOIs (Kayser et al, 1985; Liebowitz et al, 1984). Some have argued that many of these patients are, in fact, bipolar II (Akiskal, 1982), which may explain their preferential responsiveness to MAOIs over TCAs (see below; Kupfer and Spiker, 1981; Himmelhoch et al, 1982).

The irony of prescribing antidepressants is that these potentially dangerous agents are prescribed for those most at risk of taking them in an overdose attempt. Therefore, they should only be prescribed when one is certain of the presence of an affective disorder, and the proper dosage should be given in order to maximize the benefit/risk ratio. As an example of the risk involved, treatment of borderline personality disorder patients with amitriptyline actually resulted in an *increase* in suicidal threats and ideation (Soloff et al, 1986a). Finally, the amount prescribed at any one time should be limited, and patients should be encouraged to discard outdated prescriptions so that the temptation to resort to overdose is minimized. There is evidence that those at greatest risk for engaging in suicidal behavior are most likely to have outdated prescriptions on hand (Robin and Freeman-Browne, 1968).

Bipolar Affective Disorder

A high proportion (17–22 percent) of adult (Barraclough et al, 1972) and adolescent (Brent et al, 1986b) suicide victims have bipolar disorder. Barraclough and associates (1972) observed that if these bipolar suicide victims had received lithium, suicide in this proportion of patients might have been prevented. Studies of patients attending lithium clinics support this view (insofar as the rates of suicide among these high risk patients are much lower than one would expect), leading some to posit that lithium and the attendant clinical support services offer a protective effect (Jamison, 1986; Blumenthal and Kupfer, 1986a). This in turn suggests that strategies such as marital and individual therapy, which improve medication compliance, are an integral part of the prevention of suicide among bipolar patients (Blumenthal and Kupfer, 1986a; Miklowitz et al, 1986).

However, some bipolar patients do not respond to lithium, particularly those who present with a mixed state (Himmelhoch and Garfinkel, 1986). Patients with a chronic mixed state are more likely to be abusing drugs and alcohol, so that the substance abuse problem needs to be resolved before effective pharmacoprophylaxis can take place (Himmelhoch and Garfinkel, 1986). In addition, other antimanic agents may need to be added to lithium, such as carbamazepine, valproate, or verapamil in order to attain a euthymic state (Himmelhoch and Garfinkel, 1986). Other strategies to augment the efficacy of lithium prophylaxis include maintenance of proper sleep hygiene (for example, avoiding circadian disruptions and sleep deprivation) (Wehr et al, 1987) and education of the patient and significant others as to the early signs of mania and depression, so that extreme mood swings and functional impairment can be averted (Miklowitz et al, 1986).

The avoidance of either rapid cycling or a mixed state is important insofar as there is evidence that the presence of a mixed state and/or rapid change in polarity are both significant risk factors for completed suicide (Fawcett et al, 1987). Since the TCAs may be more likely to induce rapid cycling or a mixed state in bipolar depressed patients (Wehr and Goodwin, 1979), MAOIs may be preferable to tricyclic antidepressants (Himmelhoch et al, 1982; Kupfer and Spiker, 1981). Furthermore, it is important to monitor thyroid function in patients on lithium maintenance, as the hypothyroidism due to chronic use of lithium can contribute to rapid cycling and render pharmacotherapy ineffective (Cowdrey et al, 1983).

Schizophrenia

Given that the typical profile of the schizophrenic suicide victim is a person who finds that they cannot realize their high premorbid aspirations due to their illness, it is clear that supportive therapy is important, particularly in the early stages of the disorder. Psychoeducational family therapy, which teaches family members to avoid critical statements to schizophrenic patients, has been shown to prevent relapses during the first year after onset (Hogarty et al, 1986). Therefore, such psychoeducational treatment should be considered a powerful augmenter of neuroleptic treatment.

Several other treatment approaches may decrease the high risk of suicide in this population. First, this disorder is frequently complicated by drug and alcohol abuse, which has been shown to increase the rates of symptomatic relapse (Alterman et al, 1980, 1984; Negrete et al, 1986), and perhaps (though currently unproven) noncompliance and suicidal behavior. Second, there have been several case reports and clinical studies linking akathisia with depressive symptoms, suicide, and suicidal behavior (Drake and Ehrlich, 1985; Marder et al, 1984; Shear et al, 1983; Spohn et al, 1985), so that recognition and prompt pharmacologic amelioration of this condition by use of the lowest possible dose of neuroleptic should always be attempted. In fact, there is now strong clinical and pharmacologic evidence that lower doses of neuroleptics than are currently in vogue are just as effective in treating psychotic symptoms and are also much less likely to provoke extrapyramidal and akathetic side effects (Marder et al, 1984; van Putten et al, 1984; van Putten and Marder, 1986).

In addition, depressed and disturbed affect regulation are frequently part of the picture of schizophrenia, particularly after the psychosis has resolved (McGlashan and Carpenter, 1976; Siris et al, 1981). This observation had led some clinician-researchers to call for the treatment of depressive symptomatology with antidepressants in schizophrenic patients. Both Prusoff and colleagues (1979) and Siris and associates (1985) found beneficial effects of adding an antidepressant to a neuroleptic maintenance regimen. In the latter report, the most methodologically rigorous to date, 28 schizophrenic patients on maintenance neuroleptic medication, who also met Research Diagnostic Criteria (RDC) for major or minor depression and were all free of akathisia or extrapyramidal system side effects, were randomly assigned to antidepressant or placebo. An improvement in mood in the antidepressant treated group was noted, *without* an associated increase in thought disorder. Therefore, addition of an antidepressant to neuroleptic medication in schizophrenic patients who show additional signs of depression should be considered.

Treatment of Alcohol and Substance Abuse

Individuals who abuse alcohol are much more likely to engage in suicidal behavior than are normal controls (Aarens and Roizen, 1977). It has been estimated that 15 percent of alcoholics eventually commit suicide (Miles, 1977). Problems with alcohol are found in 40 percent of suicide completers, and 25 to 30 percent of completers are reported to have been intoxicated at the time of death (Barraclough et al, 1974; Brent et al, 1987; Ford et al, 1979; James, 1966; Robins et al, 1959). Therefore, it is likely that proper treatment of alcohol abuse will reduce the risk of suicide in this population. However, treatment studies of alcoholism have not examined the relationship between treatment outcome and subsequent suicidal behavior, with the exception of the incidental finding of Welu (1977) that among suicide attempters who received more intense outreach and follow-up, a diminution in alcohol intake occurred that was related to a reduction in recidivism. One other study reports on a four-year follow-up of 922 adult alcoholics, and found a lower mortality rate due to suicide, accidents, and homicide combined among long-term abstainers compared to nonabstainers (Polich et al, 1981). Unfortunately, the mortality due to suicide alone, specifically, was not reported. Thus the efficacy of treatment for alcoholism in relation to subsequent suicidal behavior has not been evaluated but appears to be a fruitful area of inquiry. Even less is known about the relation between treatment outcome for substance abuse and subsequent risk for suicide, although given the high prevalence of this disorder among suicide victims (Rich et al, 1986), it is likely that effective treatment of substance abuse will reduce the risk for suicide in these patients. Therefore, it is relevant that psychotherapy focused on drug abuse may prevent relapse of opiate abuse in opioid addicts (Kosten et al, 1986; Rounsaville et al, 1986). Proper diagnosis and treatment of comorbid psychiatric disorders in alcohol and substance abusing patients may improve treatment outcome insofar as poor response to alcohol and drug rehabilitation is related to the severity of psychopathology *other* than substance use disorder (McClellan et al, 1983; Rounsaville et al, 1986).

Research

Meta-analytic approaches or longitudinal studies of large cohorts will be required to assess the efficacy of different treatment approaches to the prevention of suicide, given the rarity of this outcome even in psychiatric samples. In addition, researchers should target for study variables proximal to suicide with the view that if these precursors (for example, suicidal ideation and behavior) can be prevented, then so can suicide. As an example, Fawcett and colleagues (1987) recently demonstrated that bipolar patients who experience recent or rapid changes in polarity in episode are at high risk for suicide. Therefore, research on the etiology, treatment, and prevention of these phenomena in bipolar patients are likely to prevent suicide. Research into the optimal pharmacologic and psychotherapeutic management of the major psychiatric disorders, as well as elucidation of the psychosocial and biological risk factors for suicide and suicidal behavior, will greatly enhance the likelihood that the suicide rate in psychiatric patients can be reduced.

CONCLUSIONS

The proper identification, assessment, and treatment of psychiatric disorders remains a cornerstone of the prevention of suicide in psychiatric patients. Improved methods of casefinding are important insofar as many psychiatrically ill suicide victims never receive proper psychiatric treatment. An accurate diagnostic assessment with respect to primary and comorbid psychiatric disorder, alcohol and drug abuse, personality disorders, and attendant medical disorders is a necessary precursor to appropriate treatment. Additional general principles for the treatment of patients at high risk for suicide include: provision of hope (particularly in newly diagnosed cases), proper assessment and mobilization of the families of these patients in order to improve compliance and decrease the chance of relapse, proper use of inpatient hospitalization, and restriction of the availability of lethal agents. Specific somatic treatments appear to be helpful in reducing the risk of relapse in the affective disorders and schizophrenia, but psychosocial treatments, both alone and in combination with pharmacotherapy, appear to augment compliance and decrease the rate of relapse over pharmacotherapy alone. Research using either large multicenter-based cohorts followed longitudinally, or meta-analytic strategies to focus on suicidality as an outcome, may be helpful in elucidating which treatments are most effective in the prevention of suicide in psychiatric patients.

REFERENCES

Aarens M, Roizen R: Alcohol and suicide, in Alcohol, Casualties, and Crime. Edited by Aarens M, Cameron T, Roizen R, et al. Special report prepared for the NIAAA, Contract No. (ADM) 281-76-0027. Berkeley, Social Research Group, University of California, 1977

Abramowitz EZ, Baker AH, Fleischer S: Onset of depressive crises and the menstrual cycle. Am J Psychiatry 1982; 139:475-478

Adams KS, Bonchong A, Steiner D: Parental loss and family stability in attempted suicide. Arch Gen Psychiatry 1980; 39:1081-1085

Akiskal HS: Factors associated with incomplete recovery in primary depressive illness. J Clin Psychiatry 1982; 43:255-271

Akiskal HS, Downs J, Jordan P, et al: Affect disorder in referred children and younger siblings of manic-depressives. Arch Gen Psychiatry 1985; 42:996-1003

Alterman AI, Erdlen FR, McClellan AT, et al: Problem drinking in hospitalized schizophrenic patients. Addict Behav 1980; 5:273-276

Alterman AI, Ayre FR, Williford WO: Diagnostic validation of conjoint schizophrenia and alcoholism. J Clin Psychiatry 1984; 45:300-303

Asberg M: Neurotransmitter monoamine metabolites in the cerebrospinal fluid as risk factors for suicidal behavior. Paper presented to the NIMH Conference on Youth Suicide, Bethesda, MD, May, 1986

Asberg M, Traskman L, Thoran P: 5-HIAA in the cerebrospinal fluid: a biochemical suicide predictor. Arch Gen Psychiatry 1976; 33:1193-1197

Asberg M, Nordstrom P, Traskman-Bendz L: Cerebrospinal fluid studies in suicide: an overview, in Psychobiology of Suicidal Behavior. Edited by Mann JJ, Stanley M. New York, Annals of the New York Academy of Sciences, 1986

Avery D, Winokur G: Suicide, attempted suicide, and relapse rates in depression. Arch Gen Psychiatry 1978; 35:749-753

Bancroft J, Backstrom T: Premenstrual syndrome. Clin Endocrinol 1985; 22:313-336

Barraclough B: Suicide prevention, recurrent affective disorder and lithium. Br J Psychiatry 1972; 121:391-392

Barraclough B: Suicide and epilepsy, in Epilepsy and Psychiatry. Edited by Reynolds EH, Trimble MR. Edinburgh, Churchill Livingstone, 1981

Barraclough B, Bunch J, Nelson B, et al: A hundred cases of suicide: clinical aspects. Br J Psychiatry 1974; 125:355-373

Beardslee W, Bemporad J, Keller M, et al: Children of parents with major affective disorder: a review. Am J Psychiatry 1983; 140:825-832

Beck AT, Schuyler D, Herman J: Development of suicidal intent scales, in The Prediction of Suicide. Edited by Beck AT, Resnick HLP, Lettieri DJ. Bowie, Maryland, Charles Press, 1974

Beck AT, Weissman A, Lester D, et al: The measurement of pessimism: the hopelessness scale. J Consult Clin Psychol 1974b; 42:861-865

Beck AT, Kovacs M, Weissman A: Hopelessness and suicidal behavior: an overview. JAMA 1975; 234:1146-1149

Beck AT, Beck R. Kovacs M: Classification of suicidal behaviors, I: quantifying intent and medical lethality. Am J Psychiatry 1979a; 132:285-287

Beck AT, Kovacs M, Weissman A: Assessment of suicidal intention: the scale for suicide ideation. J Consult Clin Psychol 1979b; 217:343-352

Beck AT, Steer R, Kovacs M, et al: Hopelessness and eventual suicide: a 10-year prospective study of patients hospitalized with suicidal ideation. Am J Psychiatry 1985; 142:559-563

Behar D, Winokur G, Berg CJ: Depression in the abstinent alcoholic. Am J Psychiatry 1984; 141:1105-1107

Bellack AS, Hersen M, Himmelhoch J: Social skills training compared with pharmacotherapy and psychotherapy in the treatment of unipolar depression. Am J Psychiatry 1981; 138:1562-1566

Bennett R, Hughs GR, Bywaters EG, et al: Neuropsychiatric problems in systemic lupus erythematosus. Br Med J 1972; 4:342-345

Bibb JL, Chamblis D: Alcohol use and abuse among diagnosed agoraphobics. Behav Res Ther 1986; 24:49-58

Blackburn I, Bishop S, Glen A, et al: The efficacy of cognitive therapy in depression: a treatment trial using cognitive therapy and pharmacotherapy, each alone and in combination. Br J Psychiatry 1981; 139:181-189

Blumenthal SJ, Kupfer DJ: Generalizable treatment strategies for suicidal behavior. Ann NY Acad Sci 1986a; 487:327-340

Blumenthal SJ, Kupfer DJ: Overview of early detection and treatment of strategies for suicidal behavior in young people. Paper presented at the Conference on Prevention of Youth Suicide, June 11–13, Oakland, California, 1986b

Boyd JH: The increasing rate of suicide by firearms. N Engl J Med 1983; 308:313-317

Boyd JH, Moscicki EK: Firearms and youth suicide. Am J Public Health 1986; 76:1240-1242

Brent D: Overrepresentation of epileptics in a consecutive series of suicide attempters seen at a children's hospital, 1978–1983. J Am Acad Child Psychiatry 1986; 25:242-246

Brent D: Correlates of the medical lethality of suicide attempts in children and adolescents. J Am Acad Child Psychiatry 1987; 26:87–89

Brent D, Perper JA, Allman C: Alcohol, firearms, and suicide among youth: temporal trends in Allegheny County, PA, 1960–1983. JAMA 1987; 3369-3372

Brent D, Kalas R, Edelbrock C, et al: Psychopathology and its relationship to suicidal ideation in childhood and adolescence. J Am Acad Child Psychiatry 1986a; 25:666-673

Brent D, Perper JA, Kolko D, et al: A comparison of adolescent suicide victims and suicidal inpatients. Paper presented at the American Academy of Child and Adolescent Psychiatry, Los Angeles, October, 1986b

Brent D, Crumrine P, Varma R, et al: Phenobarbital and major depressive disorder among children with epilepsy. Pediatrics (in press)

Bromet EJ, Dew MA, Brent D: Suicide Prevention: A Review. (Contract No. 85M059146401S). Washington, DC, Center for Affective Disorders, National Institute of Mental Health, 1985

Brown GW, Harris TD: Social Origins of Depression: A Study of Psychiatric Disorder in Women. London, Tavistock Publications; New York, Free Press, 1978

Brown G, Goodwin F, Ballenger J, et al: Aggression in human correlates with cerebrospinal fluid amino metabolites. Psychiatry Res 1979; 1:131-139

Brown G, Ebert M, Goyen P, et al: Aggression, suicide and serotonin: relationships to CSF metabolites. Am J Psychiatry 1982a; 139:741-746

Brown RP, Frances A, Kocsis JH, et al: Psychotic vs. nonpsychotic depression: comparison of treatment response. J Nerv Ment Dis 1982b; 170:635-637

Cadoret RJ, Troughton E, O'Gorman TW, et al: An adoption study of genetic and environmental factors in drug abuse. Arch Gen Psychiatry 1986; 43:1131-1136

Campbell PC: Suicide among cancer patients. Connecticut Health Bulletin 1966; 80:207-212

Carlson G, Cantwell D: Suicidal behavior and depression in children and adolescents. J Am Acad Child Psychiatry 1982; 21:361-368

Chandler JM, Reed TE, DeJong RN: Huntington's chorea in Michigan. Neurology 1960; 10:148-153

Chowdhury N, Hicks RC, Kreitman N: Evaluation of an after-care service for parasuicide (attempted suicide) patients. Soc Psychiatry 1973; 8:67-81

Clayton PJ, Lewis CE: The significance of secondary depression. J Affective Disord 1981; 3:25-35

Clayton PJ, Desmarais L, Winokur G: A study of normal bereavement. Am J Psychiatry 1968; 125:168-178

Clayton PJ, Herjanic M, Murphy GE, et al: Mourning and depression: their similarities and differences. Can J Psychiatry 1974; 19:309-312

Clum G, Patsiokas A, Luscomb R: Empirically based comprehensive treatment program for parasuicide. J Consult Clin Psychol 1979; 47:937-945

Cohen-Sandler R, Berman AL, King RA: Life stress and symptomatology: determinants of suicidal behavior in children. J Am Acad Child Psychiatry 1982; 21:178-186

Corbett JA, Trimble MR: Epilepsy and anticonvulsant medication, in Developmental Neuropsychiatry. Edited by Rutter M. New York, Guilford Press, 1983

Cowdrey RW, Wehr TA, Zis AP, et al: Thyroid abnormalities associated with rapid-cycling bipolar illness. Arch Gen Psychiatry 1983; 40:414-420

Davidson J, Pelton S: Forms of atypical depression and their response to antidepressant drugs. Psychiatry Res 1986; 17:87-95

Davidson J, Miller R, Strickland R: Neuroticism and personality disorder in depression. J Affective Disord 1985; 8:177-182

deMontigny C, Cournoyer G, Morissette R, et al: Lithium carbonate addition in tricyclic antidepressant-resistant unipolar depression. Arch Gen Psychiatry 1983; 40:1327-1334

Dew MA, Bromet EJ, Brent D, et al: A quantitative literature review of the effectiveness of suicide prevention centers. J Consult Clin Psychol 1987; 55:239-244

Dewhurst K, Oliver JE, McKnight AL: Socio-psychiatric consequences of Huntington's disease. Br J Psychiatry 1970; 116:255-258

Deykin EY, DiMascio A: Relationship of patient background characteristics to efficacy of pharmacotherapy in depression. J Nerv Ment Dis 1972; 155:209-215

DiMascio A, Weissman MM, Prusoff BA, et al: Differential symptom reduction by drugs and psychotherapy in acute depression. Arch Gen Psychiatry 1979; 36:1450-1456

Dorpat T, Ripley H: A study of suicide in the Seattle area. Compr Psychiatry 1960; 1:349-359

Dorpat TL, Anderson WF, Ripley HS: The relationship of physical illness to suicide, in Suicidal Behaviors. Edited by Resnick LP. Boston, Little, Brown, 1968

Downing RW, Rickels: Predictors of response to amitriptyline and placebo in three outpatient treatment settings. J Nerv Ment Dis 1973; 156:109-129

Drake RE, Cotton PG: Depression, hopelessness and suicide in chronic schizophrenia. Br J Psychiatry 1986; 148:554-559

Drake RE, Ehrlich J: Suicide attempts with akathisia. Am J Psychiatry 1985; 142:499-501

Drake RE, Gates C, Cotton PG, et al: Suicide among schizophrenics: who is at risk? J Nerv Ment Dis 1984; 172:613-617

Drye RC, Goulding RL, Goulding ME: No-suicide decisions: patient monitoring of suicidal risk. Am J Psychiatry 1973; 130:170-174

Dyer JAT, Kreitman N: Hopelessness, depression and suicidal intention in parasuicide. Br J Psychiatry 1984; 144:127-133

Edman G, Asberg M, Levander S, et al: Skin conductance habituation and cerebrospinal fluid 5-hydroxyindoleacetic acid. Arch Gen Psychiatry 1986; 43:586-593

Egeland J, Sussex J: Suicide and family loading for affective disorders. JAMA 1985; 254:915-918

Ettlinger R: Evaluation of suicide prevention after attempted suicide. Acta Psychiatr Scand 1975; 260:1-124

Evenson R, Waite J, Holland R: Admission decisions in the psychiatric emergency room. Compr Psychiatry 1983; 24:90-93

Farberow NL, Schneidmen ES, Leonard CV: Medical bulletin 9: suicide among general medical and surgical hospital patients with malignant neoplasms. Washington, DC, Dept. of Medicine and Surgery, Veterans Administration, February, 1963

Fawcett J, Sheftner W, Clark D, et al: Clinical predictors of suicide in patients with major affective disorders. Am J Psychiatry 1987; 144:35-40

Flood RA, Seager CP: A retrospective examination of psychiatric case records of patients who subsequently committed suicide. Br J Psychiatry 1968; 114:443-450

Ford AB, Rushforth NB, Rushforth NM, et al: Violent death in a metropolitan county, II: changing patterns in suicides (1959-1974). Am J Public Health 1979; 69:459-464

Fourestie V, de Lignieres B, Roudot-Thoroval, et al: Suicide attempts in hypoestrogenic phases of the menstrual cycle. Lancet 1986; 2:1357-1360

Fowler RC, Tsuang MT, Kronfol Z: Communication of suicidal intent and suicide in unipolar depression. J Affective Disord 1979; 1:219-225

Fox BH, Stanek EJ, Boyd SC, et al: Suicide rates among cancer patients in Connecticut. J Chronic Dis 1982; 35:89-100

Frank E, Kupfer DJ: Psychotherapeutic approaches to the treatment of recurrent unipolar depression: work in progress. Psychopharmacol Bull 1986; 22:558-563

Frank E, Prien RF, Kupfer DJ, et al: Implications of noncompliance on research in affective disorders. Psychopharmacol Bull 1985; 21:37-42

Fras I, Litin EM, Pearson JS: Comparison of psychiatric symptoms in carcinoma of the pancreas with those in some other intra-abdominal neoplasms. Am J Psychiatry 1967; 123:1553-1562

Friedman AS: Interaction of drug therapy with marital therapy in depressive patients. Arch Gen Psychiatry 1975; 32:619-637

Friedman IM: Alcohol and unnatural deaths in San Francisco youths. Pediatrics 1985; 76:191-193

Gerson S, Bassuk E: Psychiatric emergencies: an overview. Am J Psychiatry 1980; 137:1-11

Gibbons JS, Butler J, Urwin P, et al: Evaluation of a social work service for self-poisoning patients. Br J Psychiatry 1978; 133:111-118

Goldberg EL: Depression and suicidal ideation in the young adult. Am J Psychiatry 1981; 138:35-40

Goldney RD, Katsikitas M: Cohort analysis of suicide rates in Australia. Arch Gen Psychiatry 1983; 40:71-74

Gould MS, Shaffer D: The impact of suicide in television movies: evidence of imitation. N Engl J Med 1986; 315:690-694

Greer S: The relationship between parental loss and attempted suicide: a controlled study. Br J Psychiatry 1974; 110:698-705

Greer S, Bagley C: Effect of psychiatric intervention in attempted suicide: a controlled study. Br Med J 1971; 1:310-312

Griest J, Griest T: Antidepressant treatment. Baltimore, Williams & Wilkins, 1979

Griffin SJ, Friedman MJ: Depressive symptoms in propranolol users. J Clin Psychiatry 1986; 47:453-457

Guze SB, Robins E: Suicide and primary affective disorders. Br J Psychiatry 1970; 117:437-438

Haas GL, Glick FD, Spencer JH, et al: The patient, the family and compliance with post-hospital treatment for affective disorders. Psychopharmacol Bull 1986; 22:999-1005

Halbreich U, Endicott J: Premenstrual depressive changes. Arch Gen Psychiatry 1983; 40:535-542

Harris JC, Carol CA, Rosenberg LA, et al: Intermittent high dose corticosteroid treatment in childhood cancer: behavioral and emotional consequences. J Am Acad Child Psychiatry 1986; 25:120-124

Hawton K, Catalon J: Attempted Suicide. A Practical Guide to Its Nature and Management. Oxford, Oxford University Press, 1982

Hawton K, O'Grady, Osborn M, et al: Adolescents who take overdoses: their characteristics, problems and contacts with helping agencies. Br J Psychiatry 1982b; 140:118-123

Hawton K, Fagg J, Marsack P: Association between epilepsy and attempted suicide. J Neurol Neurosurg Psychiatry 1980; 43:168-170

Hawton K, Bancroft J, Catalon J, et al: Domiciliary and outpatient treatment of self-poisoning patients by medical and non-medical staff. Psychol Med 1981; 11:169-177

Hawton K, Cole D, O'Grady J, et al: Motivational aspects of deliberate self-poisoning in adolescents. Br J Psychiatry 1982a; 141:286-291

Hawton K, Osborn M, O'Grady J, et al: Classification of adolescents who take overdoses. Br J Psychiatry 1982c; 140:124-131

Hellerstein D, Frosch W, Koenigsberg HW: The clinical significance of command hallucinations. Am J Psychiatry 1987; 144:219-221

Heninger GR, Charney DS, Sternberg DE: Lithium carbonate augmentation of antidepressant treatment: an effective prescription for treatment-refractory depression. Arch Gen Psychiatry 1983; 40:1335-1342

Hillard JR, Ramm D, Zung WWK, et al: Suicide in a psychiatric emergency room population. Am J Psychiatry 1983; 140:459-462

Himmelhoch JM, Garfinkel ME: Sources of lithium resistance in mixed mania. Psychopharmacol Bull 1986; 22:613-620

Himmelhoch JM, Detre TP, Kupfer DJ, et al: Treatment of previously intractable depression with tranylcypromine and lithium. J Nerv Ment Dis 1972; 155:216-220

Himmelhoch JM, Fuchs CA, Symons BJ: A double-blind study of tranylcypromine treatment of major anergic depression. J Nerv Ment Dis 1982; 628-634

Hirsch SR, Walsh C, Draper R: The concept and efficacy of the treatment of parasuicide. Br J Clin Pharmacol 1983; 15:189S-194S

Hogarty GE, Anderson CM, Reiss DJ, et al: Family psychoeducation, social skills training, and maintenance chemotherapy in the aftercare treatment of schizophrenia. Arch Gen Psychiatry 1986; 43:633-642

James IP: Blood alcohol levels following successful suicide. J Stud Alcohol 1966; 27:23-29

Jamison KR: Suicide and bipolar disorders. Ann NY Acad Sci 1986; 487:301-315

Janicak P, Davis J, Gibbons R, et al: Efficacy of ECT: a meta-analysis. Am J Psychiatry 1985; 142:297-302

Johnson GF, Hunt G: Suicidal behavior in bipolar manic-depressive patients and their families. Compr Psychiatry 1979; 20:159-164

Kaplan RD, Kottler DB, Frances AJ: Reliability and rationality in the prediction of suicide. Hosp Community Psychiatry 1982; 33:212-215

Kayser A, Robinson DS, Nies A, et al: Response to phenelzine among depressed patients with features of hysteroid dysphoria. Am J Psychiatry 1985; 142:486-488

Keith-Spiegel P, Spiegel DE: Affective states of patients immediately preceding suicide. Psychiatry Res 1967; 5:89-93

Keller MB, Shapiro RW, Lavori PW, et al: Recovery in major depressive disorder. Arch Gen Psychiatry 1982a; 39:905-910

Keller MB, Shapiro RW, Lavori PW, et al: Relapse in major depressive disorder. Arch Gen Psychiatry 1982b; 39:911-915

Keller MB, Beardslee WR, Dorer DJ, et al: Impact of severity and chronicity of parental affective illness on adaptive functioning and psychopathology in children. Arch Gen Psychiatry 1986; 43:930-937

Keller MB, Lavori PW, Endicott J, et al: "Double-depression": two-year follow-up. Am J Psychiatry 140:689-694, 1983

Kellermann AL, Reay DT: Protection or peril? an analysis of firearms-related deaths in the home. N Engl J Med 1986; 314:1557-1560

Kennedy P: Efficacy of a regional poisoning treatment centre in preventing further suicidal behavior. Br Med J 1972; 4:255-257

Kerr TA, Schapira K, Roth M: The relationship between premature death and affective disorders. Br J Psychiatry 1969; 115:1277-1282

Kirstein L, Weissman MM: Utilization review of treatment for suicide attempters: chart review as patient care evaluation. Am J Psychiatry 1975; 132:851-855

Klein DF: Anxiety reconceptualized. Compr Psychiatry 1980; 21:411-427

Klerman GL, Hirschfeld RM: Treatment of depression in the elderly. Geriatrics 1979; 34:51

Knop J, Fisher A: Duodenal ulcer, suicide, psychopathology and alcoholism. Acta Psychiatr Scand 1981; 63:346-355

Kosten TR, Rounsavile BJ, Kleber HD: A 2.5 year follow-up of depression, life crises, and treatment effects on abstinence among opioid addicts. Arch Gen Psychiatry 1986; 43:733-738

Kovacs M, Beck AT: The wish to die and the wish to live in attempted suicides. J Clin Psychol 1977; 33:361-364

Kovacs M, Rush J, Beck A, et al: Depressed outpatients treated with cognitive therapy or pharmacotherapy: a one year follow-up. Arch Gen Psychiatry 1981; 38:33-39

Kreitman N: The coal gas story. United Kingdom suicide rates, 1960–1971. British Journal of Social and Preventive Medicine 1976; 30:86-93

Kreitman N, Smith P, Tan E: Attempted suicide as language: an empirical study. Br J Psychiatry 1970; 116:465-473

Kupfer DJ, Spiker DG: Refractory depression: prediction of nonresponse by clinical indicators. J Clin Psychiatry 1981; 42:307-312

Lerner JA, Mrazek DA, Strunk RC: Prednisone use is associated with psychiatric disturbance in asthmatic children. Paper presented at the Annual Meeting of the American Academy of Child Psychiatry, Los Angeles, 1986

Lester D: Seasonal variation in suicidal deaths. Br J Psychiatry 1971; 118:627-628

Lester D, Murell ME: The influence of gun control laws on suicidal behavior. Am J Psychiatry 1980; 137:121-122

Lester D, Murrell ME: The preventive effect of strict gun control laws on suicide and homocide. Suicide Life Threat Behav 1982; 12:127-138

Liberman RP, Eckman T: Behavior therapy vs insight-oriented therapy for repeated suicide attempters. Arch Gen Psychiatry 1981; 38:1126-1130

Liebowitz MR, Quitkin FM, Stewart JW, et al: Phenelzine vs. imipramine in atypical depression; a preliminary report. Arch Gen Psychiatry 1984; 41:669-677

Ling MHM: Side effects of corticosteroid therapy: psychiatric aspects. Arch Gen Psychiatry 1981; 38:471-477

Linkowski P, Maertelaerd V, Mendlewicz J: Suicidal behavior in major depressive illness. Acta Psychiatr Scand 1985; 72:233-238

Linnoilla M, Virkkunen M, Scheiner M, et al: Low cerebrospinal fluid 5-hydroxyindole-acetic acid concentration differentiates impulsive from non-impulsive violent behavior. Life Sci 1983; 33:2609-2614

Lishman WA: Organic Psychiatry: The Psychological Consequences of Cerebral Disorder. Oxford, Blackwell Scientific Publications, 1978

Lonnqvist J, Niskanen P, Rinta-Manty R, et al: Suicides in psychiatric hospitals in different therapeutic eras: a review of the literature and own study. Psychiatria Fennica 1974; 265-273

Loranger AW, Oldham JM, Rusalcoff LM, et al: Personality Disorder Examination: A Structured Interview for Making DSM-III Axis I Diagnoses (POE). White Plains, NY, The New York Hospital–Cornell Medical Center, Westchester Division, 1984

Louhivouri KA, Hakama M: Risk of suicide among cancer patients. Am J Epidemiol 1979; 109:59-65

Mackay A: Self-poisoning: a complication of epilepsy. Br J Psychiatry 1979; 174:277-282

Mackenzie TB, Popkin MK: Suicide in the medical patient. Int J Psychiatry Med 1987; 17:3-22

Marder SR, Van Putten T, Mintz J, et al: Costs and benefits of two doses of fluphenazine. Arch Gen Psychiatry 1984; 41:1025-1029

Markush RE, Bortolucci AA: Firearms and suicide in the United States. Am J Public Health 1984; 74:123-127

Martin R, Cloniger R, Guze SB, et al: Mortality in a follow-up of 500 psychiatric outpatients, II: case-specific mortality. Arch Gen Psychiatry 1985; 42:58-66

Matthews W, Barabas G: Suicide and epilepsy: a review of the literature. Psychosomatics 1981; 22:515-524

McGlashan TH, Carpenter WY Jr: Post-psychotic depression in schizophrenia. Arch Gen Psychiatry 1976; 33:231-241

McLean PD, Hakistian AR: Clinical depression: comparative efficacy of outpatient treatments. J Consult Clin Psychol 1979; 47:818-836

McLellan AT, Luborsky L, Woody O, et al: Predicting response to alcohol and drug abuse treatments. Arch Gen Psychiatry 1983; 40:620-625

Miklowitz DJ, Goldstein MJ, Nueckterlein KH, et al: Expressed emotion, affective style, lithium compliance, and relapse in recent onset mania. Psychopharmacol Bull 1986; 22:628-632

Miles C: Conditions predisposing to suicide: a review. J Nerv Ment Dis 1977; 164:231-246

Montgomery S, Montgomery D, Rani S, et al: Maintenance therapy in repeat suicidal behavior: a placebo controlled trial. Proceedings of the 10th International Congress for Suicide Prevention and Crisis Intervention, Ottawa, Ontario, June 1979

Montgomery SA, Roy D, Montgomery DB: The prevention of recurrent suicidal acts. Br J Clin Pharmacol 1983; 15:183S-188S

Morson RJ, Lyon JL: Proportional mortality among alcoholics. Cancer 1975; 36:1077-1079

Morrison JR: Suicide in a psychiatric practice population. J Clin Psychiatry 1982; 43:348-352

Motto J: Suicide attempts: a longitudinal view. Arch Gen Psychiatry 1965; 13:516-520

Motto J: Suicide prevention for high-risk persons who refuse treatment. Suicide Life Threat Behav 1976; 6:223-230

Murphy GE: Clinical indication of suicidal risk. Arch Gen Psychiatry 1972; 27:356-359

Murphy GE, Wetzel RD: Family history of suicidal behavior among suicide attempters. J Nerv Ment Dis 1982; 170:86-90

Murphy GE, Armstrong JW, Hermele SL, et al: Suicide and alcoholism: interpersonal loss confirmed as a predictor. Arch Gen Psychiatry 1979; 36:65-69

Murphy GE, Simons AD, Wetzel RD, et al: Cognitive therapy and pharmacotherapy: single and together in the treatment of depression. Arch Gen Psychiatry 1984; 41:33-41

Nayha S: The biseasonal incidence of some suicides: experience from Finland by marital status, 1961-1976. Acta Psychiatr Scand 1983; 67:32-42

Negrete JC, Knapp WP, Douglas DE, et al: Cannabis affects the severity of schizophrenic symptoms: results of a clinical survey. Psychol Med 1986; 16:515-520

Nelson JC, Mazure CM: Lithium augmentation in psychotic depression refractory to combined drug treatment. Am J Psychiatry 1986; 143:363-366

Otto U: Suicidal acts by children and adolescents: a follow-up study. Acta Psychiatr Scand (suppl) 1972; 233:1-123

Pallis DJ, Barraclough BM, Levey AB, et al: Estimating suicide risk among attempted suicide, I: the development of new clinical scales. Br J Psychiatry 1982; 141:37-44

Pallis DJ, Gibbons JS, Pierce DW: Estimating suicide risk among attempted suicides, II: efficiency of predictive scales after the attempt. Br J Psychiatry 1984; 144:139-148

Parker G, Walter S: Seasonal variation in depressive disorders and suicidal deaths in New South Wales. Br J Psychiatry 1982; 140:626-632

Patterson WM, Dohn HH, Bird J, et al: Evaluation of suicidal patients: the SAD persons scale. Psychosomatics 1983; 24:343-346

Paykel ES: Stress and Life Events. National Institutes of Mental Health Conference on Youth Suicide. Bethesda, MD, May 1986

Paykel ES, Hallowell C, Dressler DM, et al: Treatment of suicide attempters: a descriptive study. Arch Gen Psychiatry 1974a; 31:487-491

Paykel ES, Myers JK, Lindenthal JJ, et al: Suicidal feelings in general population: a prevalence study. Br J Psychiatry 1974b; 124:460-469

Paykel ES, Prusoff BA, Myers JR: Suicide attempts and recent life events: a controlled comparison. Arch Gen Psychiatry 1975; 32:327-337

Paykel ES, Parker RR, Penrose RJ, et al: Depressive classification and prediction of response to phenelzine. Br J Psychiatry 1979; 134:572-581

Paykel ES, Fleminger R, Watson JP: Psychiatric side effects of antihypertensive drugs other than reserpine. J Clin Psychopharmacol 1982; 2:14-39

Pfeffer CR: Parental suicide: an organizing event in the development of latency-age children. Suicide Life Threat Behav 1980; 11:43-50

Pfeffer CR: Suicidal behavior in children: a review with implications for research and practice. Am J Psychiatry 1981; 138:154-159

Pfeffer CR, Conte HR, Plutchik R, et al: Suicidal behavior in latency-age children: an empirical study. J Am Acad Child Psychiatry 1979; 18:679-692

Pfeffer CR, Conte HR, Plutchik R, et al: Suicidal behavior in latency-age children: an empirical study; an outpatient population. J Am Acad Child Psychiatry 1980; 19:703-710

Pfeffer CR: Family characteristics and support systems as risk factors for youth suicidal behavior. Paper presented at the National Institute of Mental Health Conference on Youth Suicide, Bethesda, MD, May 1986

Pfohl B, Stangl D, Zimmerman M: Structured interview for the DSM-III personality disorders (SIDP). Iowa City, University Medical Center, Dept. of Psychiatry, 1983

Phillips DP, Carstensen LL: Clustering of teenage suicides after television news stories about suicide. N Engl J Med 1986 315:685-689

Pierce DW: Predictive validation of a suicide intent scale. Br Psychiatry 1981; 139:391-396

Pokorny AD: Characteristics of forty-four patients who subsequently committed suicide. Arch Gen Psychiatry 1960; 2:314-323

Pokorny AD: A follow-up of 618 suicidal patients. Arch Gen Psychiatry 1966; 14:1109-1116

Pokorny AD: Prediction of suicide in psychiatric patients. Arch Gen Psychiatry 1983; 40:249-257

Polich J, Armor D, Bracker H: The course of alcoholism: four years after treatment. New York, Wiley, 1981

Pottenger M, McKennon J, Paine L, et al: The frequency and persistence of depressive symptoms in the alcohol abuser. J Nerv Ment Dis 1978; 166:562-569

Prien RF, Kupfer DJ: Continuation drug therapy for major depressive episodes: how long should it be maintained? Am J Psychiatry 1986; 143:18-23

Prusoff BA, Williams DH, Weissman MM, et al: Treatments of secondary depression in schizophrenia. Arch Gen Psychiatry 1979; 36:569-575

Quitkin FM, Rifkin A, Kaplan J, et al: Phobic anxiety syndrome complicated by drug dependence and addiction: a treatable form of drug abuse. Arch Gen Psychiatry 1972; 27:159-162

Quitkin FM, Schwartz D, Liebowitz MR, et al: Atypical depressives: a preliminary report of antidepressant response and sleep patterns. Psychopharmacol Bull 1982; 18:78-80

Rich CL, Young D, Fowler RC: San Diego Suicide Study, I: young vs. old subjects. Arch Gen Psychiatry 1986; 43:577-582

Robbins D, Conroy R: A cluster of adolescent suicide: is suicide contagious? J Adolesc Health Care 1983; 364:253-255

Robin AA, Freeman-Browne DL: Drugs left at home by psychiatric inpatients. Br J Psychiatry 1968; 3:424-425

Robins E, Murphy GE, Wilkinson RM, et al: Some clinical considerations in the prevention of suicide based on a study of 134 successful suicides. Am J Public Health 1959; 49: 888-898

Roose SP, Glassman AH, Walsh T, et al: Depression, delusions, and suicide. Am J Psychiatry 1983; 140:1159-1162

Rosenthal NE, Sack DA, Gillin JC, et al: Seasonal affective disorder. Arch Gen Psychiatry 1984; 41:72-80

Rounsaville BJ, Kosten TR, Weissman MM, et al: Prognostic significance of psychopathology in treatment of opiate addicts. Arch Gen Psychiatry 1986; 43:739-745

Roy A: Risk factors for suicide in psychiatric patients. Arch Gen Psychiatry 1982a; 39: 1089-1095

Roy A: Suicide in chronic schizophrenia. Br J Psychiatry 1982b; 141:171-177

Roy A: Family history of suicide. Arch Gen Psychiatry 1983; 40:971-974

Rush A, Beck A, Kovacs M, et al: Comparative efficacy of cognitive therapy and pharmacotherapy of depressed outpatients. Cognitive Therapy Research 1977; 1:17-37

Rutter M, Quinton D: Parental psychiatric disorder: effects on children. Psychol Med 1984; 14:853-880

Ryan ND, Puig-Antich J, Ambrosini P, et al: The clinical picture of major depression in children and adolescents. Arch Gen Psychiatry (in press)

Schotte DE, Clum CA: Problem-solving skills in suicidal psychiatric patients. J Consult Clin Psychol 1987; 55:49-54

Schuckit MA: Alcoholism and affective disorder: diagnostic confusion, in Alcoholism and Affective Disorders: Clinical, Genetic, and Biochemical studies. Edited by Goodwin DW, Erickson CF. New York, SP Medical & Scientific Books, 1979

Schulsinger R, Kety S, Rosenthal D, et al: A family study of suicide, in Origins, Prevention, and Treatment of Affective Disorders. Edited by Schou M, Stromgren E. New York, Academic Press, 1979

Sergent TS, Lockshin MD, Klempner MS, et al: Central nervous system disease in systemic lupus erythematosus—therapy and prognosis. Am J Med 1975; 58:644-654

Shaffer D: Suicide in childhood and early adolescence. J Child Psychol Psychiatry 1974; 15:275-291

Shaffer D, Fisher P: The epidemiology of suicide in children and young adolescents. J Am Acad Child Psychiatry 1981; 20:545-565

Shaffer D, Gould M, Trautman P: Suicidal behavior in children and young adults. Paper presented at the Psychobiology of Suicidal Behavior Conference. New York, September 1985

Shafii M, Carrigen S, Whittinghill JR, et al: Psychological autopsy of completed suicide in children and adolescents. Am J Psychiatry 1985; 142:1061-1064

Shafii M: Psychological autopsy study of suicide in adolescents. Paper presented at the Child Depression Consortium, St. Louis, MO, October 1986

Shear MK, Frances A, Weiden P: Suicide associated with akathisia and depot fluphenazine treatment. J Clin Psychopharmacol 1983; 3:235-236

Siegel K, Tuchel P: Rational suicide and the terminally ill cancer patient. Omega 1984-1985; 15:263-269

Simons AP, Garfield SL, Murphy GE: The process of change in cognitive therapy and pharmacotherapy. Arch Gen Psychiatry 1984; 41:45-51

Simons AP, Murphy GE, Levine JL, et al: Cognitive therapy and pharmacotherapy for depression—sustained improvement over one year. Arch Gen Psychiatry 1986; 43: 43-48

Siris SG, Endicott J: Post-psychotic depressive symptoms in hospitalized schizophrenic patients. Arch Gen Psychiatry 1981; 38:1122-1123

Siris SG, Rifkin A, Reardon GT, et al: A trial of adjunctive imipramine on post-psychotic depression. Psychopharmacol Bull 1985; 21:114-116

Soloff PH, George A, Nathan RS: Paradoxical effects of amitryptiline on borderline patients. Am J Psychiatry 1986a; 143:1603-1605

Soloff PH, George A, Nathan RS: Progress in pharmacotherapy of borderline disorders: a double-blind study of amitryptiline, haloperidol, and placebo. Arch Gen Psychiatry 1986b; 43:691-697

Spitzer RL, Williams JBW, Gibbon M: Structured Clinical Interview for DSM-III-R Personality Disorders (SCID-II). New York, Biometrics Reserach Department, New York State Psychiatric Institute, October 15, 1986

Spohn HE, Coyne L, LaCoursiere R, et al: Relation of neuroleptic dose and tardive dyskinesia to attention, information-processing, and psychophysiology in medicated schizophrenics. Arch Gen Psychiatry 1985; 42:849-859

Stallone F, Dunner DL, Ahean J, et al: Statistical prediction of suicide in depressives. Compr Psychiatry 1982; 21:381-387

Starkman MN, Schteingart DE, Schork MA: Depressed mood and other psychiatric manifestations of Cushing's syndrome: relationship to hormone levels. Psychosom Med 1981; 43:3-18

Steiner J: A questionnaire study of risk-taking in psychiatric patients. J Med Psychol 1972; 45:365-373

Steinmetz JL, Lewinsohn PM, Antonuccio DO: Prediction of individual outcome in a group intervention for depression. J Consult Clin Psychol 1983; 51:331-337

Strayhorn JM Jr: Foundations of Clinical Psychiatry. Chicago, Year Book Medical Publishers, 1982

Strober M, Carlson G: Bipolar illness in adolescents with major depression: clinical, genetic and psychopharmacological predictors in a three- to four-year prospective follow-up investigation. Arch Gen Psychiatry 1982; 39:549-555

Targum SD: Neuroendocrine challenge studies in clinical psychiatry. Psychiatric Annals 1983; 13:385-395

Thase ME, Kupfer DJ: Characteristics of treatment resistant depression, in Special Treatments for Resistant Depression. Edited by Zohar J, Belmaker R. Great Neck, NY, PMA Publishing Corp., 1987

Topol P, Reznikoff M: Perceived peer and family relationships, hopelessness and locus of control as factors in adolescent suicide attempts. Suicide Life Threat Behav 1982; 12:141-150

Tsuang MT: Risk of suicide in the relatives of schizophrenics, manics, depressives, and controls. J Clin Psychiatry 1983; 44:396-400

Tsuang M, Dempsey G, Fleming J: Can ECT prevent premature death and suicide in "schizoaffective" patients? J Affective Disord 1979; 1:167-171

Tuckman J, Youngman WF: a scale for assessing suicide risk for attempted suicide. J Clin Psychol 1968; 24:17-19

van Praag H, Plutchik R: An empirical study of the "cathartic" effect of attempted suicide. Psychiatry Res 1985; 16:123-130

van Putten T, Marder SR: Low dose treatment strategies. J Clin Psychiatry 1986; 47(Suppl):12-16

van Putten T, May PRA, Marder SR: Akathisia with haloperidol and thiothixene. Arch Gen Psychiatry 1984; 41:1036-1039

Vandivort DS, Locke BZ: Suicidal ideation: its relationship to depression, suicide and suicide attempt. Suicide Life Threat Behav 1979; 9:205-218

Virkkunen M: Attitude to psychiatric treatment before suicide in schizophrenia and paranoid psychoses. Br J Psychiatry 1976; 128:47-49

Viskum K: Ulcer, attempted suicide and suicide. Acta Psychiatr Scand 1975; 51:221-227

Wehr TA, Goodwin FR: Rapid cycling in manic-depressives induced by tricyclic antidepressants. Arch Gen Psychiatry 1979; 36:555-559

Wehr TA, Sack DA, Rosenthal NE: Sleep reduction as a final common pathway into the genesis of mania. Am J Psychiatry 1987; 144:201-204

Weissman MM, Fox K, Klerman GL: Hostility and depression associated with suicide attempts. Am J Psychiatry 1973; 130:450-459

Weissman MM, Klerman GL, Paykel ES, et al: Treatment effects on the social adjustment of depressed patients. Arch Gen Psychiatry 1974; 30:771-778

Weissman MM, Prusoff BA, Klerman GL: Personality and the prediction of long-term outcome of depression. Am J Psychiatry 1978; 135:797-800

Weissman MM, Prusoff BA, Dimascio A, et al: The efficacy of drugs and psychotherapy in the treatment of acute depressive episodes. Am J Psychiatry 1979; 136:555-558

Weissman MM, Klerman GL, Prusoff BA, et al: Depressed outpatients results one year after treatment with drugs and/or interpersonal psychotherapy. Arch Gen Psychiatry 1981; 38:51-55

Weissman MM, Prusoff BA, Merikangas K: Is delusional depression related to bipolar disorder? Am J Psychiatry 1984; 141:892-893

Welner A, Welner Z, Fishman R: Psychiatric inpatients: eight- to 10-year follow-up. Arch Gen Psychiatry 1979; 36:698-700

Welu TC: A follow-up program for suicide attempters: evaluation of effectiveness. Suicide Life Threat Behav 1977; 7:17-30

Wender PH, Kety SS, Rosenthal D, et al: Psychiatric disorders in the biological and adoptive families of adopted individuals with affective disorders. Arch Gen Psychiatry 1986; 43:923-929

Wetzel RD: Hopelessness, depression, and suicidal intent. Arch Gen Psychiatry 1976; 33:1069-1073

Zuckerman DM, Prusoff BA, Weissman MM, et al: Personality as a predictor of psychotherapy and pharmacotherapy outcome for depressed outpatients. J Consult Clin Psychol 1980; 48:730-735

Zung WNK, Green KL: Seasonal variation of suicide and depression. Arch Gen Psychiatry 1974; 30:89-91

Chapter 17

Suicidal Behavior among Children and Adolescents: Risk Identification and Intervention

by Cynthia R. Pfeffer, M.D.

In 1984, suicide was the second leading cause of death among 15- to 24-year-olds in the United States, with an average of one young person committing suicide every 1¾ hours. The epidemic of youth suicide, apparent for the last two decades, has created national alarm. Newspaper reports have increased public awareness of the problem and stimulated a strong impetus to understand and treat suicidal youngsters. From a public health perspective, prevention of youth suicide can be accomplished by identifying and then decreasing factors associated with greatest risk. This chapter will emphasize these issues and discuss clinical perspectives for prevention of youth suicide.

RISK FACTORS

A risk factor is an epidemiological term that indicates a variable associated with an increased probability of a particular outcome. Currently, there is relatively little research information on risk factors for youth suicide. Most data, although relatively sparse, address risk for nonfatal suicidal acts among adolescents and young adults. In this regard, data have not been collected systematically enough to answer the important question, Are the risk factors for youth suicide similar to those for individuals who express suicidal ideas or for those who carry out nonfatal suicidal acts? With this question in mind, the following sections will present information separately for youth suicide and nonfatal suicidal behavior and, when possible, comparisons will be made.

Suicide Rates and Demographic Risk Factors

In 1984, approximately 5,026 people aged 15 to 24 years committed suicide, which accounts for a suicide rate of 12.5 per 100,000 population (National Center for Health Statistics, 1986b). In fact, this suicide rate exceeds that of 12.4 per 100,000 for all ages. Violent deaths—accidents, suicide, and homicide—are the leading causes of death in the youth age group and account for 76.3 percent of all deaths for youth. Among all deaths for the youth age group, suicide accounts for 12.9 percent of deaths, a percentage that far exceeds the 1.4 percent of suicidal deaths for all ages (the total number of suicides for all ages in 1984 was 29,286). These facts indicate that suicide among teenagers and young adults is a major mental health problem.

Trends over the last few decades show that suicide rates for 15- to 24-year-olds have been increasing dramatically. For example, between 1960—when the youth suicide rate was 5.2 per 100,000 population, and 1984—when the youth suicide rate was 12.5 per 100,000 population, there has been an almost 2.5-fold increase in youth suicide (Mental Health, United States, 1985). The most striking increase is for young white males, a group whose suicide rates are the highest of all youth groups. The next highest rates are for nonwhite males, followed by white females and then nonwhite females. In contrast to the high suicide rates for 15- to 24-year-olds, suicide rates among 5- to 14-year-olds are the lowest of all age groups. In 1984, 232 children aged 5 to 14 years old committed suicide, which amounts to a rate of 0.7 per 100,000 population. Nevertheless, this rate reflects a significant increase over the rate of 0.3 per 100,000 population in 1960 (Mental Health, United States, 1985).

In the last few decades, the increases in youth suicide rates parallel increases for other risk factors among youth, including depression (Klerman et al, 1985), family divorce rates (National Center for Health Statistics, 1986a), and use of firearms as a suicide method (Boyd and Moscicki, 1986). However, there is no definitive explanation accounting for the rise in youth suicide and the relatively low suicide rates for preadolescents.

Three approaches have been proposed to explain the increases in youth suicide rates. Holinger and Offer (1982) suggested that there is a positive correlation between youth suicide rates and changes in the proportion of adolescents in the United States population. These authors suggested that factors related to competition, failure to achieve goals, and social isolation are important stressors that are especially prominent when there are more adolescents and young adults in the population at a given time. These factors lead to despair, hopelessness, and expression of suicidal impulses.

Another model, which has been studied in the United States, Canada, and Australia emphasizes the relation between youth suicide and birth cohort effects (a birth cohort is defined as a group of people who were born in a specific time period; for example, people born between 1950 and 1955 can be considered to be a birth cohort) (Hellon and Solomon, 1980; Murphy and Wetzel, 1980; Solomon and Hellon, 1980; Goldney and Katsikitis, 1983). These studies indicate that as age increases among the individuals in a given birth cohort, so does the suicide rate. In addition, the suicide rates for people born in more recent cohorts are higher than for those born in earlier cohorts. For example, the suicide rate of 2.5 per 100,000 population is lower for 15- to 19-year-olds who were born between 1930 and 1934 than the suicide rate of 7.2 per 100,000 population for the 15- to 19-year-olds who were born between 1955 and 1959 (Murphy and Wetzel, 1980). The results of these three studies are consistent: For each successive birth cohort, there is a higher suicide rate in certain age groups than in the same age groups for the preceding cohort. This model suggests that whatever the cause for this cohort effect, it appears to take hold early in life and appears to last (Murphy and Wetzel, 1980).

A third population study related suicide methods to youth suicide rates. Boyd and Moscicki (1986) showed that for 15- to 24-year-olds there has been a dramatic increase in suicide rates associated with firearms as a suicide method. While the suicide rates for all other methods have increased, suicide resulting from the use of firearms has increased most dramatically. Specifically, between 1933 and 1982, the suicide rates using firearms increased 3 times faster than the suicide rates using other methods in the 15- to 19-year-old group, and 10 times faster in the 20- to 24-year-old group. This study, therefore, suggests that firearms account for most of the increase in suicide rates for this age group. Furthermore, such facts are important in suggesting that suicide can be reduced by limiting the availability of firearms.

In summary, United States epidemiologic data point out increasing suicide rates for adolescents and young adults during the last few decades. From a demographic perspective, youth who are most at risk are white males. However, the national statistics are not specific enough to indicate whether there is an especially high risk for suicide among certain demographic groups of our population. For example, some American Indian groups have very high suicide rates. Furthermore, although it is clear that the number of nonfatal suicidal acts far outnumber completed suicides, the actual prevalence of suicide attempts among adolescents and young adults is not known. What has been recognized, however, is that females attempt suicide more frequently than males.

Psychological Risk Factors for Youth Suicide

Information about psychological risk factors for suicide among adolescents and young adults, although relatively scant, has been derived from record reviews and psychological autopsy methods. Follow-up studies also have provided data about early risk factors for suicide and incidence of suicide in designated populations.

In the first published study of youth suicide, Shaffer (1974) highlighted psychological risk factors of 30 young adolescent suicide victims who were 12 to 14 years old at the time of death. In this record review study of youth suicide occurring in England and Wales between 1962 and 1968, there was a high prevalence (80 percent of the sample) of psychiatric disorders involving affective and/or antisocial symptoms. Seventeen percent of the sample had only antisocial symptoms, 57 percent had antisocial and affective symptoms, 13 percent had only affective symptoms, and 13 percent had neither type of symptomatology. Forty-six percent of the youngsters had previous suicidal ideas or attempts; this figure was considered an underestimate. Four types of personality characteristics were clearly evident: paranoid type, impulsive type, uncommunicative type, and perfectionist–self-critical type. There were also some adolescents who could not be classified into personality types because of insufficient information in the records.

In contrast to the previous study, two psychological autopsy investigations of adolescent suicide used comparison groups that provided information about factors that specifically distinguished the suicide victims from the control adolescents. Shafii and associates (1985) used the psychological autopsy method of interviewing friends, relatives, teachers, and other contacts, and gathered written reports of teenagers, aged 12 to 19, who committed suicide in Jefferson County, Kentucky, from 1980 to 1983. They compared the clinical characteristics of the teenagers who committed suicide to those of nonsuicidal teenagers who were matched for sex, age, social status, and race to the suicide victims. Of the 20 teenagers who committed suicide, 95 percent were white and 90 percent were male. The psychological factors that were associated with suicide were: presence of previous suicidal ideas or acts; drug or alcohol abuse; and antisocial behavior. Furthermore, as an indicator of psychiatric problems, the suicide victims, as compared to the nonsuicidal controls, had significantly greater histories of psychiatric treatment. In fact, 95 percent of the suicide victims, in contrast to

48 percent of the controls, had at least one *Diagnostic and Statistical Manual of Mental Disorders, Third Edition* (DSM-III) (American Psychiatric Association, 1980) pyschiatric disorder (Holden, 1986). Symptoms of depression were prominent in 76 percent of the suicide victims compared to 24 percent of the controls. Approximately 65 percent of the suicide victims, compared to 24 percent of the controls, appeared to have inhibited personalities characterized by loneliness, extreme quietness, lack of close friends, and extreme sensitivity. This study also suggested that suicide attempters do not seem to be a distinct group from those who commit suicide. This conclusion was based on the fact that a relatively high percentage of the suicide victims showed previous suicidal tendencies. For example, 85 percent of the group of suicide victims, compared to 18 percent of the controls, expressed previous suicidal ideas, and 40 percent had made a prior suicide attempt compared to 6 percent of the controls.

Preliminary data from a larger psychological autopsy study of 160 teenagers, who were younger than age 19 when they committed suicide in the New York area, corroborate many of the findings of Shafii and his group. However, in this study, Shaffer (Holden, 1986) and colleagues noted that the majority of the victims, who were males, did not meet the *DSM-III* criteria for a depressive disorder. However, symptoms of dysphoria were present in many. Shaffer noted that there were three pominent psychological patterns and that each of these patterns was present in approximately one-third of the sample. One pattern was characterized by impulsiveness, another pattern by a compulsive–perfectionistic personality, and a third group by no specific pattern. As also shown in Shafii's study, Shaffer found that antisocial symptoms, previous history of suicidal tendencies, and drug abuse were prominent among the suicide victims. An additional feature of Shaffer's study is the presence of two control groups that were matched for age, sex, and race to the suicide victims. One control group was of suicide attempters and the other control group was of normal adolescents. The results of these comparisons will elucidate whether there are distinctions between adolescents who commit suicide and those who attempt suicide. In this way, it may become clearer whether suicidal behavior among youth occurs on a continuous spectrum, or whether there is, in fact, a distinction between fatal and nonfatal suicidal acts. Furthermore, the results will also indicate how different these teenage suicide victims and attempters are from normal adolescents.

Another issue is whether there are distinctions between younger and older suicide victims; an issue that is especially relevant in view of the dramatic increase of youth suicide. Rich and colleagues (1986) gathered extensive clinical data by means of psychological autopsy methods on 133 consecutive suicides under the age of 30 and on 150 consecutive suicides aged 30 years and older in the San Diego County, California, area. Althouth there were many similarities, such as that 90 percent of the two suicide groups were psychiatrically ill, the main distinctions between the two groups were that the younger suicide victims compared to the older victims had more substance abuse disorders, fewer affective and organic disorders, and more antisocial personality disorders. Presence of drug abuse and antisocial personality disorders in the younger suicide victims agrees with the results of studies on adolescent suicide victims by Shafii and associates (1985) and Shaffer and associates (Holden, 1986).

Psychological Risk Factors for Nonfatal Suicidal Behavior

Unlike studies of adolescent suicide in which subjects are drawn from all suicides in a given community, research on adolescent nonfatal suicidal behavior has used primarily clinical populations. There are almost no data about psychological risk factors for nonfatal suicidal behavior among adolescents in the general population. As a result, it is not possible to compare directly the findings of studies of nonfatal suicidal behavior with studies of adolescent suicide. Nevertheless, studies about adolescent nonfatal suicidal behavior have used a variety of populations ranging from psychiatric inpatients, incarcerated juvenile delinquents, and adolescents enrolled in emergency room settings. These studies illustrate trends that are consistently found in many of these populations and, in this way, make it possible to draw general inferences about psychological features of adolescents and young adults who exhibit nonfatal suicidal behavior.

The most consistent finding across different populations is the association of depressive symptoms and/or *DSM-III* major depressive disorder and suicide attempts. For example, Robbins and Alessi (1985) reported that in a sample of 64 consecutively admitted adolescent psychiatric inpatients, aged 13 to 18, six patients made medically serious suicide attempts as rated on the Schedule for Affective Disorders and Schizophrenia (SADS). Eighty-three percent of the 6 patients who made a serious suicide attempt had a diagnosis of major depressive disorder, and 17 percent had a diagnosis of dysthymic disorder. Significant associations between major depressive disorder and suicidal behavior in adolescent and preadolescent psychiatric inpatients were noted by others (Pfeffer, 1986b).

Other diagnoses found frequently among psychiatric inpatients with suicide attempts were drug and alcohol abuse and borderline personality disorder (Friedman et al, 1983; Pfeffer et al, 1986a). Friedman and colleagues (1983) studied 53 young psychiatric inpatients and found that among 36 patients with depression and borderline personality disorder, 92 percent made one or more suicide attempts, and that 6 percent of these attempts resulted in death. The percentage (78 percent) of patients with depression and borderline personality disorder who attempted or completed suicide was significantly higher than the percentage (60 percent) of suicide attempters with depression and other Axis II disorders. This study suggests that there is a synergistic effect for the coexistence of major depression and borderline personality disorder for nonfatal as well as fatal suicide attempts among youth.

Although further systematic exploration is needed, the relations among depression, suicide attempt, and hopelessness have been evaluated among child and adolescent suicide attempters. The findings of Kazdin and associates (1983) for 66 preadolescent psychiatric inpatients agree with those of Dyer and Kreitman (1984) for 120 adult psychiatric inpatients. Each study suggested that greater degrees of hoelessness were evident among patients with suicide attempts than among nonsuicidal subjects. Furthermore, suicidal intent was more consistently correlated with hopelessness than with depression. The importance of the relation between hopelessness and suicidal risk was emphasized by Beck and his group (1985) in their study of 207 adult psychiatric inpatients who had suicidal ideation. Five to 10 years later, 14 patients committed suicide. Of all variables studied at the time of the index hospitalization, only hopelessness and pessimism predicted the eventual suicides. However, these predictors suffered from the usual problem of relatively high sensitivity but poor specificity.

Strong evidence for the relation between antisocial behaviors and suicide attempts has been identified, especially among adolescent delinquents (Miller et al, 1982). Alessi and associates (1984) found that 68 percent of a sample of 71 incarcerated juvenile offenders had suicidal tendencies, with the more serious suicidal behavior occurring in the subjects with major depressive disorder or borderline personality disorder. The prevalence of these psychiatric disorders in the delinquent suicidal adolescents is similar to that found among suicidal adolescent inpatients.

When adolescents admitted to hospital emergency services for suicide attempts are studied, it is found that a large number are admitted for drug overdoses (Garfinkel et al, 1982; Hawton et al, 1982; Taylor and Stansfeld, 1984a). Common psychological characteristics of these teenagers are that they have dysphoric mood, aggressiveness and/or hostility, and frequent problems with peers. Furthermore, they appear to be reacting to a crisis situation. In addition, a significant number of these suicidal youngsters have a current medical illness such as asthma or juvenile arthritis. Finally, although types of psychiatric disorders are not evaluated systematically in these samples, the suicidal youngsters appear to have more psychiatric symptoms than the nonsuicidal controls.

Follow-Up Studies

Other avenues of research have provided additional data about early predictors of suicide for adolescents and young adults. These studies are primarily follow-up investigations. Three features stand out, with regard to outcome, of adolescents and young adults at risk for suicidal behavior:

1. Previous suicidal behavior predicts future suicidal behavior.
2. Certain DSM-III diagnoses are associated with future suicide.
3. There are characteristic early psychosocial features associated with suicide.

The most consistent finding is that adolescent suicide attempters frequently repeat their suicidal acts. Table 1 presents follow-up studies of youth suicide attempters who have gone on to commit suicide.

Table 1 indicates that the number of follow-up studies involving suicidal behavior are relatively few. Among the short-term follow-up studies (Stanley and Barter, 1970; Cohen-Sandler et al, 1982a; Goldacre and Hawton, 1985), there is a low incidence of suicide. However, Stanley and Barter (1970) noted that 50 percent of the 38 psychiatrically hospitalized suicide attempters in their study repeated a suicide attempt within the time of the 1.75-year follow-up assessment period. With regard to other psychological features, the repeat suicide attempters in that study, compared to those adolescents who had no posthospitalization suicide attempts, had less adequate peer relationships, were less likely to be living with their parents, and had more social agency contacts. Similar results about social relationships were found by Cohen-Sandler and colleagues (1982b). Goldacre and Hawton (1985) found that most of the adolescents who made a repeat suicide attempt did so within the first few months of the initial hospitalization. Approximately 9.5 percent of the 2,492 patients repeated a suicide attempt within the follow-up study. In addition, the repetition rates of suicide attempts were higher

Table 1. Follow-up Studies of Suicidal Youth

Study	Subjects	Follow-up Period (years)	Suicide at Follow-up N (%)
Short-term studies:			
Stanley and Barter (1970)	38 psychiatric inpatients, age 10–21, suicide attempters	1.75	0 (0)
Cohen-Sandler et al (1982a)	20 suicidal psychiatric inpatients, aged 5–14	0.5–3; mean, 1.5	0 (0)
Goldacre and Hawton (1985)	2,492 medically hospitalized patients, aged 12–20, for self-intended overdoses	1–5; mean, 2.8	6 (0.3)
Long-term studies:			
Otto (1972)	1,547 medical and psychiatric patients, aged 12–20, suicide attempters	15	67 (4.3)
Paerregaard (1975)	27 psychiatric patients, aged 0–19, suicide attempters; and 98 psychiatric patients, aged 20–29, suicide attempters	10	0 (0) of the 0–19-year-olds; 8 (3) of the 20–29-year-olds
Nardini-Maillard and Ladame (1980)	130 medical inpatients, aged 0–20, suicide attempters	10	5 (4.0)
Angle et al (1983)	10 male and 37 female psychiatric inpatients, aged 12–18, self-intended overdoses	9	0 (0)
Motto (1984)	122 male psychiatric inpatients; aged 10–19, suicide attempters	4–10; mean, 7	11 (9.0)

among the girls than the boys in the 12- to 15-year-old group, but they were higher among the boys than the girls in the 16- to 20-year-old age group.

The long-term follow-up studies, ranging from approximately 9 to 15 years, indicate that suicide occurs in approximately 0 to 9 percent of the original samples of suicide attempters. Otto (1972) noted that compared to a group of nonsuicide attempters, adolescent suicide attempters have a much higher suicide rate within 10 to 15 years after an initial suicide attempt. He found that the greatest risk for suicide occurs during the first two years after the suicide attempt. This finding is not in agreement with the short-term follow-up studies described above, where suicide was very infrequent. Otto also reported that most of the suicide attempters used the same method to commit suicide as they used in their initial suicide attempt. In a very systematic follow-up of 122 male suicide attempters, Motto (1984) recorded a suicide rate of 1.3 percent per year during the mean follow-up time of seven years. In comparison to the initially hospitalized suicide attempters who subsequently did not commit suicide, Motto reported that those who committed suicide had the following characteristics at the time of hospitalization for the initial suicide attempt:

1. communication of intent to commit suicide
2. fear of losing one's mind or fear of a rare disease
3. seeking help before the attempt
4. hypersomnia
5. mixed or negative attitude to an interviewer
6. hopelessness
7. ability to communicate with others
8. psychomotor retardation
9. adequate financial resources

This study suggests that adolescents who committed suicide acknowledged feeling ill, were unpredictable in their utilization of help, had vegetative signs of depression such as hypersomnia and psychomotor retardation as well as hopelessness, and had adequate resources to carry out a suicidal act. Although alcohol and drug abuse and broken homes may have been prominent in the entire group of 122 suicide attempters, these factors, which have been found in other studies of youth suicide victims (Schaffer, 1974; Shafii et al, 1985), did not distinguish those who committed suicide from those who did not commit suicide.

Finally, Welner and colleagues (1979) provided the most specific information about psychiatric disorders in inpatient adolescents who commit suicide. In this 8- to 10-year follow-up study of 110 psychiatric inpatients aged 12–19, 77 were followed up. The main finding was the poor prognosis of patients with adolescent onset bipolar disorder. Twenty-five percent (three male patients) of these subjects committed suicide. These patients committed suicide by hanging, jumping, and shooting 2½, 8, and 10 years, respectively, after their hospitalization. Among the 13 schizophrenic patients, two males committed suicide by shooting themselves 8 to 10 years after hospitalization. Among the 16 patients with unipolar depression, 1 female carried out a fatal overdose with antidepressants and alcohol. There were no suicides among the remaining patients who had antisocial personality disorder, alcoholism, and undiagnosed or no known psychiatric disorder. This study highlighted the important relation between affective disorders and schizophrenia among youth with subsequent suicide. In fact, the seriousness and chronicity of psychological and psychosocial morbidity of children and adolescents with affective disorders has been highlighted by a number of other recent investigations (Pfeffer, 1986b).

Family Risk Factors

There is strong evidence that environmental and interpersonal factors play a role in risk for youths' suicidal behavior. The few studies of youth suicide indicate that suicide is often precipitated by an immediate interpersonal crisis. Shaffer (1974), in a study of 30 suicide victims aged 12 to 14, found that just before the suicide, 36 percent of the youngsters experienced a disciplinary crisis; 23.3 percent had a dispute with a peer or a boyfriend/girlfriend; 10 percent had an argument with a parent; and 33 percent had a variety of other immediate stressful events. The effects of these experiences were to intensify feelings in the youngster of humiliation, fear, rejection, inadequacy, and despair. Furthermore, 55 percent of the children lived in families in which one or more persons had either consulted a psychiatrist or had been treated for emotional problems. Shafii and associates (1985) provided supportive evidence in their study of 20 youth suicides who were compared to a nonsuicidal comparison group. In that study, the environmental variables that were associated with the suicides were: exposure to parental, peer or relative suicidal ideas, threats, attempts and/or suicide; parental emotional problems; parental absence; and evidence of physical abuse.

More extensive data about environmental variables are available from studies of nonfatal youth suicidal behavior and suicides among adults. These studies provide more detailed insights and amplify upon the trends reported for youth suicide. These studies indicate that loss of social supports due to parental psychopathology, marital discord, and family break-up are key factors. The stresses of suicidal youngsters often are experienced chronically and at an early time of life (Pfeffer, 1986a).

An important issue is to define the types of family psychopathology and the mechanisms by which they have their effects upon suicidal behavior in youth (Pfeffer, 1986a). Clarity in the relations between suicidal behavior in youth and such features as modeling behavior, identification, and genetic underpinnings is needed. Nevertheless, regardless of the genetic–constitutional forces, a youngster growing up in a family with serious psychopathology is at risk.

Most intriguing is the prevalence of suicidal behavior within families. Three approaches have been used to delineate this: family studies of suicide, twin studies, and adoption studies. All have been carried out in adult populations so that relations for youth suicide are not specified. Studies of families indicate a relation between suicide in an index subject and a high incidence of suicide in the family (Murphy and Wetzel, 1982; Roy, 1983; Tsuang, 1983; Egeland and Sussex, 1985). Twin studies comparing incidence of suicide among monozygotic and dizygotic twins have not been fruitful in indicating a genetic predisposition to suicide (Kallmann et al, 1949; Bertelsen et al, 1977). Finally, studies of adoptees who committed suicide, who were compared to subjects who did not, suggests a significant incidence in suicide in the biological relatives of adoptees who committed suicide (Schulsinger et al, 1979). This finding suggested the possibility of a genetic factor for suicide that is independent of psychiatric condition.

Nevertheless, these findings must be considered tentative because of methodological features of this study, especially the nature of selection of the sample in which it is possible that adoptive relatives are inherently healthier than biological relatives. Thus, Kety (1983) suggested that "it is clear that genetic factors play a significant role in suicide" (p. 112). However, the major conclusion that can be drawn from current research data is that "genetic factors contribute significantly but not exclusively" to suicide (p. 113).

Suicidal behavior among youth has been associated with chronic emotional illness, especially among the parents (Pfeffer, 1986a). Such emotional disorders include parental depression, substance abuse, and suicidal behavior. A number of developmental issues should be considered that suggest relations between suicidal behavior among youth, youth affective disorders, and family affective disorders. Recent research indicates that parental depression increases risk for depression in children and adolescents (Cytryn et al, 1982; Beardslee et al, 1983). Furthermore, other factors that increase risk for depressive disorders in children and adolescents are a degree of familial loading for psychiatric illness, parental assortative mating, parental recurrent depression, and age of onset of parental affective disorders (Weissman et al, 1984a; Weissman et al, 1984b). Finally, in a study that compared 194 children aged 6 to 18 years, of parents who had a major depressive disorder (with 82 normal children), it was determined that 6.5 percent of the children of depressed parents reported suicidal ideas, and 0.9 percent of the children of depressives attempted suicide (Weissman et al, 1984a). There was no suicidal ideation and no suicidal acts among the normal children. Thus, children with relatives who are severely depressed are at increased risk for suicidal behavior.

Assessment of family interactions of parents who are severely depressed has indicated that there are numerous adverse effects on the personality development, symptoms, and behavior of the children. These effects are evident when the children are very young and exhibit difficulty in maintaining friendly social interactions, in sharing, and in modulating hostile impulses (Pfeffer, 1986a). The disturbances appear to increase in severity as the children get older. When parental functioning is appraised, it is notable that depressed parents are less attentive to their children's health needs and report more negative attitudes toward their children. Keller and colleagues (1986) evaluated some of these issues in great detail. Their study of 72 children, aged 6 to 19 years, with at least one parent who had suffered from a depressive disorder, aimed to evaluate specific parental variables and the risk for the children of developing psychiatric disorders. The study found that severe and chronic depression in the parents was associated with poor adaptive functioning and an increase in psychopathology among the children. In fact, the first episode of major depressive disorder in the children always followed an episode of depression in at least one parent. Furthermore, if the parents had a poor relationship with each other, the children had impaired adaptation. Maternal depression was associated with increased psychopathology in the children but there was no association between paternal depression and the children's psychopathology. The results of this study suggest that serious attention be given to documenting family psychiatric disorder, especially affective disorders, as a means of recognizing children who may be at risk for psychopathology, depression, and suicidal behavior.

Another issue of parent–child disturbed interactions involves child abuse.

Deykin and associates (1985) found that a history of child abuse is associated with subsequent suicide attempts in adolescents. In this study, 159 adolescents aged 13 to 17, treated in an emergency room for attempted suicide, were matched on age and sex to teenagers who were not suicidal but required emergency treatment. The records of the Massachusetts Department of Social Services were reviewed for evidence of child abuse during the time before the index suicide attempts. The results indicated that the suicide attempters were three to six times more likely to have had contact with the Social Service Department for Child Abuse. Other reports also indicate an association between child abuse and suicidal behavior in children and adolescents (Pfeffer, 1986a). Another association between attempted suicide and child abuse involves mothers who attempt suicide. Hawton and colleagues (1985) studied 114 mothers treated in the emergency room for attempted suicide. Forty-five of these subjects were compared to 45 mothers from the general population and to 64 mothers considered to be at risk for depression. Records from the Child Abuse Bureau were used to identify child abuse. The results indicated that no mothers from the general population had evidence of abuse. Twenty percent of the mothers who attempted suicide showed evidence of child abuse before the suicide attempt. Furthermore, the incidence of child abuse was greater in the attempted suicide mothers (15.8 percent) before the attempt than in the mothers at risk for depression (4.7 percent). Among the total of 114 mothers who attempted suicide, 29.8 percent abused their children. The main findings of this study point out the degree of serious child care problems among mothers who make suicide attempts. However, the study was unable to specify factors that distinguish those mothers who attempt suicide and who were at risk for child abuse from those who attempt suicide but have no evidence of child abuse.

In summary, the studies described for family risk factors of suicidal behavior are consistent in the type of factors found. Family stresses from marital discord, loss of involvement with the child from parental separation/divorce, death, and serious parental psychopathology are notable risk indicators for suicidal behavior among youth. From the perspective of suicide prevention, the results of these investigations imply that early recognition of family stress and parental psychopathology involving suicidal behavior, affective disorders, and child abuse may provide an opportunity for early intervention.

Sociocultural Risk Factors: Imitative Suicidal Behavior

Phenomena that apparently have special impact on suicidal behavior in youth involve imitation of suicidal behavior. Shafii and associates (1985) found that adolescent suicide victims have previous experience with a relative or a friend who exhibited suicidal tendencies. They noted that "exposure to suicide or suicidal behavior of relatives and friends appears to be a significant factor in influencing a vulnerable young person to commit suicide" (p. 1,064). A number of "clusters" of suicide such as those occurring in Plano, Texas, and Westchester County, New York, was a sign that imitation may have occurred. An example, on a large scale, is the epidemic of youth suicide in Micronesia (Rubinstein, 1983). The rapid increase in adolescent male suicide after World War II in Micronesia seemed to be a cohort effect related to the disintegration of communal village social organization, which shifted the adolescent socialization processes into the nuclear family. The stresses among familial generations appeared to be the main factor for the increased incidence of male suicide, which also had extensive imitative underpinnings.

Relations have been identified between youth suicide, news reporting, and other media presentations about suicide. Phillips and Carstensen (1986) found that there was a significant increase in teenage suicide within 7 days after a television news broadcast about suicide. The increase in suicide occurred after both general information stories about suicide and after news stories about a particular suicide. Gould and Shaffer (1986) added to knowledge about the impact of media by documenting that there was an increase in youth suicide and youth suicide attempts in the greater New York area after fictional television stories about suicide. The results of these reports agree with the hypothesis that imitation plays a role in suicidal behavior among youth.

Biological Risk Factors

There is very little information about biological correlates of suicidal behavior in youth. Most research on youth has focused on depressive disorders which yielded findings related to sleep architecture, hypersecretion of cortisol, and hyposecretion of growth hormone in response to insulin induced hypoglycemia (Puig-Antich, 1983). These studies do not evaluate factors in relation to youth suicidal behavior.

Biological research for suicide has focused on studies of adult suicidal patients and has yielded findings involving serotonin functioning in cerebral frontal cortices (Mann et al, 1986) and spinal fluid (Asberg et al, 1976; Lidberg et al, 1985). Findings from suicidal subjects of a low level of serotonin metabolite, 5-hydroxyindoleacetic acid (5-HIAA) in the spinal fluid, reduced imipramine binding in the frontal cortices of suicide victims, and an increased number of post-synaptic serotonin and beta-adrenergic receptor bindings in the frontal cortices of suicide victims, have been important for the understanding of the biological factors involving suicidal behavior. Similar investigations are needed in younger populations to evaluate whether there are developmental continuities or discontinuities in these biological factors.

CLINICAL STRATEGIES FOR PREVENTION

Prevention of youth suicidal behavior can be approached from a variety of perspectives that encompass sociocultural, philosophical, political, intrapsychic, psychosocial, and biological domains. However, most psychiatrists focus in depth on the latter three. The aims of clinical strategies for prevention of suicidal behavior among youth are to reduce morbidity and mortality associated with risk factors and the suicidal episode. Clinical acumen is needed to discern the risk factors and to appreciate the seriousness of the youngster's statements about suicide. In fact, the two strongest factors impinging on the clinician's ability to work effectively with the suicidal youth are the psychiatrist's anxiety and shortcomings in carrying out a comprehensive assessment and treatment plan (Pfeffer, 1986b).

One of the greatest hopes for prevention of youth suicidal behavior is accurate prediction of which youngster is most at risk for suicide. However, although empirical research has delineated a number of high risk factors, prediction of suicide for an individual youngster is impossible (Pokorny, 1983). The best that a clinician can do is to assess the likelihood that a suicidal act will occur in the near future. Diagnosis of suicidal risk in clinical practice "typically consists of a sequence of small decisions . . . the first decision might be based on some alerting note or sign, and the decision would be to investigate further . . . the decision is not what to do for all time, but rather what to do next, for the near future" (Pokorny, 1983, p. 257).

Assessment of and intervention for a suicidal youngster must be broadly conceptualized and involves many modalities, many people, and potentially many therapeutic settings (Pfeffer, 1986a). Work with the youngster, the family, and the environment is crucial. Comprehensive discussion with the suicidal youngster is mandatory. Topics include the specific suicidal fantasies or acts, concepts of what would happen if the act was effective, the circumstances surrounding the suicidal behavior, previous experiences with suicidal behavior, motivation for suicidal behavior, experiences and concepts with death, depression and other aspects, and family and environmental situations (Pfeffer, 1986b). Simultaneously, extensive family discussion is required to appraise the family's ability to support a therapeutic process, to appreciate the seriousness of the youngster's problems, and to help keep the youngster alive.

Intervention follows from a diagnostic assessment and has an initial goal of protecting the youngster from harm. If the youngster can form a working alliance with the clinician, is committed to resolving problems and has a wish to live, it may be possible to work on an outpatient basis. This treatment plan also necessitates the assurance that the environment can provide support and predictability for the youngster. However, if the youngster is intent on carrying out a suicidal act, has severe depression, intense aggressive tendencies, and little ability to delay impulses or has poor judgment, psychiatric hospitalization may be indicated (Pfeffer et al, 1986b). Such a setting can provide constant observation and continual therapeutic work during the phase of an acute suicidal episode (Pfeffer, 1986b).

Regardless of whether the youngster is in an acute hospital setting or is able to benefit from outpatient treatment, a network of other people, who are not family but are in close contact with the youngster, must be identified and efforts made to develop avenues of communication between the clinician, the suicidal youngster, the family, and the environmental support network. Such an environmental support system can be effective in observing for signs of acute suicidal risk, in helping the youngster cope with daily experiences, and in fostering in the youngster a commitment to maintain treatment. This is especially important because suicidal youngsters often resist remaining in treatment. It has been suggested that the attitudes of the parents and other important people are quite influential in determining the likelihood that the youngster will accept the process of treatment (Taylor and Stansfeld, 1984b; Pfeffer et al, 1986b). Another treatment support that should be considered is medication to stabilize the youngster's emotional state. The most efficacious medication will be that directed toward decreasing target symptoms for psychiatric disorder. Thus, the medicine of choice, if medication is indicated, can range from major tranquilizers, antidepressants, psychostimulants, and so on. Finally, it must be recognized that, at the present time, there are no empirical treatment studies to evaluate the relative efficacies of psychodynamic, behavioral, cognitive, or biological interventions for youth suicidal behavior. This is an important area for future investigation.

CONCLUSION

Suicide, the second leading cause of death for 15- to 24-year-olds, is preventable. The most effective clinical strategies to prevent this tragedy of youth are early recognition of an impending suicidal episode with its attendant risk factors and the immediate intervention aimed to protect the youngster from harm. Although empirical research has not yet provided comprehensive information about youths who commit suicide, many risk factors exist: severe depression, antisocial symptoms, experience with other suicidal people, previous personal suicidal episodes, alcohol and drug abuse, and family disruption from marital discord and parental psychopathology. Factors related to imitation that promote "epidemic" youth suicides require further evaluation. Research into biological risk factors and efficacy of treatment for suicidal behavior among youth is needed. Finally, any approach that will be useful in decreasing access to lethal suicide methods, such as firearms or drugs, is a practical approach to the prevention of youth suicide.

REFERENCES

Alessi NE, McManus M, Brickman A, et al: Suicidal behavior among serious juvenile offenders. Am J Psychiatry 1984; 141:286-287

American Psychiatric Association: Diagnostic and Statistical Manual of Mental Disorders, Third Edition (DSM-III). Washington, DC, American Psychiatric Association, 1980

Angle CR, O'Brien TP, McIntire MS: Adolescent self-poisoning: a nine-year follow-up. Developmental and Behavioral Pediatrics 1983; 4:83-87

Asberg M, Traskman L, Thoren P: 5-HIAA in the cerebrospinal fluid: a biochemical suicide predictor? Arch Gen Psychiatry 1976; 33:1193-1197

Beardslee WR, Bemporad J, Keller MB, et al: Children of parents with major affective disorder: a review. Am J Psychiatry 1983; 40:825-832

Beck AT, Steer RA, Kovacs M, et al: Hopelessness and eventual suicide: a 10-year prospective study of patients hospitalized with suicidal ideation. Am J Psychiatry 1985; 142:559-563

Bertelsen A, Harvald B, Hauge M: A Danish twin study of manic-depressive disorders. Br J Psychiatry 1977; 130:330

Boyd JH, Moscicki EK: Firearms and youth suicide. Am J Public Health 1986; 76:1240-1242

Cohen-Sandler R, Berman AL, King RA: A follow-up study of hospitalized suicidal children. J Am Acad Child Psychiatry 1982a; 21:398-403

Cohen-Sandler R, Berman AL, King RA: Life stress and symptomatology: determinants of suicidal behavior in children. J Am Acad Child Psychiatry 1982b; 21:178-186

Cytryn L, McKnew DH Jr, Bartko JJ, et al: Offspring of patients with affective disorders, II. J Am Acad Child Psychiatry 1982; 21:389-391

Deyken EY, Alpert JJ, McNamarra JJ: A pilot study of the effect of exposure to child abuse or neglect on adolescent suicidal behavior. Am J Psychiatry 1985; 142:1299-1303

Dyer JAT, Kreitman N: Hopelessness, depression, and suicidal intent in parasuicide. Br J Psychiatry 1984; 144:127-133

Egeland JA, Sussex JN: Suicide and family loading for affective disorders. JAMA 1985; 254:915-918

Friedman RC, Arnoff MS, Clarkin JF, et al: History of suicidal behavior in depressed borderline inpatients. Am J Psychiatry 1983; 140:1023-1026

Garfinkel BD, Froese A, Hood J: Suicide attempts in children and adolescents. Am J Psychiatry 1982; 139:1257-1261

Goldacre M, Hawton K: Repetition of self-poisoning and subsequent death in adolescents who take overdoses. Br J Psychiatry 1985; 146:395-398

Goldney RD, Katsikitis M: Cohort analysis of suicide rates in Australia. Arch Gen Psychiatry 1983; 40:71-74

Gould MS, Shaffer D: The impact of suicide in television movies: evidence for imitation. N Eng J Med 1986; 315:690-694

Hawton K, O'Grady J, Osborn M, et al: Adolescents who take overdoses: their characteristics, problems and contacts with helping agencies. Br J Psychiatry 1982; 140:118-123

Hawton K, Roberts J, Goodwin G: The risk of child abuse among mothers who attempt suicide. Br J Psychiatry 1985; 146:486-489

Hellon CP, Solomon MI: Suicide and age in Alberta, Canada, 1951 to 1977: the changing profile. Arch Gen Psychiatry 1980; 37:505-510

Holden C: Youth suicide: new research focuses on a growing social problem. Science 1986; 233:839-841

Holinger PC, Offer D: Prediction of adolescent suicide: a population model. Am J Psychiatry 1982; 139:302-307

Kallman FJ, DePorte J, DePorte E, et al: Suicide in twins and only children. Am J Hum Genet 1949; 1:113-126

Kazdin AE, French NH, Unis AS, et al: Hopelessness, depression, and suicidal intent among psychiatrically disturbed inpatient children. J Consult Clin Psychol 1983; 51:504-510

Keller MB, Beardslee WR, Dorer DJ, et al: Impact of severity and chronicity of parental affective illness on adaptive functioning and psychopathology in children. Arch Gen Psychiatry 1986; 43:930-937

Kety SS: Observations on genetic and environmental influences in the etiology of mental disorder from studies on adoptees and their relatives, in Genetics of Neurological and Psychiatric Disorders. Edited by Kety SS, Rowland LP, Sidman RL, et al. New York, Raven Press, 1983

Klerman GL, Lavori PW, Rice J, et al: Birth-cohort trends in rates of major depressive disorder among relatives of patients with affective disorders. Arch Gen Psychiatry 1985; 42:689-693

Lidberg L, Tuck JR, Asberg M, et al: Homicide, suicide and CSF 5-HIAA. Acta Psychiatr Scand 1985; 71:230-236

Mann JJ, Stanley M, McBride PA, et al: Increased serotonin$_2$ and B-adrenergic receptor binding in the frontal cortices of suicide victims. Arch Gen Psychiatry 1986; 43:954-959

Mental Health, United States: Suicide in the United States: 1958-1982. Edited by Taube CA, Barrett SA. Washington, DC, DHHS Publication (ADM) 85-1378, 1985

Miller ML, Chiles JA, Barnes VE: Suicide attempters within a delinquent population. J Consult Clin Psychol 1982; 50:491-498

Motto JA: Suicide in male adolescents, in Suicide in the Young. Edited by Sudak HS, Ford AB, Rushforth NB. Boston, John Wright, PSG Inc., 1984

Murphy GE, Wetzel RD: Suicide risk by birth cohort in the United States, 1949 to 1974. Arch Gen Psychiatry 1980; 37:519-523

Murphy GE, Wetzel RD: Family history of suicidal behavior among suicide attempters. J Nerv Ment Dis 1982; 170:86-90

National Center for Health Statistics Monthly Vital Statistics Report: Advance report of final divorce statistics, 1984; 1986a; 35(6), September 25

National Center for Health Statistics Monthly Vital Statistics Report: Advance report of final mortality statistics, 1984; 1986b; 35(6), September 26

Nardini-Maillard D, Ladame FG: The results of a follow-up study of suicidal adolescents. J Adolesc 1980; 3:253-260

Otto U: Suicidal acts by children and adolescents: a follow-up study. Acta Psychiatr Scand 1972; (Suppl 233):7-123

Paerregaard G: Suicide among attempted suicides: a 10-year follow-up. Suicide 1975; 5:140-144

Pfeffer CR: Family characteristics and support systems as risk factors for youth suicidal behavior. Paper presented at the Department of Health and Human Services Secretary's Task Force on Youth Suicide, Bethesda, Maryland, 1986a

Pfeffer CR: The Suicidal Child. New York, Guilford Press, 1986b

Pfeffer CR, Newcorn J, Kaplan G, et al: Suicidal behavior in adolescent psychiatric inpatients. Paper presented at the 139th Annual Meeting of the American Psychiatric Association, Washington, DC, May 1986a

Pfeffer CR, Plutchik R, Mizruchi MS: A comparison of psychopathology in child psychiatric inpatients, outpatients and nonpatients: implications for treatment planning. J Nerv Ment Dis 1986b; 174:529-535

Pfeffer CR, Plutchik R, Mizruchi MS, et al: Suicidal behavior in child psychiatric inpatients and outpatients and in nonpatients. Am J Psychiatry 1986c; 143:733-738

Phillips DP, Carstensen LL: Clustering of teenage suicides after television news stories about suicide. N Engl J Med 1986; 315:685-689

Pokorny AD: Prediction of suicide in psychiatric patients. Arch Gen Psychiatry 1983; 40:249-257

Puig-Antich J: Neuroendocrine and sleep correlates of prepubertal major depressive disorder: current status of the evidence, in Affective Disorders in Childhood and Adolescence: An Update. Edited by Cantwell DP, Carlson GA. New York, Spectrum Publications, 1983

Rich CL, Young D, Fowler RC: San Diego Suicide Study, I: young versus old subjects. Arch Gen Psychiatry 1986; 43:577-582

Robbins DR, Alessi NE: Depressive symptoms and suicidal behavior in adolescents. Am J Psychiatry 1985; 142:588-592

Roy A: Family history of suicide. Arch Gen Psychiatry 1983; 40:971-974

Rubinstein DH: Epidemic suicide among Micronesian adolescents. Soc Sci Med 1983; 17:657-665

Schulsinger F, Kety SS, Rosenthal D, et al: A family study of suicide, in Origin, Prevention and Treatment of Affective Disorders. Edited by Schou M, Stromgren E. Academic Press, New York, 1979

Shaffer D: Suicide in childhood and early adolescence. J Child Psychol Psychiatry 1974; 15:275-291

Shafii M, Carrigan S, Whittinghill JR, et al: Psychological autopsy of completed suicide in children and adolescents. Am J Psychiatry 1985; 142:1061-1064

Solomon MI, Hellon CP: Suicide and age in Alberta, Canada, 1951 to 1977: a cohort analysis. Arch Gen Psychiatry 1980; 37:511-513

Stanley EJ, Barter JT: Adolescent suicidal behavior. Am J Orthopsychiatry 1970; 40:87-96

Taylor EA, Stansfeld SA: Children who poison themselves, I: a clinical comparison with psychiatric controls. Br J Psychiatry 1984a; 145:127-135

Taylor EA, Stansfeld SA: Children who poison themselves, II: prediction of attendance for treatment. Br J Psychiatry 1984b; 145:132-135

Traskman L, Asberg M, Bertilsson L, et al: Monoamine metabolites in CSF and suicidal behavior. Arch Gen Psychiatry 1981; 38:631-636

Tsuang MT: Risk of suicide in the relatives of schizophrenics, manics, depressives, and controls. J Clin Psychiatry 1983; 44:396-400

Weissman MM, Prusoff BA, Gammon GD, et al: Psychopathology in the children (ages 6–18) of depressed and normal parents. J Am Acad Child Psychiatry 1984a; 23:78-84

Weissman MM, Wickramaratne P, Merikangas KR, et al: Onset of major depression in early adulthood: increased familial loading and specificity. Arch Gen Psychiatry 1984b; 41:1136-1143

Welner A, Welner Z, Fishman R: Psychiatric adolescent inpatients: eight- to ten-year follow-up. Arch Gen Psychiatry 1979; 36:698-700

Chapter 18

Prevention of Suicide

by George E. Murphy, M.D.

CAN SUICIDE BE PREVENTED?

In a recent malpractice case the plaintiff alleged that a Health Maintenance Organization (HMO) had been negligent in supplying a lethal amount of a tricyclic antidepressant to a depressed patient without a physician first examining him. An expert witness stated in his deposition for the defense: "I know of no credible evidence that any treatment or other intervention has successfully prevented even a single suicide." While this statement may appear shocking at first glance, a moment's thought will show not only that this is true at present but it will always be so. The prevention of a suicide generates no data. A nonsuicide is, statistically, a nonevent. Thus, we can never prove our individual successes.

This should not be an occasion for despair, and most assuredly not a reason to conclude that our efforts are fruitless. It is not that suicides can't be prevented, but that prevention cannot be detected with any great sense of assurance. (This problem has been discussed by Murphy, 1984.) This being the case, something may yet be learned from the failure of prevention. A number of studies of completed suicides have indicated that approximately one-half of those officially recognized as having taken their own lives had been under a physician's care within a month or less of their death. The first conclusion therefore, is that suicide is a clinical problem, and the first line of defense is the doctor's office.

Suicide prevention centers, by contrast, have had previous contact with no more than three to six percent of completed suicides (Wilkins, 1970; Barraclough and Shea, 1970). While such a finding might superficially suggest that such centers are indeed highly successful, two lines of evidence suggest that this is not the case. First, it appears that the characteristics of their clientele much more closely resemble those of suicide attempters than of suicides (Murphy et al, 1969). Second, the advent of suicide prevention centers has not generally been attended by a reduction in the suicide rate (Wilkins, 1970; Wold and Litman, 1973; Barraclough et al, 1977). (For dissenting opinion, see Bagley, 1968.) Miller and colleagues (1984), however, have found and replicated an effect on the local suicide rate for young women, a group highly represented among callers to such services.

Systematic studies have shown that persons who commit suicide are all, or nearly all, clinically ill (Robins et al, 1959b; Dorpat and Ripley, 1960; Barraclough et al, 1974; Beskow, 1979; Cheynoweth et al, 1980; Rich et al, 1986). Moreover, 95 percent or more of them were psychiatrically ill at the time of their death. To further refine the point, two psychiatric illnesses account for two-thirds of the suicides: depressive illness for 40 to 50 percent and alcoholism for approximately 25 percent. The population at risk is therefore not the population at large but a rather narrow segment of it and a highly recognizable segment at that. The reliable clinical recognition of these two conditions would go a long way toward narrowing the focus of our concern.

THE PHYSICIAN'S ROLE

If the prevention of suicide is not demonstrable, perhaps we can learn from its failure. Given that one-half of suicide victims have been under a physician's care, the nature of that care may prove instructive.

In an interview study conducted with physicians who had cared for a patient who had committed suicide (Murphy, 1975a, 1975b), one striking finding was the very low frequency of *diagnosed* depressive disorder. This was found despite the fact that in a great majority of cases the physicians were able to describe symptoms of the patient that would have led readily to a diagnosis of depressive disorder. Most of the physicians had recognized depressed mood in their patients. Most of them were aware of the presence of other depressive symptoms. But clinical depressive disorder was only rarely diagnosed. There was a tendency for depressive complaints to have been treated symptomatically rather than to have been regarded syndromically. As a consequence, the diagnosis of depressive disorder was not made and the disorder was not treated.

It must be acknowledged that this study was conducted prior to the general acceptance of criterion-based diagnosis, so it is unlikely that the physicians in practice had had modern training in psychiatric diagnosis. Despite increased acceptance of the importance of systematic psychiatric diagnosis by the psychiatric community, the majority of physicians currently in practice will still have completed their training prior to the promulgation of the *Diagnostic and Statistical Manual of Mental Disorders, Third Edition, Revised (DSM-III-R)* (American Psychiatric Association, 1987). Indeed, psychiatrists themselves are not yet of a single mind with regard to this matter.

While the greatly increased prescribing of antidepressant medications in recent years attests to an increase in diagnosing depression, there are no data that can answer the question of correctness of the diagnosis or the appropriateness of antidepressant use. In a number of instances in the Murphy (1975) study, the amount of antidepressant prescribed per day was considerably below accepted therapeutic standards. In two instances, through no fault of the physician, the patient had presented so recently with a depressive syndrome that despite appropriate medicating there was simply not time enough between the beginning of treatment and the suicide for the medication to have been likely to have taken effect. In such a case, hospitalization is an option. One patient had refused further medication.

Although in retrospect one could easily say that these patients should have been hospitalized, the evidence from the physicians' records indicated that the patients had not presented as so severely depressed as to require hospitalization. There were other instances in which the patient simply denied the severity of the depression, as well as suicidal ideation, while proceeding to make suicidal plans. Obviously, in this sort of case, little can be done to prevent the suicide. However, this was a small minority of the total.

Equally important as failing to diagnose depression was the common failure of physicians to inquire about suicidal ideation. Except for the psychiatrists involved, only one physician in six was aware that his patient had suicidal thinking. Typically, the reason for this lack of information is the simple failure to inquire. It can be given as a general rule that upon making a diagnosis of depressive disorder, the physician should ask the patient about suicidal thoughts. The diagnostic inquiry is itself not complete until such questions have been asked.

Nor is it sufficient to have asked at the time of initial evaluation. Suicidal risk is coextensive with the depressive episode, so the patient's thinking must be reviewed at suitable intervals. Should the slightest doubt arise as to the patient's veracity or openness on this issue, family members can be questioned as well. Communication of suicidal thoughts has been found to be quite frequent among those who complete the act, having occurred in two-thirds or more of cases (Robins et al, 1959a; Robins, 1981). It has also been shown that patients harboring suicidal thoughts will, in most instances, tell a physician of their thoughts if they are asked (Delong and Robins, 1961).

CAN WE PREDICT SUICIDE?

As noted above, systematic studies of suicide have shown that the phenomenon is not random but is associated with identifiable factors, most notably, psychiatric diagnosis. The possibility that there are telltale characteristics other than diagnosis that would permit advance recognition of those at risk has given rise to efforts to develop predictive tests. The literature abounds with studies of suicide attempters that are aimed at identifying the potentially suicidal. These efforts have been substantially unsuccessful.

There is, indeed, an overlap. Up to one-third of suicides have a prior history of suicide attempt (Robins et al, 1959a; Rich et al, 1986). On the other hand, follow-up studies of cohorts of suicide attempters have repeatedly shown that one to two percent will commit suicide in the first year following the attempt and about one percent per year thereafter. Gradually the suicides diminish, so that a long follow-up of hospitalized cases may yield 8 to 13 percent of deaths from this cause (Stengel, 1972). While this is undeniably a high risk population, efforts to identify characteristics that distinguish the subsequent suicides from the nonsuicides within it have proved relatively nonproductive. This is so largely because suicide is a rare event. It is also the case that suicide is not a trait with a unique marker such as an identifiable gene locus. Rather, there appears to be a large and highly individual psychosocial component. There is no known pathognomonic characteristic.

The Search for Predictors

Because suicide is a rare event in the general population, occurring 12 or 13 times per 100,000 live population per year, population surveys are impractical. Enrichment strategies, such as those represented by the studies of suicide attempters, have been tried. The hope was that in a population already shown to be at increased risk for suicide, there would be enough suicides within a finite length of time to give a meaningful number of such events. From this, it was hoped that characteristics or patterns of characteristics could be found that would distinguish the suicides from the nonsuicides. Acute psychiatric hospital admissions offer a population at increased risk for suicide. Two large prospective studies illustrate the problem of clinical prediction when the base rate of the phenomenon under investigation is low.

VETERANS ADMINISTRATION HOSPITAL STUDY. Pokorny (1983) prospectively studied 4,800 consecutive first psychiatric admissions to Veterans Administration Hospitals by having them rated on a variety of assessment instruments. He then followed up the patients after four to six years. Sixty-seven of them had committed suicide. The group as a whole had a suicide rate of 279 per 100,000 per year; 12 times that of U.S. military veterans and 23 times the general civilian suicide rate. Note that even with this enrichment, the base rate is low: less than three per 1,000 persons per year. By means of stepwise discriminant analysis, Pokorny derived weighted combinations of variables. Those having the highest correlations with suicide were then used as predictor variables to attempt to identify the suicides among the population from which these variables had been obtained.

Allowing the computer to assume equal frequencies of suicide and no suicide, the program identified 35 of 63 suicides. It did so, however, at a cost of 1,200 false positives; 25 percent of the sample! This result illustrates how little difference there is in a broad range of characteristics between suicides and nonsuicides. When the computer was asked to assume the actual base rate for the sample (278 per 100,000 population), it did not identify a single suicide. There were only three false positives and the specificity rate of the test was 99.98 percent. A similar result is achieved by simply predicting no suicide in every case. This obviously is unsatisfactory from a practical standpoint, however. Since the criteria for high risk of suicide were derived from the same population upon which they were tested, this represents the best case, not an average or worst case outcome. MacKinnon and Farberow (1976) had concluded earlier on statistical grounds that the limiting accuracy of a suicide prediction schedule for Veterans Administration neuropsychiatric patients is .20, meaning that only 20 percent of patients predicted to commit suicide would actually do so.

CIVILIAN HOSPITAL STUDY. Motto (1979, 1980) employed a different strategy in searching for predictors of suicide. He started with 3,006 psychiatric admissions of patients who were considered depressed and/or suicidal. He ignored clinical diagnosis. Rather, he proposed that certain kinds of people respond in similar ways to certain constellations of stresses by resorting to suicide. He called this a clinical models approach.

He took a sophisticated methodologic step by dividing his population into an index sample and a replication sample. Predictors derived from the first sample set would be tested for utility on the second. He has reported three clinical models. One is males under 40; another is stable with forced change (Motto, 1979). The third is subjectively diagnosed alcohol abusers (no diagnostic criteria) (Motto, 1980). Note that only the alcohol abusers model bears a relationship to clinical matters. One problem with this approach is that since the models are not the sorts of things that clinicians are accustomed to looking for, nor even the sorts of things that take patients to physicians, the utility to the medical community of this approach is dubious at best.

Motto and colleagues (1985) have gone on to produce a scale for estimating risk of suicide within two years, based on the original data set of hospitalized depressed and/or suicidal patients. It is proposed to be statistically most useful in patients characterized similarly to those who provided the basis for the scale;

that is, patients admitted to a psychiatric hospital with depression and/or suicidal thinking. As with Pokorny's (1983) variables, achievement of a reasonable level of identification of true positives (say, 50 percent) is accomplished at a cost of more than 25 percent false positives. Motto appropriately cautions that clinical judgment should be given precedence over an inconsistent scale score. He further thinks the scale will be most useful to the less clinically skilled user.

Prediction versus Risk Assessment

Suicide is a rare phenomenon that shares the statistical characteristics of other rare phenomena. Tests of extraordinarily high sensitivity and specificity are required if anything is to be accomplished (Galen and Gambino, 1975). One can argue that perhaps it is simply a matter of the right questions not having been asked. Thus far, there do not appear to be any pathognomonic features exhibited by those who will subsequently commit suicide.

The fact that both of the above studies start with hospitalized patients capitalized on the clinical judgment of anonymous clinicians. The psychiatrically hospitalized population does represent a group at increased risk, as Pokorny's and Motto's data show. The fact that suicides occurred attests to the limited ability of our treatments to influence longer term outcome.

If accurate prediction is so difficult with inpatients, how much more difficult will it be with outpatients? Various authors have commented on the sharp falloff in power when a clinically derived scale is applied to a different sort of population than that from which it was derived (Pallis et al, 1982; Motto et al, 1985). It is this author's opinion that current research offers no encouragement for the belief that the assessment of a patient at a given point in time, with whatever elaborate battery of instruments, is more likely to identify persons at long-term risk than is simple clinical diagnosis. Fortunately, this is not the tragedy it might appear at first glance to be. Pokorny (1983) has pointed out that the utility of knowing that someone may, at some time later in life, terminate his or her own existence is of little clinical use. What would one do with such knowledge?

From a practical standpoint, what is needed is an assessment for the immediate future. This, in fact, is how clinicians operate. They assess the patient, make decisions about need for further assessment, increased surveillance, hospitalization, medication, and other forms of intervention. They decide how frequently the patient needs to be observed, the level of caution indicated, and so forth.

Seeing the patient through a suicidal crisis is a matter of acute clinical management rather than long-range prediction. It starts with clinical diagnosis, progresses to inquiry about suicidal ideation and hopelessness, and culminates in a treatment plan having the principal characteristic of being subject to change with updated information. The patient who is suicidal today is less likely to be suicidal one year later.

Since the population to be considered at high risk is nearly all psychiatrically ill, the problem of false positives is not what it might be under other circumstances. Every patient identified as suffering from major depressive disorder, alcoholism, schizophrenia, or organic brain syndrome is deserving of treatment, whether or not there is suicidal risk. For at least the first two of these four conditions, active treatment is quite effective. It appears that successful treatment of the underlying condition will terminate the risk of suicide, at least for the current episode.

INDICATORS OF INCREASED RISK

Affective Disorders

While the prediction of suicide in a general way is both statistically unreliable and of limited clinical use in any event, there remains the question of identifying those individuals at acutely greater risk. The diagnoses of affective disorder, alcoholism, and schizophrenia all indicate an increased lifetime risk. That risk is approximately 15 percent for affective disorder (Guze and Robins, 1970) and alcoholism (Pitts and Winokur, 1966), and approximately 10 to 13 percent for schizophrenia (Tsuang, 1978; Bleuler, 1978). But which 10 to 15 percent?

How may the high risk state be identified? Our studies of patients suffering from affective disorder who committed suicide failed to find any unusual increment of recent negative life events, with the exception that more than expected were living alone. Rich and colleagues (in press) identified a greater than expected rate of recently enforced change of living circumstances among affectively disordered suicides. Since two-thirds of the suicides had communicated their preoccupation in advance, the presence of such communication is a valuable clue. (Just how discriminating it may be would depend on how widespread suicidal communication may be among the nonsuicidal—a datum not in our possession at present.) Apart from these findings, little has emerged to distinguish the suicidal from the nonsuicidal depressed patient.

One additional finding is of possible significance, however. In an earlier study, Robins (1981) found some suicides experiencing their first depression and others with a history of prior depression who were again depressed. But there were no suicides with a prior history of depression who were not depressed at the time they took their lives. The implication of this seems clearly to be that persons with the affective disorder diathesis are at risk for suicide only when depressed.

In over 1,000 cases systematically studied from a diagnostic standpoint (Robins et al, 1959a; Dorpat and Ripley, 1960; Barraclough et al, 1974; Beskow, 1979; Chynoweth et al, 1980; Rich et al, 1986) not a single suicide has been reported in a patient who was clinically manic. It must therefore be concluded that the presence of a clinical depression is a significant risk factor and those individuals suffering from the disorder are not at risk when they are between episodes or manic.

As is well known, manics may abruptly plunge into depression. Therefore, the manic state may be followed by suicide if depression supervenes. (Data are lacking as to the suicide risk attending rapidly cycling bipolar disorder.) Reports in the literature are not in agreement as to whether bipolar affective disorder poses greater or less risk of suicide than the unipolar form. There was no instance of a history of mania having been obtained in any of 63 subjects with depressive disorder in the earliest diagnostic study (Robins, 1981). Nor was psychosis particularly common. Delusions were found in only 8 (13 percent) of these 63 suicides (Robins, 1986).

It should also be mentioned that the depression that leads to suicide is not necessarily pure. While little attention was paid to this issue in earlier studies, Rich and colleagues (1986) found reason to divide the affective disorders into major depression, atypical depressive disorder, and dysthymic disorder. As used in that study, the term atypical referred in most instances to persons in whom there was a concomitant substance abuse diagnosis (Rich, personal communication). This is substantially different—and more severe—than DSM-III-R—atypical depression.

Forty-seven (35 percent) of the 133 subjects under age 30 were given an affective disorder diagnosis. Of these, 68 percent were judged atypical, 19 percent major depression, and 13 percent dysthymic disorder. Of the 150 subjects aged 30 and older, 78 (52 percent) received an affective disorder diagnosis. Atypical affective disorder was diagnosed in 59 percent, major depression in 37 percent, and dysthymic disorder in 4 percent. Overall, therefore, 44 percent of subjects were diagnosed as suffering from an affective disorder and 62 percent of these were considered to be atypical. That some suicidal depressions are of lesser severity, or may be mixed with personality disorder features (Rich et al, 1986) or substance abuse (Murphy et al, 1979; Rich et al, in press) is a fact that has received too little attention in the literature. Without knowing the relative prevalence of pure and "impure" affective disorder, it is nevertheless clear that the depressive syndrome, alone and in various company, is the chief contributor to suicide.

Alcoholism

In contrast to depressives, the study of alcoholics has yielded a single risk factor. Murphy and Robins (1967) found that a significantly greater than chance number of suicides (32 percent) among 31 alcoholics had experienced loss of a close interpersonal relationship within six weeks or less of the time of their suicidal act. This study was replicated with an additional 50 alcoholic suicides (Murphy et al, 1979) and again, there was a significant concentration of suicides (26 percent) within six weeks of an interpersonal loss event.

Recently, Rich and associates (in press), in an extensive study of 283 suicides in San Diego, have confirmed the significantly increased frequency of recent loss in relation to suicide among alcoholics. Owing to the increasingly widespread distribution of substance abuse disorders in the last 20 years (and perhaps more so in such coastal cities as San Diego) (Fowler et al, 1986), it was possible to test whether this association of interpersonal loss to suicide was characteristic of substance abusers in general. Indeed, this proved to be the case, as might have been expected. Thirty-six percent of substance abusers were found to have experienced such loss within six weeks; 25 percent within one week of the suicide. The psychodynamics of substance abusers are much alike, regardless of the choice of substance abused.

In order to avoid circularity of argument, the above studies carefully avoided counting anticipated losses (loss events believed by the victim to be about to occur). If anticipated losses with a realistic likelihood of occurrence had been included, the proportion of such instances among the alcoholics studied by Murphy would have been approximately 40 percent. It can therefore be safely said that an important factor in anticipating increased suicidal risk among alcoholics and other substance abusers is the recognition of recent or impending loss of a close interpersonal relationship (and possibly of a forced change in living circumstances). Therefore, any steps that can be taken to provide greater emotional support for these individuals around the time of the loss may prove protective.

Schizophrenia

The number of persons diagnosed as suffering from schizophrenia is approximately 10 percent as great as for major depression. Therefore, the number of suicides identified as schizophrenic is comparatively small. Within the diagnostic group, however, the risk for suicide is about two-thirds of that in major depression. While some authors have claimed that young schizophrenics are at greater risk than older ones (Drake et al, 1985), neither Bleuler (1978) nor Rich and colleagues (1986) found evidence to support this belief. It is probable that depression complicates the majority of cases that eventuate in suicide (Cohen et al, 1964; Roy, 1982). Given the high prevalence of secondary depression in schizophrenia, it is unlikely to prove to be a particularly useful indicator, except as a reminder to the clinician to ask about suicidal thoughts and, perhaps, hopelessness.

Recently, Drake and Cotton (1986) have reported that hopelessness distinguished the schizophrenic suicides from their matched controls on the last hospitalization. "These suicide victims had shown high premorbid achievement, high self-expectations of performance, and high awareness of pathology." Drake and Cotton reach the following conclusion: "In the absence of hopelessness, depressed cases of schizophrenia are at no greater risk for suicide than non-depressed patients with schizophrenia." While the number of probands is small (15), the finding has considerable intuitive appeal. Pending further data, hopelessness appears to be a potentially useful warning signal of heightened risk.

Panic Disorder

Although studies have shown that anxiety disorders (Wheeler et al, 1950) and particularly panic disorder (Coryell et al, 1986) are associated with a suicide rate as high as 20 percent (Coryell et al, 1982), no cases of panic disorder have been identified in the large body of material thus far published. (Rich and colleagues, in 1986, identified one case of agoraphobia.) Given the close association of panic disorder and unipolar depression (Coryell et al, 1983), it is likely that the clinically more striking diagnosis of affective disorder (depression) has been more readily recognized and has preempted the diagnostic field. The risk factor is almost certainly depression in these cases. The clinician is warned to be alert to the development of a secondary depression and its life-threatening implications.

Personality Disorder

In the wake of the fairly recent acceptance by the psychiatric community of criterion-based psychiatric diagnosis, increased attention is being paid to clearer definition of personality disorders. While there is both a lack of consensus on definitions and poor separation of the various proposed subdivisions, the Axis II category has been attended to in the more recent studies of suicides. Beskow (1979) noted 12 cases of "personality disorders" among 270 Swedish male suicides. Chynoweth and associates (1980) reported four diagnoses of personality disorder among 135 consecutive suicides in Brisbane, Australia. Whether these cases were complicated by other psychiatric diagnoses is uncertain. Rich and colleagues (1986) diagnosed 14 subjects as exhibiting antisocial personality disorders and one as having a mixed personality disorder. All but one of these cases was complicated by substance abuse (Rich, personal communication; see "Comorbidity," following).

Hopelessness

Beck and co-workers (1975) have reported that hopelessness is a better predictor of suicidal thinking than is depression per se. Wetzel (1976) and Wetzel and colleagues (1980), studying suicide attempters and suicide ideators, replicated this finding. However, not everyone would agree that what is true of the thinking of suicide attempters is likely to be characteristic of suicides: the populations have only modest overlap (Murphy, 1986).

Beck and associates (1985), in a 5- to 10-year follow-up of 207 diagnostically heterogeneous inpatients with suicidal ideation, found that a hopelessness scale (Beck et al, 1974) score of 10 or greater correctly identified 10 of 11 inpatients with suicidal ideation who, within 5 to 10 years, committed suicide. While this scale distinguished "significantly" between subsequent suicides and nonsuicides, the false positive rate was given as 88.4 percent, showing this to be a highly nonspecific test for long-term prediction. (It seems likely that Beck miscalculated the false positive rate and that it was actually 49 percent.) The utility of the Hopelessness Scale for acute prediction of suicide risk among a mixed population of inpatients thinking of suicide remains insufficiently demonstrated.

Fawcett and colleagues (1987) had a larger sample and a shorter follow-up. In the Psychobiology of Depression study (Katz et al, 1979) there were 25 suicides in the first year of follow-up, 8 within 6 months. "More intense hopelessness reported on admission to the study characterized the suicide group ($p < .001$)" more than the 929 subjects who did not take their lives. Ratings were made by trained interviewers on the six-point hopelessness scale of the Schedule for Affective Disorders and Schizophrenia (SADS) (Endicott and Spitzer, 1978), rather than on Beck's (1974) Hopelessness Scale. The difference in hopelessness scores was small: 4.6 ± 0.7 for suicides versus 4.0 ± 1.3 for the remainder (Fawcett et al, 1987). While statistically significant, this difference is unlikely to be *clinically* significant, as the overlap is very large (Fawcett, personal communication). In combination with clinical depression and loss of interest and pleasure it was predictive.

There is an inevitable gap between the assessment of hopelessness and the subsequent suicide, even in so short a follow-up. Is it reasonable to assume that the hopelessness identified in the course of hospitalization has persisted uninterruptedly until the suicide? It seems more likely that the tendency to hopelessness is not shared by all depressives and that those who experience it may constitute an especially high risk group. The point seems to be made that a pervasive sense of hopelessness is a symptom not to be ignored. Similarly, while suicidal thoughts may occur fleetingly in most, if not all clinical depressions, sustained and directed suicidal thoughts are much less common and are evidence of greatly increased risk.

Comorbidity

Morrison (1982) noted among suicides in his private patient sample that there was a trend toward multiple diagnoses. He raised the question whether multiple diagnoses per se confer increased risk. Alternatively, he asked, "Do patients with two diagnoses assume the suicidal risk of the diagnosis more frequently associated with completed suicide?" The absence of reliable comorbidity data makes this a difficult question to answer with any authority. Certain diagnoses rarely appear in uncomplicated form in suicide studies. Antisocial personality disorder (ASPD) eventuating in suicide, for example, is characteristically accompanied by substance abuse (Robins et al, 1959b; Rich, personal communication). The same is true of Briquet's syndrome (DSM-III-R somatization disorder is a diluted cognate of this diagnosis) (Robins, 1981; Rich et al, 1986). These two conditions are familially related (Cloninger et al, 1975). Coryell (1981) did not find excess mortality from sucide among 72 women with Briquet's Syndrome followed up after 42 years. Comparable data for ASPD are not available at this time. It would appear likely that the suicide risk in these two diagnoses is that of substance abuse.

Approximately three-fourths of alcoholic suicides were suffering from concurrent depression (Murphy et al, 1979). Schizophrenics who commit suicide have often been noted to be depressed as well. However, population data on the prevalence of secondary depression in these two disorders are lacking. We have cited the lack of identified cases of panic disorder in suicide studies in relation to a 15 to 20 percent lifetime risk for this disorder as suggesting an association with depression. It would seem that some type of comorbidity must be operating to mask recognition of panic disorder. Secondary depression has been cited as a risk factor for suicide in organic brain syndromes.

Rich and associates (1986) listed 214 diagnoses for 122 suicides under age 30 who were given any psychiatric diagnosis. This is a mean of 2.14 diagnoses per subject. For 136 psychiatrically diagnosed suicides age 30 and over, 257 diagnoses were made; a mean of 1.89 diagnoses per subject. Thus, comorbidity is very common in suicide.

Except for Briquet's syndrome and ASPD, where comorbidity with substance abuse is the rule in suicide, it seems likely that suicide risk is principally contributed by depression. Any psychiatric illness that is complicated by depression may present a risk of suicide approximately that of depression alone. Studies of comorbidity in the general population as well as in psychiatric populations will be necessary to give a final answer on this question. In the meantime, the depressive syndrome would seem to be an even more powerful indicator than has been noted heretofore. It may also be true that hopelessness is the key component (Drake and Cotton, 1986; Wetzel, 1976; Wetzel et al, 1980; Fawcett et al, 1987).

Attempted Suicide

Twenty-two percent of the suicides in the study by Robins and colleagues (1959a) were known to have had a history of suicide attempt. Dorpat and Ripley (1960) noted a rate of 33 percent. Rich and colleagues (1986) found a history of suicide attempt in 42 percent of the suicides under age 30 and in 35 percent of those older. Follow-up studies of suicide attempters tabulated by Stengel (1972) ranged from 1 year to 14 years in samples of varying size. Important factors such as mean age and seriousness of attempt were not uniform. There was a very strong tendency to find one to two percent of suicides in the first follow-up year and one percent or less per year thereafter. Only four of 24 follow-ups were longer than 8 years. In general, the longer the follow-up, the less likely was the annual suicide rate to continue at one percent. This suggests declining probabilities over extended periods. The data presented do not permit calculation of lifetime risk.

In a 12-year follow-up of 221 previously hospitalized serious suicide attempters, Ettlinger (1964) found that 13.2 percent had committed suicide. This was the highest proportion of suicides in any of the studies cited. While Ettlinger's data would suggest a lifetime risk of suicide among suicide attempters in the neighborhood of 12–15 percent, there are statistical reasons to think it is not that high.

Estimates vary as to the ratio of suicide attempts to suicides, but it tends to cluster around 10:1 with little supporting evidence. The most careful effort to arrive at a reliable ratio was that of Parkin and Stengel (1965), who surveyed not only general and mental hospitals but physicians in the community as well. They identified, over a 2-year period, 9.7 suicide attempters who had some type of medical contact for every suicide in Sheffield, England. Attempters not identified from hospital records but seen only by a physician accounted for 14 percent of the total. The proportion seen as hospital outpatients but not admitted is unclear. It may have been as low as 11 percent or as high as 62 percent.

If we assume that the ratio of attempted suicides to suicides is indeed about 10:1 and that approximately one-half of attempters are hospitalized (this is relevant because virtually all suicide attempt studies begin with hospitalized patients), then there are about 500 hospitalized attempters for every 100 suicides. If one-third of the suicides have a history of attempted suicide, the lifetime risk of suicide in the population of hospital-admitted suicide attempters is 33/500 = 6.6 percent, or approximately one-half of that found by Ettlinger. This figure is closer to the combined experience of the other follow-up studies.

But which six to seven percent is at greatest risk? Rosen (1976), in a well presented study of 886 suicide attempters, identified 144 attempts (16 percent) as medically and/or psychiatrically serious. In a five-year follow-up the serious attempt group had double the suicide rate of the nonserious group. Medical and/or psychiatric seriousness of the attempt appears to predict (to some extent) worse things to come. Ettlinger and Wistrand (1972) found a similar ratio between serious and nonserious attempts on five-year follow-up.

Suicides are not a random sample of suicide attempters. In Rosen's (1976) report, of the 12 serious attempters who ended their own lives, 9 (75 percent) had been diagnosed as suffering from depression (one with schizophrenia as well). Alcoholism complicated three of these depressions and one, organic psychiatric disorder. Psychopathy with drug addiction was diagnosed in one case and no psychiatric diagnosis but neurotic personality was given in another.

The diagnostic distribution was not greatly dissimilar among the 22 nonserious attempters who killed themselves. Depression was diagnosed in 11 (50 percent), 1 of these with schizophrenia and sociopathic personality as well. Alcoholism was identified in 6 cases (27 percent), 5 of them as comorbidity. Various personality disorders made up most of the remainder. Thus, the major psychiatric disorders associated with suicide in this large study were those most prominent in the major studies of suicide: depression and alcoholism.

While seriousness of an attempt appears to hold some prognostic significance for fatal outcome, it is particularly important to note that the apparent triviality of an attempt is not necessarily proportional to seriousness of the risk. A small ingestion, a few scratches on the wrist or neck from a razor blade, the firing of a gun into the air or a wall, may be thought to be histrionic. Depending on underlying diagnosis, it may be a rehearsal for a truly serious assault on the self a few hours or days later.

Suicide attempt in itself may or may not identify persons at greater risk than does clinical diagnosis. It does, however, effectively bring such patients to medical attention. It is generally agreed that the more similar the diagnostic and psychosocial characteristics of an attempter to those of suicides, the greater the risk of a suicidal outcome. Suicide attempts must be taken seriously as an opportunity to assess suicide potential. Issues of importance are psychiatric diagnosis, family history, suicidal intent, method contemplated, seriousness of the act (either medically or psychiatrically), and hopelessness. While 85 to 95 percent of attempters do not go on to suicide, careful clinical assessment can be expected to identify most of those at increased risk.

STEPS TO PREVENTING SUICIDE

Diagnose

All evidence points to the fact that the physician is the most central "gatekeeper" for the prevention of suicide. The physician's first task is to diagnose, with particular attention to the presence and/or history of affective disorder, substance abuse (including alcoholism), schizophrenia, and panic disorder, as each of these conditions has been significantly linked to self-destruction. Since clinical diagnosis is uniquely the province of the physician as well as his or her first priority in patient care, it is important that this skill be well developed and used. Fortunately, the advent of criterion-based psychiatric diagnosis (Feighner et al, 1972; American Psychiatric Association, 1987) has made this a much more reliable undertaking than in the past. Regrettably, no discernible drop in suicide rates has followed.

Treat

The second step in prevention of suicide is adequate treatment of the underlying psychiatric disorder. Due to the fact that all of the psychiatric contributors to suicide produce considerable discomfort and morbidity, and that nearly all are eminently treatable, the issue of false positives is inconsequential. Treatment itself is discussed elsewhere in this volume.

Ask

To further focus on the highest risk patients in the high risk diagnoses, it is important to ask and repeatedly review the question of suicidal ideation. A stepwise approach to the issue is recommended, substantially as follows: "Do you ever wish you would go to sleep and not wake up?" "Do you ever wish you were dead?" "Do you ever think about harming yourself or taking your life?" "Have you ever made a suicide attempt?" (get details) "What have you thought of doing?"

Hospitalize

The patient who has formulated a fully lethal plan and who possesses or can readily access the means to carry it out should be admitted forthwith to a secure psychiatric facility for treatment. In the event the patient refuses hospital admission, steps should be taken to involve the family. If they cannot bring sufficient pressure to bear on the patient to accept admission, their cooperation should be sought in securing involuntary admission of the patient. On occasion, the patient will protest involvement of the family on grounds of professional confidentiality. It is my position that protection of life takes precedence over confidentiality considerations. I tell the patient this and call the family (spouse, parent, whomever) while the patient remains with me in the office. I do not want to allow the patient to go home to pack—and perhaps elope or shoot himself or herself. Failing satisfactory cooperation on the part of the family, charging them to maintain round-the-clock surveillance of the patient will often change their minds in a short time.

Limit Prescribing

In dealing with a new patient who is depressed or a longer-term patient whose depression is worsening, it is important to limit antidepressant prescriptions to a few days' supply until one is comfortable that a suicidal crisis is not in progress. In the days before benzodiazepine hypnotics, a common way for a physician to facilitate a suicide unwittingly was to prescribe a month's supply of a short- or intermediate-acting barbiturate (Murphy, 1975a). With the advent of the safer benzodiazepine hypnotics, tricyclic antidepressants (TCAs) have supplanted barbiturates as a means of suicide by ingestion. Amitriptyline currently ranks fifth among medical examiners' drug mentions, after alcohol (in combination), heroin, cocaine and codeine, while secobarbital has dropped to 13th place (Department of Health and Human Services, 1985, Table II-6, p. 72). If numbers of mentions of various tricyclic antidepressants in the top 40 substances are summed, TCAs replace cocaine as third in frequency of mentions. (It must be kept in mind that a mention is not equivalent to a cause of death. These are the cumulative drug findings by selected medical examiners and thus indicative but not conclusive.)

Remove Firearms

An important precaution whenever the slightest hint of suicidal thinking is detected is to advise the family to remove all firearms from the premises. This includes .22 calibre weapons. Firearms have long been used preferentially by men to accomplish their demise. In recent years, their popularity has gained with women: Firearms have actually supplanted drug overdose as the most common agent of death. With gunshot, the margin of opportunity for effective intervention is virtually nonexistent, in contrast to other common methods. Hanging and other forms of asphyxia, to say nothing of drug overdose, provide at least minutes in which to intervene. Locking up the guns is not enough. They must be removed from the premises.

Treat Vigorously

Hospitalization on a closed psychiatric unit, coupled with vigorous somatic treatment, remains the wisest course when dealing with an acutely suicidal patient. For the severely depressed, electroconvulsive therapy (ECT) is by far the most effective and safest treatment that we psychiatrists have at our disposal (Huston and Locher, 1948a, 1948b; Avery and Winokur, 1978; Tanney, 1986). Atypicality of the depression picture may reduce the response rate to ECT but the question must be decided on an individual basis: In what way is the depression atypical?

Antidepressant pharmacotherapy, with or without psychotherapy, is the second choice in the remaining instances, with psychotherapy alone being reserved for patients with milder depression or those prepared to remain in a secure treatment facility for many months. If substance abuse is present, a detoxification program is indicated when the patient is able to participate (that is, when not too depressed to function). For the depressed schizophrenic, antidepressant medication may be added to the antipsychotic regimen. Occasionally, ECT may be of benefit.

Follow Closely after Discharge

There is a sharp rise in the incidence of suicide in the first few weeks following discharge from the psychiatric hospital (Temoche et al, 1964; Roy, 1982). One possible reason is premature discharge. With hospital costs being what they are and psychiatric hospitalization coverage being limited as it often is, there is considerable pressure to get patients out of the hospital. While this may contribute to the suicide rate immediately after hospital discharge it is not the only factor. After being seen daily by the attending psychiatrist during the inpatient stay, it is not uncommon for patients upon discharge to be given an appointment for two to six weeks hence. The abrupt cessation of physician contact may be interpreted as rejection by the patient. Alternatively, he or she may experience a return of symptoms, and, lacking early scheduled contact with the psychiatrist, may descend rapidly into hopelessness. Close follow-up is indicated after hospital discharge, including provisions for the patient to contact easily his or her psychiatrist in the event of adverse change.

ASSESSMENT OF RISK

Of Little Help:

THE SEX OF THE PATIENT. Although men are approximately three times as likely as women to commit suicide, about twice as many women as men visit physicians. Women are also twice as likely as men to suffer from depression (Robins, et al, 1984). For these reasons there may be little difference by sex in the number of suicidal patients in the average physician's case load. The 3:1 betting odds favoring women does not provide a secure basis for prognostication.

AGE. For many years, the age-rate curve for suicide in white males rose steadily in an almost straight line. In the past 30 years, however, there has been a dramatic increase in suicide among young males. The rate for white males is now virtually flat from age 20 to age 64, rising steadily thereafter (Murphy, 1986). Of some concern is the finding that those under 30 are less likely to have seen a physician than those older (Rich et al, 1986).

MARITAL STATUS. Demographic studies show clearly that the single, the divorced, and the widowed are at statistically greater risk for suicide than are the married. The magnitude of the difference is not great, however. What these nonmarried states have in common is the lower likelihood of a firm social support system or a sense of connectedness to others. In the presence of one of the relevant psychiatric illnesses, it is advisable to inquire as to the existence and quality of emotional and/or social support. Since most of the adult population of the United States is married, the great majority of suicides are married. This is substantially less true for those under 30, who, interestingly enough, may be *less* likely to be living alone (Rich et al, 1986).

COMMUNICATION OF SUICIDAL THOUGHTS AS SUCH. A great many people, perhaps the majority, have fleeting thoughts of suicide. In and of itself, such a thought may reflect fear, anger, frustration or other negative emotion. It is only in the context of certain psychiatric illnesses that suicidal thinking takes on grave significance. The circumstances giving rise to the self-destructive impulse are important to determine, as well as the degree of evolution of a suicide plan and the availability of the means under consideration.

Consider Serious

CLINICALLY DEPRESSED. As the single greatest contributor to suicide, a diagnosis of affective disorder, depressed, must keep the clinician alert to the development of serious suicidal intent. Depression complicating another illness has the same potential.

SUICIDE ATTEMPT IN A PERSON OVER AGE 35. Suicide attempt is predominantly the province of the young. When it occurs in later years, it is usually associated with more serious psychopathology, particularly depression or substance abuse. In general, the closer the resemblance of the suicide attempter's diagnostic and psychosocial profile to that of described suicides, the greater the risk.

SELF-ORIENTED REASON FOR DEATH WISH. The typical suicide attempter wants something from others. When the wish to die relates to an internal state only—hopelessness, a profound sense of guilt, or pain—it closely resembles the truly presuicidal state. In general, the greater this resemblance, the greater the risk.

ABSENCE OF IMMEDIATE PRECIPITANT OF SUICIDAL THINKING. Depending on diagnosis, a suicide attempt or threat in the immediate wake of an upsetting event is sometimes an expression of anger, frustration, or spite. In the absence of such a precipitant, the same considerations apply as in the immediately preceding item. While the absence of a precipitant in relation to suicidal thoughts is ominous, the presence of such a circumstance is no indication of inconsequentiality of the risk. In the presence of interpersonal disruption the risk is increased in substance abusers.

SUICIDAL COMMUNICATION IN AFFECTIVE DISORDER. When suicidal thinking reaches the point where it spills over spontaneously into everyday discourse, it is likely to have become a preoccupation. Risk is accordingly likely to be high. Reports of family members concerning this behavior should be taken with great seriousness.

LETHAL METHOD CONSIDERED AND AVAILABLE. A depressed young woman replied to my inquiry as to suicidal thinking the following way: "For the last three mornings I have gone down to the railroad overpass near my apartment and timed when the morning freight train comes by. I'm thinking of jumping in front of the train." I arranged for her immediate hospitalization where she received ECT and secured a complete remission of her depression. The means of suicide under consideration was not a common one, but it could be expected to be lethal and was certainly available.

RECENTLY CHANGED BEHAVIOR. This calls for a diagnostic evaluation. The most important cause to be considered is the advent or worsening of a depression and its attendant risk for suicide. A recent behavior change in an alcoholic may be evidence of the development or worsening of a depression. Most alcoholics who commit suicide are depressed as well (Murphy et al, 1979). Worsening of behavior in the young may represent the onset or worsening of depression. Suicide is more often impulsive in the young, rather than planned. Follow closely.

RECENT OR IMPENDING INTERPERSONAL LOSS IN SUBSTANCE ABUSER. One-third or more of substance abusers taking their own lives have experienced this type of loss within six weeks of their suicide (Murphy and Robins, 1967; Murphy et al, 1979; Rich et al, in press).

SCHIZOPHRENIA. The lifetime risk of suicide in schizophrenia is 10 to 13 percent. Data on the comorbidity and complicating factors relating to this outcome are thin. Few cautions can be given with any degree of confidence. It seems likely that a suicide attempt, a secondary depression, and particularly the advent of hopelessness are clues to increased risk.

HOPELESSNESS. As a state of mind in any of the above circumstances, hopelessness is likely to indicate increased risk for suicide.

REFERENCES

American Psychiatric Association, Committee on Nomenclature and Statistics: Diagnostic and Statistical Manual of Mental Disorders, Third Edition, Revised. Washington, DC, American Psychiatric Association, 1987

Avery D, Winokur G: Suicide, attempted suicide and relapse rates in depression. Arch Gen Psychiatry 1978; 35:749-753

Bagley C: The evaluation of a suicide prevention scheme by an ecological method. Soc Sci Med 1968; 2:1-14

Barraclough BM, Shea M: Suicide and Samaritan clients. Lancet 1970; 2:686-870

Barraclough B, Bunch J, Nelson B, et al: A hundred cases of suicide: clinical aspects. Br J Psychiatry 1974; 125:355-373

Barraclough BM, Jennings C, Moss JR: Suicide prevention by the Samaritans: a controlled study of effectiveness. Lancet 1977; 2:237-238

Beck AT, Weissman A, Lester D, et al: The measurement of pessimism: the Hopelessness Scale. J Consult Clin Psychol 1974; 42:861-865

Beck AT, Kovacs M, Weissman A: Hopelessness and suicidal behavior: an overview. JAMA 1975; 234:1146-1149

Beck AT, Steer RA, Kovacs M, et al: Hopelessness and eventual suicide: a 10-year prospective study of patients hospitalized with suicidal ideation. Am J Psychiatry 1985; 142:559-563

Beskow J: Suicide and mental disorder in Swedish men. Acta Psychiatr Scand 1979; (suppl. 277):138

Blueler M: The Schizophrenic Disorders. New Haven, Yale University, 1978

Cheynoweth R, Tonge JI, Armstrong J. Suicide in Brisbane—a retrospective psychosocial study. Austr NZ J Psychiatry 1980; 14:37-45

Cloninger CR, Reich T, Guze SB: The multifactorial model of disease transmission, III: familial relationship between sociopathy and hysteria. Br J Psychiatry 1975; 127:23-32

Cohen S, Leonard CV, Farberow NL, et al: Tranquilizers and suicide in the schizophrenic patient. Arch Gen Psychiatry 1964; 11:312-321

Coryell W: Diagnosis-specific mortality: primary unipolar depression and Briquet's syndrome (somatization disorder). Arch Gen Psychiatry 1981; 38:939-942

Coryell W, Noyes R, Clancy J: Excess mortality in panic disorder: a comparison with primary unipolar depression. Arch Gen Psychiatry 1982; 39:701-703

Coryell W, Noyes R, Clancy J: Panic disorder and primary unipolar depression: a comparison of background and outcome. J Affective Disord 1983; 5:311-317

Coryell W, Noyes R Jr, House JD: Mortality among outpatients with anxiety disorders. Am J Psychiatry 1986; 143:508-510

Delong WB, Robins E: The communciation of suicidal intent prior to psychiatric hospitalization: a study of 87 patients. Am J Psychiatry 1961; 117:695-705

Department of Health and Human Services, U.S. Public Health Service, Alcohol, Drug Abuse, and Mental Health Administration: National Institute on Drug Abuse Statistical Series. Series G, Number 16. Semiannual Report. January–June 1985. Washington, DC, U.S. Government Printing Office, 1985

Dorpat TL, Ripley HS. A study of suicide in the Seattle area. Compr Psychiatry 1960; 1:349-359

Drake RE, Cotton PG. Depression, hopelessness and suicide in chronic schizophrenia. Br J Psychiatry 1986; 148:554-559

Drake RE, Gates C, Whitaker A, et al: Suicide among schizophrenics: a review. Compr Psychiatry 1985; 26:90-100

Endicott J, Spitzer RL: A diagnostic interview: the Schedule for Affective Disorders and Schizophrenia. Arch Gen Psychiatry 1978; 35:837-844

Ettlinger R: Suicides in a group of patients who had previously attempted suicide. Acta Psychiatr Scand 1964; 40:363-378

Ettlinger R: Evaluation of suicide prevention after attempted suicide. Acta Psychiatr Scand 1975; (suppl 260)

Ettlinger R, Wistrand M: Somatic sequelae, in Suicide and Attempted Suicide. Edited by Waldenstrom J, Larsson, T, Ljungstedt N. Stockholm, Nordiska Bokhandelns Forlag, 1972

Fawcett J, Scheftner W, Clark D, et al: Clinical predictors of suicide in patients with major affective disorders: a controlled prospective study. Am J Psychiatry 1987; 144:35-40

Feighner JP, Robins E. Guze SB, et al: Diagnostic criteria for use in psychiatric research. Arch Gen Psychiatry 1972; 26:57-63

Fowler RC, Rich CL, Young D: San Diego suicide study, II: substance abuse in young cases. Arch Gen Psychiatry 1986; 43:962-965

Galen RS, Gambino SR: Beyond Normality: The Predictive Value and Efficiency of Medical Diagnoses. New York, John Wiley & Sons, 1975

Guze SB, Robins E: Suicide and primary affective disorders. Br J Psychiatry 1970; 117:437-438

Huston PE, Locher LM. Involutional psychosis: Course when untreated and when treated with electric shock. Arch Neurol Psychiatry 1948a; 59:385-394

Huston PE, Locher LM: Manic depressive psychosis: course when treated and untreated with electric shock. Arch Neurol Psychiatry 1984b; 60:37-48

Katz MM, Secunda SK, Hirschfeld RMA, et al: NIMH clinical research branch collaborative program on the psychobiology of depression. Arch Gen Psychiatry 1979; 36:765-771

MacKinnon DR, Farberow NL: An assessment of the utility of suicide prediction. Suicide Life Threat Behav 1976; 6:86-91

Miller HL, Coombs DW, Leeper JD, et al: An analysis of the effects of suicide prevention facilities on suicide rates in the United States. Am J Public Health 1984; 74:340-343

Morrison JR: Suicide in a psychiatric practice population. J Clin Psychiatry 1982; 43:348-352

Motto JA: The psychopathology of suicide: a clinical model approach. Am J Psychiatry 1979; 136:516-520

Motto JA: Suicide risk factors in alcohol abuse. Suicide Life Threat Behav 1980; 10:230-238

Motto JA, Heilbron DC, Juster RP: Development of a clinical instrument to estimate suicide risk. Am J Psychiatry 1985; 142:680-686

Murphy GE: The physician's responsibility for suicide, I: an error of commission. Ann Intern Med 1975a; 82:301-304

Murphy GE. The physician's responsibility for suicide, II: errors of omission. Ann Intern Med 1975b; 82:305-309

Murphy GE: The prediction of suicide: why is it so difficult? Am J Psychother 1984; 38:341-349

Murphy GE: Suicide and attempted suicide, in The Medical Basis of Psychiatry. Edited by Winokur G, Clayton P. Philadelphia, W.B. Saunders, 1986

Murphy GE, Robins E: Social factors in suicide. JAMA 1967; 199:303-308

Murphy GE, Wetzel RD, Swallow CS, et al: Who calls the suicide prevention center: a study of 55 persons calling on their own behalf. Am J Psychiatry 1969; 126:314-324

Murphy GE, Armstrong JW, Hermele SL, et al: Suicide and alcoholism: interpersonal loss confirmed as a predictor. Arch Gen Psychiatry 1979; 36:65-69

Pallis DJ, Barraclough BM, Levey AB, et al: Estimating suicide risk among attempted suicides, I: the development of new clinical scales. Br J Psychiatry 1982; 141:37-44

Parkin D, Stengel E: Incidence of suicidal attempts in an urban community. Br Med J 1965; 2:133-138

Pitts FN Jr, Winokur G: Affective disorder, VII: alcoholism and affective disorder. J Psychiatr Res 1966; 4:37-50

Pokorny AD: Prediction of suicide in psychiatric patients. Arch Gen Psychiatry 1983; 40:249-257

Rich CL, Young D, Fowler RC: San Diego suicide study, I: young vs old subjects. Arch Gen Psychiatry 1986; 43:577-582

Rich CL, Fowler RC, Fogarty LA, et al: San Diego suicide study, III: relationships between diagnoses and stressors. Arch Gen Psychiatry (in press).

Robins E. The Final Months: A Study of the Lives of 134 Persons who Committed Suicide. New York, Oxford University Press, 1981

Robins E: Psychosis and suicide. Biol Psychiatry 1986; 21:665-672

Robins E, Gassner S, Kayes J, et al: The communication of suicidal intent: a study of 134 consecutive cases of successful (completed) suicide. Am J Psychiatry 1959a; 115:724-733

Robins E, Murphy GE, Wilkinson RH, et al: Some clinical considerations in the prevention of suicide based on a study of 134 successful suicides. Am J Public Health 1959b; 49:888-899

Robins LN, Helzer JE, Weissman MM, et al: Lifetime prevalence of specific psychiatric disorders in three states. Arch Gen Psychiatry 1984; 41:949-958

Rosen DH: The serious suicide attempt: five-year follow-up study of 886 patients. JAMA 1976; 235:2105-2109

Roy A: Suicide in chronic schizophrenia. Br J Psychiatry 1982; 141:171-177

Stengel E: A survey of follow-up examinations of attempted suicides, in Suicide and Attempted Suicide. Edited by Waldenstrom J, Larsson T, Ljungstedt N. Stockholm, Nordiska Bokhandelns Forlag, 1972

Tanney BL: Electroconvulsive therapy and suicide. Suicide Life Threat Behav 1986; 16:198-222

Temoche A, Pugh RF, MacMahon B: Suicide rates among current and former mental institution patients. J Nerv Ment Dis 1964; 138:124-130

Tsuang MT: Suicide in schizophrenics, manics, depressives, and surgical controls. Arch Gen Psychiatry 1978; 35:153-155

Wetzel RD: Hopelessness, depression and suicide intent. Arch Gen Psychiatry 1976; 33:1069-1073

Wetzel RD, Margulies T, Davis R, et al: Hopelessness, depression and suicide intent. J Clin Psychiatry 1980; 41:159-160

Wheeler EO, White PD, Reed EW, et al: Neurocirculatory asthenia (anxiety neurosis, effort syndrome, neurasthenia): a twenty-year follow-up study of 173 patients. JAMA 1950; 142:878-889

Wilkins J: A follow-up study of those who called a suicide prevention center. Am J Psychiatry 1970; 127:73-79

Wold CI, Litman RE: Suicide after contact with a suicide prevention center. Arch Gen Psychiatry 1973; 28:735-739

Afterword

by J. John Mann, M.D., and Michael Stanley, Ph.D.

Suicide is a major cause of mortality in the United States. Some psychiatrists have found a certain comfort in the notion that although their patients are in distress and experience emotional pain, they do not suffer from a potentially fatal illness. However, epidemiological studies paint a very different picture. The rate of suicide as a percentage of all causes of death in psychiatric patients is approximately 20 percent in manic-depressive patients; 15 percent in alcoholic patients; 15 percent in patients with a depressive disorder; and 10–13 percent in schizophrenics. The importance of suicide as a cause of death in psychiatric patients is easily overlooked unless a systematic long-term follow-up is carried out. The longer the follow-up, the higher the rate of suicide that is found, indicating that many suicides are not detected by clinicians simply because they lose contact with the patient. The patient who is no longer coming for treatment is assumed to have found treatment elsewhere or to have merely dropped out of treatment. The possibility of suicide is often overlooked.

Having recognized the magnitude of the problem, the next step is to develop guidelines for determining who is at risk. The task is very difficult precisely because although the carefully reviewed list of risk factors provided by Hirschfeld and Davidson describes most suicide victims, it also describes many more patients who will never commit suicide. Cohen (1986) has summarized the problem. If we take the highest suicide risk groups (past attemptors, depressive disorders, and so on) the prevalence rate is about one to two percent per year. Assume the availability of a hypothetical superpredictor with a sensitivity of 90 percent (detects 9 out of 10 patients who will commit suicide) and a specificity of 90 percent (9 out of 10 patients predicted to suicide will do so). This predictor is far better than any currently available but is still very inadequate. The problem is that the base rate of suicide is very low even in the highest risk groups. If we assume a suicide rate of one percent per year (the rate in the general population is about 12 in 100,000, which is approximately 0.01 percent) and then apply our superpredictor, the false positive rate of our predictor would be 92 percent! In other words, if we screened 10,000 cases, the predictor would designate 1,080 as potential suicides, of whom 990 would *not* commit suicide.

As pessimistic as the situation may seem, there is another practical aspect to consider. We now know that almost all of these 1,080 patients will be suffering from a serious psychiatric disorder (see Chapters 14 and 16). Psychiatric treatment of these patients is therefore indicated on grounds *in addition* to suicide prevention and such treatment does not represent a "wasted" effort.

Robins and Kulbok describe major shifts in the segments of the population at the greatest risk for suicide. In 1950, the suicide rate in the 15- to 24-year-old group was one-tenth that of those 75 years or older. In 1980, that ratio of older versus younger suicide rates had dropped to only 3.6 to 1. Why had the rate dropped so dramatically in the age groups 45–70 years and risen markedly in males under the age of 45 years? Clearly the genetic factors had not changed significantly. The explanation lies in the environment. One possible explanation for the decline in the suicide rate in the 45- to 70-year-old group is the availability and improved method of use of more effective antidepressant medications for depressive disorders. The increase in suicide rate in the under 40-year-old group is largely confined to men, suggesting a specific vulnerability in men to changing psychosocial risk factors.

Availability of method may play some role in suicide rates. There was a decline in the suicide rate associated with the detoxification of cooking gas. There have been reports of a link between the increase in suicide rates in young males and the increased availability of handguns in the United States. As a general rule, the more difficult it is to find the means with which to commit suicide, the greater the possibility of a therapeutic intervention. This approach argues for restricting the availability of handguns and for wrapping each pill of a potentially lethal medication individually in foil so as to reduce the possibility of impulsive suicides. Unfortunately, there is *another* significant group of suicides that are carried out after careful planning. Such planned suicides are less likely to be significantly reduced in number by making the means of suicide more difficult to obtain.

Certain medical illnesses (particularly those with a central neurological component involving the brain) are associated with higher suicide rates. Examples of such illnesses are Huntington's disease and Acquired Immune Deficiency Syndrome (AIDS), and they require vigilance for suicide risk on the part of the physician. Moreover, study of the specific biological effects on the brain of these illnesses may provide further clues as to the biological correlates of suicide.

A risk factor of substantial research and ultimately clinical significance is the genetic predisposition for suicide. The existence of a genetic risk factor for suicide has been established by twin, family, and adoption studies. The presence of such a genetic factor raises the possibility that psychological or biological traits may ultimately be detected that may prove to be of diagnostic value. It means that the best predictor of suicide, namely, a previous suicide attempt, may also be viewed as evidence for this genetic predisposition. The same holds true for a family history of suicide, which had often been regarded as a risk factor that operated psychologically but now may also be interpreted as a biological risk factor.

Evidence is also presented by Drs. Hirschfeld and Davidson in Chapter 14, as well as by Dr. Brent and colleagues in Chapter 16, for the impact of personality disorders on suicide risk. Moreover, it appears a higher risk for suicide exists in patients who suffer from both an Axis I and certain Axis II diagnoses in whom comorbidity appears to represent *separate additive risks* for suicide. Such separate additive risks could operate by both psychological and biological mechanisms. The biological and psychological mechanisms or traits may be partly genetic in origin, including the traits that comprise the personality disorder.

A correlation has been established between reduced serotonergic function and violent suicide. This relationship appears to hold true across diagnostic boundaries, and the data are reviewed in detail in Chapter 15. Low levels of 5-hydroxy-indoleacetic acid (5-HIAA), the major metabolite of serotonin, have been found in the cerebrospinal fluid (CSF) of patients making violent suicide attempts compared to nonattemptors with the same diagnosis. This finding holds true for depressive disorders, schizophrenia, and personality disorders. Several studies of postmortem brain tissue have shown lower levels of 5-HT or 5-HIAA, as well as alterations in serotonin receptors, consistent with reduced serotonin activity and compensatory postsynaptic receptor supersensitivity. Neuroendocrine studies have found a relationship between blunted serotonergic responsiveness and suicidal acts. Data from CSF studies suggest that impaired serotonergic activity may be a *trait*. This trait may be a phenotypic expression of the genetic risk factor for suicide.

There are therapeutic implications of these changes. If the serotonergic system's function is diminished in patients at risk for suicide, then it may be *hypothesized* that enhancing serotonergic function, pharmacologically or by electroconvulsive therapy (ECT), should reduce suicide risk. Antidepressants that inhibit serotonin reuptake, such as chlomipramine, imipramine, fluoxetine, or amitriptyline; inhibit monoamine oxidase, such as phenelzine; and increase serotonin turnover, such as lithium, should be of therapeutic value in reducing suicide risk regardless of whether the suicidal patient is suffering from a depressive *or* a nonaffective disorder such as schizophrenia or a personality disorder. This important treatment corollary of the serotonin hypothesis of suicide remains to be tested in a controlled study.

The choice of the antidepressant should be based on safety, especially given the risk of an overdose. Newer antidepressants such as fluoxetine have a safety advantage over tricyclics in the case of overdose.

In constructing a model that describes suicide, it is clear that several causal and facilitatory factors must be considered. No single factor is sufficient alone. There are psychological and biological traits (at least partly inherited) that place certain individuals at risk. These individuals may never actually experience suicidal ideation or make an attempt unless some other factors come into play. Such additional factors may include alcoholism, a depressive illness, schizophrenia, divorce, a physical illness, among others. Mitigating factors such as a family support system, psychiatric intervention, or recognition on the part of the patient of a need for help must also be considered.

Figure 1 attempts to describe this multifactorial model of suicide. It distinguishes between state and trait effects and emphasizes the multifactorial contribution to the endpoint of a suicidal act.

From this model it is possible to develop treatment strategies. It may be hypothesized that interventions that ameliorate some, but not all, factors will avert the danger of suicide. This is fortunate since it is unlikely that any treatment plan for an individual patient will identify and be able to treat any more than some of the factors contributing to suicide risk.

It is within this overall plan that Drs. Brent and colleagues and Dr. Murphy set out to provide some guidelines for treatment and prevention. Only guidelines are offered because, to date, no specific intervention has been shown to prevent suicide in a controlled prospective study. Thus, treatment suggestions are basically hypothetical, although at a practical level, they will also be beneficial for the Axis I and Axis II disorders associated with suicidal risk. Since these disorders contribute to risk, their treatment should reduce the risk for suicide.

What about the specific management of the suicide risk? This involves several pragmatic steps that include: 1) remove all possible means for committing suicide; 2) maintain increased surveillance of the suicidal patient; 3) activate support systems; and 4) maximize opportunity for patients to discuss their suicidal feelings and their perceived causes of such feelings with a qualified mental health

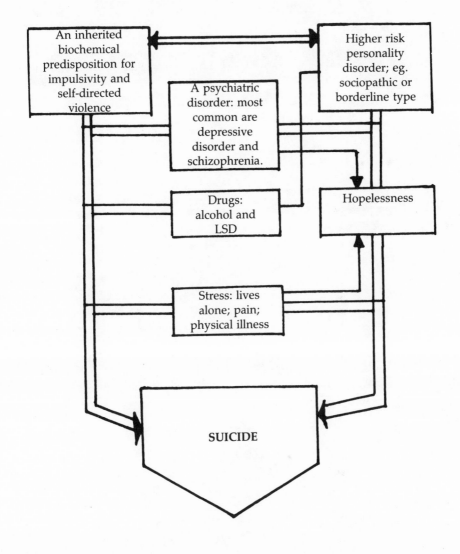

Figure 1. A psychobiological model of suicide.

professional. Psychiatrists should admit patients to the hospital if in doubt about their safety. Prediction of risk is difficult but that does not preclude the need for a careful evaluation. Ultimately, although these suggestions seem to make good sense, they will all require careful scientific evaluation by prospective controlled studies. How to conduct such studies may present an ethical challenge to psychiatry because studies of the effectiveness of any treatment in preventing suicide will involve large numbers of patients and carries the risk of suicide in the "placebo" group. However, given the high rate of mortality due to suicide in psychiatric patients, and the absence of any scientifically proven effective treatments, we cannot afford to wait. Psychiatry must face this therapeutic challenge now.

REFERENCES

Cohen J: Statistical approaches to suicidal risk factor analysis, in Psychobiology of Suicidal Behavior. Edited by Mann JJ, Stanley M. New York, Annals of the New York Academy of Sciences, 1986.

IV

Electroconvulsive Therapy

IV

Electro-convulsive Therapy

Section IV

Electroconvulsive Therapy

Foreword

by Robert M. Rose, M.D., and Harold Alan Pincus, M.D., Section Editors

If one were to ask almost any practicing psychiatrist what is the most controversial, currently utilized treatment in our profession, it is almost certain that the answer would be electroconvulsive therapy (ECT). It is also probable that the reasons given for this continuing controversy, should this also be inquired after, would differ, ranging from perceptions of lack of efficacy, to questions persisting about possible brain damage, concerns about its intrusive, even demeaning nature, along with a perspective of its being more punitive than therapeutic, not to mention concerns about its legality. This list is neither complete nor overly dramatic in capturing the ambivalence about ECT in our profession. In 1978 an APA survey of members reported that one-third of us felt "generally opposed" or "more opposed than favorable" to its use.

Of course, the ultimate utility of any particular form of treatment in medicine must be assessed by a consideration of the data regarding efficacy, indications, side effects, and so on. It is our intent in this section to provide a systematic description of the current literature to assist clinicians in making informed decisions about the use of this procedure.

Importantly, because of the still widespread concerns about the appropriateness of ECT, its being the focus of attack by several patient advocacy groups, we have attempted in this introduction to place ECT in some historical perspective, including some discussion of the origins of the controversy surrounding its use.

We have been tremendously assisted in our review of ECT by the occurrence two years ago of a Consensus Development Conference on Electroconvulsive Therapy, organized by the Office of Medical Applications of Research (OMAR) of the National Institutes of Health (NIH), and jointly sponsored by NIH and the National Institute of Mental Health (NIMH).

These consensus conferences are designed specifically to examine important and controversial issues in medicine, with the goal of achieving a consensus statement from a panel of scientists and clinicians, but also including legal and public representatives. Input is solicited from the audience, along with presentations from experts in the field, and the resulting consensus statement is not only published in the archival literature (see the *Journal of the American Medical Association,* 1985, for the ECT statement), but was also mailed to 21,000 persons and institutions.

One of the editors of this section (RMR) chaired the conference and the other of us (HAP) was instrumental in the planning process for it. The intensity of the controversy that still surrounds ECT became very clear to us, along with some appreciation of how painfully held are the memories of ECT for some individuals.

The panelists participating in the conference were also impressed with the need for our profession to pursue two crucial goals. The first was to attempt to communicate the value of ECT for certain, selected patients, along with a second parallel task of establishing appropriate, widely disseminated, and consistently utilized guidelines for the administration of ECT.

This section can be viewed as an elaboration and further extension of the answers to the five questions that were addressed in the final consensus statement:

1. What is the evidence that ECT is effective for patients with specific mental disorders?
2. What are the risks and adverse effects of ECT?
3. What factors should be considered by the physician and patient in determining if and when ECT would be an appropriate treatment?
4. How should ECT be administered to maximize benefits and minimize risks?
5. What are the directions for future research?

The answers to these questions—how useful is it and for which patients; how to do it; what are the risks to be avoided; how it may work; as well as what are the current relevant legal and ethical issues—are well covered in this section.

ECT is first and foremost a convulsive therapy. The use of an electric current to induce a seizure is primarily a matter of ease and safety of administration compared to chemical induction. This is relevant, as some concern still exists relating to the use of electricity in the minds of the public, and perhaps even among some professionals ("frying the brain," "shocking therapy," and so on). It is also the basis of some of the persistent concerns that are voiced regarding brain damage, for which there is no clear, consistent evidence. The evidence leading to this conclusion of the consensus panel is well reviewed by Dr. Gary S. Sachs and Dr. Alan J. Gelenberg in Chapter 22.

However, it is essentially impossible to prove that something never happens, as we are restricted to the limits of sensitivity of our current techniques and instruments. Nevertheless, it is fair to conclude that the induction of seizure activity by the use of brief pulsed or sinusoidal current, as is done in ECT, does not cause brain damage. Similarly, the occurrence of seizures per se is not a cause of brain tissue injury.

Despite any clarification of the essential quality of ECT involving induction of a convulsive episode, we are unlikely to free ourselves from the stigma attached to this form of treatment by merely emphasizing the essential underlying physiological event. Besides, even many psychiatrists still utilize the term "electroshock therapy" or EST. We must look elsewhere to address the intensity and persistence of the controversy.

ECT evolved in the 1930s in the context of the development of various forms of somatic therapy intended to help those with major disabling neuropsychiatric disorders. Wagner-Jauregg had developed malarial fever therapy for the treatment of neurosyphilis, for which he received the Nobel Prize in 1927. Somewhat later, Moniz developed the technique of prefrontal lobotomy, for which he was also awarded the Nobel Prize. A Hungarian neuropsychiatrist, Ladislas Meduna, attempted to utilize what was felt at the time to be a clinical antagonism between epilepsy and dementia praecox. He believed that the induction of seizures might be clinically efficacious in altering the course of this illness. He utilized metrazol for seizure induction, which was modified by Cerletti and Bini in Italy in 1938 with their use of electric current. Also at this time convulsive therapy was found to be effective in patients with melancholia. Curare began to be used in 1940 in an attempt to reduce the incidence of fractures that too often occurred with unmodified, intense seizure activity. Indoklon was also used after World War II for seizure induction, but gradually was replaced by electroconvulsive therapy.

It must be recalled that the late 1930s, the 1940s, and the early 1950s was an era essentially without any other form of clearly effective therapy for major depression, mania, or schizophrenia. There was insulin coma, prefrontal lobotomy, and ECT. There were no neuroleptics, no tricyclic antidepressants, and no lithium. So in the 1940s ECT began to be used, and used extensively. Perhaps the overly rapid embracing of this new, seemingly most effective treatment, and the intensity of enthusiasm for it can be judged from the highly critical comment on ECT use from the GAP report of 1947. This report cautioned against its excessive and indiscriminate use by some psychiatrists. This was only seven years following its introduction into the United States.

Part and parcel of this excessive and, at times, clearly inappropriate use, was the practice that developed of utilizing ECT to control unwanted, bothersome, or even socially undesired behavior in certain patients. This practice, no matter how circumscribed, was crucial in sowing the seeds of controversy about ECT, and contributed to its being viewed by a not insignificant portion of the public as more a form of punishment than a useful therapeutic treatment.

Our understanding of the evolution of the controversy has been helped enormously by the scholarly review undertaken by Professor David Rothman (Rothman, 1985) as a background paper prepared for presentation at the ECT Consensus Development Conference. In this discussion of the nature of the controversy over ECT practices we have borrowed heavily from his paper, entitled "ECT: The Historical, Social, and Professional Sources of the Controversy."

One may quarrel with the depiction of violent, unmodified seizures following administration of ECT to the hero in the film *One Flew Over the Cookoo's Nest*. One may also be concerned with its continuing powerful message of how ECT was used so inappropriately, and worry about how frightened anyone who views this poignant film might become if, after viewing it, and in need of treatment, they were told of how beneficial ECT could be for them. At the same time, however, one cannot dismiss a major issue this film so intensely projects. It was not used for treating any specific illness, though one might argue about McMurphy's "sociopathy." Its primary purpose was control, to diminish or eliminate his undesirable, disruptive, and clearly highly inconvenient behavior. And, of course, as part of its use to control, there was no attempt to request informed consent, nor was any such need ever hinted at.

This theme of ECT being used so coercively is most coincident with the assertions of many of psychiatry's most vocal critics, such as Szasz, along with some patient groups such as the Network Against Psychiatric Assault (NAPA). They claim the essential function of psychiatry is to control, not treat.

As pointed out by Klerman (1985) in his introduction to the consensus conference on the use of various somatic treatments for psychiatric illness, this perspective of psychiatry's role as primarily an agent for social control extends beyond individual critics or antipsychiatry patient groups. It can be viewed as an outgrowth of labeling theorists in sociology and social psychology, who emphasized the negative social consequences of being labeled mentally ill.

In any event, it is clear that ECT became and continues to function as a lightning rod and a key rallying point by psychiatry's critics against what they perceive as the most egregious tool utilized by us to manipulate those not complying with society's expectations, or those that are just "out of control."

Unfortunately, there are significant elements of truth to the assertion that ECT was used at times primarily for control, which comes from the profession itself. Rothman quotes a study reported in 1950 about the use of ECT on chronic patients in California. "Our goals were not curative; they were limited to the level of improved ward behavior." Aggressive patients were started on daily ECT until they became manageable, and the researchers stated that they judged ECT a success because the "physical labor of attendants was cut in half." Rothman continues to point out that the line between managing a patient and punishing a patient is very thin, and concludes that this issue is clearly a most important one in the unfortunate development of ECT's reputation as a punishment.

Given these historical problems in ECT use, it is also important and relevant to point out that the consensus statement and authors of this section emphasize that ECT is a safe and effective treatment primarily for major depression, mania, and, in certain circumstances, for schizophrenia. It is not intended for treatment of a variety of other problems, such as alcoholism, other addictions, personality disorders, dysthymic or anxiety states, and certainly not to be employed as a technique for behavioral control, which can be viewed as emphasizing and utilizing the side effects of ECT; that is, acute confusional state and memory loss, which can and should be minimized with proper techniques.

Rothman and others have pointed to another major issue that contributes significantly to the ECT controversy. This relates to the absence of clearly articulated guidelines and regulations to implement such guidelines. There are certain risks to ECT treatment, and there are clear strategies available to minimize the occurrence of such risks; these are well outlined in Chapter 21, by Dr. Max Fink. However, there is evidence that there exists considerable variability in the skill and sophistication employed in giving ECT in this country, probably not very dissimilar to what was found in the national survey in Great Britain conducted and reported by Pippard and Ellam (1981). They reported that approximately one-quarter of ECT centers in England were "unsatisfactory" or had "very serious shortcomings." In addition, they found that 41 percent of the physicians usually present during ECT treatment sessions had only minimal training, and supervision was usually lax.

It also can be persuasively argued that ECT treatment has many similarities to other, highly effective medical and surgical interventions, yet there is a general absence of peer oversight committees, such as tissue audit committees, to review operative procedures. Thus, in its endorsement and support of ECT treatment, the consensus panel also emphasized the need for the dissemination of appropriate guidelines.

The panel believes it is imperative that appropriate mechanisms be established to ensure proper standards and monitoring of ECT. Hospitals and centers using ECT should establish review committees modeled on other medicosurgical review committees and should formulate rules and regulations to govern privileging of physicians giving the treatments. (JAMA, p. 2107)

There is another major problem associated with the continuing controversy surrounding ECT. While initially there was excessive use of ECT, currently there is evidence to suggest that ECT is not available to all those who might benefit. In a recent article Thompson and Blaine (1987), in reviewing ECT use in the United States, found in 1980 that between 4.6 and 4.9 percent of psychiatric patients admitted to general hospitals received ECT, but only 0.3 percent of patients in state and county mental hospitals received ECT. The interpretation that the poor and disadvantaged, who are most often patients in the state hospitals, are less likely to receive ECT is further bolstered by their observation that:

> Nonwhite admissions were much less likely to receive ECT than were white admissions, even when the number of admissions of whites and nonwhites was controlled for. In some types of facilities, almost no people of color received ECT—for example, the sample of state mental hospital patients in 1980 did not include a single nonwhite patient who received ECT (Thompson and Blaine, p. 560).

It is hard to imagine that there was not a single nonwhite patient with endogenous, drug resistant, major depression in a state hospital during all of 1980 who might not have benefited significantly from ECT. It is also reasonable to conclude that the administrators responsible for setting policy in many state institutions have been reluctant to utilize ECT, given the intensity of controversy and the large number of state legislatures (37) that have rules on the books regarding ECT use. However, as reviewed by Winslade, there has been some change in attitude, both judicial and legislative, regarding ECT so as to permit its use when medically indicated.

If we are successful as a profession in informing ourselves about its efficacy, indications, side effects, the importance of the informed consent process, as well as the appropriate techniques to be employed in administering ECT, it is highly likely that we will not only see substantially less legislative involvement, but also we will be able to provide this important treatment to all who can benefit from its often dramatic and even life-saving effects.

REFERENCES

Consensus Conference: Electroconvulsive therapy. JAMA 1985; 254:2103-2108

Klerman GL: The use of somatic treatments for psychiatric illnesses: program and abstracts, Consensus Development Conference on ECT. Washington, DC, OMAR NIH, 1985

Pippard J, Ellam L: Electroconvulsive treatment in Great Britain, 1980. London, Gaskell, 1981

Rothman D: ECT: the historical, social and professional sources of the controversy: program and abstracts, Consensus Development Conference on ECT. Washington, DC, OMAR NIH, 1985

Thompson JW, Blaine JD: Use of ECT in the United States in 1975 and 1980. A J Psychiatry 1987; 144:557-562

Chapter 19

Mechanisms of Action of Electroconvulsive Therapy

by Harold A. Sackeim, Ph.D.

Electroconvulsive therapy (ECT) is often regarded as the most controversial treatment used in psychiatry. Fueling the controversy is the frequently repeated criticism that we are ignorant of how ECT works, both in producing therapeutic change and with respect to adverse side effects. This criticism is both correct and incorrect.

Like all other psychiatric somatic treatments, we do not have a detailed and complete understanding of the mechanisms of action of ECT. In this respect, ECT remains an empiric form of therapy. Its use is justified by its rate of therapeutic success relative to its associated side effects.

On the other hand, after 50 years of research on convulsive therapies, we can safely rule out some views as to how ECT might work. Indeed, soon after the introduction of ECT, Gordon (1948) described 50 theories of ECT mechanisms of action. Since then the list has increased considerably. Particularly early in its history, the therapeutic properties of ECT were often attributed to psychological factors, such as fear of treatment, punishment for guilt feelings, enhancement of repression, and the development of confusion and amnesia. Prior to recent neuropathological investigations (for example, Dam and Dam, 1986; Meldrum, 1986), some investigators emphasized structural brain changes, which were usually thought to be an outcome of hypoxia and cyanosis. Both historically and currently, the neurophysiological changes induced by ECT have been a source of theories concerning therapeutic and adverse effects. These 'essential' neurophysiological changes have been viewed either as a direct result of electrical stimulation of neural tissue or as a consequence of the elicitation of grand mal seizures. Neurophysiological theories have emphasized changes in the electroencephalogram (EEG), blood–brain barrier, neurometabolism, seizure duration, and seizure threshold as critical to mechanisms of action. At the biochemical level, competing theories have been offered concerning the unique importance of particular neurotransmitter and peptide systems, with debate as to whether the critical changes pertain to concentration, turnover, or receptor physiology within the relevant system. As described below, some of the progress in the field has been to determine what is not the case. We now know that many of the theories that have been offered are incorrect.

It is also true that substantive advances have been made in establishing what a comprehensive theory of ECT must take into account. At the clinical level, the conditions that benefit from ECT have been increasingly refined. The nature of side effect profiles has been explicated so that linkage to other types of organic amnesia is evident. Manipulation of technical factors in ECT, such as electrode placement, stimulus intensity, and stimulus waveform, has increasingly suggested

Supported in part by grant MH35636 from the National Institute of Mental Health.

that seizures are not all-or-none phenomena. Both the therapeutic and adverse side effects of ECT may depend in part on the conditions used to elicit seizures. Similarities and differences in the neurochemical effects of ECT and psychotropic medications have been identified. These advances provide the framework for much of the current theorizing about mechanisms of action.

THE PHENOMENA IN SEARCH OF MECHANISMS

The Nature of Efficacy

One of the difficulties in offering a view on how ECT works is the necessity of delimiting the conditions for which it is efficacious. As discussed elsewhere in this volume, the evidence has been consistent that ECT is the most powerful antidepressant agent currently available. In controlled comparative trials, ECT has consistently proven to be as effective or more effective than antidepressant medications. However, the indications for ECT are more far ranging than major depressive episodes. Retrospective and prospective studies have demonstrated marked antimanic properties (Small, 1985b). The second most common use of ECT in the United States is in treatment of schizophrenia, and controlled studies have indicated that a significant proportion of acute schizophrenic patients may manifest short-term benefit from this modality (Small, 1985a). There are a plethora of uncontrolled reports of ECT being of value in conditions as diverse as organic psychoses, toxic delirium, pernicious catatonia, delirium tremens, and some forms of intractable epilepsy (Fink, 1979).

Currently we have no way of knowing with assurance whether the mode of antidepressant action of ECT is similar to or different from its mode of action in other conditions. The breadth of clinical conditions that is posited as being responsive to ECT due to a common mode of action will often strongly influence the search for mechanisms. For example, Ottosson (1985) hypothesized that the elicitation of the full grand mal seizure has intrinsic antidepressant properties, while he viewed the antimanic effects of ECT as secondary to confusional and amnestic effects. It would be compatible with this view to search for similarities between the antidepressant mode of action of ECT and that of tricyclic antidepressants (TCAs) and monoamine oxidase inhibitors (MAOIs). In contrast, Post and colleagues (1986) suggested that a unitary mechanism may underlie ECT's efficacy in depression and mania, focusing attention on commonalities with the modes of action of other agents believed to have a similar spectrum of efficacy; that is, lithium carbonate and the anticonvulsant medications, carbamazepine and valproic acid. Given that TCAs and MAOIs are not believed to be of value in treatment of acute mania, the view advanced by Post and colleagues (1986) implies that these agents and ECT differ in how they exert antidepressant effects.

Despite this uncertainty concerning the breadth of clinical phenomena to be accounted for, much of current research on ECT mechanisms has centered on neurophysiological and neurochemical similarities between ECT and antidepressant medications (see Lerer and Shapira, 1986, for a review). For example, as described below, preclinical research on the chronic effects of electroconvulsive shock (ECS) in animals has demonstrated important similarities to the chronic effects of TCAs in enhancing the availability of norepinephrine (NE) and reducing the number and function of beta-adrenergic receptors (Kellar and Stockmeier, 1986). These findings are compatible with seminal theories regarding the role of noradrenergic function in depressive states and the action of antidepressant therapies (for example, Schildkraut, 1965). Two principle factors have limited our capacity to establish whether indeed such effects provide the biochemical substrate for ECT antidepressant properties.

First, as in the case of TCAs, the bulk of evidence implicating noradrenergic function in the pathophysiology of depression and in the effects of antidepressant somatic treatment comes from preclinical research with animals. Much of this work examines the impact of psychiatric treatments on normal mechanisms in the rat or mouse brain and generalizability to abnormal states of the human brain is hypothetical. Techniques to assess directly noradrenergic function in the human brain are still lacking and tests of the critical role of this system in contributing to human ECT response must await methodological developments.

Second, were it shown that TCAs and ECT have similar effects on human noradrenergic functioning, it would not be established that this type of effect is fundamental to ECT's antidepressant efficacy. The nagging question would remain as to why depressed patients who fail to respond to adequate trials of antidepressant medications respond at remarkably high rates to ECT (Avery and Lubrano, 1979). This clinical reality suggests either 1) that ECT at times produces the same types of neurochemical changes as TCAs but does so to a more powerful degree; 2) that TCAs and ECT share a mode of action for some patients, but, particularly for TCA-resistant patients, ECT antidepressant effects can be mediated through distinctly different systems; or 3) that the modes of action of ECT and TCAs are independent and the search for biochemical mechanisms of action should concentrate on the differences between the therapeutics and not on their similarities.

The Nature of Cognitive Side Effects

There is also heterogeneity in the cognitive side effects of ECT. There is no evidence that, generally speaking, the nature of cognitive side effects differs among diagnostic groups or among ECT clinical responders and nonresponders. However, the nature and extent of cognitive sequaelae are a function of time point during or after the course of ECT at which patients are assessed, the form of ECT administered (electrode placement, electrical dosage, stimulus waveform), the types and dosages of medications administered concomitantly with ECT, the extent of preexisting cognitive impairments, and other factors. ECT induces a profile of cognitive disturbances, the constituents of which vary in extent over time and from individual to individual.

This variability in cognitive effects suggests that a unitary mode of action for all cognitive changes is unlikely. Immediately following the seizure patients typically manifest the most severe levels of disturbance. At this time point neurological signs may be evident (for example, Babinski response). Patients will invariably experience a period of disorientation with marked attentional disturbance. At this time point, patients will have deficits in both learning and remembering new information (anterograde amnesia) and remembering information they have previously learned (retrograde amnesia). Generally speaking, the acute confusional and amnestic state following ECT will be of greater severity when the traditional bilateral (bifrontotemporal) electrode placement is used, relative to nondominant placements. There is evidence that the stimulus waveform and the intensity of the electrical stimulus may have an impact on the severity of deficits. Waveforms that are relatively inefficient in eliciting seizures, such as the sine wave, require administering substantially more electrical intensity than more efficient waveforms, such as the brief pulse. There is substantial evidence that sine wave stimuli, relative to brief pulse stimuli, are associated with greater short-term cognitive deficits. Even within a waveform, use of stimulus intensities closer to seizure threshold may be associated with less severe and shorter lasting cognitive effects (Sackeim et al, 1986b; Weiner et al, 1986b; Valentine et al, 1968).

In addition to characteristics of the electrical stimulation, other aspects of ECT procedures have an impact on cognitive sequelae. There is marked variability in the field in the doses used of short-acting barbiturate medications for ECT anesthesia. These medications have amnestic properties and there is evidence that dose of methohexital is related both to the short-term cognitive effects of ECT and to seizure duration (Miller et al, 1985). Higher barbiturate doses are associated with shorter seizure durations and more profound cognitive disturbance. Adequacy of oxygenation procedures in protecting against an hypoxic state is also believed to be critical in moderating short-term side effects.

These indications that technical factors in ECT administration impinge on the severity of short-term cognitive side effects are of clinical relevance. There is always the possibility in ECT of patients developing an organic brain syndrome. This syndrome typically manifests as a profound state of disorientation and confusion. While rarely studied empirically, the available evidence suggests that once manifest the state may last for an average of two weeks (Summers et al, 1979). A recent retrospective study on consecutive patients treated with ECT in a general hospital practice found that in over 50 percent of cases ECT was interrupted due to the development of an organic brain syndrome (Miller et al, 1986). In contrast, it is established that with attention to issues of stimulus intensity, waveform, electrode placement, and concommitant medications, manifestation of an organic brain syndrome can be a relatively rare event (Sackeim et al, 1986b).

As time from last ECT treatment increases, there is typically rapid recovery from the acute cognitive effects of treatment. With the exception of patients who develop an organic brain syndrome, it is usually the case that a few days after the ECT course patients return to pretreatment baseline or perform better on measures of orientation and attention. On tests assessing capacity to learn new information (for example, repeating back a list of words just presented), patients will also show either the same level or improved performance relative to before the start of ECT (Steif et al, 1986). This type of learning (anterograde immediate memory) is often markedly compromised during the depressed state, and improvement shortly following the course of ECT has been associated with degree of symptomatic recovery (Cronholm and Ottosson, 1961). However, if patients are assessed on their capacity to retain the information (for example, repeating back the list of words several hours later), they often display clearcut deficits. In this respect ECT results in rapid forgetting of information that has been recently learned. This pattern suggests that there is a double dissociation in the effects of depression and ECT on anterograde memory. The depressed state is characterized by difficulties in learning or the acquisition of information, but not in retaining what has been learned. In contrast, ECT will generally have no effect or results in improvement in the acquisition of information, but will produce, instead, impairment in the capacity to retain what has been learned (Steif et al, 1986).

In addition to this pattern of deficit in anterograde memory, ECT often results in retrograde memory deficits. For a period of weeks following the treatment course, patients may experience problems in remembering events from their own past or nonpersonal information that they learned prior to the start of ECT. Like the anterograde amnesia, the retrograde amnesia is usually most profound immediately following the treatment and recedes with time. The recovery from retrograde amnesia is believed to display a temporal gradient. Initially the amnesia is most dense for events that occurred during the months and years immediately prior to ECT, with less difficulty in remembering events from the more distant past. It is believed that the retrograde amnesia shrinks with time from ECT, with more remote memory improving prior to memory for events that were more proximal to the treatment (Squire, 1986).

The anterograde and retrograde memory deficits show recovery during the weeks and months following treatment. With respect to anterograde memory, there is no evidence that, for several months following the ECT course, patients are characterized by difficulties in acquiring or retaining new information. However, there is suggestive evidence that patients may have difficulties remembering events that occurred during the first several weeks following ECT and that the spottiness of memory for this time period may be permanent. During this period patients often manifest difficulties in retaining newly acquired information over delays of a few hours (anterograde delayed memory). It is likely, therefore, that the permanent loss of memory for events in the first few weeks following ECT is related to this deficit (Squire, 1986; Weiner et al, 1986b).

Similarly, there is suggestive evidence that in at least some patients the retrograde memory disturbance never recovers completely. There may be spottiness in recall for events that transpired during the first few months that preceded the ECT course. This has suggested that ECT interferes with a critical process of memory consolidation, with the most recently acquired information most vulnerable (Squire, 1986).

The technical factors that in ECT administration appear to be critical in determining the intensity of acute cognitive side effects may be of less consequence with respect to these more long-term cognitive sequelae. For example, differences between unilateral and bilateral ECT in cognitive consequences are easily demonstrated within a few days of the ECT course, but are less readily apparent within a few weeks. The rapid recovery in cognitive functioning that occurs as time from ECT increases may contribute to the difficulties in establishing such relations. It is also possible that the more long-term consequences reflect to a greater extent the effects of seizure elicitation in humans, regardless of methods of induction. This is supported by findings of similar patterns of memory deficit in patients in whom seizures are elicited by chemical convulsants (Small, 1974) or who are subject to spontaneous seizures, particularly involving the temporal lobe (Trimble and Thompson, 1986).

Despite the fact that there is no objective evidence of long-term cognitive impairments, other than the restricted amnesia for events that occurred in the months surrounding the course of ECT, a minority of former ECT patients will report substantial and wide-ranging cognitive deficits (Freeman and Kendell, 1986). The validity of these subjective complaints has been extremely difficult to determine. First, the nature of statistical inference in clinical research almost always requires the examination of groups of individuals. Unless sample sizes are extraordinarily large, isolation of iatrogenic effects that characterize a small minority is extremely difficult. Second, the methodological requirements of using psychometrically sound testing instruments to study objectively cognitive sequelae has strongly influenced the types of cognitive processes examined. For example, the most common method of quantifying anterograde memory deficit has involved asking patients to deliberately commit to memory lists of words or shapes (Steif et al, 1986). However, following ECT, patients frequently report difficulty in remembering material that they did not deliberately attempt to learn, such as where they placed their keys or what they had for dinner the night before. Until recently there has been little investigation in ECT of incidental learning and memory. Third, there is evidence that following ECT, intensity of subjective complaints about cognitive functioning is associated with level of residual symptomatology (Pettinati and Rosenberg, 1984). Given that major depression and other forms of psychopathology are associated with cognitive disturbance, to some degree subjective complaints following ECT may reflect true dysfunction that is incorrectly attributed to the treatment. Regardless of the source, increased subjective perception of cognitive disablity attributed by the patient to a treatment may be considered an iatrogenic effect of the treatment.

Generally speaking, this summary indicates that in accounting for mechanisms of action it may be helpful to parcel out three general domains of cognitive sequelae. The first pertains to the relatively acute effects of ECT that may impact broadly across a variety of intellectual functions and, when most severe, reflect an organic brain syndrome. With time these acute effects recede and patients manifest circumscribed anterograde and retrograde amnestic deficits. The amnesia is most often seen without impairment in other intellectual faculties. Third, the experience of having received ECT may alter patients' perceptions of their cognitive functioning.

CURRENT THEORIES OF THERAPEUTIC ACTION

The Role of the Seizure

Perhaps the most fundamental claims concerning the mechanisms of ECT have been that the seizure is necessary and sufficient for the antidepressant effects of the treatment, while the intensity of electrical stimulation is related to the magnitude of cognitive side effects (Ottosson, 1960, 1985). With regard to efficacy, this view stipulates that the critical therapeutic aspect of ECT is the generalized grand mal seizure and that no matter how such seizures are elicited they will have robust antidepressant properties. Indeed, were this view correct the search for mechanisms should concentrate on the biochemical changes that are intrinsic to seizure elicitation.

There is a large body of evidence that supports this view. A series of studies contrasted the therapeutic effects of traditional ECT with sham ECT. In sham treatment, all the procedures of traditional ECT are followed, including general anesthesia and application of electrodes to the head, but no current is passed. In general this set of studies found that traditional ECT resulted in superior short-term clinical outcome over sham ECT (see Crow and Johnstone, 1986; Sackeim, 1986, for reviews). The fact that patients in these trials were blind to whether they were receiving sham or traditional ECT also rules out a number of psychological accounts of the efficacy of ECT. Theories that related efficacy to hypothesized patient beliefs that ECT was a punishment, or to presumed therapeutic properties of the ECT ritual—scheduled treatments, repeated experiences of unconsciousness, and so on—are incompatible with the results of the sham versus traditional ECT studies.

Fewer studies have contrasted the efficacy of ECT with that of delivering subconvulsive intensities of electrical stimulation. This work, while subject to methodological limitations, nonetheless has suggested that therapeutic effects were more robust when full seizures are elicited than when electrical stimulation is applied without producing seizures (Fink et al, 1958; Ulett et al, 1956). In a different vein, the relative efficacy of traditional ECT has also been contrasted with that of convulsive therapies using chemical agents to induce full seizures. This work generally found that the therapeutic properties of electrical and chemical seizure induction were equal, with perhaps less marked cognitive side effects when chemical induction was used (Small, 1974). Therefore, again it appeared that the seizure was fundamental in accounting for antidepressant effects.

The study reported by Ottosson (1960) was the most critical in establishing this view. Ottosson contrasted efficacy and side effects in three groups. One group received a traditional form of bilateral ECT, using a relatively robust electrical stimulus. A second group received the same form of ECT, but with a greater intensity of electrical stimulation. The third group received the same type of ECT as the first group, but were also administered lidocaine prior to application of the electrical stimulus. Lidocaine has anticonvulsant properties and the neural seizure discharge was aborted to one-third its typical duration in the lidocaine group. Comparison of the first and second group allowed for examining the role of electrical intensity on efficacy, and comparison of the first and third groups allowed for examining the role of the seizure discharge, holding electrical intensity constant. Ottosson found that the first and second groups were essentially equivalent in improvement in depressive symptoms, whereas efficacy was reduced in the third group. In contrast, cognitive side effects, particularly the capacity to retain information over a delay, were more pronounced in the second group, which received the highest intensity of stimulation. Therefore, it appeared that characteristics of the electrical stimulus were largely irrelevant to efficacy, as long as full generalized seizures were elicited. On the other hand, it appeared that intensity of electrical stimulation was related to cognitive sequelae.

These investigations not only had profound impact on views concerning the mechanisms of action of ECT, but were also highly relevant to clinical practice. Based on this evidence one would think that the way to maintain strong clinical efficacy and to minimize cognitive side effects would be to insure that patients have full generalized seizures and to use the least intense electrical stimulus possible to produce such seizures. Indeed, this position was explicitly adopted in the recent NIH Consensus Development Conference statement on ECT, ". . .

the lowest amount of electrical energy to induce an adequate seizure should be used" (Rose, 1985).

Recent studies have seriously questioned, however, whether the generalized seizure is both necessary and sufficient for the antidepressant effects of ECT. Following the original view, Sackeim and colleagues (1987a) designed a titration procedure to individualize ECT stimulus intensity to just above seizure threshold for individual patients. Using this method, a marked difference in efficacy was observed between bilateral and unilateral nondominant ECT (Sackeim et al, in press). Approximately 70 percent of the low dosage bilateral group were considered clinical responders compared to only 28 percent of the unilateral nondominant group. Low dosage unilateral nondominant ECT was remarkably weak in therapeutic properties, even though full grand mal seizures were elicited in this condition, which were equal in duration to those produced by low dosage bilateral ECT. Sackeim and colleagues (in press) suggested that stimulus intensity has an impact on the efficacy of ECT and that at low intensity unilateral nondominant ECT loses much of its therapeutic potential.

Related to these findings, Robin and De Tissera (1982) contrasted three forms of bilateral ECT: a high intensity sine wave group, a high intensity brief pulse group, and a low intensity brief pulse group. The low intensity group showed inferior efficacy. Interpretation of this study was complicated by the fact that the three groups differed not only in stimulus intensity but also stimulus waveform. Recently, Robin and associates (1987) and Sackeim (1987) presented preliminary findings from ongoing studies that address the intensity issue directly. In both studies higher levels of stimulus intensity appear to augment ECT clinical response.

These findings, coupled with prior reports (for example, Cronholm and Ottosson, 1963), have prompted revision of the view that the elicitation of the grand mal seizure is both necessary and sufficient for antidepressant effects. It appears that seizures can be reliably elicited that meet conservative criteria for extent of generalization and duration that, nonetheless, are weak in therapeutic properties. This new research suggests that a stimulus intensity "therapeutic window" may characterize ECT. The classic study by Ottosson (1960) that led to the belief that stimulus intensity was incidental to ECT efficacy may have used stimulus intensities in all groups that were sufficiently high to be in the upper range of the putative therapeutic window (Abrams, 1986; Sackeim and Mukherjee, 1986).

This new perspective complicates the clinical practice of ECT. It suggests that the traditional indications of an adequate treatment, elicitation of a generalized seizure of at least 25 or 30 seconds in duration, may not be fully satisfactory. Further, since there is reasonable evidence that higher levels of stimulus intensity are associated with more pronounced cognitive side effects, it may be the case that the most efficacious forms of ECT result in more cognitive disturbance than less efficacious forms of treatment.

This perspective also offers new possibilities regarding investigation of mechanisms of action. The elicitation of a generalized seizure is associated with a myriad of changes in neurophysiological and biochemical parameters. These changes are so numerous that pessimism has often been expressed about the possibility of isolating the specific changes that are responsible for ECT mechanisms of action (for example, Kety, 1974). Now that it is known that full seizures can be reliably elicited that have weak therapeutic potential, there is marked interest in the research community in attempting to isolate those factors that distinguish therapeutic from nontherapeutic seizures. Such investigations may ultimately provide the clinician with a marker of what constitutes a therapeutic seizure, in addition to furthering understanding of mechanisms.

Neurotransmitter Systems

For the last 30 years dysregulation in neurotransmitter systems has been a source of hypotheses about the pathophysiology of affective disorders. Much of the force behind such hypotheses has come from animal research demonstrating altered neurotransmitter function with administration of mood stabilizing medications (TCAs, MAOIs, or lithium). Similar preclinical research has been conducted on the chronic effects of electrocerebral silence (ECS). Here a brief review is provided of what has been learned about the effects of ECS on noradrenergic, serotonergic, dopaminergic, cholinergic, and GABAergic function.

NORADRENERGIC FUNCTION. The seminal theories linking noradrenergic function to depression were based on the observation that agents that increase the postsynaptic availability of norepinephrine (for example, TCAs, MAOIs) have antidepressant effects, whereas agents that deplete NE availability may induce depression (for example, reserpine). ECS has a number of effects in common with chronic administration of TCAs in altering noradrenergic function.

Perhaps the most consistent finding concerning the biochemistry of ECS is that repeated treatment results in a decrease in the number of beta-adrenergic receptors. This reduction is progressive with repeated ECS and appears to be an adaptive down-regulation due to increased norepinephrine stimulation. The reduction appears functional in that it is associated with decreased receptor-mediated cyclic AMP production. Furthermore, the reduction in receptor number displays anatomic specificity in rat brain, as it is observed in the cortex and hippocampus, but not the striatum, cerebellum, or hypothalamus (Kellar and Stockmeier, 1986). Other preclinical findings are largely compatible with the view that ECS results in increased availability of norepinephrine, although these effects have been observed with less consistency. They include increased synthesis and turnover of NE and higher levels of tyrosine hydroxylase activity (the rate limiting enzyme). Using behavioral pharmacology methodologies, there is also evidence that ECT, like TCAs, may result in subsensitivity of presynaptic alpha-2 adrenergic receptors, although biochemical studies of alpha-2 receptor density have been inconsistent (Green and Nutt, in press).

In summary, preclinical research has shown that TCAs and ECS both result in a decreased beta-adrenergic receptor number that is believed to result from enhanced norepinephrine availability. The meaningfulness of these changes in accounting for the therapeutic action of ECT is uncertain. Methods for studying beta-adrenergic function in humans are limited. While there is evidence that acutely following ECT there is a surge in levels of plasma catecholamines, particularly epinephrine, these increases are short-lived and may be of greater relevance to the acute effects of ECT on cardiac function than to therapeutic efficacy. Studies of subacute or chronic changes in peripheral or CSF measures of catecholamines and their metabolites have been largely negative or inconsistent. Like the status of the hypothesis that reduced noradrenergic function is critical to the pathophysiology of the depressed state, the hypothesis that alterations in noradrenergic function are responsible for the antidepressant efficacy of ECT awaits the development of techniques to study human neural fluctuations in this system.

DOPAMINERGIC FUNCTION. Dopamine is less frequently suggested as a neurotransmitter influencing abnormal mood states. Rather, the role of dopamine in contributing to psychotic states is more frequently discussed. ECT is believed to be particularly effective in the treatment of psychotic depression, a condition that may manifest relatively poor response to monotherapy with TCAs or antipsychotics. Further ECT has shown marked efficacy in treatment of psychotic mania and may be of value in some forms of schizophrenia and organic psychoses (Small, 1985a, 1985b). Therefore, its impact on dopaminergic function is of interest.

A variety of studies have indicated that behaviors that are believed to be mediated by dopamine are enhanced following ECS. Locomotor responses and stereotypic behavior provoked by apomorphine and amphetamine are increased following chronic ECS. These changes might be interpreted as reflecting increased postsynaptic dopamine receptor sensitivity. However, studies of dopamine biochemistry and receptor physiology following ECS have failed to observe consistent changes. Neuroendocrine strategies (for example, growth hormone and prolactin response to apomorphine) used to examine dopaminergic tone in humans have not yielded consistent results, with the findings suggesting either increased dopaminergic function following ECT or no change (Christie et al, 1982). In attempting to integrate the behavioral and neuroendocrine data suggesting enhanced dopaminergic function following ECT and the absence of clearcut receptor changes, it has been suggested that enhanced dopaminergic function may be due to changes downstream from the postsynaptic receptor (Green and Nutt, in press).

It is noteworthy that the available evidence suggests that if ECT affects dopaminergic function it is in the direction of enhancement. This is the opposite of what would typically be thought to be the case for treatment that is effective in controlling psychotic symptomatology. This effect may be relevant to the reported beneficial impact of ECT in some cases of Parkinsonism (Fink, 1979).

SEROTONERGIC FUNCTION. Like the noradrenergic hypothesis, there is some evidence that serotonergic function is decreased in depression and that antidepressant medications redress this imbalance. The effects of ECS and TCAs on serotonergic function are particularly intriguing since at face value they are in opposite directions with regard to 5-HT2 receptor density. Antidepressant drugs (TCAs and MAOIs) result in a reduction of these receptors, while ECS results in an increase.

With chronic ECS the evidence is unclear as to whether sustained effects are obtained on brain concentration or turnover of serotonin. However, behavioral pharmacology studies have consistently indicated that, coupled with the increase in 5-HT2 receptor number, ECS results in increased responsivity to serotonin agonists (Green, 1986). Therefore, it is fairly certain that ECS produces increased serotonergic functioning. The decrease in 5-HT2 receptor density following chronic TCA administration may not be coupled with parallel behavioral subsensitivity. In fact, following such administration enhanced behavioral and electrophysiological responsivity to serotonin has been observed (De Montigny and Aghajanian, 1978).

As with other neurotransmitter systems, there is no direct evidence demonstrating that changes in serotonergic tone are critical to antidepressant effects in humans. Imipramine-binding in platelets has been suggested as a peripheral measure of central serotonergic effects. Initial evidence from human studies indicates that ECT does not have effects on this measure that are related to short-term clinical outcome (Langer et al, 1986). The opposite effects of ECS and antidepressant medications on central 5-HT2 receptor number may suggest a mechanism by which ECT has strong antidepressant properties in patients resistant to pharmacotherapy.

CHOLINERGIC FUNCTION. Alterations in cholinergic functioning have also been implicated in abnormal mood states (Janowsky et al, 1972). Cholinesterase inhibitors (for example, physostigmine) may produce rapid reduction in manic symptoms and such agents have been suggested to induce depressive symptoms in normals. There is suggestive evidence from behavioral paradigms that supersensitivity to cholinergic challenge may be a trait marker of depression (Sitaram and Gillin, 1980).

Chronic ECS in animals has been shown to result in significant but small decreases in muscarinic cholinergic receptor number in cortex and hippocampus (Lerer et al, 1983a). This is coupled with evidence of reduced brain levels of acetylcholine and choline acetyltransferase activity. In humans, there is evidence that CSF acetylcholine levels increase following ECT and spontaneous seizures (Fink, 1979). These effects may be interpreted as suggesting a reduction in cholinergic function following ECT. This is in line with behavioral pharmacology evidence that ECS results in decreased sensitivity in cataleptic response to muscarinic agonists (Green and Nutt, in press).

These effects are compatible with the view that ECT may exert antidepressant action through reduction of cholinergic supersensitivity. Problems with this view are that there is evidence that cholinergic supersensitivity characterizes depressives in remission and further, that ECT has strong antimanic properties. Typically, it would be thought that a reduction in cholinergic tone would exacerbate mania and not result in clinical improvement. Given that the cholinergic system has been strongly implicated in subserving aspects of learning and memory, the reduction of cholinergic function associated with ECS may provide a key to mechanisms underlying some of the cognitive side effects.

GABAERGIC FUNCTION. GABA is the primary mammalian inhibitory neurotransmitter and approximately one-third of neurons are GABAergic. The GABA system has also been implicated in affective disorders, as a number of studies have reported reduced CSF levels of GABA during the depressed state, and medications that are GABA-mimetic (for example, progabide) appear to have antidepressant properties (Sackeim et al, 1986a).

In animals and humans electrical induction of a seizure results in a subsequent increase in seizure threshold (Sackeim et al, 1987a). As discussed below, there is evidence relating the change in seizure threshold to the antidepressant efficacy of ECT. A series of studies by Green and colleagues suggested that ECS raises the threshold for convulsant agents that produce seizures through antagonism of GABA. ECS did not raise the threshold when seizures were evoked with a glycine antagonist or a serotonergic agonist. This suggested that ECS produces a functional increase in GABAergic activity and that the changes in seizure threshold observed with ECT are due to this effect (Green, 1986).

This view is compatible with evidence that single and repeated ECS raises concentrations of GABA in specific brain regions. However, complicating interpretation is evidence that following ECS GABA synthesis and release are reduced. These characteristics are in line with reduced GABA functioning (Green and Nutt, in press).

Two other sources of evidence may be helpful here. Recently, it has been suggested that ECS results in a substantial up-regulation of the GABA-B receptor (Lloyd et al, 1986). It was found that this effect was also shown by conventional antidepressant medications. If this pattern is replicated in future work, it will indicate that most antidepressant medications and ECS share two major effects on receptor physiology: down-regulation of the beta-adrenergic receptor and up-regulation of the GABA-B receptor.

Second, it appears that chronic administration of the GABA-mimetic agent, progabide, results in a number of the same changes in monoamine biochemistry that are associated with chronic ECS. These include up-regulation of 5-HT2 receptors, behavioral indications of supersensitivity to serotonergic agonists, and reduced behavioral sensitivity to an $alpha_2$-adrenergic receptor agonist (Green, 1986). It is well established that manipulations of GABAergic activity can alter monoamine function. That enhancement of GABAergic activity mimics some of the biological consequences of ECS is also suggestive that ECS results in increased GABAergic tone.

Peptides and Neuroendocrine Function

Another major source for theories concerning the mechanisms of action of ECT has concentrated on changes in neuromodulatory functions exerted by peptides or endocrine hormones (for example, Fink and Ottosson, 1980). Such theories are compatible with findings concerning neurotransmitter changes, since release of hormones through impact on the hypothalamus is regulated in part by monoaminergic transmission.

Various indirect sources of evidence are suggestive that changes in hypothalamic or other deep structure function are tied to ECT efficacy. It has been traditional to view vegetative or endogenous symptomatology in depression as reflecting hypothalamic dysregulation. Disturbances in sleep, appetite, libido, and diurnal rhythms are abnormalities of functions subserved in part by hypothalamic nuclei. There is some evidence that depressed patients particularly characterized by such symptoms are relatively more responsive to ECT. More directly, it is well established that subgroups of affective disorder patients present with neuroendocrinological abnormalities, as revealed by abnormal patterns of cortisol secretion, early escape from suppression of cortisol following dexamethasone, and blunted thyrotropin stimulating hormone (TSH) response to thyrotropin releasing hormone (TRH), among others.

This view is reinforced by reports that a number of peptides may be elevated in plasma immediately following seizure induction in humans. These include prolactin, beta-endorphin-like immunoreactivity, vasopressin, oxytocin, neurophysin, adrenocorticotropin (ACTH), cortisol, follicle-stimulating hormone, and luteinizing hormone (Deakin et al, 1983; Skrabanek et al, 1981; Whalley et al, 1982). For the most part changes in plasma growth hormone and TSH have not been observed and in some cases the positive changes have been inconsistent. Nonetheless, the acute changes in substances such as prolactin or in beta-endorphin-like immunoreactivity are intense in magnitude, and a number of these effects cannot be attributed solely to stress-like reactions or the impact of anesthetic agents. This pattern of ECT effects certainly suggests strong impact on hypothalamic–pituitary function.

Another source for hypotheses concerning the role of deep structures has been speculation about the nature of the seizure discharge. There is near universal agreement that a generalized seizure is necessary for the antidepressant effects of ECT. Some have argued that the generally symmetric and rapid manifestation of the cerebral seizure is centrencephalic in origin. Likewise, there is some evidence suggesting that the development of symmetric slow wave activity in the EEG during the ECT course is prognostic of good outcome. This pattern was also attributed to centrencephalic effects (Fink, 1979).

Finally, the degree of direct electrical stimulation of deep midline structures is a function in part of electrode placement. Generally speaking, current density will be greater in the hypothalamus and other deep structures with bilateral relative to unilateral ECT (Sackeim and Mukherjee, 1986). There appear to be relatively consistent data indicating that the acute prolactin surge is greater following bilateral than unilateral ECT. In the context of a continuing controversy about the relative efficacy of bilateral and unilateral ECT, it has been argued that the putative superiority of bilateral ECT is due to this greater deep structure stimulation (Abrams, 1986).

Several considerations are problematic for the view that the antidepressant efficacy of ECT is mediated by effects on the hypothalmus or the hypthalamic–adrenal–pituitary axis. After initial enthusiasm that laboratory tests of neuroendocrine function could serve as predictors of ECT clinical response, subsequent research has not been encouraging. Abnormal dexamethasone suppression test (DST) results have not been found to predict ECT outcome. Further, there is evidence that a substantial subgroup may respond to ECT without normalization from pretreatment nonsuppressor status. Indeed, some patients who respond to ECT may convert from normal suppression to abnormal nonsuppression (Devanand et al, 1987). It has also been found that regardless of clinical outcome, ECT may result in a short-term increased blunting of TSH response to TRH (Decina et al, 1987). This change is in the direction of increased abnormality.

The acute increases that are observed in plasma measures of peptides and hormones are short-lived. There is little evidence that ECT results in sustained changes in basal levels of these substances. Given that for a short period following the seizure there is increased permeability of the blood–brain barrier, it is possible that even the more acute changes are critical to efficacy. Nonetheless, with the possible exceptions of prolactin and neurophysin, there is little evidence relating the acute changes to efficacy.

Abrams (1986) has suggested that the magnitude of the prolactin surge acutely following ECT is related to antidepressant effects. This claim is of particular interest since there are data suggesting that the magnitude of the prolactin increase is related to electrode placement (unilateral versus bilateral), seizure duration, and stimulus intensity (Robin et al, 1985). The direction of these effects are that bilateral placement, longer seizures, and higher levels of stimulus intensity have been associated with larger increases. However, the data of Abrams and colleagues suggest that superior ECT outcome is associated with smaller prolactin surges, a pattern that at face value would seem disharmonious with the other suggested correlates. Others have reported no relation between prolactin changes and efficacy (for example, Deakin et al, 1983). There is one positive report associating larger neurophysin increases with positive outcome and this requires further investigation (Scott et al, 1986).

The view that ECT-induced generalized seizures emanate from a centrencephalic pacemaker has two problems. It stems from an analogy to primary generalized epilepsy. First, it may well be that ECT seizures are focal in origin with rapid spread (Sackeim and Mukherjee, 1986). This is not determined and the more appropriate analogy may be to secondary generalized epilepsy. Second, the original belief that a centrencephalic pacemaker was responsible for the widespread synchronous discharges of primary generalized epilepsy is now disputed. Particularly relevant to ECT are findings that the hippocampal neurons (particularly CA3 pyramidal cells) appear to have a low seizure threshold, capacity for sustained depolarizations and burst discharges, and, in some models, have been shown to drive epileptogenic activity (for example, Prince, 1982). Therefore, like views centering on neurotransmitter function, the role of hypothalamic stimulation in accounting for the efficacy of ECT is largely hypothetical.

Particular mention should be made concerning ECT effects on endogenous opioid peptides. Extensive preclinical research has shown that chronic ECS enhances endogenous opioid activity (see Holaday et al, 1986, for a review). Met-enkephalin concentration and synthesis increase in several brain regions and, like morphine tolerance, ECS produces increased binding of opioid ligands. There is also evidence that ECS shows cross sensitization to acute morphine challenge. Opiate antagonists have been shown to alter a number of the ictal and postictal effects of ECS, including changes in seizure threshold and extent of retrograde amnesia. Given that there is some evidence linking the endogenous opioid peptides to depressive disorder, there are further grounds for investigation in this area.

Anticonvulsant Properties

A new theory has been offered suggesting that the antidepressant effects of ECT are a consequence of its anticonvulsant properties. This view stipulates that the critical aspect of ECT is not the elicitation of the seizure, but rather the process that terminates the seizure. Seizures do not stop because the brain runs out of carbohydrate supplies or oxygen or due to neuronal exhaustion. The phenomenon of status epilepticus demonstrates that humans are capable of sustaining seizure activity for considerably longer than the typical 60 seconds observed in ECT. It is hypothesized that seizures are self-terminating due to the potentiation of an active inhibitory process, resulting in enhancement of inhibitory neurotransmission (Sackeim et al, 1983).

Several characteristics have been suggested as reflecting the anticonvulsant properties of ECT. These include 1) the progressive increase in seizure threshold; 2) the progressive decrease in seizure duration; 3) postictal reductions in regional cerebral blood flow (rCBF) and glucose metabolism and possibly the development of slow wave activity in the EEG; 4) the antagonism by ECS of the development and/or expression of "kindled" seizures and the utility of ECT in some cases of intractable epilepsy; and 5) the increased functional activity of inhibitory neurotransmitters and peptides.

As noted, in humans and animals, electrically induced seizures raise the threshold for subsequent seizures. This effect is progressive throughout the ECT course and there is initial evidence that forms of ECT that fail to raise threshold or do so only weakly have diminished antidepressant effects (Sackeim et al, 1987b). Seizure duration typically decreases during the ECT course. There is some evidence that higher levels of stimulus intensity may accelerate the duration decrease (Robin et al, 1987; Sackeim, 1987). The ictal state is hypermetabolic and during the seizure cerebral glucose and oxygen consumption and cerebral blood flow may increase by a few hundred percent. However, it appears that like the interictal state in focal epilepsy, perfusion and metabolic reductions characterize the postictal pattern following ECT. These changes are regional in nature and differ for unilateral and bilateral ECT (Ackermann et al, 1986; Prohovnik et al, 1986; Silfverskiold et al, 1986). It would not be unexpected that metabolic reductions and slowing in the EEG were related. There have been inconsistent data relating the development of EEG slowing to efficacy (Volavka, 1974). In animal models of amygdala kindling, ECS has shown as strong or superior anticonvulsant properties relative to traditional anticonvulsant medications (Post et al, 1986). There are clinical reports of ECT reducing the frequency of spontaneous seizures in patients with medication-resistant epileptic disorders (for example, Caplan, 1946; Sackeim et al, 1983). The ECT induced increase in seizure threshold undoubtedly has a biochemical basis. It has been shown that when CSF is taken from an animal that has received ECS and is injected into the ventricular system of a naive animal, seizure threshold in the host can be raised. This effect can be blocked by opioid antagonism (Holaday et al, 1986). As described above, GABAergic changes have also been implicated in the seizure threshold effects of ECT, as have changes in levels of endogenous MAOI.

This view of the mechanisms of action of ECT suggests that it may share a therapeutic spectrum with anticonvulsant medications. The fact that some anticonvulsants have been shown to have antidepressant and/or antimanic properties is compatible with this perspective. This perspective may also aid in explaining why ECT, rather than promoting a kindling phenomenon in humans, does not result in posttreatment seizure disorders.

Like the other hypotheses raised regarding ECT efficacy, this view remains largely speculative. Ultimately its validity could be tested by determining whether conditions which block the anticonvulsant properties of ECT also block its efficacy. A corollary of this view is the hypothesis that psychiatric conditions responsive to ECT involve heightened levels of neural excitability in particular functional brain systems (Flor-Henry, 1986; Sackeim et al, 1986a). However, initial evidence from brain imaging studies have generally not revealed increased levels of rCBF or glucose metabolism in depressed patients (Post et al, 1987; Sackeim et al, 1987c).

CURRENT THEORIES OF COGNITIVE SEQUELAE

As described earlier, the more long-term cognitive effects of ECT resemble the profile of classic amnesia. While other intellectual functions are unaltered or improved, patients often display transient and restricted retrograde and anterograde memory deficits in the weeks following the ECT course. The nature of this amnesia resembles that observed with insult to medial temporal structures; that is, the hippocampal formation and amygdala (for example, Squire, 1986). Critical to understanding mechanisms of action, the extent of global cognitive impairment following ECT is not associated with the extent of therapeutic improvement. This suggests that the neurobiological mechanisms and/or the anatomic loci related to therapeutic efficacy and those related to global memory disturbance are distinct.

Neuropathology

Some have interpreted the acute and more long-term cognitive effects of ECT as indicating that the treatment produces brain damage. The transient nature of the major cognitive effects would mitigate against this view. However, the possibility of irreversible structural damage must be examined closely. There is evidence suggesting that ECT can produce permanent gaps in memory for some events that occurred in the period immediately prior to and following the treatment course, and a small minority of patients report more extensive impairment (Squire, 1986). Also of concern are the facts that hippocampal sites that appear critical to the type of amnesia manifested following ECT have low seizure threshold, and are particularly likely to show cell loss and gliosis in patients with a history of frequent spontaneous seizures and in animal epilepsy models.

The neuropathological findings from autopsy studies in former ECT patients and from experimental animal models have recently been reviewed by Dam and Dam (1986), Meldrum (1986), and Weiner (1984). Although limited in number of investigations, there does not appear to be evidence from postmortem studies linking neuronal cell loss to current clinical ECT practice. Investigations with animal models have been more definitive. For instance, Dam and colleagues (1981) administered unmodified ECS 3 times a day for 50 days to rats. Brains were perfusion fixed 2 or 12 weeks following the last ECS. Pyramidal cell counts in hippocampal fields showed no differences relative to controls, while the same histological techniques demonstrated cell loss in epilepsy patients with frequent seizures.

Considerable progress has been made in identifying the metabolic and molecular substrates for cell death consequent to seizures. Under conditions in which oxygenation is maintained, the minimum time for experimental status epilepticus to result in cell death appears to be 25 to 30 minutes. This effect is believed to depend on both sustained metabolic increases in the vulnerable neurons and agonist–receptor interactions that trigger dissipative fluxes of sodium and calcium ions across postsynaptic membranes (Siesjo et al, 1986). There is strong agreement that the minimal conditions that are necessary for observing cellular necrosis in experimental seizure models do not apply to the human ECT circumstance.

Neurophysiology

There has been limited investigation of the neurophysiological correlates of ECT cognitive effects. Manipulations of ECT technique provide strong indications that this is likely to be a fruitful area of inquiry.

Bilateral and unilateral ECT differ markedly in short-term cognitive sequelae. Unilateral nondominant ECT produces greater disruption of nonverbal relative to verbal memory and is generally associated with more rapid recovery of orientation in the immediate postictal period compared to unilateral dominant or bilateral ECT. Unilateral dominant ECT is associated with greater verbal than nonverbal impairment. Bilateral ECT produces both verbal and nonverbal memory impairment and may do so to a greater degree than either type of unilateral ECT (Sackeim et al, 1986b; Squire, 1986).

Current density paths are a function of electrode placement and current density is considerably greater over the side of the brain ipsilateral to unilateral stimulation. Attributing the electrode placement pattern to current path effects is also compatible with research examining manipulations of stimulus intensity and stimulus waveform. There are animal and human data indicating that anterograde and retrograde memory deficts are enhanced by increased stimulus intensity (for example, Weiner et al, 1986b). Therefore, it is possible that direct effects of current on neural tissue largely determine the profile and extent of short-term cognitive impairment.

However, an alternative to this position is equally plausible. Manipulations of stimulus parameters may alter the nature of the seizure discharge and subsequent postictal metabolic and EEG changes. Even though generalized seizures are elicited with unilateral ECT, ictal EEG activity is often asymmetric during and following the seizure. Likewise, the postictal reductions in rCBF show different topographic organization for bilateral and unilateral ECT (Prohovnik et al, 1986). There is also suggestive evidence that manipulations of stimulus intensity and/or waveform affect the extent of subsequent slow wave activity in the EEG (Weiner et al, 1986a).

It is expected that a treatment modality that results in suppression of regional metabolic activity has notable cognitive side effects. No study has yet attempted to correlate regional metabolic measures with cognitive alterations. However, a few attempts to link the development of slow wave activity in the EEG to extent of global memory impairment had positive findings (for example, Stromgren and Jensen, 1975). One might expect that over the next few years attempts to map topographically the EEG and metabolic effects of ECT will be productive in establishing relations with impairments in specific cognitive domains.

Neurochemistry

Investigation of the biochemical effects of ECT has concentrated more on issues related to efficacy than on cognitive side effects. This is somewhat surprising given that ECS is the primary animal model for human amnesia and several classes of agents have been shown to attenuate or ameliorate ECS-induced amnesia. Often these agents have been used with limited success in human clinical trials in attempts to reverse cognitive deficits associated with Alzheimer's disease and other dementias. There have been relatively few attempts to moderate pharmacologically the cognitive consequences of human ECT.

It can be argued that the core deficit underlying the anterograde and retrograde amnesia produced by ECT is a dysfunction in memory consolidation. For a period extending to months or years after encoding, information is vulnerable to loss, since the process of consolidation is not yet complete. Memories that are more remote in time are less vulnerable. If consolidation is interfered with, recently acquired information may be permanently lost.

There is a substantial body of evidence that indicates that drugs that reversibly inhibit protein synthesis interfere with long-term, but not short-term, memory (Davis and Squire, 1984). The cognitive effects of ECT indicate selective disruption of long-term memory. One of the characteristic effects of seizure elicitation in animals and man is reversible inhibition of protein synthesis (for example, Siesjo et al, 1986). Therefore, at face value one might suspect that ECT transiently disrupts the neuronal plasticity mechanisms necessary for maintenance of long-term memories. However, there has not been an attempt to link, directly, the effects of ECT on measures of protein synthesis with cognitive parameters.

A number of the effects of ECT on neurotransmitter and peptide systems may also be related to cognitive sequelae. Although there is evidence suggesting that ECT results in cholinergic down-regulation, there has been limited investigation of the utility of cholinergic-agonists in reversing ECT cognitive effects. Enhanced endogenous opioid activity has been related to ECS-induced retrograde amnesia, but a limited clinical trial using naloxone to block these effects had negative findings (Nasrallah et al, 1986). The peptide vasopressin has been claimed to modulate learning and memory in animal models and there are conflicting findings concerning the clinical utility of the administration of the synthetic analogue of vasopressin in ECT patients in reversing cognitive deficits (for example, Lerer et al, 1983b). Various nootropic agents, or putative metabolic enhancers, have shown encouraging results in preclinical trials in attenuating ECS-induced amnesia. The one human ECT trial to date with such an agent also observed beneficial effects (Ezzat et al, 1985).

SUMMARY AND FUTURE DIRECTIONS

In the last few years considerable progress has been made in detailing neurobiological effects of ECT. A fundamental limitation in investigating mechanisms of action has been the lack of research strategies for determining which of these effects is most critical for issues of efficacy or side effects. In clinical research a common practice has been to compare neurobiological parameters in patients who have responded to ECT with those who have not. This approach follows the intrinsic assumption that ECT exerts different biological effects in patients who differ in clinical outcome. Particularly given the high rate of response to ECT, this assumption is highly questionable. It may be more likely that nonresponders are characterized by different pathophysiologies for which the changes induced by ECT are not helpful.

The field, however, is now facing the possibility that generalized seizures can be reliably elicited with weak therapeutic properties. This complicates the practice of ECT as the previously accepted marker of effective treatment, the elicitation of a generalized seizure of a minimum duration, may not be sufficient. This possibility will likely result in a new search for additional markers of effective treatment. Further, the understanding of mechanisms has always been handicapped by the fact that the plethora of neurobiological changes that accompany seizure elicitation make it difficult to sort out which are important and which are irrelevant. In determining what constitutes fully therapeutic seizures the search for mechanisms of action will surely be advanced.

REFERENCES

Abrams R: A hypothesis to explain divergent findings among studies comparing the efficacy of unilateral and bilateral ECT in depression. Convulsive Therapy 1986; 2:253-258

Ackermann RF, Engel J Jr, Baxter L: Positron emission tomography and autoradiographic studies of glucose utilization following electroconvulsive seizures in humans and rats. Ann NY Acad Sci 1986; 462:263-9

Avery D, Lubrano A: Depression treated with imipramine and ECT: the DeCarlos study reconsidered. Am J Psychiatry 1979; 136:559-562

Caplan G: Electrical convulsion therapy in treatment of epilepsy. J Ment Sci 1946; 92:783-793

Christie JE, Whalley LJ, Brown NS, et al: Effect of ECT on the neuroendocrine response to apomorphine in severely depressed patients. Br J Psychiatry 1982; 140:268-73

Cronholm B, Ottosson J-O: Memory functions in endogenous depression: before and after electroconvulsive therapy. Arch Gen Psychiatry 1961; 5:193-199

Cronholm B, Ottosson J-O: Ultrabrief stimulus technique in electroconvulsive therapy, II: comparative studies of therapeutic effects and memory disturbance in treatment of endogenous depression with the Elther ES electroshock apparatus and Siemens Konvulsator. J Nerv Ment Dis 1963; 137:268-276

Crow TJ, Johnstone EC: Controlled trials of electroconvulsive therapy. Ann NY Acad Sci 1986; 462:12-29

Dam A, Dam M: Quantitative neuropathology in electrically induced generalized seizures. Convulsive Therapy 1986; 2:77-91

Dam M, Hertz M, Bolwig T, et al: The number of hippocampal neurons and Purkinje cells in rats after electrically-induced seizures, in Advances in Epileptology XII: Epilepsy International Symposium. Edited by Dam M, Gram L, Penry JK. New York, Raven Press, 1981

Davis H, Squire L: Protein synthesis and memory. Psychol Bull 1984; 96:518-559

Deakin JF, Ferrier IN, Crow TJ, et al: Effects of ECT on pituitary hormone release: relationship to seizure, clinical variables and outcome. Br J Psychiatry 1983; 143:618-624

Decina P, Sackeim HA, Kahn D: Effects of ECT on the TRH stimulation test. Psychoneuroendocrinology, 1987

De Montigny C, Aghajanian GK: Tricyclic antidepressants: long-term treatment increases responsivity of rat forebrain neurons to serotonin. Science 1978; 202:1303-1306

Devanand D, Decina P, Sackeim HA, et al: Serial dexamethasone suppression tests in initial suppressors and nonsuppressors treated with electroconvulsive therapy. Biol Psychiatry 1987; 22:463-472

Ezzat D, Ibraheem M, Makhawy B: The effect of piracetam on ECT-induced memory disturbances. Br J Psychiatry 1985; 147:720-721

Fink M: Convulsive Therapy: Theory and Practice. New York, Raven Press, 1979

Fink M, Ottosson JO: A theory of convulsive therapy in endogenous depression: significance of hypothalamic functions. Psychiatry Res 1980; 2:49-61

Fink M, Kahn R, Green M: Experimental studies of the electroshock process. Diseases of the Nervous System 1958; 19:113-118

Flor-Henry P: Electroconvulsive therapy and lateralized affective systems. Ann NY Acad Sci 1986; 462:389-97

Freeman CP, Kendell RE: Patient's experiences of and attitudes to electroconvulsive therapy. Ann NY Acad Sci 1986; 462:341-52

Gordon H: Fifty shock therapy theories. Military Surgery 1948; 103:397-401

Green AR: Changes in gamma-aminobutyric acid biochemistry and seizure threshold. Ann NY Acad Sci 1986; 462:105-19

Green AR, Nutt D: Psychopharmacology of repeated seizures: possible relevance to the mechanism of action of electroconvulsive therapy (ECT), in Handbook of Psychopharmacology. Edited by Iversen LL, Iversen SD, Snyder SH. New York, Plenum (in press)

Holaday JW, Tortella FC, Long JB, et al: Endogenous opioids and their receptors: evidence for involvement in the postictal effects of electroconvulsive shock. Ann NY Acad Sci 1986; 462:124-39

Janowsky D, El-Yousef M, Davis J, et al: A cholinergic-adrenergic hypothesis of mania and depression. Lancet 1972; 2:6732-6735

Kellar KJ, Stockmeier CA: Effects of electroconvulsive shock and serotonin axon lesions on beta-adrenergic and serotonin-2 receptors in rat brain. Ann NY Acad Sci 1986; 462:76-90

Kety S: Biochemical and neurochemical effects of electroconvulsive shock, in Psychobiology of Convulsive Therapy. Edited by Fink M, Kety S, McGaugh J, et al. Washington, DC, Winston & Sons, 1974

Langer SZ, Sechter D, Loo H, et al: Electroconvulsive shock therapy and maximum binding of platelet tritiated imipramine binding in depression. Arch Gen Psychiatry 1986; 43:949-52

Lerer B, Shapira B: Neurochemical mechanisms of mood stabilization: focus on electroconvulsive therapy. Ann NY Acad Sci 1986; 462:366-75

Lerer B, Stanley M, Demetriou S, et al: Effect of electroconvulsive shock on muscarinic cholinergic receptors in rat cerebral cortex and hippocampus. J Neurochem 1983a; 41:1680-1683

Lerer B, Zabow T, Egnal N, et al: Effect of vasopressin on memory following electroconvulsive therapy. Biol Psychiatry 1983b; 18:821-824

Lloyd K, Pilc A, Leroux B, et al: ECT, antidepressants, and the $GABA_B$ receptor, in Biological Psychiatry 1985. Edited by Shagass C, Josiassen RC, Bridger WH, et al. New York, Elsevier, 1986

Meldrum BS: Neuropathological consequences of chemically and electrically induced seizures. Ann NY Acad Sci 1986; 462:186-93

Miller AL, Faber RA, Hatch JP, et al: Factors affecting amnesia, seizure duration, and efficacy in ECT. Am J Psychiatry 1985; 142:692-6

Miller ME, Siris SG, Gabriel AN: Treatment delays in the course of electroconvulsive therapy. Hosp Community Psychiatry 1986; 37:825-7

Nasrallah HA, Varney N, Coffman JA, et al: Opiate antagonism fails to reverse post-ECT cognitive deficits. J Clin Psychiatry 1986; 47:555-6

Ottosson J-O: Experimental studies of the mode of action of electroconvulsive therapy. Acta Psychiatrica Neurologica Scandinavica 1960; 35(Suppl 145):1-141

Ottosson J-O: Use and misuse of electroconvulsive treatment. Biol Psychiatry 1985; 20:933-46

Pettinati HM, Rosenberg J: Memory self-ratings before and after electroconvulsive therapy: depression- versus ECT-induced. Biol Psychiatry 1984; 19:539-48

Post RM, Putnam F, Uhde TW, et al: Electroconvulsive therapy as an anticonvulsant: implications for its mechanisms of action in affective illness. Ann NY Acad Sci 1986; 462:376-88

Post RM, DeLisi L, Holcomb H, et al: Glucose utilization in the temporal cortex of affectively ill patients: positron emission tomography. Biol Psychiatry 1987; 22:545-553

Prince D: Epileptogenesis in hippocampal and neocortical neurons, in Physiology and Pharmacology of Epileptogenic Phenomena. Edited by Klee MR, Lux HD, Speckman E-J. New York, Raven Press, 1982

Prohovnik I, Sackeim HA, Decina P, et al: Acute reductions of regional cerebral blood flow following electroconvulsive therapy: interactions with modality and time. Ann NY Acad Sci 1986; 462:249-62

Robin A, De Tissera S: A double-blind controlled comparison of the therapeutic effects of low and high energy electroconvulsive therapies. Br J Psychiatry 1982; 141:357-66

Robin A, Binnie CD, Copas JB: Electrophysiological and hormonal responses to three types of electroconvulsive therapy. Br J Psychiatry 1985; 147:707-12

Robin A, Montagu J, Jolley A, et al: Rising trends and current policy, presented at the International Conference on New Directions in Affective Disorders, Jerusalem, 1987

Rose R: Consensus conference: electroconvulsive therapy. JAMA 1985; 254:2103-2108

Sackeim HA: The efficacy of electroconvulsive therapy. Ann NY Acad Sci 1986; 462:70-5

Sackeim HA: Stimulus intensity and electrode placement: efficacy and side effects, presented at the International Conference on New Directions in Affective Disorders, Jerusalem, 1987

Sackeim HA, Mukherjee S: Neurophysiological variability in the effects of the ECT stimulus. Convulsive Therapy 1986; 2:267-276

Sackeim HA, Decina P, Prohovnik I, et al: Anticonvulsant and antidepressant properties of electroconvulsive therapy: a proposed mechanism of action. Biol Psychiatry 1983; 18:1301-10

Sackeim HA, Decina P, Prohovnik I, et al: Dosage, seizure threshold, and the antidepressant efficacy of electroconvulsive therapy. Ann NY Acad Sci 1986a; 462:398-410

Sackeim HA, Portnoy S, Neeley P, et al: Cognitive consequences of low-dosage electroconvulsive therapy. Ann NY Acad Sci 1986b; 462:326-340

Sackeim H, Decina P, Portnoy S, et al: Studies of dosage, seizure threshold, and seizure duration in ECT. Biol Psychiatry 1987a; 22:249-268

Sackeim H, Decina P, Prohovnik I, et al: Seizure threshold in ECT: effects of sex, age, electrode placement and number of treatments. Arch Gen Psychiatry 1987b; 44:355-364

Sackeim HA, Prohovnik I, Apter S, et al: Regional cerebral blood flow in affective disorders: relations to phenomenology and effects of treatment, in Cerebral Dynamics, Laterality, and Psychopathology. Edited by Flor-Henry P, Gruzelier J. New York, Elsevier, 1987c

Sackeim HA, Decina P, Kanzler M, et al: The efficacy of titrated, low dosage ECT: effects of electrode placement. Am J Psychiatry (in press)

Schildkraut J: The catecholamine hypothesis of affective disorders: a review of supporting evidence. Am J Psychiatry 1965; 122:509-522

Scott AI, Whalley LJ, Bennie J, et al: Oestrogen-stimulated neurophysin and outcome after electroconvulsive therapy. Lancet 1986; 1:1411-4

Siesjo BK, Ingvar M, Wieloch T: Cellular and molecular events underlying epileptic brain damage. Ann NY Acad Sci 1986; 462:207-23

Silfverskiold P, Gustafson L, Risberg J, et al: Acute and late effects of electroconvulsive therapy: clinical outcome, regional cerebral blood flow, and electroencephalogram. Ann NY Acad Sci 1986; 462:236-48

Sitaram N, Gillin J: Development and use of pharmacological probes of the CNS in man: evidence of cholinergic abnormality in primary affective illness. Biol Psychiatry 1980; 15:925-955

Skrabanek P, Balfe A, Webb M, et al: Electroconvulsive therapy (ECT) increases plasma growth hormone, prolactin, luteinising hormone and follicle-stimulating hormone but not thyrotropin or substance P. Psychoneuroendocrinology 1981; 6:261-7

Small J: EEG and neurophysiological studies of convulsive therapies, in Psychobiology of Convulsive Therapy. Edited by Fink M, Kety S, McGaugh J, et al. Washington, DC, Winston & Sons, 1974

Small J: Review: efficacy of electroconvulsive therapy in schizophrenia, mania, and other disorders, I: schizophrenia. Convulsive Therapy 1985a; 1:263-270

Small J: Review: efficacy of electroconvulsive therapy in schizophrenia, mania, and other disorders, II: mania and other disorders. Convulsive Therapy 1985b; 1:271-276

Squire LR: Memory functions as affected by electroconvulsive therapy. Ann NY Acad Sci 1986; 462:307-14

Steif BL, Sackeim HA, Portnoy S, et al: Effects of depression and ECT on anterograde memory. Biol Psychiatry 1986; 21:921-30

Stromgren L, Jensen P: EEG in unilateral and bilateral electroconvulsive therapy. Acta Psychiatr Scand 1975; 51:340-360

Summers W, Robins E, Reich T: The natural history of acute organic mental syndrome after electroconvulsive therapy. Biol Psychiatry 1979; 14:905-912

Trimble MR, Thompson PJ: Neuropsychological and behavioral sequelae of spontaneous seizures. Ann NY Acad Sci 1986; 462:284-92

Ulett G, Smith K, Gleser G: Evaluation of convulsive and subconvulsive shock therapies utilizing a control group. Am J Psychiatry 1956; 112:795

Valentine M, Keddie K, Dunne D: A comparison of techniques in electroconvulsive therapy. Br J Psychiatry 1968; 114:989-996

Volavka J: Is EEG slowing related to the therapeutic effect of convulsive therapy?, in Psychobiology of Convulsive Therapy. Edited by Fink M, Kety S, McGaugh J, et al. Washington, DC, Winston & Sons, 1974

Weiner RD: Does electroconvulsive therapy cause brain damage? The Behavioral and Brain Sciences 1984; 7:1-54

Weiner RD, Rogers HJ, Davidson JR, et al: Effects of electroconvulsive therapy upon brain electrical activity. Ann NY Acad Sci 1986a; 462:270-81

Weiner RD, Rogers HJ, Davidson JR, et al: Effects of stimulus parameters on cognitive side effects. Ann NY Acad Sci 1986b; 462:315-25

Whalley LJ, Rosie R, Dick H, et al: Immediate increases in plasma prolactin and neurophysin but not other hormones after electroconvulsive therapy. Lancet 1982; 2:1064-8

Chapter 20

Indications for Use of Electroconvulsive Therapy

by Richard D. Weiner, M.D., Ph.D.,
and C. Edward Coffey, M.D.

Lifesaver; last resort; vestige of past abuses: These are all terms that have been applied to electroconvulsive therapy (ECT). For 50 years this treatment modality has tossed through the violent seas of controversy—extolled by its admirers and vilified by its foes. But despite this history of controversy, ECT has survived. Though annual utilization rates for ECT have continued to decline year after year as our pharmacopia of psychotropic alternatives rises, the psychiatric use of electrically induced seizures remains with us. The main reason for this persistence—this failure to fade away into the halls of oblivion alongside insulin coma and the other "great physiodynamic therapies" of yore—is simply that ECT works.

The task of this chapter will be to present a summary of what is known and what is not known about the indications for ECT: In whom does it work? How well does it work? And, to the extent possible on the basis of efficacy considerations alone, when should it be used? We will focus first upon the use of ECT in depressive disorders, mania, and schizophrenia, as these areas remain the primary clinical indications (Consensus Conference, 1985). Following this, brief outlines will be given regarding indications for ECT; the use of ECT in special populations; the implications of ECT technique upon efficacy; and, finally, the issue of contraindications to ECT. As we shall see, rather than a panacea or cure-all, ECT is merely a tool—a powerful tool—which, when used appropriately and selectively, can help to bring about therapeutic change.

ECT IN DEPRESSIVE DISORDERS

Very soon after the development of convulsive therapy, it was discovered that this treatment modality was particularly potent in cases of severe depressive illness. Since the early 1940s, literally hundreds of research and clinical reports have attempted to delineate the role of ECT in the treatment of depression. Recent reviews of this work have been provided by the American Psychiatric Association (1978), Fink (1979), Scovern and Kilmann (1980), Kendell (1981), Taylor (1982), and Siris and colleagues (1982).

Because the terms major depression and melancholia (American Psychiatric Association, 1980; Keller, Chapter 9 in this volume) are actually quite new to the psychiatric nomenclature, it is often impossible to transform diagnoses from earlier studies into the more modern frame of reference. Even in present times, significant differences in the nature and interpretation of diagnostic criteria exist on a worldwide basis. Because of this confounding, the efficacy data for major depression of different types will, of necessity, be presented together. Discriminations among major depressive subtypes will then be discussed separately in the context of predictive factors.

ECT in Major Depressive Disorders

ECT VERSUS INACTIVE TREATMENT. The earliest studies considering the efficacy of ECT in depressive disorders were retrospective in nature, contrasting response rates to ECT with those of patients who did not receive this treatment modality. In all cases, diagnostic entry criteria were broad, treatment assignments were clinically open, and only global outcome ratings were included. Still, despite obvious methodologic flaws, these investigations served to establish in the minds of most clinicians that ECT was indeed highly effective in depressive illness. Using more contemporary diagnostic criteria, Avery and Winokur (1977) compared the acute therapeutic outcome of 318 patients with unipolar or bipolar major depression, treated between 1959 and 1969, with that of a roughly clinically comparable group of 75 who had received no active somatic treatments. With respect to their findings, these investigators reported that ECT was more likely to be associated with both marked improvement (49 versus 25 percent), as well as significant or greater improvement (89 versus 60 percent). Even more recently, Black and colleagues (1987a) presented similar findings in a subsequent series from the same institution.

In addition to retrospective data, a large number of prospective studies compared the efficacy of ECT with that of inactive treatment. Of studies done in the absence of double blind procedures, two large multicenter trials (Greenblatt et al, 1964; Medical Research Council, 1965) stand out because of their size and because they compared the efficacy of ECT not only against placebo but against active psychopharmacologic antidepressant therapy as well (see below). In each of these studies, ECT was significantly more effective in inducing both a marked and a significant or greater response than the placebo.

Studies involving a simulated, or sham, ECT procedure offer the most convincing data for clarification of the efficacy of ECT in major depression. Because sham ECT investigations are difficult to carry out due to both methodological and ethical factors, the size of experimental and control groups has typically been relatively small (ranging between 4 and 40), a feature which makes a reported advantage for ECT even more impressive. In terms of both size and experimental design, three particular studies stand out. The first of these investigations randomly assigned 70 hospitalized depressed patients, all meeting contemporary American and British criteria for endogenicity, to a series of eight real or sham ECT treatments (Johnstone et al, 1980). As in other sham ECT studies, both subjects and raters were blind to subject group assignment. By the end of the treatment course, subjects receiving real ECT were significantly more improved than those receiving sham ECT, with reductions in Hamilton Depression Rating Scale scores of 69 versus 55 percent. This relatively high level of improvement with sham ECT resulted in a copious correspondence directed toward a number of methodological issues, including the possibility that the subject population was not clinically typical. Following the acute treatment phase, clinical outcome was followed for a six-month period, during which time subjects received further treatment of various sorts, including ECT, at the discretion of their attending psychiatrists. Not surprisingly, intergroup differences in depressive symptomatology rapidly disappeared over this time period.

Several years later, Brandon and colleagues (1984) carried out a sham ECT controlled study in a group of 77 depressed patients clinically referred for ECT, 69 of which met British criteria for major depressive disorder. Reduction in symptomatology was once more significantly greater in the real ECT group at both 2 and 4 weeks after treatment onset, particularly at the latter time period, where there was a 67 percent reduction in Hamilton scores for real ECT versus 28 percent for sham ECT. This study is notable in that it included a sizable fraction of all clinical ECT referrals from a large catchment area, indicating that its findings are especially relevant to clinical practice situations.

In an even more recent investigation, Gregory and associates (1985) randomly assigned 69 subjects meeting British criteria for major depressive disorder to either real or sham ECT. Hamilton Depression Scale ratings performed after the sixth treatment revealed a highly significant therapeutic advantage for real ECT that was nearly identical to that reported by Brandon and colleagues. Following the sixth treatment, subjects were allowed to continue on real ECT in an open fashion, with those initially assigned to sham ECT receiving a greater number of additional treatments. In addition, all five of the subjects who terminated the series because of rapid clinical improvement were in the real ECT group.

Supporting the advantage for real ECT over sham ECT described above are the results of studies which assigned sham ECT failures to a series of real ECT. In each such investigation, the sham ECT nonresponders were found to respond as well to real ECT as did subjects who initially received the latter, though in no case were these assignments carried out or assessed on a blind basis.

ECT VERSUS ACTIVE TREATMENT.   A rather large body of data exists which is germane to the efficacy of ECT compared with psychopharmacologic treatment alternatives. This literature shall be considered in three groups: ECT versus tricyclic antidepressant agents (TCAs); ECT versus monoamine oxidase inhibitors (MAOIs); and ECT versus the combination of TCAs and antipsychotic drugs (APs).

In reviewing 19 studies comparing ECT with TCAs, Siris and co-workers (1982) found a significant advantage for ECT in nine, a trend in ECT's favor in six, no trend in either direction in two others, and an advantage for TCAs in the two final reports (both in "neurotic" depression [see below]). On the basis of a meta-analysis involving the results of six prospective controlled comparison studies, Janicak and colleagues (1985) calculated that ECT was 20 percent more likely to produce a therapeutic response than TCAs ($p < 0.001$).

This extent of therapeutic advantage for ECT over TCAs is quite close to that reported by larger, retrospective investigations. Nearly all such studies found ECT to be significantly more effective than TCAs, with a mean advantage of 23 percent for marked improvement and 19 percent for at least significant improvement. While these favorable results must be viewed with caution, given the fact that TCA dosages in many of the applicable studies were often not at what are now considered adequate levels, prospective studies incorporating daily drug dosages of at least 200 mg per day have all reported a significant therapeutic advantage for ECT. In addition, studies comparing ECT plus drug placebo versus sham ECT plus a TCA (150–300 mg/day) have also reported significantly better therapeutic effects with ECT.

Siris and associates (1982) reviewed 12 investigations that compared the therapeutic effects of ECT and MAOIs in the treatment of major depression, finding ECT significantly more effective in eight, and a trend in that direction in two others. Janicak and colleagues (1985) estimated a therapeutic advantage of 45 percent for ECT over MAOIs based on a meta-analysis of four studies that included response rates.

There have been numerous reports that, at least for delusional depression, the addition of antipsychotic agents to antidepressant drugs greatly improves the degree of therapeutic response over the latter given alone (see Chapter 10 in this volume). Unfortunately, only a modest number of studies have compared the efficacy of this combination therapy with ECT, and none of these has been prospective in design (Kroessler, 1985). Available data suggest a high response rate with both ECT and combined pharmacotherapy groups, but do not allow any conclusion as to whether either modality is more effective. Still, there is some suggestive evidence that marked improvement may be greater with ECT, and also that failure to respond to combination pharmacotherapy does not preclude a response to ECT (see below).

ECT COMBINED WITH DRUGS. A large number of investigations, including some of a prospective nature, have, for the most part, concluded that antidepressant pharmacologic supplementation during the ECT course does not offer any additional benefit (Siris et al, 1982). In some cases, notably lithium and l-tryptophan, the combination may even be associated with lessened efficacy. A recent report that concurrent use of yohimbine (which augments down-regulation of beta-adrenergic receptors) speeds up clinical improvement (Sachs et al, 1986) remains to be replicated. As might be expected, benzodiazepines, which raise seizure threshold, interfere with therapeutic outcome. The use of antipsychotic medication with ECT has not been studied systematically, but does appear to be necessary sometimes, particularly early in the treatment course of an agitated psychotic patient. In all decisions as to whether a given psychopharmacologic agent should be combined with ECT, the potential for additional risk should be considered (see Chapter 21 in this volume).

DEPRESSIVE SUBTYPES. As already mentioned, variability in diagnostic criteria has plagued attempts to clarify definitively the relative effectiveness of ECT in various depressive subtypes. The preceding discussion of ECT in major depression pertains to the following *Diagnostic and Statistical Manual of Mental Disorders, Third Edition, Revised (DSM-III-R)* syndromes: major depression and bipolar disorder, depressed type. These conditions have been subjected to a variety of diagnostic subtypings, both within the *DSM-III-R* framework and elsewhere. Based upon available data, the present discussion shall focus upon the following subtypes of major depression: melancholia, primary versus secondary, unipolar versus bipolar, and involutional. In addition, the role of ECT in a separate *DSM-III-R* type of depressive disorder, dysthymia, will also be considered.

The issue of the effectiveness of ECT in melancholic versus nonmelancholic major depression is unfortunately intertwined with that of major depression versus dysthymia. While *DSM-III-R* admirably makes such diagnostic distinctions quite clear, the same cannot be said to be true of the ECT literature, where, in effect, nonmelancholic major depression is sometimes combined with melancholia, and at other times is lumped together with dysthymia. Still, enough diagnostically precise data exist to allow the conclusions that ECT is highly effective in the presence of endogenous features (that is, mainly in the melancholic population), and that it is relatively ineffective in "neurotic/reactive" depression (that is, in a predominantly dysthymic population). Still, it must be kept in mind that a major depressive episode can be superimposed upon an underlying dysthymic disorder. Although this double depression has not yet been the subject of systematic investigation, it is likely that ECT is of at least some benefit.

Major depression in patients with dysthymia is one example of a depressive subtype that has been termed "secondary depression." Secondary depression consists of a major depressive episode which is superimposed upon either a pre-existing mental disorder or a chronic debilitating medical illness. The issue of the effectiveness of ECT in primary versus secondary depression has been investigated in only a retrospective, uncontrolled fashion (Zorumski et al, 1986). Such studies are, however, relatively consistent in reporting significantly higher response rates with primary depression. In terms of specific underlying illnesses, depression in patients with generalized anxiety disorder is believed to be relatively refractory to ECT, while depressed patients with chronic pain syndrome seem to show improvement with this treatment modality.

Most studies focusing upon the efficacy of ECT in unipolar versus bipolar depressed patients have failed to find a difference (Black et al, 1986), though, again, the applicable data have not been well controlled. The few reports of efficacy differences favor the unipolar group. Involutional melancholia is a depressive subtype that appears late in life and is generally linked to life changes inherent in the senescent period. There are very little objective data available as to the efficacy of ECT for this condition, although anecdotal claims of good results abound.

Predictors of Response

Attempts to formulate valid and reliable predictors of ECT response have been common throughout the history of this treatment modality (Fink, 1979; Scovern and Kilmann, 1980; Taylor, 1982; Hamilton, 1982). Potential areas of importance have included clinical symptomatology, history of present illness, personality traits, demographic factors, family history, and a host of biological factors. While some studies have considered potential predictors on an individual basis, others have endeavored, on the basis of discriminant or factor-analytic procedures, to implement composite predictive indices. Unfortunately, most work in this area was done at a time when ECT was a first-line treatment, and does not, therefore, necessarily apply to the question of more contemporary clinical relevance, namely: "In whom is ECT likely to be more effective than antidepressant drugs?"

The most widely used and, in a relative sense, the most successful predictive index is the Newcastle ECT Predictor Index, which incorporates factors dealing with both endogenous symptomatology and relevant personality characteristics (see below). As with other such measures, absence of predictive power beyond that of simple diagnostic classification has limited the utility of predictive indices to research protocols, where they serve as a means of establishing equivalence among experimental groups.

Of all the individual response predictors investigated, the most promising is the presence of delusions. Though ECT is clearly more effective in such cases than placebo, antidepressant drugs or antipsychotic agents, it remains to be established whether it is more effective than combination pharmacotherapy. In a recent review of 17 studies, Kroessler (1985) reported response rates in delusional depressed patients of 34 percent for TCAs, 51 percent for APs, 77 percent for TCA/AP, and 82 percent for ECT. Still, there is suggestive evidence that there may be differences in quality of remission between ECT and AD/APs. Nelson and Bowers (1978), for example, found that even though they were able to obtain a positive response of 92 percent of the delusional depressives with combination drug therapy, in only 38 percent of the cases was a complete remission achieved.

Overall severity of symptomatology has also been implicated as having prognostic significance, with a majority of investigators reporting significantly greater improvement in severely impaired subjects. Still, one cannot rule out the possibility that this finding may be related to the fact that greater initial severity by its nature is associated with a rating bias in the direction of higher change scores with treatment. Suicidal ideation has often been considered a clear indication for ECT (Consensus Conference, 1985). In practice, the advantages for ECT in acutely suicidal patients are probably secondary to its rapid and complete action in treating the underlying depression, rather than to any specific suicidolytic action.

As already mentioned, ECT appears to have lessened efficacy in patients with pre-existing generalized anxiety disorder. Similarly, the presence of intense and pervasive symptoms of anxiety in association with the depressive episode has been reported to be a poor prognostic sign. On the other hand, motor retardation and, to a lesser degree, agitation, have been claimed to be positively associated with ECT response. Personality traits represent yet another situation in which the clinical presentation may have a bearing upon the extent of therapeutic improvement with ECT. Traits which seem to be associated with a good ECT response are high use of denial, psychological rigidity, and tendency to avoid introspection (Fink, 1979). It is tempting to speculate that such individuals might possibly respond better to ECT because of its enhancement of their ability to utilize repression as a defense. Negative prognostic indicators include hysteric personality, hypochondriasis, and borderline syndrome (Taylor, 1982).

In addition to factors related to symptomatologic presentation and personality traits, the manner in which the present depressive episode has evolved is also of potential prognostic significance. Sudden onset and short duration have both been reported to be associated with a good response to ECT. A history of antidepressant drug failure within the present episode may or may not significantly affect the likelihood of a therapeutic response to subsequent ECT. Conditions where ECT is particularly potent, both in an absolute sense and compared with antidepressant drugs, appear to be least likely to show a decrement in efficacy in the wake of drug failure. Focusing upon this issue, De Carolis and colleagues evaluated the effects of ECT in 437 depressed patients who failed to show significant improvement with 200 to 350 mg of imipramine given for at least 25 days (Avery and Lubrano, 1979). Overall, 72 percent of drug nonresponders went on to remission with ECT. With respect to depressive subtypes, the figures ranged from around 85 percent for melancholic, delusional, and "severe" cases, to only 25 percent for dysthymic patients.

Research directed toward the discovery of biological response predictors for

ECT has been likened to the search for the Holy Grail. Although a number of biological measures may be more or less specific for certain diagnostic subgroups, none so far have consistently improved predictive accuracy for ECT response beyond that achieved by diagnostic factors alone (Fink, 1982; Hamilton, 1982). The most highly investigated of these tools, at least in recent years, has been the dexamethasone suppression test (DST). In a number of initial studies, the DST was observed to be highly predictive of positive ECT response, with nonsuppression of cortisol to an exogenous dexamethasone load associated with an excellent response to ECT. There were even data suggesting that normalization presaged early relapse (Albala et al, 1981). Later studies, however, have demonstrated that electrically induced seizures have a confounding effect upon cortisol regulation, and that this effect appears to be opposite to that associated with therapeutic outcome (Devanand et al, 1987).

Maintenance ECT

It is generally accepted that a course of ECT does not in itself prevent a depressive relapse at some later point in time. The consistent demonstration that prophylactic use of antidepressant therapy following completion of the ECT course is highly successful in limiting relapse (typically 20 percent versus 50 percent for a six-month follow-up period) has made continuation therapy a standard procedure (Siris et al, 1982). This type of follow-up management is particularly important in the first few months post-ECT, as the incidence of symptomatologic recurrence is much greater during this period.

Occasionally, patients are intolerant of the side effects of prophylactic medications (often a reason why they came to ECT in the first place), or these agents do not prevent recurrence of the illness. In such cases continuation therapy with ECT may provide a successful option for maintenance treatment (Chapter 21 in this volume). There are little hard data on the relative efficacy and safety of maintenance ECT, however, and the precise schedule of administration has not been studied. Still, a sizable number of practitioners believe that in selected cases maintenance ECT, typically on an outpatient basis, can be an effective and safe means to help prevent relapse.

The Role of ECT in Depression

As discussed above, ECT is a highly effective treatment of major depression, particularly in the presence of melancholia and/or delusions. The availability of antidepressant and antipsychotic drugs, however, has been associated with a marked decline in ECT utilization. At least in the United States, most psychiatrists prefer, when possible, to carry out a trial of such agents prior to consideration of ECT. In part this is because ECT tends to be viewed by mental health professionals and patients alike as a powerful though complicated and invasive procedure. Still, the longer response latency to the onset of significant therapeutic effects with drugs, typically two to four weeks versus one to two weeks with ECT, combined with the probable lower certainty of eventual response, both act to make ECT a more attractive first-line intervention in cases requiring an early response. Potential characteristics of such a patient population include inadequate nutritional intake, active suicidal ideation, and uncontrollable agitation or psychosis. Other indications for primary use of ECT are cases in which drug toxicities are perceived as presenting an unacceptable level of risk (see

Chapter 10) or where a strong history of positive response to ECT is present. A growing tendency by third-party carriers to require shorter hospital stays suggests that economic considerations may also play a role in this decision process in the future.

ECT IN MANIA

Optimistic reports of the efficacy of convulsive therapy in mania first began to appear in 1939 (Fink, 1979). Schiele and Schneider (1949) reviewed 16 early papers dealing with the use of ECT in mania, covering a total of 466 patients. They found that 62 percent of these patients were considered "recovered," while a total of 80 percent were listed as at least "improved." However, because some of the index patients would probably now be diagnosed as schizoaffective, or even frankly schizophrenic, these figures may even represent an underestimate of ECT's therapeutic effect in mania.

More recent reviews of the efficacy of ECT in mania have tended to yield estimates for therapeutic recovery closer to 75 percent (Fink, 1979; Taylor, 1982; Small, 1985a). In a retrospective investigation of ECT in mania, McCabe (1976) found that ECT induced a "marked improvement" in 82 percent of manic patients as opposed to only 36 percent for those receiving neither ECT nor pharmacologic treatment. More recently, Black and colleagues (1987b) reported similar retrospective results for 438 hospitalized manics, with marked recovery in 78 percent of those given ECT versus 37 percent for patients receiving neither ECT nor lithium. This latter study also allowed the opportunity for a comparison, albeit on a retrospective basis, of ECT versus lithium-treated patients, with marked recovery present in only 62 percent of the latter group (lithium levels of at least 0.9 meq/L for at least two weeks). This finding supports the view that the relative therapeutic potency of ECT for acute management of manics is at least that of lithium, if not even greater.

Still, methodological inadequacies inherent in retrospective investigations point to the need for prospective comparisons of ECT versus lithium. Recently taking on this rather herculean task, Small and co-workers (1986) have already reported, for the first 21 subjects in a prospective study involving random assignment and equivalent doses of antipsychotic agents for both groups, that ECT does in fact appear to be more effective than lithium. In addition, during the follow-up phase of their study, with both subject groups maintained on lithium, Small and colleagues have so far found a longer duration of remission in the ECT-treated group.

While the resolution of the efficacy of ECT versus lithium awaits further study, it is also important to realize that contemporary use of ECT in mania is, to probably even a greater degree than use of ECT in major depressive disorder, a secondary treatment. In this regard, more than 50 percent of Black and colleagues' series of ECT-treated manics were lithium nonresponders during the index episode. Similarly, a preliminary report from a separate ongoing prospective study in medication failures (Mukerjee et al, 1986) is also consistent with a high remission rate with ECT in such a population. A first-line use of ECT in mania can be reserved either for highly agitated patients who are intolerant to antipsychotic agents, or for patients with established or anticipated toxicity to antimanic drugs.

As in depressive disorders, mania is a recurrent condition, and, whenever possible, prophylactic therapy is strongly indicated following induction of a clinical remission. While continuation or maintenance therapy is typically pharmacologic, maintenance ECT has been observed in uncontrolled trials to be successful for this purpose.

ECT IN SCHIZOPHRENIA AND ALLIED DISORDERS

From the late 1930s to the late 1950s, when effective psychopharmacologic alternatives became available, convulsive therapy was, for many psychiatrists, the treatment of choice for schizophrenia. During that time period, widespread use allowed major inroads to be made in assessing the role for ECT in these conditions. As with affective disorders, however, this determination was confounded by considerable variability regarding diagnoses, with diagnostic entry criteria often allowing the inclusion of subjects who would now more likely be diagnosed as schizophreniform disorder, schizoaffective disorder, psychotic depression, secondary major depression, and mania. As much as possible, this review will attempt to discuss the use of ECT in schizophrenia and associated conditions in the context of contemporary diagnostic nomenclature (American Psychiatric Association, 1987). This analysis will include a focus upon schizophrenic subtypes as well as upon response predictors. Other sources of information on ECT in schizophrenia have been provided by Fink, 1978; Salzman, 1980; and Small, 1985b.

ECT in Schizophrenia

As defined in *DSM-III-R* a diagnosis of schizophrenia requires at least a six-month continuous period of functional impairment. This fact serves to relegate some patients who would previously have been diagnosed as "acute schizophrenia" to a separate diagnosis, schizophreniform disorder (see below). This is an important distinction, as acute versus chronic typology is an important consideration in terms of therapeutic outcome with ECT. Schizophrenia, as now defined, implies either a chronic or subchronic course. In effect, such categorizations subsume not only the old "chronic" schizophrenia category, but also some "acute" schizophrenic presentations as well, particularly since the timing of disease onset to prodromal symptomatology is a modern concept.

ECT VERSUS NO ACTIVE TREATMENT.   Early studies of ECT in schizophrenia were generally large, clinically open in design, broad in entry criteria, and poorly controlled. Given these caveats, such studies typically reported claims of significant improvement in 50 to 70 percent of patients following a course of 12 to 20 ECT, as opposed to 10 to 30 percent with no active treatments (Fink, 1978). In point of fact, "improvement" often consisted of nonspecific effects, such as discharge from the hospital, while application of more careful means of assessment suggests that true remission in such patients was a far less common outcome.

The first major indication that ECT might not be quite as effective in schizophrenia as had been believed came with the results of two sham ECT controlled investigations in the 1950s, both of which were carried out in largely chronic populations (Miller et al, 1953; Brill et al, 1959). In each case ECT was not found to be more effective than simulated ECT. Still, advocates of ECT in chronic schizophrenia countered these findings by claims that intensive, or "regressive"

ECT, consisting of one or two treatments given daily over a period of weeks, was necessary in such cases. This argument was based upon the hypothesis that the attainment of a profound organic state would allow a therapeutic "reprogramming" to take place. The elicitation of such dense delirious states, as one might expect, was in time proven to be countertherapeutic.

Other, later, investigations focused upon the use of ECT in subchronic (that is, ill less than two years) populations. The most widely known of these is the Camarillo Study (May, 1968). In this study, which involved random assignment to drug-treated groups as well (see below), it was established on a variety of measures that ECT was indeed more effective than no active treatment. Similar findings were later reported as well by Small and co-workers (1982).

ECT VERSUS ANTIPSYCHOTIC DRUGS. The discovery of chlorpromazine as an effective antipsychotic agent in the mid-1950s sparked a number of comparisons with ECT. Early retrospective studies of this type concluded that antipsychotics (APs) were as effective as ECT, though, again, diagnostically diverse study populations were involved. In their comparisons of ECT and APs in subchronically ill schizophrenics, both May (1968) and Small and colleagues (1982) observed an even greater acute improvement with drugs than with ECT.

ECT PLUS ANTIPSYCHOTIC DRUGS. Numerous studies have considered the combined effects of ECT and APs in schizophrenia. Though findings have been mixed, it is generally believed that combined treatment is more effective than that of either ECT or APs alone (Salzman, 1980; Small, 1985b). Smith and associates (1967) observed more rapid and extensive benefit in chronic patients with 12 ECT treatments supplemented by chlorpromazine 400 mg per day than occurred with chlorpromazine alone (mean dose of 655 mg per day). In subchronic patients, Small and co-workers (1982) reported a potentiating effect of ECT plus AP (650 mg chlorpromazine-equivalent [cpz-eq] given daily), as compared with either APs (913 mg cpz-eq per day) or ECT alone.

Additional data concerning the effects of combined ECT and APs in schizophrenics with a subchronic course has come from sham ECT controlled trials. In the first of these studies, Taylor and Fleminger (1980) found that at four weeks following onset of treatments, schizophrenics receiving true ECT plus a standardized AP dosage (approximately 300 mg cpz-eq per day) were rated globally as significantly more improved than those given sham ECT plus the same standardized AP dosage. Still, given the fixed, and relatively low, AP dosage used, this study does not allow the conclusion that an ECT/AP combination is necessarily more efficacious than a more active AP dosing regimen. To some extent, this issue was considered by Janakiramaiah and colleagues (1982), who compared combined ECT plus AP versus AP alone at two AP dosage levels (300 and 500 mg per day of chlorpromazine). The results of this study suggest that the advantage for combined therapy over APs indeed appears to be a function of AP dosage, with patients receiving 500 mg doses of chlorpromazine responding as well as those given combined treatment.

A third sham ECT trial was carried out by Brandon and associates (1985) in a population that probably included some schizophreniform subjects in addition to those with schizophrenia. In this latter investigation, subjects were allowed to remain on their maintenance AP dosage (mean of around 300 mg cpz-eq per day), thus making the study more akin to an ECT versus no active treatment comparison protocol. As expected, subjects in the true ECT groups showed greater improvement by the end of the four-week acute treatment phase than those receiving sham ECT.

SCHIZOPHRENIC SUBTYPES. A quite consistent finding throughout the ECT/ schizophrenia literature is the relatively high remission rate claimed for catatonic schizophrenia (Salzman, 1980). This is interesting given the continued controversy over whether catatonics are schizophrenic at all or whether they instead represent an atypical subtype of mood disorder. The observation that it is only "acute" catatonia that responds to ECT (Miller et al, 1953) is compatible with this perspective, but, at the same time, also suggests that a more classically schizophrenic chronic form of catatonia occurs as well. There have been mixed claims concerning the efficacy of ECT in paranoid schizophrenia. A possible reason for these conflicting findings is that, particularly during the early portions of the disease course, significant depressive or even manic symptomatology may be present (Taylor and Fleminger, 1980). As will be discussed below, such symptoms appear in themselves to be associated with greater likelihood of improvement with ECT, and also raise the issue of diagnostic overlap with mood disorders. Disorganized, undifferentiated, and residual subtypes of schizophrenia are generally applicable to more chronically impaired individuals and have not been reported to be subject to improvement with ECT.

RESPONSE PREDICTORS. As already noted, a major predictor of response to ECT in schizophrenia is duration of course of illness. The longer the course, the less the chance of a therapeutic response and the longer the series of ECT that must be given to produce any such beneficial effect (Fink, 1978; Salzman, 1980; Small, 1985b). An acute onset of illness, particularly when superimposed upon an adequate premorbid state, was observed as far back as Meduna's original pentylenetetrazole studies to be a good prognostic sign.

Symptomatologic features are also useful in predicting response to ECT. The presence of depression is clearly a good prognostic indicator. In their retrospective series of schizophrenics given ECT, for example, Folstein and co-workers (1973) concluded that only the presence of affective disturbance was associated with a good ECT response. In addition to the occurrence of affective symptomatology itself, overt depressive and manic episodes can also be seen in schizophrenics. In a controlled prospective study addressing this issue, Greenblatt and colleagues (1964) found that ECT was more effective than antidepressant agents or drug placebo, but also observed that the occurrence of marked improvement was less than that seen with nonschizophrenic depressed subjects. The presence of Schneiderian first rank symptoms appears to have an opposite effect upon ECT prognosis than does the existence of affective disturbance. Similarly, the predominance of so-called negative symptoms, which are especially common with residual schizophrenia, generally augers a poor response to ECT.

The matter of whether nonresponse to APs during the present episode affects the likelihood of response to ECT has not been well studied. Friedel (1986) makes an appeal for the use of such management, presenting anecdotal data concerning nine mainly chronic schizophrenics who had not responded to thiothixene. In 8 cases, a combination of ECT (mean of 14 treatments) plus thiothixene 30–60 mg per day was said to elicit a complete remission. In a largely acutely schizophrenic population of 276 patients who had failed to respond to APs in cpz-eq doses of less than 1,000 mg per day, Wells (1973) reported a good response in 37 percent of cases, and at least moderate effects in 75 percent, to ECT (mean of 7 treatments), which was at times combined with APs. Still, the incorporation of schizoaffective and probably schizophreniform diagnoses as well, along with the high incidence of severe depression as the most prominent symptom (54 percent), make it impossible to extend this finding to classical schizophrenia.

MAINTENANCE ECT. As with mood disorders, schizophrenia is a disease marked by intermittent relapses or, as is more often the case, exacerbations. Despite numerous claims to the contrary, there is no consistent evidence that a course of ECT, regardless of its success in inducing a remission or alleviating symptomatology, has a significant impact upon long-term outcome. Because of this situation, maintenance AP therapy is nearly always indicated, although the risk of tardive dyskinesia has prompted some psychiatrists to recommend AP usage only during and shortly after periods of decompensation in schizophrenics with long interepisode intervals. The use of maintenance ECT (see Chapter 21) has for several decades been advocated by some practitioners, though its utilization appears to have diminished considerably over time. Whether concern over tardive dyskinesia will eventually result in a reassessment of the prophylactic value of maintenance ECT remains unclear.

THE ROLE OF ECT IN SCHIZOPHRENIA. ECT is not the treatment of choice in schizophrenia. Patients with a subchronic course may respond to ECT, particularly if affective or catatonic disturbances are present. The use of AP supplementation of ECT does appear to have a potentiating effect upon at least those patients with a subchronic course. Whether this finding can be extended to psychotic episodes of chronically ill individuals remains open to further clarification. There are suggestive data that combined ECT and AP therapy may be beneficial in AP nonresponders, though the incidence and extent of improvement in such cases has not yet been established. There is no evidence that residual schizophrenic symptomatology responds to ECT. A course of ECT may, however, be useful in patients who cannot tolerate the use of APs, at least in the doses necessary for acute treatment of a schizophrenic decompensation. In addition, the growing concern in recent years regarding tardive dyskinesia with APs also seems to be resulting in a more favorable view of ECT as a treatment alternative.

ECT in Schizophreniform Disorder

There are no studies that specifically address the issue of ECT in schizophreniform disorder. This is because, until quite recently, this condition was included in what was loosely termed "acute" schizoprenia. Still, the largely positive findings reported by investigations involving the use of ECT in acute cases suggest that at least a moderate improvement may be seen in 70 to 75 percent of such individuals (Wells, 1973; Fink, 1978). Again, the likelihood of improvement appears to be dependent, at least in part, upon symptomatologic factors as described above for schizophrenia.

ECT in Schizoaffective Disorder

Schizoaffective disorder exists as a phenomenologic entity without clear etiologic support as a distinct disease process. Still, epidemiologic work has suggested that schizoaffective disorder may actually be more akin to mood disorders than to schizophrenia. Not surprisingly, in this regard, patients with schizoaffective disorder respond to ECT better than do all other categories of schizophrenics except for acute catatonics. Wells (1973) reported a good response to ECT in 40 percent of mainly depressed schizoaffective cases, and at least a moderate response in 85 percent. In a three-month prospective survey of ECT use in Great Britain, Pippard and Ellam (1981) reported quite similar findings, with 57 percent good response and at least a fair response in 93 percent. Again, whether such attractive response rates will hold up to the scrutiny of controlled investigation remains to be established.

EFFICACY OF ECT IN OTHER DISORDERS

As stated in the 1985 NIH Consensus Development Conference report on ECT, "there are no controlled studies supporting the efficacy of ECT for any conditions other than . . . delusional and severe depression, acute mania, and certain schizophrenic syndromes." In spite of this statement, a large number of clinical reports have suggested that ECT may prove beneficial in a variety of other mental and systemic disorders. Still, the general applicability of these claims is made uncertain by the predominantly anecdotal nature of such reports, coupled with the general tendency to publish positive, rather than negative, findings.

Mental Disorders

ORGANIC MENTAL SYNDROMES. Specific therapy for organic mental syndromes should always be directed at the underlying medical disorder when possible. Frequently, however, there is also a need for symptomatic control of the emotional and behavioral manifestations associated with the condition. In particular, ECT has been used to manage the confusion, clouded consciousness, behavioral agitation, and disturbances of thought and mood characteristic of delirium. Causes of delirium in which ECT has been reported to offer a safe and effective form of symptomatic relief include drug intoxications/poisonings with bromide, lead, barbiturates, amphetamine, cannabis, lysergic acid diethylamide (LSD), and alcohol; drug withdrawal from alcohol and barbiturates; head trauma; epilepsy; systemic infections such as pneumonia, rheumatic fever, cholecystitis; metabolic disturbances such as uremia; central nervous system infections such as meningitis, encephalitis and neurosyphilis; multiple sclerosis, lupus cerebritis, and degenerative disorders of the brain such as Alzheimer's disease and Pick's disease. In many of these patients, improvement can be seen regardless of any effects upon the underlying disease process. In some cases, improvement can be observed following as few as one to four ECT treatments, although in other instances as many as 12 treatments may be required.

Other organic mental syndromes that have responded to ECT include akinetic states associated with pellagra, and psychosis induced by hallucinogens, steroids, and pernicious anemia. Several reports have indicated that ECT may also be effective in ameliorating the severe and even life-threatening symptoms of lethal catatonia. Thus, catatonia secondary to renal transplant, typhoid fever, and fever of unknown origin have been reported to respond to ECT, even after a variety of drug therapies proved ineffective. Neuroleptic malignant syndrome may be considered a particularly virulent form of lethal catatonia that is associated with exposure to neuroleptic medications. Again, several reports of patients with this condition have suggested that ECT may be efficacious either alone or following partial improvement with dantrolene and/or dopamine agonists.

Affective symptoms such as depression and mania may also accompany a variety of systemic and brain disorders. Whether these mood disturbances represent organic affective disorders, or simply the coexistence of two separate illnesses, is not always clear. Whatever the relationship of the affective symptoms to the organic disease process per se, ECT has been reported to alleviate affective symptoms associated with endocrinopathies, autoimmune disorders, pellagra, pernicious anemia, carcinoma, multiple sclerosis, cerebral palsy, cerebral vascular disease, epilepsy, and degenerative brain diseases such as Alzheimer's disease, Parkinson's disease, and Huntington's disease.

CHRONIC PAIN. In certain types of "atypical" depression, the predominant symptomatology may be somatic; for example, a pain syndrome or hypochondriasis. There have been several reports that ECT may be helpful in patients with chronic pain and various other types of somatic dysfunction, though it has been suggested that the beneficial effects of ECT in such cases is a result of its thymoleptic properties rather than a specific analgesic effect per se. Still, the potentiating effects of ECT upon endogenous opioid systems indicate a need for further research.

OTHER MENTAL DISORDERS. ECT has been used in some patients with eating disorders (anorexia nervosa, bulimia), but has generally only been found to be effective when there is also a major affective disorder present. Historically, ECT has also been reported in the management of obsessive-compulsive disorders, though this use appears to have largely disappeared, presumably because of a lack of compelling evidence of its benefit. Still, recent findings that some obsessive-compulsive patients exhibit dexamethasone suppression test (DST) and rapid eye movement (REM) latency changes similar to those observed in major depression have suggested the possibility of an ECT-response subgroup. There is no evidence that ECT is effective in the treatment of anxiety, somatoform, or dissociative disorders, or in the management of character disorders (American Psychiatric Association, 1978; Taylor, 1982), although, as discussed above, an associated depressive illness may sometimes respond to ECT.

Physical Disorders

A number of reports have suggested that the neurobiological changes associated with ECT may actually directly benefit a number of underlying organic disorders (Weiner and Coffey, 1987). Specifically, conditions such as panhypopituitarism, hypothyroidism, and mild glucose intolerance have been reported to improve with ECT. The movement disturbances of Parkinson's disease and tardive dyskinesia have, at times, also been reduced following ECT. In addition, the anticonvulsant properties of ECT have in the past led to its use in the control of seizures in a few patients with intractable epilepsy.

THE USE OF ECT IN SPECIAL POPULATIONS

Children and Adolescents

There are no controlled studies of the efficacy and safety of ECT in children. Bender (1973) has described her extensive experience with 59 children under 12 with "schizophrenia" who were treated with ECT. The "quality of remission" was described as better in those patients than in a non-ECT treated group, although there was little difference in long-term "social adjustment" (40 percent versus 32 percent, respectively). In a report on 23 psychotic children, Hift and colleagues (1960) found no benefit from ECT treatment after two years. Case reports have produced conflicting results, though it has been reported that children and adolescents with clear evidence of major depression or mania who have failed drug therapy may experience a successful remission with ECT. At present, extremely little use is made of ECT in children and young adolescents, though many practitioners consider older adolescents to be in an "adult" category.

Pregnancy

Because of the possible adverse effects of psychotropic medications on the unborn fetus, ECT has been considered by some a preferred treatment for mood disorders during pregnancy. Numerous reports have found ECT to be safe and effective in all three trimesters of pregnancy, and to be well tolerated by both the mother and the fetus. Monitoring of maternal arterial blood gases has revealed that adequate PaO_2 and $PaCO_2$ levels are maintained during the treatments. Likewise, Doppler ultrasonography of fetal heart rate has demonstrated no evidence of fetal distress during the course of ECT. Still, some authors have recommended that the use of ultrasonography, uterine muscle dynamometry, and maternal blood gases be considered, particularly for high-risk patients during the latter half of the pregnancy (Wise et al, 1984).

The Elderly

The role of ECT in the treatment of depression in the elderly is becoming an increasingly important topic given the present rising proportion of this age group. Further, the incidence of depression may increase with age and its prognosis in the elderly may be worse with respect to both morbidity and mortality. The use of drug therapy in the depressed geriatric population can be problematic given their sensitivity to medication side effects and the frequency of concurrent medical illness.

Despite a large anecdotal clinical experience, surprisingly little hard data exist on the use of ECT in the elderly (Weiner, 1982a). With respect to efficacy, some retrospective studies in the depressed elderly have observed a high response rate while others have not. Only two prospective studies exist. As part of a larger study comparing the effects of different types of electrode placements (see below) in a varied age group, Heshe et al (1978) found no overall significant differences in clinical improvement between patients older and younger than 60 years. In another prospective study of differing electrode placements, Fraser and Glass (1980) observed a "good or moderate" response in 83 percent of depressed subjects aged 64 to 86. As with clinical efficacy, there is a paucity of data concerning the risks of ECT in the elderly, though there is probably an increased likelihood of both systemic complications and encephalopathic side effects (see Chapter 22 in this volume). In addition, the use of ECT in this age group often requires modification of both medication for underlying systemic illnesses as well as the ECT procedure itself (see Chapter 21).

Patients with Severe Medical Illness

The use of ECT in medically ill patients is increasing, and as such may be associated with certain risks and precautions which have implications for ECT treatment technique (Weiner and Coffey, 1987; Chapter 22 in this volume). Given these increased risks, use of ECT in these patients must be preceded by well documented clinical justification and maximal medical therapy of the underlying systemic illness. Again, where appropriate, consideration should be given to modification of the ECT procedure so as to minimize the level of risk.

CENTRAL NERVOUS SYSTEM DISEASE. The use of ECT in patients with primary organic mental syndromes has been discussed above. As noted, ECT may be effective in managing the organic affective and behavioral disturbances associated with both delirium and dementia. A careful neurologic evaluation is always indicated in patients with such conditions, in order to clarify the etiology and to delineate lesions which may create an increased risk for ECT. While not well studied, ECT also appears to be an effective therapy for susceptible nonorganic mental disorders (including depressive pseudodementia) in patients with dementia, cerebrovascular disease, epilepsy, myasthenia gravis, as well as those with indwelling ventricular shunts and skull defects. Such patients may be at greater risks from the encephalopathic side effects of ECT, in addition to other adverse sequelae, but in many cases such effects can be minimized by judicious modifications in the ECT procedure (Weiner and Coffey, 1987). In patients with increased intracranial pressure from intracerebral mass lesions, or with very recent stroke or unstable cerebral aneurysm, the ictal and acute postictal cerebrovascular and intracranial pressure fluctuations associated with ECT may lead to cerebral herniation and/or intracerebral bleeding. Here too, in the unusual event that the patient's clinical status dictates the need for intervention with ECT in spite of such normally overriding concerns, these ECT-related physiologic fluctuations can be significantly attenuated by antihypertensive agents, steroids, diuretics, and/or hyperventilation.

CARDIOVASCULAR DISEASE. The ECT procedure is associated with marked, though transient, increases in blood pressure, pulse, and cardiac output, along with a variety of brief disturbances in cardiac rhythm (see Chapter 22). These effects are associated with significantly higher cardiac morbidity in patients with preexisting cardiac disease. In patients with ischemic heart disease, morbidity may be reduced with preoxygenation, muscular relaxation, and pretreatment with nitroglycerin and adrenergic receptor blockade (Weiner and Coffey, 1987). In situations involving very recent myocardial infarction or unstable angina, however, an appreciable level of risk may remain, resulting in a need for an increased level of clinical justification for ECT. With respect to cardiac arrhythmias, it should be noted that some antiarrhythmic agents may be problematic during ECT, either because of slowing the metabolism of succinylcholine (quinidine and digitalis), or shortening seizure duration (lidocaine). The typical transient surges in blood pressure with ECT are well tolerated by most patients, though excessive and prolonged hypertension during ECT increases the morbidity from certain other medical conditions (for example, aneurysm, intracerebral masses, hypercoagulable states). In such latter cases, pharmacologic attenuations of blood pressure may be desirable.

OTHER DISORDERS. Bronchopulmonary disease may predispose to hypoxia and laryngospasm during ECT, and all such patients should be adequately preoxygenated and receive bronchodilator therapy where appropriate. Because of reports of status epilepticus with elevated theophylline levels, careful monitoring of this agent is indicated. The routine use of muscle relaxant drugs has obviated the risk of musculoskeletal complications from ECT, even in patients with severe musculoskeletal disease. While some reports have claimed that ECT may exert a beneficial effect on mild diabetes mellitus, patients with insulin-dependent diabetes require careful monitoring during ECT. Although the transient sympathetic activation that occurs during ECT could theoretically provoke a "thyroid storm" in patients with hyperthyroidism, in practice this can be prevented by the use of beta-adrenergic blocking agents. Likewise, anticoagulant therapy has reduced the risk of emboli being dislodged during ECT in patients with thrombophlebitis. In such cases, heparin is the preferred anticoagulant, as it has a short half-life, its action can be readily reversed by protamine, and its metabolism is not affected by anesthetic agents used with ECT. Patients with acute closed-angle glaucoma may be at risk because of the transient increase in intraocular pressure during ECT. Further, the metabolism of succinylcholine may be prolonged by drugs used in treating glaucoma, especially long-acting organophosphorus anticholinesterases (for example, echothiopate).

IMPLICATIONS OF ECT TECHNIQUE UPON EFFICACY

Stimulus Electrode Placement

In the late 1950s, Lancaster and associates (1958) reported that seizures generated by electrodes placed over the nondominant hemisphere (ULND ECT) produced significantly less cognitive dysfunction than the standard bifrontotemporal arrangement (BL ECT). The same authors also noted that even though the two types of electrode placement did not significantly differ in therapeutic response as monitored by objective ratings, there was a subjective belief that the clinical improvement engendered with ULND ECT was not as pervasive as that engendered with BL ECT. Since the time of this initial report, numerous studies comparing ULND with BL ECT have been carried out. These investigations have established without a doubt the existence of lessened cognitive impairment with ULND ECT (see Chapter 22). At the same time, however, they have not resolved the issue of whether ULND ECT is as effective as BL ECT (d'Elia and Raotma, 1975; Welch, 1982; Janicak et al, 1985; Overall and Rhoades, 1986; Pettinati et al, 1986; and Abrams, 1986a).

DEPRESSIVE DISORDERS. D'Elia and Raotma (1975) were the first to review the relative efficacy of ULND versus BL ECT in depressive disorders. A total of 29 published comparisons were considered, 14 of which were interpreted as showing equal efficacy, 12 as indicating ULND to be "somewhat less effective," 1 with ULND as "decidedly ineffective," and the remaining 2 with ULND "somewhat more effective" than BL ECT. Since 1975, an additional 12 comparison studies have been reported, bringing the total to 41; with 19 showing no difference in efficacy on the basis of electrode placement, 18 favoring BL ECT (in 6 cases to a significant degree), and 2 favoring ULND ECT. In studies reporting greater efficacy with BL ECT, this determination has been on the basis of at least one of the following occurrences: lower responder rate, less improvement on depression rating scales, larger number of treatments, and more rapid relapse. A smaller number of investigations have considered the relative efficacy of dominant unilateral ECT. In all cases ULD was either equivalent to or less potent than NDUL or BL ECT, with studies reporting lower effectiveness predominating. Although the relatively small amount of data available does not allow complete resolution of this issue, there appears to be very little use of ULD in depression in recent years.

Various explanations have been offered for the discrepancies between studies investigating ULND as opposed to BL efficacy. An analysis of the characteristics of individual investigations indicates that absence of efficacy differences is probably not an artifact of small group size, since negative results were reported by some of the largest series. Similarly, outcome measures employed by such investigations appear to be no less sensitive than those used in studies with positive findings. The possibility that a differential effectiveness on the basis of diagnostic, symptomatologic, or other subject-related factors could account for interstudy variability must also be considered. Still, even though there is evidence that the relative efficacy of ULND ECT may be affected by certain subject characteristics (see below), studies with apparently similar subject populations have reported quite opposite findings.

One area that does appear to relate to efficacy differences, however, is the type of unilateral electrode placement used (see Chapter 21). Unilateral placements in which the interelectrode distance is relatively short (for example, Lancaster et al, 1958) are associated with a number of phenomena suggesting that the induced seizures are either minimally suprathreshold or poorly generalized. These effects, which include missed, abortive, highly asymmetrical, or even frankly unilateral seizures, along with the presence of grossly asymmetrical interictal electroencephalographic (EEG) slowing, have all been reported to be related to lessened therapeutic response. Stimulus dosing is another technical factor that appears to impinge upon the efficacy of ULND versus BL ECT. Malitz and colleagues (1986) have recently shown, for example, that with barely suprathreshold stimuli, an extremely large advantage with respect to attainment of responder status (70 versus 28 percent) exists for BL ECT.

A final factor that may contribute to the presence of an efficacy advantage for BL ECT has to do with whether a fixed or open number of ECT treatments were administered. If claims that a greater number of ECT treatments are required for remission with ULND ECT are true, then evaluation of clinical outcome after a fixed number of treatments would be expected to favor BL ECT. Still, though this effect may be operative in some cases (Pettinati et al, 1986), it cannot explain an advantage for BL ECT in the larger group of studies which utilized an open number of treatments.

Given the uncertainties delineated above for the efficacy of ULND versus BL ECT, several attempts have been made to establish predictors for response to one electrode placement or the other. Black and co-workers (1986) retrospectively investigated this issue in the context of unipolar versus bipolar major depressive episodes, finding no therapeutic advantage for either type of electrode placement. In a separate retrospective series, Small and associates (1985) concluded, however, that patients with hypomanic symptomatology, regardless of primary psychiatric diagnosis, responded better to BL ECT. This finding is particularly interesting, given the situation with regard to ULND versus BL ECT in mania (see below).

In addition to these diagnostic and symptomatologic factors, several other studies have reported that the relative efficacy of ULND ECT diminishes with age. Proponents of this view have tied this finding to the known increase in seizure threshold that occurs with age. Still, it is unlikely that such an effect is present with widely spaced parietofrontotemporal electrodes, since seizure threshold in this case is actually lower than that with BL ECT.

On the whole, the data summarized above suggest that with optimum technique ULND ECT is probably as effective, or at least is nearly as effective, as BL ECT in treating most cases of major depression. Given that ULND ECT is safer than BL ECT, at least in terms of cerebral toxicity (see Chapter 22), a growing number of clinicians are indicating a preference for ULND ECT. One clinical "compromise" that was recently advocated by Abrams and Fink (1974) is to start all but the most clinically urgent cases on ULND ECT, switching nonresponders to BL ECT after five to seven treatments. While some investigators have claimed great success with the use of such a procedure, positive results have so far only occurred in the hands of those who have reported ULND ECT to be of less overall effectiveness. In any event, this situation awaits resolution on the basis of a controlled prospective study of ULND nonresponders.

MANIA. Very recent data concerning ULND versus BL ECT in mania are of great interest given contemporary hypotheses regarding the role of hemispheric laterality in mood disorders (see Chapter 19 in this volume). Although a retrospective analysis by Black and colleagues (1987b) failed to observe any efficacy differences, two preliminary reports from ongoing prospective investigations have both favored BL over ULND (Mukerjee et al, 1986; Milstein et al, 1987). Because of these tentative findings, some clinicians are already turning to BL ECT as the electrode placement of choice in mania, though, again, the data cannot yet be considered conclusive.

SCHIZOPHRENIA. Interestingly, schizophrenia is the only major diagnostic indication for ECT for which there is no controversy over ULND versus BL ECT efficacy, with all studies to date reporting a therapeutic equivalence between these two treatment types.

Stimulus Waveform

The electrical waveform used with ECT varies considerably between ECT devices. The sine wave stimulus, which requires a relatively high amount of electrical charge or energy to produce a seizure, has given way in recent years to the brief-pulse waveform, which is associated with considerably less cerebral toxicity (see Chapters 21 and 22). Efficacy studies have consistently demonstrated an equivalence between pulse and sine wave stimuli, except in cases where the pulses are extremely brief (Weiner, 1982b). This latter difference, which is reminiscent of the lessened efficacy of ULND ECT with short interelectrode distances, probably reflects the occurrence of incompletely generalized seizures. Uncontrolled reports of pulse ECT nonresponders improving with sine wave treatments have been difficult to interpret because of a confounding of waveform effects with those of both electrode placement and stimulus dosing (Price and McAllister, 1986). Given the available data, the preferential use of pulse stimuli appears justified, as long as ultra-brief pulses are avoided and intensity dosing effects are taken into consideration.

Frequency and Number of Seizures

FREQUENCY OF ECT TREATMENTS. In the United States, ECT treatments are typically administered at a frequency of three per week, with one seizure induced per treatment, whereas in many other countries the administration rate is twice per week (Chapter 21). Occasionally, this pattern is altered either because of unacceptable encephalopathic side effects (treatments reduced in frequency or number) or because of a particularly urgent need for a rapid response in acutely and severely ill patients. Despite nearly a half-century of experience, however, an optimum schedule of ECT administration has yet to be defined.

With respect to clinical efficacy, no differences were observed between twice and three times weekly ULND ECT was recently found to be as effective as three times weekly ECT in a four-week prospective trial in 18 depressed inpatients conducted by McAllister and associates (1986). Sand-Stromgren (1975) found no therapeutic difference between ULND ECT given twice weekly as opposed to 4 times weekly in a retrospective review of 102 depressed patients, though the 4 per week group was associated with both a more rapid response and a larger number of treatments. Sand-Stromgren also reported that the 4 ECT per week group did not show any additional memory impairment, as opposed to McAllister and colleagues (1986), who found greater transient nonverbal memory dysfunction with three ULND ECT per week than with two per week. The possibility that a more rapid response can be safely accomplished with frequent ULND ECT runs counter to the findings from older investigations using daily BL ECT, largely in schizophrenic populations, where, as noted above, claims for increased benefit were counterbalanced by severe degrees of induced cerebral impairment. The above studies, though flawed by either retrospective nature or the inclusion of only small numbers of subjects, indicate the need for further, more definitive investigation of the apparent risk/benefit tradeoff present with variations in frequency of ECT administration.

MULTIPLE-MONITORED ECT (MMECT). This is a technique whereby multiple seizures are induced during a single ECT session (see Chapter 21). A remission may be induced in fewer treatment sessions with MMECT, though a larger number of seizures is usually administered. Well controlled studies of MMECT remain to be carried out, however, and are of particular importance given claims that the technique may be associated with greater systemic and encephalopathic side effects.

NUMBER OF ECT TREATMENTS. In clinical practice, the number of ECT treatments administered during a course of therapy should be determined on an individual basis by the nature of the response. There is no scientific justification for delivering a fixed, predetermined number of ECT treatments or for using additional treatments "to consolidate" the therapy once maximal benefit has been obtained, particularly since larger numbers of treatments are associated with greater confusion and cognitive impairment. Once clinical improvement has plateaued the treatments can be stopped. The precise number of ECT treatments required to induce a remission remains unclear, however, and, as noted above, may depend in part on treatment technique. In affective disorders, catatonia, and deliria, the range is from 6–10 treatments; in nonaffective schizophrenia 10–20 treatments may sometimes be required (Fink, 1979). The number of treatments that should be given in the absence of a significant therapeutic response is debatable, though many clinicians will administer up to 8–12 in refractory cases of depression and mania.

Seizure Duration

It has generally been held that elicitation of a generalized tonic-clonic seizure provides the basis for the therapeutic effects of ECT and that brief (< 25 sec) electrically induced seizures are less effective than those of greater duration. Whether there exists a relationship between either mean or total cumulative seizure duration and clinical outcome has not been established, however. In practice, positive claims for the latter have been confounded by the issue of whether individual seizures have been adequate in duration. Another reason for caution in the use of seizure duration as a measure of the "adequacy" of ictal response are recent data suggesting that under some conditions seizures of equivalent duration may not have equivalent therapeutic potency (Malitz et al, 1986).

CONTRAINDICATIONS TO ECT

We believe that there are no absolute contraindications to ECT, only conditions for which there is increased risk. Of greatest concern, as mentioned above, are patients with increased intracranial pressure secondary to intracerebral masses, along with individuals with markedly fragile myocardial vascular status and those with leaky or otherwise unstable aneurysms. As with any therapy, the potential benefits of ECT must be weighed against the risks of treatment, and this evaluation is especially critical for patients with these conditions. Still, modifications in treatment technique can often attenuate these risks (Weiner and Coffey, 1987). In addition, it is also important to remember that other treatment alternatives, including taking no action at all, each carry their own associated morbidity and mortality. Unfortunately, such treatment alternatives tend to be of high risk in most situations for which appreciable risks for ECT are also present.

REFERENCES

Abrams R: Is unilateral electroconvulsive therapy really the treatment of choice in endogenous depression?, In Electroconvulsive Therapy: Clinical and Basic Research Issues. Edited by Malitz S, Sackeim HA. Ann NY Acad Sci 1986; 462:50-55

Abram R, Fink M: The present status of unilateral ECT: some recommendations. J Affective Disord 1984; 7:245-247

Albala AA, Greden JF, Taraka J, et al: Changes in serial dexamethasone suppression tests among unipolar depressives receiving electroconvulsive treatment. Biol Psychiatry 1981; 16:551-560

American Psychiatric Association Task Force on ECT: Electroconvulsive Therapy. Task Force Report #14. Washington, DC, American Psychiatric Association, 1978

American Psychiatric Association: Diagnostic and Statistical Manual of Mental Disorders, Third Edition. Washington, DC, American Psychiatric Association, 1980

American Psychiatric Association: Diagnostic and Statistical Manual of Mental Disorders, Third Edition, Revised. Washington, DC, American Psychiatric Association, 1987

Avery D, Lubrano A: Depression treated with imipramine and ECT: the DeCarolis study reconsidered. Am J Psychiatry 1979; 136:549-562

Avery D, Winokur G: The efficacy of ECT and antidepressants in depression. Biol Psychiatry 1977; 12:507-523

Bender L: The life course of children with schizophrenia. Am J Psychiatry 1973; 130: 783-786

Black DW, Winokur G, Nasrallah A: ECT in unipolar and bipolar disorders: a naturalistic evaluation of 460 patients. Convulsive Therapy 1986; 2:231-237

Black DW, Winokur G, Nasrallah A: The treatment of depression: electroconvulsive therapy vs. antidepressants: a naturalistic evaluation of 1,495 patients. Compr Psychiatry 1987a; 28:169-182

Black DW, Winokur G, Nasrallah A: Treatment of mania: a naturalistic study of electroconvulsive therapy vs. lithium in 438 patients. J Clin Psychiatry 1987b; 48:132-139

Brandon S, Cowley P, McDonald, et al: Electroconvulsive therapy: results in depressive illness from the Leicestershire trial. Br Med J 1984; 288:22-25

Brandon S, Cowley P, McDonald C, et al: Leicester ECT trial: results in schizophrenia. Br J Psychiatry 1985; 146:177-183

Consensus Conference: Electroconvulsive therapy. JAMA 1985; 254:2103-2108

Brill NQ, Crumpton E, Eiduson S, et al: Relative effectiveness of various components of electroconvulsive therapy. Archives of Neurology and Psychiatry 1959; 81:627-635

d'Elia G, Raotma H: Is unilateral ECT less effective than bilateral ECT? Br J Psychiatry 1975; 126:83-89

Devanand DP, Decina P, Sackeim HA, et al: Serial dexamethasone suppression tests in initial suppressors and non-suppressors treated with electroconvulsive therapy. Biol Psychiatry 1987; 22:463-472

Fink M: Is ECT a useful therapy in schizophrenia?, in Controversy in Psychiatry. Edited by Brady JP, Brodie HKH. Philadelphia, WB Saunders Co, 1978

Fink M: Convulsive Therapy—Theory and Practice. New York, Raven Press, 1979

Fink M: Predictors of outcome in convulsive therapy. Psychopharmacol Bull 1982; 18: 50-57

Folstein M, Folstein S, McHugh PR: Clinical predictors of improvement after electroconvulsive therapy of patients with schizophrenia, neurotic reactions, and affective disorders. Biol Psychiatry 1973; 7:147-152

Fraser RM, Glass IB: Unilateral and bilateral ECT in elderly patients. Acta Psychiatr Scand 1980; 62:13-31

Friedel RO: The combined use of neuroleptics and ECT in drug resistant schizophrenic patients. Psychopharmacol Bull 1986; 22:929-930

Greenblatt M, Grosser GH, Wechsler H: Differential response of hospitalized depressed patients to somatic therapy. Am J Psychiatry 1964; 120:935-943

Gregory S, Shawcross CR, Gill D: The Nottingham ECT study: a double-blind comparison of bilateral, unilateral and simulated ECT in depressive illness. Br J Psychiatry 1985; 146:520-524

Hamilton M: Prediction of the response of depressions to ECT, in Electroconvulsive Therapy: Biological Foundations and Clinical Applications. Edited by Abrams R, Essman WB. New York, SP Medical and Scientific Books, 1982

Heshe J, Roder E, Theilvarrd A: Unilateral and bilateral ECT: a psychiatric and psychological study of therapeutic effect and the side effects. Acta Psychiatr Scand (Suppl) 1978; 275:1-180

Hift E, Hift S, Spiel W: Results of shock therapy in schizophrenics in childhood. Schweizer Archiv for Neurologie, Neurochirurgie und Psychiatrie 1960; 86:256-272

Janakiramaiah N, Channabasavanna SM, Murthy NS: ECT/chlorpromazine combination versus chlorpromazine alone in acute schizophrenic patients. Acta Psychiatr Scand 1982; 66:464-470

Janicak PH, Davis JM, Gibbons RD, et al: Efficacy of ECT: a meta-analysis. Am J Psychiatry 1985; 142:297-302

Johnstone EC, Lawler P, Stevens M, et al: The Northwick Park Electroconvulsive Therapy Trial. Lancet 1980; 2:1317-1320

Kendell RE: The present status of electroconvulsive therapy. Br J Psychiatry 1981; 139: 265-283

Kroessler D: Relative efficacy rates for therapies of delusional depression. Convulsive Therapy 1985; 1:173-182

Lancaster NP, Steinhart RR, Frost I: Unilateral electroconvulsive therapy. J Ment Sci 1958; 104:221-227

Malitz S, Sackeim HA, Decina P, et al: The efficacy of electroconvulsive therapy: dose–response interactions with modality, in Electroconvulsive Therapy: Clinical and Basic Research Issues. Edited by Malitz S, Sackeim HA. Ann NY Acad Sci 1986; 462:56-64

May PR: Treatment of Schizophrenia. New York, Science House, 1968

McAllister DA, Perri MG, Jordan RC, et al: Effects of ECT given two versus three times weekly. Psychiatr Res 1987; 21:63-69

McCabe MS: ECT in the treatment of mania: a controlled study. Am J Psychiatry 1976; 133:688-691

Medical Research Council: Clinical trial of the treatment of depressive illness. Br Med J 1965; 1:881-886

Miller DH, Clancy J, Cumming E: A comparison between unidirectional current non-convulsive electrical stimulation given with Reiter's machine, standard alternating current electroshocks (Cerletti Method), and pentothal in chronic schizophrenia. Am J Psychiatry 1953; 109:617-620

Milstein V, Small JG, Klapper MH, et al: Uni- versus bilateral ECT in the treatment of mania. Convulsive Therapy 1987; 3:1-9

Mukherjee S, Sackeim HA, Lee C, et al: ECT in treatment resistant mania, in Biological Psychiatry 1985. Edited by Shagass C, Josiassen RC, Bridgen WH, et al. Amsterdam, Elsevier Science Publishing Co., 1986

Nelson JC, Bowers MB: Delusional unipolar depression—description and drug response. Arch Gen Psychiatry 1978; 35:1321-1328

Overall JE, Rhoades HM: A comment on the efficacy of unilateral versus bilateral ECT. Convulsive Therapy 1986; 2:245-261

Pettinati HM, Mathisen KS, Rosenberg J, et al: Meta-analytical approach to reconciling discrepancies in efficacy between bilateral and unilateral electroconvulsive therapy. Convulsive Therapy 1986; 2:7-17

Pippard J, Ellam L: Electroconvulsive treatment in Great Britain. Br J Psychiatry 1981; 139:563-568

Price TRP, McAllister TW: Response of depressed patients to sequential unilateral nondominant brief-pulse and bilateral sinusoidal ECT. J Clin Psychiatry 1986; 47:182-186

Sachs GS, Pollack MH, Brotman AW, et al: Enhancement of ECT benefit by yohimbine. J Clin Psychiatry 1986; 47:508-510

Salzman C: The use of ECT in the treatment of schizophrenia. Am J Psychiatry 1980; 137:1032-1041

Sand-Stromgren L: Therapeutic results in brief-interval unilateral ECT. Acta Psychiatr Scand 1975; 52:246-255

Schiele BC, Schneider RA: The selective use of electroconvulsive therapy in manic patients. Diseases of the Nervous System 1949; 10:291-297

Scovern AW, Kilmann PR: Status of ECT: a review of the outcome literature. Psychol Bull 1980; 87:260-303

Siris SG, Glassman AH, Stetner F: ECT and psychotropic medication in the treatment of depression and schizophrenia, in Electroconvulsive Therapy: Biological Foundations and Clinical Applications. Edited by Abrams R, Essman WB. New York, Spectrum Publications, 1982

Small JG: Efficacy of electroconvulsive therapy in schizophrenia, mania and other disorders, II: mania and other disorders. Convulsive Therapy 1985a; 1:271-276

Small JG: Efficacy of electroconvulsive therapy in schizophrenia, mania and other disorders, I: schizophrenia. Convulsive Therapy 1985b; 1:263-270

Small JG, Milstein V, Klapper MH, et al: ECT combined with neuroleptics in the treatment of schizophrenia. Psychopharmacol Bull 1982; 18:34-35

Small JG, Small IF, Milstein V, et al: Manic symptoms: an indication for bilateral ECT. Biol Psychiatry 1985; 20:125-134

Small JG, Milstein V, Klapper MH, et al: Electroconvulsive therapy in the treatment of manic episodes, in Electroconvulsive Therapy: Clinical and Basic Research Issues. Edited by Malitz S, Sackeim HA. Ann NY Acad Sci 1986; 462:37-49

Smith K, Surphils WRP, Gynther MD, et al: ECT-chlorpromazine and chlorpromazine compared in the treatment of schizophrenia. J Nerv Ment Dis 1967; 144:284-290

Taylor MA: Indications for ECT, in Electroconvulsive Therapy, Biological Foundations and Clinical Applications. Edited by Abrams A, Essman WB. New York, SP Medical and Scientific Books, 1982

Taylor P, Fleminger JJ: ECT for schizophrenia. Lancet 1980; 1:1380-1384

Weiner RD: The role of ECT in the treatment of depression in the elderly. J Am Geriatr Soc 1982a; 30:710-712

Weiner RD: The role of stimulus waveform and therapeutic and adverse effects of ECT. Psychopharmacol Bull 1982b; 18:71-72

Weiner RD, Coffey CE: Use of electroconvulsive therapy in patients with severe medical illness, In Treatment of Psychiatric Disorders in Medical–Surgical Patients. Edited by Stoudemire A, Fogel B. New York, Grune and Stratton, 1987

Welch CA: The relative efficacy of unilateral nondominant and bilateral stimulation. Psychopharmacol Bull 1982; 18:68-70

Wells DA: Electroconvulsive therapy for schizophrenia: a ten-year survey in a university hospital psychiatry department. Compr Psychiatry 1973; 14:291-298

Wise MG, Ward SC, Townsend-Parchman W, et al: Case report of ECT during high-risk pregnancy. Am J Psychiatry 1984; 141:99-101

Zorumski CF, Rutherford JL, Burke WJ, et al: ECT in primary and secondary depression. J Clin Psychiatry 1986; 47:298-300

Chapter 21

Convulsive Therapy: A Manual of Practice

by Max Fink, M.D.

Convulsive therapy is technically complex and labor intensive. It was introduced by Ladislas Meduna into psychiatry in 1934 for the treatment of dementia praecox. Its efficacy in treating affective disorders was quickly recognized, and by the 1940s, convulsive therapy was a mainstay in the treatment of psychotic patients. The widespread use of psychotropic drugs in the 1960s replaced both convulsive and insulin coma therapies. The gradual recognition that the pharmacotherapies are neither as safe nor as effective as had been anticipated, and the increasing recognition of therapy-resistant syndromes, has led many clinicians to consider, again, convulsive therapy. Such a return to usage has been encouraged by a better delineation of its indications, a greater understanding of the therapeutic process, improved instruments, extensive trials with different electrode placements and electric currents, and answers to the vexing question, "Is a seizure really necessary for therapeutic efficacy?"

Because its use was not encouraged in the decades between 1960 and 1980, few psychiatrists were trained in this complex therapy. The attitude developed, and was widely taught in medical training centers, that electroconvulsive therapy (ECT) was a "last resort therapy" and its use limited to patients who had failed to improve with other therapies. Indeed, in some jurisdictions, such an attitude was codified in law and in institutional rules. Our present practice differs considerably from that of the 1960s, and even from the practices described in the 1978 report of the American Psychiatric Association Task Force on Electroconvulsive Therapy. This chapter describes present practice. (Citations are kept to a minimum. Readers seeking more detailed information are directed to the following reviews and texts: American Psychiatric Association, 1978; Fink, 1979; Fraser, 1982; Abrams and Essman, 1982; Glenn and Weiner, 1985; Taylor et al, 1985; Abrams, in press; and recent volumes of the journal *Convulsive Therapy*.) In addition, two recent reviews of the anesthesia in ECT are particularly helpful: those by Gaines and Rees (1986) and Selvin (1987).

PRETREATMENT PROCEDURES

Indications for Use

Convulsive therapy is ordinarily reserved for patients so ill as to warrant hospitalization. It is most effective in patients with severe affective disorders, both

Aided, in part, by grants from the International Association for Psychiatric Research, Inc., St. James, New York 11780.
I am grateful for the many suggestions of Dr. Richard Abrams, who reviewed this chapter in its preparation.

unipolar and bipolar, especially when accompanied by psychosis. It is effective in the schizophreniform psychoses and syndromes of catatonia; among elderly patients who are affectively ill and who have failed to respond to conventional antidepressant treatments, or who have been intolerant of their side effects; among patients who are suicidal or suffering from severe inanition or delirium; among medically ill patients, especially those with severe cardiovascular disorders, who need constant monitoring of treatments; among pregnant women with various severe psychiatric illnesses, such as melancholia or mania, where the risks of teratogenicity preclude the general use of psychoactive drugs; and among patients with confusional syndromes which may be a reflection of a severe depressive disorder, described as "pseudodementia" or "reversible dementia" (Bulbena and Berrios, 1986; McAllister and Price, 1982). More specific indications are described in detail in Chapter 20.

"Absolute" and "relative" contraindications to the use of ECT are often described. When treatment of a psychiatric condition is sufficiently compelling, as when patients are suicidal, debilitated, or starving, the "absolute contraindications" are set aside and ECT is considered a prudent intervention. Such interventions include treatment of patients with recent myocardial infarction, recent cerebrovascular accident, intracranial mass lesion, or cerebral vascular malformation. Patients with serious medical conditions are considered high risk cases, requiring special expertise on the part of therapists. The prudent physician will not treat patients with these conditions with any therapy of any risk, unless the need is compelling. But when compelled, as when ECT is the alternative of least risk, treatments have been given. At such times, the skill of the psychiatrist and that of the anesthesiologist should determine the outcome.

Consent

Convulsive therapy is seen as a "controversial" treatment, and both patients and their families are often confused as to why it is recommended (Consensus Conference, 1985). Indeed, concerns about its application may be voiced as strenuously from the therapist's peers and co-workers as from lay persons. The information that is shared with the patient and the family and its presentation are central to a good outcome and good management. It is no longer acceptable for the patient to sign a single sentence form for consent giving permission to the hospital staff for all therapies, and assuming that such general consent is valid for ECT. Our practice is to provide each patient with a detailed explanation of the ECT process—what it entails, its risks and benefits, and our understanding of its mechanism of action. This information is provided in the consent form (Appendix A) which is discussed with the patient and members of the family by a knowledgeable member of the treatment team. This discussion is accompanied by viewing a videotape describing the benefits and risks of the treatment and demonstrations of actual treatment (Somatics, 1986). The viewing of a videotape, produced in our own facility, has been very useful not only in assuring 'informed' consent, but in meeting our institutional, legal, and ethical concerns. Details of standard consent practices are described in Chapter 23.

Medical Examinations

When consent is obtained, the medical history and physical examination are reviewed. Many patients referred for ECT need continuing therapies for debilitating medical conditions, such as hypertension, arrhythmias, diabetes, and arthritis, which may increase the risk of anesthesia. Therapies for these conditions should be optimized and consultation with the patient's physician is often useful. Some recent reviews describe the management of patients with special medical conditions (Kalinowsky et al, 1982; Regestein and Reich, 1985; Weiner and Coffey, in press; Abrams, in press) or neurological conditions (Dubovsky, 1986; Hsiao et al, 1987).

A dental examination is useful, particularly in older patients, to determine the presence of loose teeth or dentures. When such are present, treatment should be considered before ECT. The anesthesiologist is asked to meet with the patient and to review the medical record.

There are no tests specifically required before ECT. Spine x-rays are no longer routinely obtained. In patients who have had prior courses of ECT, or in whom a disorder of the spine is suggested by the medical history, dorsal spine x-rays are done. (If done prior to treatment, spine x-rays are usually repeated after the course of therapy.) A pretreatment electrocardiogram (ECG) is usually requested in patients with a history of cardiovascular disease or in those over the age of 40 years. Electroencephalogram (EEG), computerized tomography (CT) scan, or neuropsychological assessment are not routine examinations; these should be requested when the patient's history or examination raise questions for which these procedures may be helpful.

For a few years, there was a wave of enthusiasm that the dexamethasone suppression test (DST) may be a useful guide to treatment, but recent findings have not been reassuring, and such interest has waned (Fink et al, 1987).

'CLEARANCE.' In some institutions, medical 'clearance' for ECT is requested of consultants. It is unclear what is expected of the physicians. The decision to administer ECT is clearly to be made by the attending psychiatrist based on the severity of the patient's illness, treatment history, and a risk–benefit analysis of the available psychiatric therapies. The most one can expect of consultants is a better understanding and an optimization of the patient's medical condition, especially treatment for any associated medical conditions. To ask for 'clearance for ECT,' as if medical consultants have special experience or training required to judge the safety of a procedure as complex as ECT, is to ask more than most consultants can answer. Such practice should not be condoned.

Drug Interactions

Since patients receive various medications for anesthesia, drug–drug interactions must be considered. The regular use of *benzodiazepines* or barbiturates for nighttime sedation may raise seizure thresholds, making inductions more difficult. On this basis, some authors preclude their routine use and taper the dosages of these medications before treatment. Others limit their use to short-acting compounds such as oxazepam. Some anti-arrhythmics, notably *lidocaine*, raise seizure thresholds (Hood and Mecca, 1983) and substitutes such as propranolol should be considered. *Theophylline* may increase the duration of seizures, including the development of prolonged seizures, especially when administered at high levels (Peters et al, 1984). Patients with glaucoma may continue their medications, unless they are receiving *echothiopate*, which should be discontinued (Sibony, 1985). Similarly, diabetic patients should continue their medications, although dosages may need to be modified on ECT treatment days. For patients with epilepsy, some authors decrease anti-epileptic medications, especially *phenytoin* and *phenobarbital*. Such practice is not necessary, although the electrotherapist should be aware that seizure thresholds may be elevated and special maneuvers may be necessary to assure an adequate seizure (see below).

The concurrent use of psychotropic drugs and ECT is a complex issue. For tricyclic antidepressants and monoamine oxidase inhibitors, there is no evidence of a synergistic therapeutic action. As cardiovascular risks are enhanced with the use of *tricyclic antidepressant* drugs, especially in elderly patients, and therapeutic efficacy may be reduced; combined use is not recommended and dosages of tricyclic drugs are tapered during ECT. Concerns have been expressed that the recent use of *monoamine oxidase inhibitors* (MAOIs) will increase the risks of hypertension in ECT, and some authors recommend that treatment be deferred until MAOI use has been suspended for two weeks. Neither Freese (1985) nor Remick and colleagues (1987) found evidence to support this practice. *Lithium* use has been shown to increase the risks of an organic mental syndrome and prolonged apnea, and most therapists reduce dosages rapidly when ECT is being considered. For *neuroleptic* drugs there may be a synergism in action, particularly in the treatment of manic and schizophrenic patients. These medications are usually maintained during the course of ECT. Some reports of cardiovascular complications and death when *reserpine* was used with ECT suggests that such combined use is hazardous. There is little information as to the safety of the concurrent use of anticholinergic drugs, so that most therapists use these substances only when clearly necessary.

TREATMENT PROCEDURES

As ECT is usually given with barbiturate-succinylcholine anesthesia, an intravenous infusion line is established with dextrose in water or normal saline. Various physiologic monitors are assured: blood pressure by cuff; ECG by three leads; and frontal EEG. For the electric stimulation, the skin over the two stimulation sites is cleansed by a fat solvent (ethyl acetate, alcohol, or acetone). In unilateral ECT, one electrode is usually placed in the hair. Occasionally, it is necessary to clip a circle of hair, about 2 cm in diameter, to allow good contact. The electrodes are applied using a small amount of electrode conducting jelly. The impedance of the circuit is checked, and the contact of the electrodes adjusted to an impedance within the ECT manufacturer's specifications. For bilateral electrode placement, the electrodes are placed on both temples. For unilateral electrode placement, one electrode is placed on a temple, about midway between the outer canthus of the eye and the meatus of the ear. Many locations for the second electrode over the homolateral scalp have been proposed (Figure 1). As there is little therapeutic advantage for one locus over another, the d'Elia location is ordinarily preferred, as it induces a seizure with lower electrical dosage (Ermin et al, 1979; d'Elia, 1970).

With facilities to maintain an airway assured, intravenous *methohexital* (0.5 to 1.0 mg/Kg) is given as a bolus. If cuff monitoring and unilateral electrode placement is used, a blood pressure cuff is inflated on an ipsilateral extremity and intravenous *succinylcholine* (0.5 to 1.5 mg/Kg) is given. The degree of motor paralysis is tested by the knee jerk, foot withdrawal to stroking the sole of the foot, or response to a nerve stimulator. Oxygenation is maintained throughout.

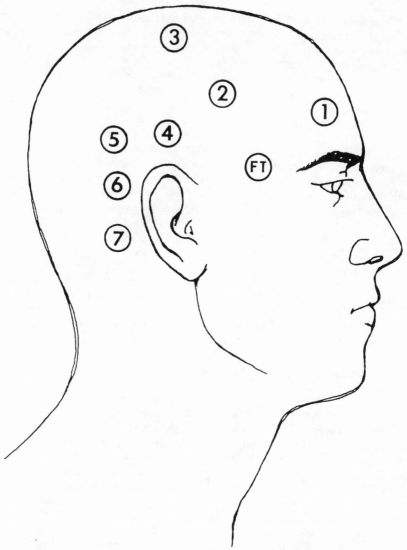

Figure 1. Electrode positions for unilateral ECT. The common fronto–temporal electrode (FT) is located midway between the outer canthus of the eye and the meatus of the ear. Second electrode position varies according to different authors (see Fink, 1979). The location marked 3 is the d'Elia position—slightly to the right of the vertex.

When motor reactions are obtunded, a bite-bloc or mouthguard is inserted and the treatment given.

Some physicians use *pentothal* (3mg/Kg) instead of methohexital, but pentothal is associated with greater cardiovascular abnormalities, especially in patients with preexisting cardiovascular disease, and is not recommended (Pitts, 1982). For severely disturbed patients, in whom it is difficult to maintain an intravenous line, intramuscular *ketamine* (6 to 10 mg/Kg) may be useful (McInnes and James, 1972). For elderly patients in whom it is difficult to induce a seizure, *etomidate* (0.15 to 0.30 mg/Kg) may be helpful since it does not raise seizure thresholds (Christensen et al, 1986).

Intravenous *atropine* (0.6 to 1.2 mg) or *glycopyrrolate* (0.2 to 0.4 mg) are recommended as preanesthetic medication to reduce the vagal effects of the seizure, especially in patients with cardiovascular disorders (Miller et al, 1987). Some authors emphasize the administration of atropine intramuscularly (30 to 90 minutes before treatment) or intravenously (5 minutes before treatment) to reduce salivation (Pitts, 1982).

A concern in the treatment is the immediate effect of the seizure on blood pressure and heart rate. Both hypertension and hypotension occur, as does transient heart block and irregular heart rhythms (Gerring and Shields, 1982; Dec et al, 1985). These effects ordinarily require no intervention, as they spontaneously normalize by the end of the seizure.

For patients with established hypertension, intervention may be warranted. The first maneuver is to dissolve one or two nitroglycerine tablets (0.3 to 0.6 mg) under the tongue, two to four minutes prior to treatment. If hypertension is severe, or blood pressure control critical, the rapid acting ganglionic blocking agent, trimethaphan camsylate (Arfonad) drip is used. Trimethaphan (250 mg or 5 ml) is mixed in 250 ml dextrose/water. The drip needle is inserted into the intravenous line, and blood pressure is titrated by a continuous drip. Blood pressure is monitored and reduced to a systolic pressure of 100 to 120 mm Hg before stimulation. During and immediately after the seizure, blood pressure is monitored and the blood pressure maintained below 180 mm Hg. Occasionally, hypotension will ensue immediately after the seizure; this is usually transient and stimulants should not be administered; we prefer to allow the blood pressure to reestablish itself.

For patients with persistent dysrhythmia, efforts are usually made to optimize the clinical status. In patients requiring ECT, treatment is usually given with attention to cardiac monitoring. Both lidocaine and phenytoin are generally not used, as the rise in seizure threshold may complicate seizure induction.

For patients with a history of malignant hyperthermia, or those who develop fever with treatment, succinylcholine may be replaced by *curare* (3 to 6 mg/Kg) or *atracurium* (0.5 mg/Kg) (Dwersteg and Avery, 1987; Hicks, 1987).

Seizure Induction

The appearance of a bilateral grand mal seizure is the hallmark of an effective induction. Subconvulsive or sham treatments are clearly less effective (Palmer, 1981; Kiloh, 1985). The most recent reports of the Northwick Park, Leicestershire, and Nottingham studies conclude that there is a distinct therapeutic advantage for treatments with induced grand mal seizures compared to those given sham treatments, both in patients with depression and in those with schizophrenia (Johnstone et al, 1980; Brandon et al, 1984, 1985; Gregory et al, 1985).

The principal risk of convulsive therapy remains cognitive impairment. Impairment is usually described for the time of the illness and the events associated with the treatments, but there are some patients who continue to describe loss of memories to events earlier than the time of the illness (Malitz and Sackeim, 1986). Cognitive impairment results, in part, from the type and amount of electrical energy and the path of the electric currents used.

CURRENT TYPE.   Two current types are in use in United States instruments—sinusoidal (Medcraft B-24) and brief pulse (MECTA, Thymatron, Medcraft B-25). Seizures induced with sinusoidal currents usually use higher amounts of total energy and elicit greater cognitive and EEG effects than those induced with brief pulse currents. While there is some question whether the efficacy of seizures induced by the two currents are equal, and clinical trials are in progress, there is a widespread acceptance of the use of brief pulse current instruments for routine use (Malitz and Sackeim, 1986).

The lesser cognitive effects of brief pulse currents were thought to result from the lower total energy used. As a consequence, the use of low total energy has been a recent aim of therapists. Treatments using threshold energies were tested, and were found to be less effective than when treatments were given with suprathreshold stimulation (Malitz and Sackeim, 1986). Lowered efficacy was particularly apparent with unilateral electrodes. But, if high induction energies are used, patients exhibit greater cognitive deficits. Present knowledge suggests that the induction energy should be substantially above threshold, but not so high as to be accompanied by excess cognitive deficits or prolonged seizures. What is the prudent therapist to do? Practice varies; we use the cuff monitored seizure duration as a guide. When seizure durations are between 25 and 40 seconds, we generally increase the dosage of the stimulation for the next treatment by 10 percent; when seizure duration is longer than 90 seconds, we reduce the dosage by about 10 percent for the next treatment.

ELECTRODE PLACEMENT.   Cognitive impairment is less with unilateral electrode placement than with bilateral (Horne et al, 1985), and in the belief that the efficacy of unilateral and bilateral treatments was equal, unilateral placement was generally recommended (American Psychiatric Association, 1978). However, recent studies demonstrate greater efficacy for seizures using bilateral placements than those using unilateral, and the general recommendations have been modified (Abrams et al, 1983; Abrams, 1986). There are many observers, however, who contend that the efficacy of treatments through unilateral electrode placements, when properly done, are equally effective to those in which bilateral electrode placements have been used (Strömgren, 1984; Horne et al, 1985).

PRESENT PRACTICE.   Seizure inductions with unilateral electrode placement over the nondominant hemisphere and brief pulse currents at higher than threshold intensity are generally recommended for all affectively ill patients, except the most suicidal or most severely ill and those with mania, in whom bilateral treatments are preferred (Abrams and Fink, 1984; Milstein et al, 1987). Bilateral treatments are also recommended in the most severely ill, and in those who have not responded within five to six treatments (Price, 1981; Abrams et al, 1983; Abrams and Fink, 1984; McAllister et al, 1985).

Seizure Monitoring

It is customary to record heart rate and blood pressure during seizures. For high risk and elderly patients, ECG monitoring is advisable. *Oximeters* may be helpful to assure adequate oxygenation during the treatment and recovery period. And *nerve stimulation monitors* are used when the determination of full paralysis is required (Baker, 1986; Coffey et al, 1986).

SEIZURE DURATION. This is observed using a number of physiologic events—the motor aspects of the seizure, EEG, and heart rate. For the motor aspects, a *cuff method* is used (Fink and Johnson, 1982). Before the injection of succinylcholine, a blood pressure cuff is inflated above the systolic pressure in a limb, usually homolateral to the electrode placement in unilateral ECT (to assure a bilateral seizure). This prevents paralysis of the muscles by succinylcholine and allows timing of the observed tonic and clonic movements. EEG monitors are now components of some ECT devices which allow the measurement of seizure duration either in a paper record (MECTA) or an audible monitor (THYMATRON). *Tachycardia* accompanies most seizure inductions, and seizure durations may be determined by palpation or from an ECG monitor (Larson et al, 1984).

When multiple monitors are used, the shortest duration is measured in the motor seizure. Cardiac acceleration is generally longer, by about 10 percent; and EEG durations are longer still, varying from 10 percent to many times the motor seizure duration. A principal reason for EEG monitoring is the frequent induction of a prolonged EEG seizure after the motor convulsion has terminated (Greenberg, 1985). EEG seizure durations longer than 180 seconds are considered *prolonged*, and warrant interruption by intravenous methohexital (30 to 80 mg) or intravenous diazepam (2.5 to 7.5 mg).

From time to time, it is difficult to determine whether a grand mal seizure has occurred, and in such instances, the determination of *plasma prolactin* levels may be helpful. Plasma prolactin is released by grand mal seizures, with a peak effect about 20 minutes postseizure (Swartz, 1985).

"ADEQUATE SEIZURE." An "adequate seizure" is conventionally defined as one with a duration greater than 25 seconds in peripheral monitoring; with bilateral cerebral generalization as evinced by bilateral tonic and clonic components; perhaps with a postseizure period of electrical silence, usually defined by an abrupt EEG seizure termination. An adequate seizure results from the interaction of patient's age, degree of anesthesia, type and dosage of electrical current, and electrode placement.

The amount of energy necessary to induce a seizure increases with age, and is generally higher in men than in women. Thresholds are higher for bilateral electrode placements than they are for unilateral. Thresholds rise during the course of therapy. It is necessary, therefore, for the therapist to monitor seizures for adequacy. From time to time, seizure durations remain short and seizures are considered "inadequate" despite changes in electrical dosage, electrode placement, and, even, electrical current form. In such instances, therapists first check the fit of the electrodes, assuring an adequate contact (low impedance) between electrodes and the patient. Dosages of barbiturate anesthetic may be reduced, or etomidate may be used instead of methohexital. If seizure durations remain short, augmentation by an analeptic agent may be tried. Pentetrazol augmentation using an intravenous bolus of 500 to 800 mg pentetrazol, 60 to 90 seconds before the electrical induction, is useful. Or, an intravenous bolus of caffeine sodium benzoate (500 to 750 mg), 5 to 10 minutes before seizure induction, may be successful (Shapira et al, 1985).

POST-SEIZURE MONITORING. The recovery period is a time of continued risk for the patient, and observation should be continued by trained personnel able to manage impaired airways and changes in cardiovascular status. Monitoring of skin color, blood pressure, heart rate, respiratory rate, and alertness continues through the postseizure recovery period, until the patient is returned to his or her room. It is useful to develop a simple scale of orientation and tests of aphasia during recovery, to determine whether the organic features are prolonged or aphasia prominent. In such instances, a change in electrode placement may be considered.

Number and Frequency of Seizures

Both the frequency and numbers of treatments are defined by clinical progress. It is conventional in the United States to treat patients three times a week, while, in Great Britain, the pattern is twice weekly. Affectively ill patients show some improvement, usually in the relief of vegetative symptoms or in mood, within four to five treatments. When such changes are not observed, electrode placement or current type should be changed. In severely ill patients, particularly those in manic delirium, daily treatments are useful. Some authors find two treatments in one induction helpful (Swartz and Mehta, 1986); while others describe multiple treatments in one session—up to six seizures with one anesthesia—as being more effective and reducing the period of incapacity (Maletzky, 1986). The evidence that such modifications are more effective and as safe as conventional ECT is not compelling.

The number of treatments averages 7 to 9 for patients with severe affective disorders, and from 12 to 20 for patients with mania and therapy resistant psychosis. The end-point of a course is defined by relief of the patient's symptoms.

Continuation Therapy

In psychoactive drug treatments, therapy is generally continued for months. Indeed, despite such continuation, many affectively ill patients relapse. In the ECT process, continuation with antidepressant drugs or lithium has been shown to reduce relapse rates when compared with no continuation or with sedative drugs (Fink, 1979; Coppen et al, 1981). Continuation therapy with weekly or biweekly ECT was a regular feature of practice in the 1950s (Karliner and Wehrheim, 1965). It is reasonable to assume that the same factors that require continuation in drug therapies will also require continuation with ECT. Unfortunately, the data are not available to provide an adequate guideline. In patients who rapidly relapse after a course of therapy, some practitioners continue ECT at weekly and biweekly intervals, proceeding to monthly intervals (Fraser, 1982; Taylor et al, 1985).

FACILITIES FOR ECT

Staffing

Psychiatrists administering ECT should be qualified, by preceptorship and experience, to assume responsibility for this complex treatment. The complexities of ECT no longer allow a cavalier attitude that accepts the least qualified intern or resident as competent to manage ECT procedures. It is a reflection of the inherent safety of ECT and the tolerance of our patients for seizures that more reports of adverse effects do not fill the medical and legal literature. There is no accreditation procedure for ECT practice, so it is the responsibility of each medical center to establish guidelines for the proficiency of physicians responsible for ECT (Moscarillo, 1986; Fink, 1986, 1987). In addition to the psychiatrist, a trained nurse and nursing assistant with experience in intensive care and resuscitation are usually required.

The administration of anesthesia, even for a procedure as short as ECT, requires skill in airway management and, occasionally, in resuscitation after cardiac or respiratory failure. Anesthesiologists and nurse–anesthetists are usually qualified in these practices and, in major institutions, especially in those equipped to treat high-risk cases, their skills should make them part of the treatment team (Fink, 1985).

Facilities

ECT is best given in a suite consisting of a treatment room and a recovery area on the psychiatric treatment unit. The use of operating rooms invariably inhibits the proper use of ECT. It is neither required by the procedure nor does it facilitate the proper treatment of patients. Such a requirement usually reflects the dogmatism of the anesthesiologist or the antagonism of an administration to psychiatric practice as well as the use of ECT.

The treatment room needs medical supplies (Appendix B); a source of oxygen and means for its delivery; and monitoring instruments for blood pressure, heart rate, and ECG. Modern ECT instruments usually include devices for EEG monitoring. The recovery room should be similarly equipped for oxygen delivery, maintenance of airways, and monitoring of cardiovascular measures.

ECT equipment has undergone many modifications and there is little justification for the continued use of equipment designed or built prior to 1980. Institutions using ECT should have at least two ECT instruments available, and they should require semiannual engineering tests to assure that the instruments meet safety standards. Since each instrument now available in the United States meets recently set standards, the selection is based on the optional features of each instrument. An evaluation of two principal instruments is available (Nilsen et al, 1986).

Record Keeping

ECT is a repeated treatment, so that records are helpful in optimizing the treatment of individual patients. Records should include anesthetic doses and adjuvant drugs; seizure induction parameters (instrument, dose, time, electrode placement); seizure duration measurements; blood pressure; and notes as to untoward events (Appendix C). In addition to the records maintained on the patient charts, a duplicate treatment room record should be kept to assist in treating patients readmitted after relapse.

Educational Materials

For patients, the Consensus Development Conference Statement (1985); the experiences of a patient titled "Holiday of Darkness" by Endler (1982); and the American Psychiatric Association Task Force Report (1978) are helpful. A videotape made especially for patients and their families provides a useful resource for consent (Somatics, 1986).

For professionals, the texts cited in the introduction should be part of their library. Instruction manuals and videotapes on treatment practice accompany most ECT instruments, and additional videotapes for professionals are available (Somatics, 1986). The journal *Convulsive Therapy* (New York, Raven Press) is a source of case and research material, especially about high risk cases. Subscribers and authors may also avail themselves of a citation service and hotline for consultation.

REFERENCES

Abrams R: Is unilateral electroconvulsive therapy really the treatment of choice in endogenous depression? Ann NY Acad Sci 1986; 462:50-55

Abrams R: Electroconvulsive Therapy. New York, Oxford University Press (in press)

Abrams R, Essman WB (Eds): Electroconvulsive Therapy. Biological Foundations and Clinical Applications. New York, Spectrum Publications, 1982

Abrams R, Fink M: The present status of unilateral ECT: some recommendations. J Affective Disord 1984; 7:245-247

Abrams R, Taylor MA, Faber R, et al: Bilateral vs. unilateral electroconvulsive therapy: efficacy in melancholia. Am J Psychiatry 1983; 140:463-465

American Psychiatric Association. Electroconvulsive Therapy. Task Force Report #14. Washington, DC, American Psychiatric Association, 1978

Baker NJ: Electroconvulsive therapy and severe osteoporosis: use of a nerve stimulator to assess paralysis; case report. Convulsive Therapy 1986; 2:285-288

Brandon S, Cowley P, McDonald C, et al: Electroconvulsive therapy: results in depressive illness from the Leicestershire trial. Br Med J 1984; 288:22-25

Brandon S, Cowley P, McDonald C, et al: Leicester ECT trial: results in schizophrenia. Br J Psychiatry 1985; 146:177-183

Bulbena A, Berrios GE: Pseudodementia: facts and figures. Br J Psychiatry 1986; 148:87-94

Christensen P, Kragh-Sorenson P, Sorenson C, et al: EEG-monitored ECT: a comparison of seizure duration under anesthesia with etomidate and thiopentone. Convulsive Therapy 1986; 2:145-150

Coffey CE, Weiner RD, Kalayjian R, et al: Electroconvulsive therapy in osteogenesis imperfecta: issues of muscular relaxation; case report. Convulsive Therapy 1986; 2:207-211

Consensus Conference: Electroconvulsive therapy. JAMA 1985; 254:103-108

Consensus Development Conference Statement: Electroconvulsive Therapy 5 (#1). Washington, DC, USDHEW, 1985

Coppen A, Abou-Saleh MT, Milln P, et al: Lithium continuation therapy following electroconvulsive therapy. Br J Psychiatry 1981; 139:284-287

Dec GW, Jr, Stern TA, Welch C: The effects of electroconvulsive therapy on serial electrocardiograms and serum cardiac enzyme values: a prospective study of depressed hospitalized inpatients. JAMA 1985; 253:2525-2529

d'Elia G: Unilateral electroconvulsive therapy. Acta Psychiatr Scand 1970; (Suppl 215): 5-98

Dubovsky SL: Using electroconvulsive therapy for patients with neurological disease. Hosp Community Psychiatry 1986; 37:819-824

Dwersteg JF, Avery DH: Atracurium as a muscle relaxant for electroconvulsive therapy in a burned patient: case report. Convulsive Therapy 1987; 3:49-53

Endler NS: Holiday of Darkness. New York, John Wiley & Sons, 1982

Erman MK, Welch CA, Mandel MR: A comparison of two unilateral ECT electrode placements: efficacy and electrical energy considerations. Am J Psychiatry 1979; 136:1317-1319

Fink M: Convulsive Therapy: Theory and Practice. New York, Raven Press, 1979

Fink M: Anesthesia in electroconvulsive therapy (Editorial). Convulsive Therapy 1985; 1:155-157

Fink M: Training in convulsive therapy (Editorial). Convulsive Therapy 1986; 2:227-230

Fink M: New technology in convulsive therapy: a challenge in training. Am J Psychiatry 1987; 144:1195-1198

Fink M, Johnson L: Monitoring duration of ECT seizures: 'cuff' and EEG methods compared. Arch Gen Psychiatry 1982; 39:1189-1191

Fink M, Gujavarty K, Greenberg LB: Serial dexamethasone suppression tests and clinical outcome in ECT. Convulsive Therapy (in press)

Fraser M: ECT: A Clinical Guide. Chichester, John Wiley, 1982

Freese KJ: Can patients safely undergo electroconvulsive therapy while receiving mono-amine oxidase inhibitors? Convulsive Therapy 1985; 1:190-194

Gaines GY, Rees DI: Electroconvulsive therapy and anesthesia considerations. Anesthesia Analgesia 1986; 1345-1356

Gerring JP, Shields HM: The identification and management of patients with a high risk for cardiac arrhythmias during modified ECT. J Clin Psychiatry 1982; 43:140-143

Glenn MD, Weiner RD: Electroconvulsive Therapy: A Programmed Text. Washington, DC, American Psychiatric Press, Inc., 1985

Greenberg LB: Detection of prolonged seizures during electroconvulsive therapy: a comparison of electroencephalogram and cuff monitoring. Convulsive Therapy 1985; 1:32-37

Gregory S, Shawcross CR, Gill D: The Nottingham ECT study: a double-blind comparison of bilateral, unilateral and simulated ECT in depressive illness. Mapperley Hospital, Nottingham. Br J Psychiatry 1985; 146:520-524

Hicks FG: ECT modified by atracurium: case report. Convulsive Therapy 1987; 3:54-59

Hood DD, Mecca RS: Failure to initiate electroconvulsive seizures in a patient pretreated with lidocaine. Anesthesiology 1983; 58:379-381

Horne RL, Pettinati HM, Sugerman AA, et al: Comparing bilateral to unilateral electro-convulsive therapy in a randomized study with EEG monitoring. Arch Gen Psychiatry 1985; 42:1087-1092

Hsiao JK, Messenheimer JA, Evans DL: ECT and neurological disorders: a review. Convulsive Therapy 1987; 3:121-136

Johnstone EC, Deakin JFW, Lawler P, et al: The Northwick Park electroconvulsive treatment trial. Lancet 1980; 2:1317-1320

Kalinowsky LB, Hippius H, Klein HE: Biological Treatments in Psychiatry. New York, Grune & Stratton, 1982

Karliner W, Wehrheim HK: Maintenance convulsive treatments. Am J Psychiatry 1965; 121:113-115

Kiloh LG: The trials of ECT. Psychiatr Dev 1985; 3:205-218

Larson G, Swartz C, Abrams R: Duration of ECT-induced tachycardia as a measure of seizure length. Am J Psychiatry 1984; 141:1269-1271

Maletzky BM: Conventional and multiple-monitored electroconvulsive therapy: a comparison in major depressive episodes. J Nerv Ment Dis 1986; 174:257-264

Malitz S, Sackeim H (Eds): Electroconvulsive Therapy: Clinical and Basic Research Issues. Ann NY Acad Sci 1986; 462:1-424

McAllister TW, Price TRP: Severe depressive pseudodementia with and without dementia. Am J Psychiatry 1982; 139:626-629

McAllister TW, Price TRP, Ferrell RB: Bilateral sinusoidal ECT following poor response to five unilateral brief-pulse ECTs. J Clin Psychiatry 1985; 46:430-431

McInnes EJ, James NM: A comparison of ketamine and methohexital in electroconvulsive therapy. Med J Aust 1972; 1:1031-1032

Miller ME, Gabriel A, Herman G, et al: Atropine sulphate premedication and cardiac arrhythmia in electroconvulsive therapy (ECT). Convulsive Therapy 1987; 3:10-17

Milstein V, Small JG, Klapper MH, et al: Uni- versus bilateral ECT in the treatment of mania. Convulsive Therapy 1987; 3:1-9

Moscarillo FM: Electrotherapy certification. Convulsive Therapy 1986; 2:129-131

Nilsen SM, Willis KW, Pettinati HM: Initial impression of two new brief-pulse electro-convulsive therapy machines: instrument review. Convulsive Therapy 1986; 2:43-54

Palmer RL: Electroconvulsive Therapy: An Appraisal. New York, Oxford University Press, 1981

Peters, SG, Wochos DN, Peterson GC: Status epilepticus complicating electroconvulsive therapy in the presence of theophylline. Mayo Clin Proc 1984; 59:568-570

Pitts FN: Medical physiology of ECT, in Electroconvulsive Therapy: Biological Foundations and Clinical Applications. Edited by Abrams R, Essman WB. New York, Spectrum Publications, 1982

Price TRP: Unilateral electroconvulsive therapy for depression (letter). N Engl J Med 1981; 304:53

Regestein QR, Reich P: Electroconvulsive therapy in patients at high risk for physical complications. Convulsive Therapy 1985; 1:101-114

Remick RA, Jewesson P, Ford RWJ: MAO inhibitors in general anesthesia: a re-evaluation. Convulsive Therapy 1987; 3:196-203

Selvin BL: Electroconvulsive therapy—1987. Anesthesiology 1987; 67:367-385

Shapira B, Zohar J, Newman M, et al: Potentiation of seizure length and clinical response to electroconvulsive therapy by caffeine pretreatment: a case report. Convulsive Therapy 1985; 1:58-60

Sibony PA: ECT risks in glaucoma (Letter). Convulsive Therapy 1985; 1:283-284

Somatics, Inc: Informed ECT for Health Professionals. Videotape. 24 min. (910 Sherwood Drive, Lake Bluff, IL 60044.), 1986

Somatics, Inc: Informed ECT for patients and families. Videotape. 22 min. (910 Sherwood Drive, Lake Bluff, IL 60044), 1986

Strömgren LS: Is bilateral ECT ever indicated? Acta Psychiatr Scand 1984; 69:484-490

Swartz C: Characterization of the total amount of prolactin released by electroconvulsive therapy. Convulsive Therapy 1985; 1:252-257

Swartz CM, Mehta RK: Double electroconvulsive therapy for resistant depression: case report. Convulsive Therapy 1986; 2:55-57

Taylor M, Sierles FS, Abrams R: General Hospital Psychiatry. New York, Free Press, 1985

Weiner RD, Coffey CE: Use of electroconvulsive therapy in patients with severe medical illness, in Treatment of Psychiatric Disorders in Medical–Surgical Patients. Edited by Stoudemire A, Fogel R. New York, Grune & Stratton (in press)

Appendix A

CONSENT FOR ELECTROTHERAPY

I, _____ , M.D.
(and _____ , M.D.) recommend
electrotherapy (brain stimulation, electroconvulsive therapy) for your present mental
symptoms. These treatments have been given to thousands of mentally ill patients since
1938, with many improvements in the treatments and greater success in helping patients
since then.

Treatments are given in the mornings before breakfast, in a specially equipped treatment
room. You will be attended by an anesthetist, a nurse, and a physician.

A needle will be placed in your vein (like you may have had when samples were taken
for blood tests) and an anesthetic will be injected. You will become drowsy and fall asleep.
Other medicines will be given to relax your muscles. The anesthetist will help you breathe
with pure oxygen through a mask.

The treatment is given while you are asleep. Momentary electric currents are passed
through electrodes on the scalp to stimulate the brain. When the brain is stimulated, there
are muscular contractions for up to a minute, but with proper relaxation, the contractions
are barely measurable.

The treatments take only a few minutes. You are then moved to the recovery room
where you will gradually wake up as after a deep sleep. You may feel groggy, probably
have some muscular aches like after a lot of exercises, and some headache. You will return
to your room, usually within an hour of the treatment. You may be hungry and will be
given your breakfast and you will spend the rest of the morning on the ward with your
nurse or attendant.

Treatments are given every other day for up to 12 treatments. Many patients improve
rapidly and require fewer treatments, some require more than 12, but these will not be
given without another discussion with you and your family.

There are some risks in the treatment. To provide safe anesthesia, the treatments are
given in a room where special equipment and supplies for your protection are available.
Patients often become confused, and may not know where they are when they awaken.
This may be frightening, but the confusion usually disappears within a few hours. Memory
for recent events may be disturbed, and dates, names of friends, public events, telephone
numbers and addresses may be difficult to recall. In most patients, the memory difficulty
(amnesia) is gone within four weeks after the last treatment, but in about 1 in 200 patients,
the problems remain for months and even years. Death is a rare complication, occurring
once in 40,000 treatments. Equally uncommon with modern anesthesia are bone fractures,
broken or lost teeth, and spontaneous seizures after the treatment is over, but these may
occur.

You may discontinue the treatments at any time, although you will be encouraged to
continue until an adequate course is completed.

I, _____ , have read this description

of the treatments and these have been explained to me by _____ .

I agree to have the treatments and understand that Dr. _____
will be the physician in charge of my treatment.

_____

Dated: _____
Witness: _____
Agreed: _____
Relationship to Patient: _____

Appendix B

RECORD OF ELECTROCONVULSIVE THERAPY

PATIENT NAME: _____   APPARATUS: _____

PATIENT AGE: _____   PLACEMENT: _____

PSYCHIATRIC DX: _____   MEDICATIONS: _____

MEDICAL DX: _____

TOTAL CUFF TIME: _____   TOTAL EEG TIME: _____

TREATMENT #									
DATE									
STIMULUS #									
METHOHEXITAL									
SUCCINYLCHOLINE									
OTHER MEDS									
BI/UNI LATERAL									
THYMATRON % ENERGY									
MECTA FREQUENCY									
PULSE WIDTH									
STIM. DURATION									
MEDCRAFT VOLTAGE									
FIT CUFF DURATION									
FIT EEG DURATION									
PRE STIM B/P									
POST STIM B/P									
POST STIM B/P									
POST STIM B/P									

RECOMMENDED:

Appendix C

Equipment for ECT

ECT Instruments (2)
Sphygmomanometer (2)
Stethoscope
Oxygen, and bag for delivery
Airways, assorted sizes
Mouthguards (bite-blocks), soft rubber, autoclavable
Nerve stimulator
Intubation set
Electrocardiogram and defibrillator
Suction apparatus
Infusion sets (assorted): glucose in water, glucose in saline
Syringes and needles (assorted)
Disposable EEG electrodes

Medical Supplies

Required for regular use:
  Atropine sulphate
  Diazepam
  Glycopyrrolate
  Methohexital
  Nitroglycerine tablets
  Succinylcholine

Drugs for occasional use:
  Atracurium
  Caffeine sodium benzoate
  Calcium chloride
  Ephedrine
  Epinephrine
  Etomidate
  Hydralazine
  Ketamine
  Labetalol hydrochloride
  Lanoxin
  Lidocaine
  Neosynephrine
  Propranolol
  Trimethaphan camsylate (Arfonad)

Chapter 22

Adverse Effects of Electroconvulsive Therapy

by Gary S. Sachs, M.D., and Alan J. Gelenberg, M.D.

Over the five decades of experience with convulsive therapies in psychiatry, sufficient data have been accumulated to establish near universal consensus on two general issues: their efficacy as a treatment for major depression, and their major adverse effect—perturbation of central nervous system (CNS) function. More specific consideration of electroconvulsive therapy- (ECT) induced CNS dysfunctions results in progressively narrower consensus on issues of the specific functions affected, the severity, the duration, and the pathophysiological basis for the perturbations. This reflects the complexity introduced into the research by factors that do not readily lend themselves to objective measurement. Among these factors are patient characteristics, the psychiatric condition being treated, other concurrent medical conditions, prior treatment history, and the specific treatment parameters. Given the variability introduced by these factors, agreement about the common expectable CNS effects is surprisingly broad. The 1978 American Psychiatric Association task force report on ECT discussed CNS adverse effects and suggested that modifications of the treatment technique, such as variation in electrode placement and stimulus waveform, could maintain efficacy while reducing adverse effects. In this chapter we will review subsequent literature on ECT-induced adverse effects and, as the data permit, we will consider the influence of stimulus parameters.

ACUTE CONFUSIONAL STATE

Regardless of etiology, generalized seizure activity is followed by a period of time during which the patient is acutely confused. Within modern ECT practice, this time period usually is less than an hour, during which there is sequential return of orientation to person, then place, and, finally, to time. Also, during this time period patients may experience varying degrees of anxiety and agitation, which tend to resolve as reorientation is achieved. Especially with an increased number of treatments, some patients may develop a more severe confusional state, which can be prolonged and may include symptoms of psychosis. Even in such cases, it is exceedingly rare for the confusional state to last longer than a few days. We found no report of permanent confusional states following ECT.

Several studies have considered the nature of the confusional state and the influence of treatment variables on its course. Daniel and Crovitz (1986b) reported on disorientation in 30 depressed male inpatients randomly assigned to receive brief pulse right unilateral (N=8), sinusoidal right unilateral (N=6), brief pulse bilateral (N=8), or sinusoidal bilateral (N=8) ECT. They monitored electroencephalogram (EEG) and rated the degree of postictal suppression as an index of seizure generalization and evaluated posttreatment orientation at intervals of 15, 30, and 45 minutes, and 1, 2, 6, 24, and 48 hours. Using 12 questions to assess orientation, the authors compared orientation scores for treatment 3 with orientation scores for treatment 8 and found highly significant advantages of unilateral versus bilateral treatment, and for brief pulse versus sinusoidal ECT. Patients treated with unilateral sinusoidal ECT reoriented significantly more slowly than those treated with bilateral brief pulse ECT. Over the course of treatment the investigators observed a cumulative increase in time to achieve full orientation in all treatment groups. Furthermore, interictal disorientation (demonstrated by comparing the number of errant responses made to orientation questions prior to treatment 3 to the number of errors made prior to treatment 8) occurred significantly more frequently in patients receiving bilateral or sinusoidal stimulation.

Ratings of postictal EEG suppression correlated with the duration of postictal disorientation after treatments 3 and 8, but the authors' hypothesis that this correlation would be independent of the stimulant current dosage (in milliamperes) was not supported. Multiple regression analysis showed an interaction between degree of postictal EEG suppression and electrical dosage in relation to duration of disorientation, which exceeded the effects of either factor independently. The investigators observed that the period of acute confusion following ECT consisted not only of disorientation and memory impairment, but also clouded consciousness and generalized EEG slowing. Therefore, they offered the hypothesis that ECT causes a period of true delirium, whose length and severity in a given patient depend on electrode placement and stimulus waveform. The authors suggest that the CNS dysfunction results from biochemical alterations produced by a "complex interaction between electrical and seizure variables."

Sackeim and colleagues (1986b) used a method of low-dose ECT titrated to just over seizure threshold in a study of 49 depressed patients randomly assigned to unilateral (N = 25) or bilateral (N = 24) constant current, bidirectional, square-wave ECT. Beginning with a stimulus rarely convulsant, patients were restimulated at a greater pulse frequency every 40 seconds until a seizure occurred. Recovery measures included time elapsed from stimulus to eye opening, spontaneous respiration, and full orientation (defined by correct response to four of five questions asking name, place, age, day, and date of birth). Using these criteria, 95.8 percent of unilaterally treated patients and 74.3 percent of bilaterally treated patients were fully oriented in less than 45 minutes. Significant correlation with patient characteristics were found only in the unilateral group, where significantly shorter orientation times were found for older, female, and those patients having shorter seizure durations. Sackeim and colleagues suggest that the effect of these factors is obscured by the effects attributable to bilateral treatment. Despite wide variability in seizure threshold (the absolute amount of electricity necessary to provoke a seizure), it was not found to be related to any measure of recovery in either group. Thus, when dosage is titrated to just above seizure threshold, the absolute dosage does not appear to be related to recovery of orientation. The cumulative pattern was evaluated by contrasting duration of disorientation for the first two treatments with duration of disorientation for the last two treatments. No change was detected in the bilateral group. Significant improvement was found in the unilateral group, where initially full reorientation was achieved in 11.72 minutes, and after the last two treatments reorientation was achieved in 4.03 minutes. This implies that at least cumulative disorientation is avoidable and is not the inevitable accompaniment of convulsive therapy.

MEMORY IMPAIRMENT

Memory impairment, once thought to be the mechanism by which ECT relieved depression, is clearly the most worrisome and most controversial sequel of electrically induced seizures. As with acute postictal confusion, epileptics experience a parallel amnestic syndrome consisting of retrograde (failure of recall for events prior to the seizure) and anterograde amnesia (loss of ability to form new memories). Reports of severe and prolonged amnestic syndromes are not uncommon in cases of poorly controlled epilepsy. Therefore, though similar reports relating to severe and prolonged amnestic syndromes to treatment and ECT are anecdotal, they cannot be ignored.

The length and significance of the period for which memory is permanently lost or new memories cannot be made is at the core of medical investigation, ethical debate, and political action related to ECT. As is the trend for other serious adverse effects, reports of ruinous amnestic syndromes following ECT seem to have diminished since the introduction of modern technique, especially hyperoxygenation. Of nearly equal concern, and despite modern refinements, a significant percentage of patients complain that their memories are never as good. It is hard, therefore, to specify with certainty when either retrograde or anterograde amnesia has ended. Research on ECT-induced memory impairment may be divided into two major categories: 1) studies categorizing the type and extent of memory impairment, and 2) studies comparing various stimulus parameters. After summarizing interesting recent research in each category, we will consider some of the factors which complicate this important research.

Research on the extent and type of memory impairment primarily seeks to document the kinds of memory impairment which might be indistinguishable from that known to be secondary to depression itself or determine the course of memory complaints. By and large, the former is done by devising objective tests to evaluate different aspects of memory, and the latter by surveys of subjective complaints. When comparing results from these different study paradigms a discrepancy is obvious. As we shall see below, objective memory tests tend to show that patients are back to their pre-ECT baseline at times when a disturbingly large percentage report subjective memory impairment.

The only available prospective study with follow-up as long as three years found that nearly one-half of the patients treated with bilateral ECT still have memory complaints. In this study Squire and Slater (1983) made comparison of patients receiving bilateral ECT (N = 30), right unilateral ECT (N = 28), and depressed patients treated without ECT (N = 19). The instruments employed included the Squire Self-Rating Scale of memory function, an 18-item survey on which patients rated various aspects of memory on a scale of −4 (worse than before) to +4 (better than ever before). All subjects also constructed time lines representing time periods for which they felt their memory was poor. These tests were administered approximately one week before treatment and one week after ECT for the bilateral and unilateral treatment groups; at seven months after treatment for the ECT groups; and at seven months postdischarge for the non-ECT group. At baseline all patient groups reported a similar degree of subjective memory impairment, and on the time line they reported their recall was poor for a period, on average, of five months before treatment. After one week of treatment, subjective rating showed the bilateral group reporting significantly worsened memory ($p < 0.05$). (The non-ECT group was not tested at this time.) By seven months the bilateral group showed an improvement in their memory complaints, reflected by a score only seven percent as high as the difference from baseline to posttreatment week one. The unilateral group experienced further improvement but still had scores reflecting subjective memory impairment with respect to their implied nondepressed baseline. The non-ECT group reported a significant sense of improvement compared to their implied nondepressed baseline. At seven months posttreatment, the bilateral group gave a median estimate of retrograde amnesia of two years, but this decreased to six months at the three-year rating. Median anterograde amnesia estimates improved from three months to two months over the interval between the seven-month and the three-year follow-up. The data suggest a return of learning capacity, but a permanent loss of at least some memories formed during a period several months before and after treatment.

Most interesting among the findings were comparisons among the 31 patients who received bilateral treatment. At three years posttreatment, 55 percent complained that treatment resulted in their memory being not as good as the memory of other people the same age. This group, and the 45 percent not reporting memory impairment, did not differ in age or number of treatments, and they reported similar duration of impairment on their time lines. Since most of these subjects had participated in other studies with objective tests performed at six months posttreatment, it was possible to compute Z scores and compare their results across a variety of tests. Based on these objective tests, no significant difference was detected. Follow-up interview at three years did, however, find the memory complainers reporting that ECT was significantly less helpful.

Squire and Slater draw the following conclusions regarding the persistence of memory complaints: 1) Conditions existing prior to treatment could persist or recur, therefore producing an association between memory complaints and ECT's perceived lack of effectiveness. 2) Since the bilateral treatment group reports a pattern of amnesia similar to that experienced one week after treatment, persistence of memory complaints might reflect a lingering tendency to question whether memory had ever fully recovered. 3) Memory complaints after bilateral treatment usually refer to the failure to recover memories around the time of treatment, rather than impairment of recent memory or incapacity for new learning. 4) Squire and Slater found "no basis for supposing that ECT causes permanent loss of memory function beyond what is represented by the time line data . . ." (p. 7). Such conclusions must be viewed as tentative because the small sample size and possible insensitivity of the objective tests limit the power of this study to detect clinically significant impairment.

Another major shortcoming of the above study is the absence of depression ratings. Pettinati and Rosenberg (1984) administered the Beck Depression Inventory (BDI) and the Hamilton Rating Scale (HRS) for depression along with the Squire Self-Rating Scale of Memory Function (SSRS) to 28 depressed patients randomly assigned to bilateral or unilateral ECT. SSRS scores correlated with severity of depression on the BDI and HRS, both pre- and posttreatment. Both groups had improved mean scores for every one of the 18 items. Squire has asserted that the first nine items are sensitive to ECT effects and the last nine items to effects of depression. On the first half of the scale, the improvement for the bilateral group reached significance on two items, which is considerably less ($p < 0.005$) than the significant improvement on seven out of the nine items achieved by the unilateral group. On the second nine items, no significant difference was found. In this study, bilateral patients show less improvement than unilateral patients on subjective memory surveyed within 24 hours of their fifth ECT. In the previous study by Squire, patients were surveyed beginning one week after receiving 5–21 treatments. Thus, the lack of impairment in patients studied by Pettinati and Rosenberg may be attributable to their patients receiving fewer treatments and/or being tested prior to their having as much opportunity to experience their memory as impaired.

Freeman and associates (1980b) recruited subjects (N = 26), who attributed permanent unwanted effects to ECT. These subjects were compared to noncomplaining ECT patients and to normal controls on a battery of 19 cognitive tests and on several symptom rating scales. Compared to controls the ECT patients as a single group performed significantly worse on eight of the tests, but significant differences were not found between the complaining and noncomplaining ECT groups. After analysis of variance, taking into account level of medication, degree of depression, symptom rating scale scores, age, and social class, significant differences remained on only three tests and just missed significance on a fourth. These tests were, respectively, logical memory, face name, verbal learning, and personal remote memory. Beyond the group mean effects, detailed consideration was given to individual patients for whom test scores indicated a degree of impairment typical of organic brain disease. Of the 11 patients mentioned, the impairment was thought to be attributable to alcohol in two, large doses of medication in two, and clinical depression in three patients. This left four patients without other known possible causes for their impairment. The authors offer two possible explanations for this. "First, is that ECT does indeed cause some lasting impairment of memory in a small proportion of people who receive it. The second is that ECT complainers (in this study) were simply people whose memory came in the lower half of the normal range, or had mild impairment of memory for other reasons, and mistakenly attributed these failings to the treatment they had received years before" (Weeks et al, 1980b, p. 22).

In another study, Squire and co-workers (1981) assessed retrograde amnesia in 43 patients treated with bilateral ECT. Recall for either public events, television shows, or personal history were assessed prior to treatment, after the fifth treatment, one week after completing treatment, and seven months after completing treatment. Recall of public events was impaired after the fifth treatment and one week after completing treatment, but by seven months was not measurably different from pre-ECT scores. Recall of television shows aired for only one season allowed estimation of the extent of retrograde amnesia. Statistical analysis showed selective impairment for recall of shows one to two years prior to treatment. This was most severe after the fifth treatment and had recovered to some extent when tested one week after treatment. At seven months performance was significantly better than after the fifth treatment, and not significantly different from performance prior to treatment.

Autobiographical memory, perhaps the most important memory function, may be tested by recall of personal events. Prior to treatment, 10 ECT patients and 7 control patients with depressive disorders were asked 10 questions designed to elicit details of personal memory. Of the 10 questions, 6 related to events occurring more than 3 years before treatment, and 3 related to events occurring from 1 week to 3 years prior to treatment. Blind raters established scores based on the numbers of details provided. The questions were repeated at two testing intervals: one close to the time of treatment (after treatment five or one week after the course of treatment), and the other at about seven months after treatment.

Prior to treatment, controls and ECT patients produced an equivalent number of responses. At the first test period, controls spontaneously recalled 89 percent of the details correctly, while ECT patients were only able to recall 64 percent. Seven months later on retesting there was no significant difference from baseline scores.

Persistence of significant memory deficit is demonstrable, however, if the three questions relating to recent events are considered separately. Consistent with the findings from the time line data presented above, there is objective evidence of continuing impairment for memories close to the time of treatment. Most of the observed deficit was in response to the question asking about events occurring on the date of admission (2–36 days before treatment). No difference was found, however, for the question asking about events occurring the Christmas before last. Interestingly, subjects were asked about the familiarity of items omitted from their spontaneous responses. Given such a reminder, controls in all cases acknowledged the familiarity of the previously presented details. ECT patients, when prompted, failed to recognize the material as familiar 39 percent of the time. Just over one-half of such failures related to events occurring on the day of admission. This perhaps informs us that the nature of persistent amnesia following ECT is patchy, with progressively fewer and smaller gaps for time periods more distant from the time of treatment. This suggests that ECT inconsistently and incompletely disrupts the ongoing processes by which memories are transformed from an unstable intermediate to a permanent form.

The American Psychiatric Association task force report on ECT cites several studies which found equivalent memory impairment during and immediately after comparable courses of ECT and flurothyl-induced seizures, but greater improvement at later testing for flurothyl treated patients. Therefore, testing at a later time demonstrated that stimulus characteristics may contribute to the duration and severity of amnesia in a manner distinguishable from the seizure itself. Daniel and Corvitz (1986a) demonstrated an opposite impact of varying testing time. They found a greater magnitude of detectable differences among bilateral, nondominant unilateral, and dominant unilateral electrode placement in studies which tested patients 22 minutes or less after ECT, versus patients tested 23 minutes or more from the last seizure. Presentation of memory tasks 10 minutes or less before seizure induction also enhanced the differences among treatment groups. Thus, extrapolation from data collected early after treatment is hazardous.

Recent reviews confirm the claims that nondominant unilateral ECT (NDU) is associated with less amnesia than bilateral treatment (Daniel and Crovitz, 1986b; Fromm-Auch, 1982; Horne et al, 1981). In 20 of 22 studies reviewed by Fromm-Auch (1982), NDU ECT resulted in improved or unchanged verbal memory regardless of the number of treatments. Other interesting trends were found: Nonverbal memory appears to deteriorate over the first one to four NDU treatments, but improves significantly after a minimum of five NDU treatments. Bilateral and dominant unilateral ECT are associated with worsening or no significant change in both verbal and nonverbal function.

On tests of verbal memory the superiority of NDU is well established, but on nonverbal memory tests the data are less clear. These tests presumably reflect impairment of nondominant hemisphere function. Some studies, however, showing less nonverbal memory impairment, are flawed because the tests assumed to measure nonverbal memory (for example, geometric designs) can actually be performed by the dominant hemisphere if the test material is easily encoded verbally. Also, some studies suffer from failure to establish which hemisphere is, in fact, dominant. Despite the methodological problems, the available studies suggest that NDU-ECT is no worse and may be better than BIL-ECT on tests of nonverbal memory.

It may be that factors other than the number of hemispheres stimulated or the laterality of the stimulated hemisphere account for the differential memory effects of BIL and UL-ECT. As Daniel and Crovitz (1986b) point out, the current denisty pattern for BIL is much more anterior than that produced by most UL electrode placements. Therefore, differences in memory may reflect anterior versus posterior effects rather than NDU versus BIL. This suggests a regional rather than hemispheric influence on ECT induced amnesia. Alternative unilateral electrode placements producing different patterns of amnesia would support this argument. Comparing the memory impairment from NDU placements, d'Elia (1981) found fronto–frontal placement superior to temporo–parietal placement for retrograde but not anterograde memory. While this could be taken as supporting the concept of a local rather than a hemispheric disturbance as the cause for retrograde amnesia, it contradicts the anterior versus posterior hypothesis.

Another strategy in reducing memory impairment is to use a lower energy stimulus. By delivering electrical energy in volleys of brief pulses, the energy required to induce a seizure is reduced by 50 percent or more compared to a sine wave stimulus. Daniel and Crovitz (1986a) found serious flaws in four of five studies reporting less memory impairment in patients given brief pulse ECT. Of the three studies reviewed without such flaws, two using bidirectional brief pulse failed to detect significant differences. The third, using ultrabrief pulse unidirectional stimulation, found less retrograde amnesia compared to unidirectional sine wave stimulation. Perhaps this can be accounted for by the fact that these brief pulse patients received, on average, a third the dose of electrical energy received by the sine wave group.

Squire and Zouzounis (1986) tested brief pulse and sine wave patient groups on two verbal and one nonverbal memory test. On all tests brief pulse ECT produced less severe anterograde amnesia than sine wave ECT during the first hour after treatment, but no advantage for brief pulse was found beyond the first hour. The study design was naturalistic in that clinicians administered ECT in doses that reliably produced seizures rather than attempting to determine individual seizure thresholds. This leaves open the possibility that a true and more persistent difference was missed because both types of stimulation were given at suprathreshold doses.

Other attempts to minimize ECT's amnestic effects include pretreatment with memory enhancing drugs. Ezzat and colleagues (1985) pretreated 15 ECT patients with piracetam and gave 15 similar patients routine ECT. Their Wechsler memory test scores at baseline were the same, but on repeat testing three days after the fifth treatment, the patients receiving piracetam scored significantly better ($p < 0.01$). In animal and some human studies, compounds such as vasopressin and hydergine show some promise of memory protection (Partap et al, 1984).

In summary, ECT causes a variety of memory effects measurable by techniques currently available. ECT reverses the memory acquisition deficit associated with depression and at least temporarily impairs memory retention. Subjective and objective tests show bilateral electrode placement results in more anterograde and retrograde amnesia than unilateral placement. Following a standard course of bilateral treatment, patient's subjective estimates and objective testing show that retrograde amnesia is patchy and shrinks over time from the last treatment to a period of about six months. Memories for the time period immediately before and after treatment are the most likely to be permanently lost. Defining a precise end point for these iatrogenic amnestic syndromes is difficult because patients cannot reliably distinguish between normal memory failures and those resulting from the persistent effects of ECT, and the subjective experience of a time period for which they have amnesia. The finding of less satisfaction with treatment results among those complaining of persistent memory impairment despite the lack of differences on objective testing between complainers and noncomplainers is consistent with both the idea that those less satisfied might complain in the absence of a true deficit, and the idea that those more satisfied might fail to report a true deficit.

BRAIN DAMAGE

Does modern ECT cause permanent brain damage? The answer to this question can only be given with the caveat, within the limitation of the technology currently available for detecting such damage. Prior to the introduction of modified ECT techniques, animal studies and occasional autopsy reports from patients who died during a course of ECT provided evidence of structural brain damage. Some of this brain damage is the result of the very rare occurrence of gross vascular accidents in high risk patients, and is not a point of controversy. Debate instead focuses on whether in routine cases ECT causes irreversible damage to brain tissue such as petechial hemorrhage, gliosis, and neuronal death. The three major strategies thus far employed to detect such changes are histological examination of brain tissue, brain imaging, and detection of brain tissue damage markers in the peripheral circulation. Histological studies focus on complications encountered by epileptics. At autopsy the brains of patients who experienced an episode of prolonged status epilepticus show a characteristic pattern of cell death. Quantitative studies show reduced hippocampal cell counts in epileptics suffering two or more seizures per month for thirty years (Dam, 1980). Meldrum's (1986) review of the consequences of chemically and electrically induced seizures reported no evidence of brain damage in animal studies when the seizures lasted less than two hours. Dam and Dam (1986) made quantitative studies of nonepileptic rats given electrically induced seizures 3 times daily for 50 days, and epileptic gerbils whose seizures were provoked by handling. Despite the large number of electrically induced seizures, rats showed no decrease in neuronal density compared to controls. The gerbils experienced fewer seizures, but had reduced hippocampal and cerebellar cell counts. Dam and Dam propose that the neuronal death in the gerbils resulted from exhaustion caused by occult hippocampal seizure activity in the apparent interictal period. This suggests that neuronal death may be more a complication of the disease epilepsy than a consequence of isolated seizures per se.

Further assurance comes from a case report of normal neuropathological finding on postmortem examination of an 89-year-old woman treated with 1250–2050 bilateral ECT between 1944 and 1970 (Lippmann et al, 1985). Negative results from histological studies must be viewed with great caution because aritfacts introduced in the process of harvesting, fixing, and staining specimens may mask smaller true effects.

Computed tomography (CT) offers a means of in vivo comparison. Studies employing this technique search for atrophy and increased ventricular size (the presumed consequences of repeated subtle injury), because the resolution of currently available technology is insufficient to detect more immediate pathology such as tiny hemorrhages. One study found increased atrophy in those schizophrenic patients who had been treated with ECT (Weinberger et al, 1979). Another study found increased frontal atrophy correlated with the number of ECT treatments received by a sample of depressed patients (Calloway et al, 1981). The significance of such findings is questionable because these same findings reportedly occur in association with schizophrenia and affective disorder (Weinberger et al, 1979). In the absence of prospective studies, two retrospective studies used more clinically relevant controls. Given the early reports (Friedberg, 1977) of localized edema, gliosis, and petechial hemorrhage beneath electrode cites, differential rates of pathological finding would be expected comparing the hemispheres ipsilateral and contralateral to unilateral ECT. Kendell (1983) reported on 12 patients who received large numbers of unilateral ECT. No association was found between laterality of stimulus and CT findings. Kolbeinsson and associates (1986), using normal controls and non-ECT treated depressives, found both patient groups had significantly more atrophy and higher ventricular/brain (V/B) ratios compared to normals. This study found no regional differences and no correlation with number of treatments. There was, however, a nonsignificant trend for more atrophy and higher V/B ratios in the ECT treated versus non-ECT treated depressives.

Recently, very sensitive radioimmunoassay techniques have been applied to detecting circulating markers of brain tissue injury. Myelin basic protein constitutes 30 percent of the myelin sheath and is specific to the CNS. Higher levels of myelin basic protein immunoreactivity are found after head trauma, stroke, and neurosurgical procedures. Patients (N = 13) receiving an average of 16 unilateral treatments were sampled before and after each treatment. No significant changes were found in any of the 13 patients individually or for the patients as a group compared to normal controls (Hoyle et al, 1984). Brain-type creatine phosphokinase levels (CPK BB) are elevated in the serum following a variety of CNS insults, including prolonged seizures, stroke, and head trauma. Mean concentration of CPK BB in samples taken before ECT (N = 31) were not significantly different from those obtained one, two, or six hours after a single bilateral ECT. There was no difference in mean CPK BB for those patient samples at the first treatment versus those sampled at later treatments (Webb et al, 1984). Individual results, however, included two patients having sustained rises of greater than 2.0 ng/ml. This is a change consistent with brain damage. One patient had a sustained fall of equal magnitude, and the authors note such variation is within the range expected by chance alone given the number of observations made.

Though the above studies are not completely reassuring, it is not possible to find substantial support for those who portray modified ECT as permanently damaging the brains of patients who receive it. As with studies on memory impairment, group means may cloud the more salient issue of individual susceptibility to adverse effects. Also, the inability to know the actual dose of electricity delivered to the brain seriously hampers research on electrically induced structural damage.

SPONTANEOUS SEIZURES

The new occurrence of spontaneous seizures—days, weeks, or even years after a course of convulsive therapy—raises the fear of a causal relationship between seizure induction and later development of seizure disorders. Most reports in the early literature involve other convulsive techniques, schizophrenic patients, lack baseline EEGs, and have no appropriate controls.

Even more recent studies addressing the epidemiology of spontaneous seizures following ECT provide conflicting results. Devinski and Duchowny (1983) reviewed the literature from 1938–1980 and found 19 studies reporting 81 well documented cases of seizures after convulsive therapy. Eight of these studies provided follow-up sufficient to allow data pooling for 5,593 patients, and a calculated incidence of new seizures of 114 per 100,000. This result is five times higher than the incidence reported for an age-matched nonpsychiatric population. Since many clinicians suspect modern techniques have lowered the incidence of tardive seizures, the authors calculated an incidence for those patients treated with modern modified ECT. In this group, 3 of 104 patients developed spontaneous seizures, yielding an incidence of 192 per 100,000. In a prospective study, however, Blackwood (1980) found no increased prevalence of seizure disorders following ECT. Small and co-workers (1981) assembled extensive prospective EEG and clinical data on 1,000 psychiatric inpatients, 12 percent of whom reported a seizure. ECT had been administered to 20 percent of the total patient sample, but was not found to lead to a higher incidence of tardive seizures than for patients given other treatments.

Given the association of affective symptoms and epilepsy, it is possible that patients with undiagnosed epilepsy, especially those with complex partial seizures, might be treated with ECT before having their first clinically apparent seizure. Thus, it is hard to draw a cause–effect conclusion from the epidemiological data. Nonetheless, until conclusive evidence to the contrary is available, it seems prudent to consider ECT a risk factor for the development of subsequent seizure disorders.

Three mechanisms might underlie the development of spontaneous seizures following ECT: 1) a seizure focus developing at the site of the ECT-induced brain tissue scars; 2) a seizure disorder developing secondary to impairment of natural seizure-inhibiting mechanisms; and 3) a seizure focus developing secondary to the process of kindling. Given the rarity of tardive seizures, and the possibility of individual variation in susceptibility to each of these mechanisms, it is impossible to rule in or out any of these possibilities. By considering the evidence supporting each of these mechanisms we can, however, make some assessment of their likely relative contributions to the purported development of tardive seizures. We shall summarize the evidence for each mechanism in reverse order.

"Kindling" refers to the process by which repeated subthreshold stimulation applied to an area of the brain transforms that area from normal tissue into a spontaneously discharging seizure focus. Over the course of this transformation, successive stimulations result in a progressive decrease in the seizure threshold and progressive increase in duration of electrical afterdischarge. The limbic structures, particularly the amygdala, are more sensitive to this process than cortical structures, but at any site kindling does not take place with continuous stimulation or if the interval between stimuli exceeds a certain maximum. Also, the number of stimulations given at this interval must exceed some minimum. ECT involves application of a superthreshold stimulus, given at a rate of usually 2–3 per week, and the treatment course usually consists of less than 20 stimulations. During such a course there is a progressive increase in the seizure threshold and shortening of seizure duration. In animal studies, Post and Ballenger (1981) report ECT is a powerful inhibitor of the kindling process. As Sackeim and colleagues report (1986a), humans with prior seizure disorders experience a decreased frequency of seizures following ECT. Therefore, none of the available evidence suggests that ECT kindles seizure foci.

Details of the natural mechanisms of seizure inhibition are incompletely understood. Cerebellar Purkinje cells are known to be involved in at least one such mechanism. Therefore, evidence of ECT-induced loss of these cells would suggest this as a possible etiology of tardive seizures. We know of no studies addressing the issue of cerebellar Purkinje cell loss in patients experiencing tardive seizures, and in the above section on brain damage, no evidence was found showing this as a routine consequence of ECT. Yet it remains possible that the cell loss associated with aging may be accelerated in certain psychiatric syndromes, and that ECT further exacerbates this loss.

A lack of evidence of ECT-generated CNS scarring does not rule out the possibility that very rarely ECT-induced injuries ripen into seizure foci. This mechanism is thought to account for seizure disorders which develop years after the head trauma or other CNS insults.

In summary, the association between modern ECT and tardive seizures is not clear. Assuming there is an increased incidence of seizure disorders in patients receiving ECT does not necessarily imply that ECT was causal in the development of seizure disorders. Of the mechanisms considered above, kindling is least consistent with the actual observations in ECT patients. The other mechanisms are less easily dismissed given the rare and sporadic occurrence of tardive seizures, but even for these mechanisms no evidence exists to prove their relevance to patients receiving modern ECT. Alternative explanations may be justified in some cases. These include increased likelihood of occult seizure disorder in the population coming to ECT, frequent use of multiple medications which lower the seizure threshold, and, in rare cases of single seizures occurring within hours of treatment, generalization of persistent ECT-induced seizure activity after the seizure-suppressing effects of anesthesia are lost.

SYSTEMIC ADVERSE EFFECTS

Adverse systemic effects associated with modern ECT arise from the seizures and the drugs used to modify the seizures. The use of barbiturate anesthesia, neuromuscular blockade, anticholinergic agents, and hyperoxygenation has reduced reported rates of significant complications from as high as 40 percent to rates between 0.46 and 0.045 percent. The American Psychiatric Association's task force reported the mortality rate for ECT as 0.03 percent per patient treated (American Psychiatric Association, 1978). These rates are comparable to those reported for barbiturate anesthesia alone, and often cited in support of claims that ECT is the safest procedure requiring general anesthesia. Despite the low incidence of serious systemic consequences, a knowledge of the systemic effects and their mechanisms is important so that patients most at risk can be recognized, and practitioners can be prepared to manage those complications that require intervention.

The most common complications in the past—fractures (mostly vertebral)—have been virtually eliminated by the use of muscle relaxants such as succinylcholine, which prevents the extreme musculoskeletal stress associated with intense seizure activity. The applied current itself may directly stimulate contraction of the oral musculature, and can lead to jaw fracture, damaged dentition, and oral lacerations. Use of a mouth guard and proper airway management can greatly reduce such problems, as well as protect against the extremely rare occurrence of laryngospasm associated with the use of anesthesia.

Now the most common systemic complications are cardiovascular, which, according to the American Psychiatric Association task force report, account for 67 percent of deaths related to ECT. Perpheralization of seizure activity from parasympathetic and sympathetic centers in the brain produce powerful effects on the heart and blood vessels. With application of the stimulus, excess vagal activity produces a transient bradycardia and hypotension. Succinylcholine also enhances cholinergic activity, but anticholinergic drugs such as atropine greatly moderate these effects. The onset of seizure activity brings increased sympathetic drive, which produces a period of elevated blood pressure and tachycardia.

Though dysrhythmias are reported in as many as 30 percent of patients receiving ECT under general anesthesia, such dysrhythmias are usually transient, seldom require intervention, and only rarely produce permanent sequelae (Price, 1986). As with most of the CNS effects discussed above, there remains the question of whether the observed dysrhythmias and ischemic changes represent a toxic effect of ECT generally, or a relative risk determined by individual susceptibility. Gerring and Shields (1982) found, in their review of 42 patients treated with ECT, that the 12 patients who developed ischemic or arrhythmic complications came entirely from the subgroup of 17 patients with known cardiac disease. In this subgroup of 17 cardiac patients (16 had an abnormal electrocardiogram [ECG] and 13 were on digitalis just prior to treatment), the complication rate was 70 percent. As the authors state, "four of the complications in the series were life-threatening, while the rest were largely asymptomatic arrhythmias. . . . The complications were scattered throughout the entire treatment course and were not localized to the initial one or two treatments" (Gerring and Shields, 1982, p. 141). Treatment techniques included use of thiopental anesthesia, and higher than usual doses of atropine and succinylcholine may account for some of the complications; but the rate of serious complication—4 out of 42 (9.5 percent) for the entire series, or 4 out of 17 (23.5 percent) with cardiac disease—is worrisome. The authors suggest use of methohexital instead of thiopental and offered precautionary guidelines for high risk patients: 1) medical clearance from an internist or cardiologist familiar with the complications of ECT; 2) cardiac monitoring immediately before, during, and for 10–15 minutes after ECT; 3) presence at the time of treatment of personnel trained in emergency resuscitation techniques; 4) ECG reading before each treatment; and 5) frequent electrolytes for patients on diuretics or digitalis.

Dec and colleagues (1985) prospectively studied serial ECG and cardiac enzymes in 29 patients, including 7 with known cardiovascular disease. They collected data four to six hours after each of the first three treatments and report no new ECG changes and no cardiac enzyme elevations. Their patients were older (74 years compared to 51 in the study mentioned above), but they report using methohexital anesthesia, succinylcholine at unspecified dose, and no atropine.

Differences in study design may account for the different observed rates of significant cardiac complications. Also, the small sample size in both studies might have distorted the result in both cases. The available evidence supports the view that patients with prior cardiac disease are at greater risk for ECT-related cardiac effects, and that even high risk cases can be managed with appropriate caution. There is no evidence that ECT is directly injurious to the myocardium, but studies of direct electrical brain stimulation suggest any deleterious effect of ECT on the ECG may be secondary to stimulation of those brain centers that directly influence cardiac function and/or result from cardiac toxicity of ECT premedications.

As Price (1986) states, endocrine effects of ECT are numerous, but rarely clinically significant. There are, however, reports of altered insulin requirements in ECT-treated diabetics. While the change in insulin requirement has been reported to be both diabetogenic and diabetolytic, no definitive studies have been reported. In the absence of such studies clinicians administering ECT should be aware of the need to closely monitor the blood glucose and tailor the dosage of hypoglycemic agents to the needs of diabetic patients treated with ECT.

SUMMARY

The most frequent adverse effects of modified ECT involve perturbation of CNS function, and serious cardiovascular complications represent a significant immediate risk in patients with prior heart disease. Unilateral nondominant ECT produces briefer periods of confusion and less memory impairment than bilateral ECT. Brief pulse may offer similar advantages over sine wave stimulation. Studies claiming prophylactic effects of medications such as piracetam encourage further modification in technique and suggest that therapeutic and adverse effects are separable. The data on ECT-induced seizure disorders are unclear and any increased incidence may reflect factors of patient susceptibility. Though present studies are not completely reassuring, our review found no clear statistical evidence of permanent damage to brain structure or function. Studies with small samples lack sufficient power to confidently rule out the occurrence of infrequent adverse effects. Conversely, the consistent absence of detectable pathology allows us to estimate with some confidence that the incidence of an undetected event lies below some finite limit. We suggest future research reports state the level of confidence of any negative findings.

REFERENCES

American Psychiatric Association. Electroconvulsive Therapy. Task Force Report #14. Washington, DC, American Psychiatric Association, 1978

Blackwood DHR, Cull RE, Freeman CPL, et al: A study of the incidence of epilepsy following ECT. J Neurol Neurosurg Psychiatry 1980; 43:1098-1102

Calloway SP, Dolan RJ, Jacoby RJ, et al: ECT and cerebral atrophy: a computed tomographic study. Acta Psychiatr Scand 1981; 64:442-445

d'Elia G: The effect of fronto–frontal and temporo–parietal unilateral ECT on retrograde memory. Biol Psychiatry 1981; 16:55-59

Dam AM: Epilepsy and neuronal loss in the hippocampus. Epilepsia 1980; 21:617-629

Dam AM, Dam M: Quantitative neuropathology in electrically induced generalized seizures. Convulsive Therapy 1986; 2:77-89

Daniel WF, Crovitz HF: Acute memory impairment following electroconvulsive therapy, 1: effects of electrical stimulus wave waveform and number of treatments. Acta Psychiatr Scand 1986a: 67:57-68

Daniel WF, Crovitz HF: Disorientation during electroconvulsive therapy: technical, theoretical and neuropsychological issues. Ann NY Acad Sci 1986; 462:293-306

Daniel WF, Crovitz HG: Acute memory impairment following electroconvulsive therapy, 2: effects of electrode placement. Acta Psychiatr Scand 1986b; 67:57-68

Dec GW Jr, Stern TA, Welch C: The effects of electroconvulsive therapy on serial electrocardiograms' and serum cardiac enzymes' values: a prospective study of depressed hospitalized inpatients. JAMA 1985; 253:2525-2529

Devinsky O, Duchowny MS: Seizures after convulsive therapy: a retrospective case survey. Neurology 1983; 33:921-925

Hoyle NR, Pratt RTC, Thomas DGT: Effect of electroconvulsive therapy on serum myelin basic protein immunoreactivity. Br Med J 1984; 288:1110-1111

Ezzat DH, Ibraheem MM, Makhavy B: The effect of piracetam on ECT-induced memory dysfunction. Br J Psychiatry 1985; 147:720-721

Friedberg J: Shock treatment, brain damage, and memory loss: a neurologic perspective. Am J Psychiatry 1977; 134:1010-1014

Fromm-Auch D: Comparison of unilateral and bilateral ECT: evidence for selective memory impairment. Br J Psychiatry 1982; 141:608-613

Gerring JP, Shields HM: The identification and management of patients with a high risk for cardiac arrhythmias during modified ECT. J Clin Psychiatry 1982; 43:140-143

Horne RL, Pettinati HM, Sugerman AA, et al: Comparing bilateral to unilateral electroconvulsive therapy in a randomized study with EEG monitoring. Arch Gen Psychiatry 1981; 38:89-95

Kendell B, Pratt RT: Brain damage and ECT (letter). Br J Psychiatry 1983; 143:99-100

Kolbeinsson H, Arnaldsson OS, Petursson H, et al: Computed tomographic scans in ECT-patients. Acta Psychiatr Scand 1986; 73:28-32

Lippmann S, Manoochehr M, et al: 1250 electroconvulsive treatments without evidence of brain injury. Br J Psychiatry 1985; 147:203-204

Meldrum BS: Neuropathological consequences of chemically and electrically induced seizures. Ann NY Acad Sci 1986; 462:186-193

Partap M, Jos CJ, Dye J: Vasopressin-8-lysine in prevention of ECT-induced amnesia (letter). Am J Psychiatry 1984; 141:148

Pettinati HM, Rosenberg J: Memory self-ratings before and after anticonvulsive therapy: depression- versus ECT-induced. Biol Psychiatry 1984; 19:539-548

Post RM, Ballenger JC: Kindling models for the progressive development of behavioral psychopathology: sensitization to electrical, pharmacological, and psychological stimuli, in Handbook of Biological Psychiatry, Part 4. Edited by Van Praag HM, Lader MH, Rafaelson OT, et al. New York, Marcel Dekker, 1981

Price TRP: Systemic effects of ECT. Psychopharmacol Bull 1986; 22:475-476

Sackeim HA, Decina P, Prohovnik I, et al: Seizure threshold and the antidepressant efficacy of electroconvulsive therapy. Ann NY Acad Sci 1986a; 462:389-410

Sackeim HA, Portnoy S, Neeley P, et al: Cognitive consequences of low-dosage electroconvulsive therapy. Ann NY Acad Sci 1986b; 462:12-40

Small JG, Milstein V, Small IF, et al: Does ECT produce kindling? Biol Psychiatry 1981; 18:773-778

Squire LR: Memory functions as affected by electroconvulsive therapy. Ann NY Acad Sci 1986; 462:315-325

Squire LR, Slater PC: Electroconvulsive therapy and complaints of memory dysfunction: a prospective three-year follow-up study. Br J Psychiatry 1983; 142:1-8

Squire LR, Zouzounis JA: ECT and memory: brief pulse versus sine wave. Am J Psychiatry 1986; 143:1027-1029

Squire LR, Slater PC, Miller PL: Retrograde amnesia and bilateral electroconvulsive therapy. Arch Gen Psychiatry 1981; 38:89-95

Webb MGT, O'Donnell MP, Draper RJ, et al: Brain-type creatine phosphokinase serum levels before and after ECT. Br J Psychiatry 1984; 144:525-528

Weeks D, Freeman CPL, Kendell RE: ECT, II: patients who complain. Br J Psychiatry 1980a; 137:17-25

Weeks D, Freeman CPL, Kendell RE: ECT, III: enduring cognitive deficits? Br J Psychiatry 1980b; 137:26-37

Weinberger DR, Torrey EF, Neophytides AN, et al: Structural abnormalities in the cerebral cortex of chronic schizophrenic patients. Arch Gen Psychiatry 1979; 36:935-939

Weiner RD, Volov MR, Gianturco DI, et al: Seizures terminable and interminable with ECT. Am J Psychiatry 1980; 137:1416-1418

Weiner RD, Rodgers HJ, Davidson JR, et al: Cognitive consequences of low dose electroconvulsive therapy. Ann NY Acad Sci 1986; 462:315-325

Chapter 23

Electroconvulsive Therapy: Legal Regulations, Ethical Concerns

by William J. Winslade, J.D., Ph.D.

For 50 years electroconvulsive therapy (ECT) has provoked continuing controversy. Some psychiatrists advocate its dramatic therapeutic benefits, especially in the treatment of primary depression (Fink, 1979). Others insist that because ECT causes irreversible and severe damage to the brain, it should be entirely prohibited (Breggin, 1979). Many psychiatrists are uneasy about ECT because of its uncertain benefits, potentially harmful side effects, legal and ethical complications, and public reactions to its use. Organized psychiatry has at times questioned the use and abuse of ECT (GAP, 1947) as well as endorsed its efficacy in the treatment of certain disorders (APA, 1978; NIH, 1985). Legislators in some states have sought to drastically restrict, if not virtually prohibit, the use of ECT, while in others no special regulations have been imposed (Brakel, 1985). Similarly, although some courts have established strict limitations on its use, others have deferred to professional discretion about when ECT is medically indicated. Some psychiatric patients vigorously oppose ECT; other patients endorse it. It is no wonder that the public is confused and many psychiatrists are ambivalent about the efficacy, safety, and control of the use of ECT.

Despite the disputes and debates, however, some trends are discernible. Psychiatrists have achieved a consensus that ECT is an appropriate treatment for certain forms of depression and, perhaps, other disorders, such as acute mania and some schizophrenias (APA, 1978; NIH, 1985). Legislatures have stopped short of abolishing ECT, but have imposed bureaucratic regulations on its use. Courts have moved from narrowly restricting to cautiously permitting professional discretion about ECT's therapeutic benefits. Although some psychiatric patients and patient groups still oppose any use of ECT, many support the right of competent persons to make their own decisions about it. The present situation, then, is that ECT is a permissible treatment option for psychiatrists to recommend and for some patients to undergo. Considerable controversy still exists, however, about the extent to which ECT may be given to involuntary patients against their will.

This chapter surveys key legal and ethical issues raised by the use of ECT as a psychiatric treatment. It is argued that in ethics as well as law it is appropriate to act on the informed preferences of competent patients or of authorized representatives of incompetent patients. Criteria for determining competence play a prominent role in legal and ethical contexts. Despite recurrent disputes about ECT practices, a surprising degree of agreement in principle has emerged about the therapeutic use of ECT in the psychiatric treatment of certain disorders.

PSYCHIATRIC SELF-REGULATION OF ECT

In 1938, ECT was introduced in Italy by Ugo Cerletti as an improved technique for inducing seizures used to treat severe mental illness such as catatonia, depression, and schizophrenia. In the first report of ECT use, a seriously disabled patient obtained dramatic—rapid and substantial—benefits. It is reported that:

a schizophrenic arrived by train from Milan without a ticket or any means of identification. Physically healthy, he was bedraggled and alternately was mute or expressed himself in incomprehensible gibberish made up of odd neologisms. The patient was brought in but despite their vast animal experience there was great apprehension and fear that the patient might be damaged, and so the shock was cautiously set at 70 volts for one-tenth of a second. The low dosage predictably produced only a minor spasm, after which the patient burst into song. Cerletti suggested another shock at a higher voltage, and an excited and voluble discussion broke out among the spectators who included Bini, Longhi, Accornero, Kalinowsky, and Fleischer. All of the staff objected to a further shock, protesting that the patient would probably die. Cerletti was familiar with committees and knew that postponement would inevitably mean prolonged and possible permanent procrastination, and so decided to proceed at 110 volts for one-half second. However, before he could do so, the patient who had heard but so far not participated in the discussion sat up and pontifically proclaimed in clear Italian without hint of jargon 'Non una seconda! Mortifera!' (Not again! It will kill me!). Professor Bini hesitated but gave the order to proceed. After recovery, Bini asked the patient "What has been happening to you?" and the man replied "I don't know; perhaps I've been asleep." He remained jargon-free and gave a complete account of himself, and was discharged completely recovered after 11 complete and 3 incomplete treatments over a course of 2 months (Brandon, 1981, p. 8–9).

This fascinating report of the first human use of ECT raises many questions. Were the psychiatrists justified in giving an experimental treatment to an incompetent patient? Should the staff's objections have been heeded? Should the patient's refusal have been respected? Who had the authority to make treatment decisions? Yet, the patient reportedly recovered and did not recall the treatment. Does this matter? These questions and their implications will be discussed further below.

At this point it is sufficient to note that the use of this technological innovation to induce seizures was greeted with mixed reactions. According to Fink, "the new method soon spread to other countries and by 1939 was accepted in the United States, despite warnings against possible electrocution by the editors of the *Journal of the American Medical Association*" (Fink, 1979, p. 11).

As with any new therapy, the full scope of its effectiveness or its risks was uncertain. Years of therapeutic, but often unregulated, experimentation produced information about efficacy as well as complaints about safety, especially fractures caused during the induced seizures. With regard to therapeutic benefits, research on patients revealed that ECT was most effective in the treatment of some forms of severe depression and schizophrenia. In response to questions of safety, muscle relaxants and anesthesia are presently administered to reduce the risk of fractures. Complaints about memory loss remain, but reports about frequency and severity range from little or none to substantial.

During the era of discovery and experimentation, ECT use was regulated only by the psychiatrist clinicians and researchers. In their zeal to gain information as well as to help their patients, some psychiatrists used ECT indiscriminately and excessively (GAP, 1947). It must be remembered, however, that few effective therapies were available for seriously disabled mental patients. ECT offered often rapid results and relief from distress as well as release from hospitalization. It has also been reported that ECT was used not only for therapeutic goals, but also to control dangerous, difficult, or uncooperative patients (Rothman, 1985). Others claim that it was used punitively (Donaldson, 1976). Recent studies suggest that ECT may still commonly be used to control patients thought to be especially dangerous or difficult (Mahler et al, 1986).

In reaction to continual and increasing complaints about overuse and abuse of ECT, in 1947 the Group for the Advancement of Psychiatry issued a one-page report critical of the use of "shock therapy." The advent of pharmacotherapy in the 1950s, however, diverted attention from ECT. Drugs were celebrated as the new panacea for mental illness, and the use of ECT diminished. As information about the limited effectiveness as well as side effects of drugs began to accumulate, ECT use increased, both in conjunction with drugs and as an alternative form of treatment (Fink, 1979).

The next official response of organized psychiatry came over thirty years later with the publication in 1978 of the American Psychiatric Association's Task Force Report, *Electroconvulsive Therapy*. The Task Force surveyed the APA membership on the use of ECT, reviewed the literature on the efficacy and adverse effects, listed techniques of administration, discussed training and education as well as research, and commented on social, ethical, and legal aspects of ECT. It provided a set of recommendations corresponding to each of the areas studied. In general, the task force endorsed the therapeutic benefits of ECT for severe depression, psychoses, catatonia, and mania when drugs are ineffective or inappropriate because of medical risks. It also made extensive recommendations for informed consent procedures. The regulatory effort of the APA task force has been summarized in greater detail elsewhere (Winslade et al, 1984).

In 1985, a National Institutes of Health Consensus Development Conference issued a report that produced a cautious consensus about the appropriate use of ECT for the treatment of some forms of depression and schizophrenia.

Unregulated psychiatric practices have been increasingly scrutinized in terms of professional self-regulatory standards, while excessively restrictive legal regulations have sometimes been modified to recognize proper use of professional discretion in determining whether ECT is medically indicated. This political compromise satisfies neither the ardent opponents nor the vigorous advocates of ECT. The former still call for abolition and the latter lobby for fewer restrictions. The public and the media have displayed intermittent interest in ECT. The Joint Commission on Accreditation of Hospitals is just now instituting oversight to monitor the administration of ECT (Rothman, 1985). Familiar complaints about inadequate training and education in the use of ECT and assertions of the need for further research about its therapeutic action are reiterated, but it is uncertain whether sustained or systematic efforts will be made to remedy these problems.

LEGAL REGULATION OF ECT

ECT was first used in the United States in 1939 and the harshly critical GAP Report was published in 1947. In the 1950s, legal interest took the form of malpractice suits for the improper administration of ECT. It was reported in a

1954 law review article that insurance carriers were reluctant to cover physicians and hospitals administering ECT (Brakel, 1985). However, in 1980 Perr reported that there have been relatively few appellate court cases over a 40-year period that specifically address ECT liability. Not even all the 34 cases reviewed by Perr dealt specifically with ECT. The cases concerned a variety of allegations, including negligent care and follow-up of patients (such as falls, lack of bed rails, inadequate treatment or radiological review, inappropriate treatment of fractures), lack of or inadequate consent, and negligent administration of ECT. Although the cases reviewed displayed no pattern of liability, the majority of the cases were won by the defendant psychiatrists. Those few cases with verdicts favorable to plaintiffs (9 out of 34) included 3 cases involving falls, 5 involving fractures or failure to use muscle relaxants, and 1 involving consent issues. Other studies have also shown that malpractice liability suits concerning ECT are very rare (Slawson, 1984).

It is possible, however, that early malpractice liability cases concerning ECT were litigated successfully by plaintiffs in trial courts or settled favorably to plaintiffs and did not reach appellate courts. Perr reported that,

> [a]s of May, 1976, the 5,626 policies in the APA malpractice plan included 710 that covered EST (or approximately 12%). Such policies were charged a 50% supplemental premium. The New York Medical Society plan (1975) showed a pay-out ration 161% higher for those psychiatrists using EST as compared to those not using EST (the latter including neurologists). The Medical Society of New Jersey plan showed an even greater disparity—465%. The Insurance Service Office, a national insurance rating organization, estimated that a 75% surcharge would be appropriate. Although purportedly as low as 5% of cliams have involved EST, the high surcharge has been justified on the basis that psychiatrists who use EST seem to be involved in more legal claims; it may be that this reflects a greater legal vulnerability to this point for those who use somatic therapies compared to those who use psychotherapy and other verbal or milieu techniques. Those who use EST are also likely to be heavy users of medication; they also undoubtedly deal with a sicker population (Perr, 1980, p. 509).

Since 1976, claims resulting from the use of ECT have decreased further, perhaps because of improved techniques in the administration of ECT or because ECT use has decreased. As a result of this decrease in claims, the APA malpractice plan has dropped the surcharge for ECT.

Although concern about malpractice claims resulting from ECT use arose in the 1950s, significant legal regulation of ECT did not emerge until the mid-1970s. The California legislature passed a statute in 1974 that imposed strict limitations on the permissible use of ECT.

> California's restrictions on ECT, by far the most stringent of any state, responded to a groundswell of public criticism from such patient and ex-patient groups as NAPA (Network Against Psychiatric Assault). This legislation gave all mental patients, involuntarily as well as voluntarily hospitalized, the right to refuse electroconvulsive therapy. The history of this legislation is itself an interesting comment on legislation governing ECT. In its effort to protect vulnerable patients from forced ECT, the original California statute ran afoul of other constitutional protections of patients, such as a patient's privacy right not to have a relative or guardian apprised of the treatment, and a competent voluntary patient's right not to be given infor-

mation concerning remote risks without requesting it. The California Court of Appeals in 1976 also found that patients' due process rights were violated by the original law because of the lack of a hearing on the patient's competency and voluntariness (Senter et al, 1984). The trend in recent years has been for legislatures to pass statutes or for health administrative agencies to promulgate regulations pertaining to ECT. Most of the statutes or regulations deal generally with the right to refuse treatment or informed consent requirements. Thirty-seven states including California have either statutes or regulations governing the administration of ECT. In other states, legislation speaks to the treatment of mental patients in general but does not offer any specific guidelines for ECT. Those state provisions specifically restricting the use of ECT range between the fairly strict California statutes and Texas Regulations and the less restrictive Massachusetts and Tennessee statutes. Like California, Texas requires independent concurring opinion from psychiatrists or neurologists that ECT is appropriate and necessary, and usually requires a court hearing to determine whether involuntarily committed patients are competent to consent to or refuse ECT. Although Massachusetts gives patients the right to refuse ECT treatment, it also allows the right to be denied for good cause if the superintendent documents the denial in the treatment record. Tennessee is silent on the administration of ECT to adults, though it prohibits the use of ECT for minors unless a court order is obtained (Senter et al, 1985, pp. 12–13).

One interesting approach to regulation of ECT through legislation involved active cooperation between a state department of mental health and a state legislature. In the early 1970s the Department of Mental Health for Massachusetts was investigating a private psychiatric facility known to give ECT to many patients. Efforts to obtain help from ethics committees of appropriate professional organizations were unsuccessful. It was discovered after investigation by the department that ECT was used excessively and inappropriately, much like the abuses reported by GAP in 1947. At this point the Department of Mental Health appointed a committee of psychiatrists to develop recommendations and guidelines for ECT practices. Two state senators, however, felt that strict limitations should be imposed on the use of ECT.

> After much haggling, a compromise was finally worked out whereby the senators would abjure their right to put electrotherapy restraints into law in exchange for additional rules and regulations regarding electrotherapy to be promulgated by the department, rules that would, as a matter of fact, have the effect of law. By departmental regulation, then, shock was prohibited under 12 years of age; between 12 and 16 it would have to be approved by a two-person jury of experts in child psychiatry not attached to the facility in which the treatment was done; and for adult individuals similar approval would have to be provided for any patient receiving more than 35 shock treatments in a given year. The senators thus gained their much desired additional safeguards in the use of electroshock, whereas the department salvaged its right to monitor professional treatment through its rules and regulations. These rules, incidentally, had to be disseminated to the public and subject to public hearings before they could be modified (Greenblatt, 1978, p. 70).

A more radical approach to regulating ECT—total prohibition—was initiated by the voters of Berkeley, California. Despite the strict regulations already governing ECT in California, on November 2, 1982, the voters of Berkeley passed a referendum to prohibit the use of ECT within the city limits of Berkeley. Subsequently the Berkeley City Council enacted a City Ordinance that absolutely prohibited ECT; a violation of the ordinance was made a misdemeanor with a criminal punishment of up to six months in jail, a $500.00 fine, or both. About 1½ months after the ordinance was adopted by the City Council, a judge issued a preliminary injunction against enforcement of the ordinance. One year after the original voter referendum, the same court issued a permanent injunction against the ordinance, declaring it unconstitutional because it went beyond existing state law that permits the therapeutic use of ECT subject to strict requirements for informed consent and medical review, and because it violates the right of every psychiatric patient to choose or refuse ECT, when medically indicated, as a mode of treatment. This ruling was upheld on appeal and the California Supreme Court refused to review the appellate court judgment. Thus, ECT was only briefly and is no longer banned in Berkeley (*Northern California Psychiatric Society v. City of Berkeley, 1983*).

Although no legislation totally prohibits the use of ECT, some statutes do restrict its use in *medical* practice. For example, some statutes stipulate when ECT is an appropriate treatment; some prohibit its use in certain circumstances. Other features of legislation that directly affect medical practice are specific requirements for consultation and medical review, limitations on frequency or number of treatments, and rules regarding record keeping. Rules pertaining to competency and consent procedures, as well as due process protections when ECT is administered over the objections of involuntary patients, are more properly *legal* in nature. Yet the statutes often lack detailed legal procedures. Legislatures are willing to restrict medical discretion but are less likely to curtail judicial and administrative discretion. While this may promote flexibility, it also creates uncertainty and provides greater opportunity for subjective rulings. Psychiatrists and their legal representatives must be able to persuade judicial authorities, especially if ECT is proposed over the objections of an involuntary patient, that it is a necessary and an appropriate treatment (Winslade et al, 1984).

Court decisions as well as statutes have specifically addressed the regulation of ECT. The most significant federal court decision is *Wyatt v. Hardin*, one of a series of cases that articulated constitutional standards for the care of the mentally ill in Alabama state hospitals.

In Hardin, the court asserted that it was "not undertaking to determine which forms of treatment are appropriate in particular situations." That is, it did not plan to practice medicine. On the other hand, the question of procedural safeguards was, it said, "a fundamental legal question." Having thus established the boundary between medical and jurisprudential activity, the court proceeded to forbid some uses of ECT and established 14 rules that severely restricted its use. These ranged from consent and due process requirements to the qualifications of doctors who might recommend it and the conditions under which it could be provided (Winslade et al, 1984, p. 1350).

The *Hardin* decision stipulates several conditions as legal requirements that psychiatrists believe should be a matter of medical discretion. For example, *Hardin* prescribes that two psychiatrists experienced in the use of ECT, with the concurrence of the hospital director, must make the decision in every case that ECT is the most appropriate treatment. A physical and neurological examination is required 10 days before ECT is administered. During treatment anesthesia and muscle relaxants must be used; both a psychiatrist and an anesthesiologist must be present at the time of treatment. In addition, the *Hardin* court limits treatment to one series of 12 treatments in 12 months. Furthermore, the *Hardin* court imposed strict record-keeping requirements.

The legal procedures required by the *Hardin* ruling are also detailed. For instance,

> [t]he *Hardin* court was sensitive to the problems of competency evaluation and fashioned its resolution almost entirely in terms of that issue. It required that a competency evaluation be conducted for any patient who was a candidate for ECT and that the evaluating group be the patient's attorney, the treating psychiatrist, and the "extraordinary treatment committee." This committee is a five-member group mandated and appointed by the court, and includes at least one psychiatrist licensed in Alabama, one neurologist or specialist in internal medicine, and one attorney. If any one of the three evaluators (the patient's attorney, the treating psychiatrist, or the extraordinary treatment committee) finds the patient incompetent, then the extraordinary treatment committee must interview everyone with an interest in the case, including the patient, and then make a final decision on behalf of the patient, giving great weight to any protest made by the patient. If, on the other hand, the committee finds the patient competent, then the patient may consent to ECT. However, the committee must additionally validate the patient's consent and guarantee that it is fully informed and voluntary. Presumably, although the court decision does not specifically say so, the competent patient is also entitled to refuse ECT and the committee must guarantee that it is a free and fully informed refusal. . . .
>
> *Hardin* provides review only when the extraordinary treatment committee approves ECT for incompetent patients. In this case, the family of the patient may request court review and, when such review is held, the patient must be represented by counsel. The court specifically states that it takes this review very seriously and that "all considerations . . . against [ECT must be] adequately explored and resolved." The assumption seems to be that even when consent procedures spelled out by the court have been adhered to, special attention must be paid to claims that an error has been made. It does not, for example, also specify that all claims for use of ECT be adequately explored (Winslade, 1984, pp. 1353–1354).

The stringency of the *Hardin* rules must be seen in the light of the deplorable conditions then existing in the Alabama state hospitals. The court was responding to specific instances of abuse in 1975 reported in general terms by GAP in 1947. Since the *Hardin* decision, no other federal court has set judicial standards for the use of ECT.

State courts have dealt primarily with clarification and elaboration of legislative standards. A recent case decided by the Supreme Court of the state of Washington illustrates the current trend of courts to permit medical discretion concerning the use of ECT, but only in the context of strict attention to legislatively protected legal rights of patients (*In the Matter of Loretta Schuoler, 1986*). A chronically mentally ill patient who had been frequently hospitalized was brought to a hospital by a friend. The patient was involuntarily committed by a court for 14 days and ECT was recommended. At a hearing held the next day, two psychiatrists testified that ECT was medically indicated. The patient's attorney, however, challenged the physician's testimony, disputed the effectiveness of ECT in previous hospitalizations, and sought to introduce conflicting psychiatric evidence. Nevertheless, the trial court ordered the patient to undergo ECT at the discretion of her treating psychiatrist. A request for a stay of the order pending appeal was denied. Even though the specific issue in this case was moot because the patient in question had been given ECT, the Supreme Court of Washington ruled on the merits of the case because the questions raised are of substantial public concern.

The Washington Supreme Court, interpreting the relevant state statutes, classified the legal rights of psychiatric patients, outlined the legal procedures established to protect those rights, and specified the circumstances in which medical discretion to treat can override the preferences of an involuntarily committed patient to refuse treatment. The court pointed out that competent adults, even involuntarily committed patients, retain a right to refuse treatment. When patients are incompetent, their interest in the right to refuse treatment must be protected by a court that conducts an adequate investigation on behalf of the patient.

> In this case, both doctors testified that discussing ECT with Schuoler was futile. The court thus should have made a "substituted judgment" for Schuoler. However, the court made no attempt to inquire into the views of individuals close to the patient. The court apparently accepted Dr. McCarthy's hearsay testimony that Schuoler's family was not interested in her treatment, and the court refused to provide Schuoler's counsel sufficient time to attempt to call Schuoler's family to testify. The court made no findings about the desires of Schuoler or her family members. We conclude that the court failed to conduct the investigation necessary to make a "substituted judgment" for Schuoler (In the Matter of Loretta Schuoler, 1986).

It is permissible, however, in certain circumstances to override the involuntary patient's refusal of treatment when there is a compelling state interest, such as preserving life or preventing suicide, in doing so. The court must conduct an inquiry to determine whether ECT is medically both necessary and effective. Even if it is, the court can impose limitations on the administration of ECT in specific cases. Thus, this court, like the Hardin court, does permit judges to restrict medical discretion on behalf of the nonconsenting patient.

In addition, the Washington Supreme Court does specify certain legal rules designed to protect patient's rights to procedural due process. A burden of proof has been established that requires "clear, cogent, and convincing" evidence of the need for ECT. This is the same standard of proof necessary to justify 90-day involuntary commitments. A jury trial is not required. The important point is that the patient's attorney be given an adequate opportunity to present the case and that the judge conduct a sufficient inquiry to properly exercise discretion in making a substitute judgment on behalf of the patient. It is significant that in this case it was judicial and not medical discretion that the Washington Supreme Court held was abused. The Court concludes by pointing out that,

> treatment of the mentally ill is one of the most significant problems facing the public today. We hesitate to frustrate professionals' efforts to treat mentally ill individuals as quickly and efficiently as possible. We also acknowledge that ECT can be a useful treatment for certain patients. Nevertheless, we cannot forget the statutory and constitutional rights of individuals afflicted with poorly understood mental illnesses. We thus conclude that a court can order ECT for a nonconsenting patient only after

considering and setting forth findings on (1) the nature of the patient's desires, (2) whether the state has a significant interest in treatment, and (3) whether ECT is necessary and effective to satisfy the state interest implicated. We also conclude that a court must allow a patient's attorney adequate time to prepare for an ECT hearing. In this case the court failed to make a substituted judgment about Schuoler's desires, and abused its discretion by denying her attorney's request for a continuance (*In the Matter of Loretta Schuoler, 1986*).

Psychiatrists reading the preceding description of the legal regulations and restrictions on the use of ECT might sympathize with the sentiments of a California psychiatric resident's frustration with what appeared to be

overwhelming legal and bureaucratic approval in obtaining court approval. The legal difficulties consisted primarily of a precedent not to give court approval for ECT to patients who are unable to give informed consent; the bureaucratic difficulties entailed the confusion, disagreement and uncertainty at the administrative levels over the proper procedure . . . (Parry, 1981, p. 1128).

In the case mentioned, in the letter, the patient was transferred to another facility where, inexcusably, the patient died after being given Thorazine, to which she was allergic—as the medical record clearly indicated.

In the aftermath of this tragic case, an attempt was made to determine whether or not ECT could be given to incompetent patients in California. It was discovered that both psychiatric and legal confusion and bureaucracy could be cleared away. It was necessary, however, to educate psychiatrists about how the legal system works and to educate attorneys and judges about ECT. Psychiatrists learned that legal resistance to ECT, even for incompetent, involuntary patients, can be overcome. It required psychiatrists to participate actively in the legal process and to present adequate medical evidence. It was also helpful to educate attorneys and judges about the actual circumstances in which ECT is used and its therapeutic effects. For example, attorneys and judges visited a psychiatric hospital to learn about ECT and psychiatrists visited the court to discuss clinical issues with legal professionals. In several subsequent cases in which ECT was recommended for incompetent, involuntary patients, legal permission to administer ECT in accordance with appropriate medical discretion was quickly obtained. Psychiatrists, attorneys, and judges learned that bureaucratic obstacles and mutual distrust can sometimes be removed through rational and persistent efforts. Competent patients or the authorized representatives of incompetent patients may then decide to choose or refuse ECT.

Given that ECT has from the first been a controversial treatment, one might find it surprising that legal regulation was so slow in coming. However, it must be remembered that law is largely a conservative force in American society. Legal change occurs gradually, usually only in a piecemeal fashion, and typically after political sentiment has crystalized. So it was with ECT. Since the late 1960s 37 states have now passed legislation that specifically regulates ECT. Furthermore, the statutory regulation has created bureaucratic legal requirements—due process procedures for competency hearings, written informed consent rules, and provisions for refusal of treatment—as well as rules concerning peer review, record keeping, and reporting requirements. On the one hand, bureaucratic regulations often seem excessively restrictive, especially when they are first enacted. On the other hand, once the procedures are routinized, forms are prepared to facilitate documentation, and initial resistance is overcome, legal regulation becomes less of a burden. In California and Texas, for example, despite restrictive legislation, public mental health centers as well as private clinics have learned the bureaucratic rules and continue to use ECT when it is medically indicated. At the same time, the legal regulation of psychiatric practice does complicate, delay, and encumber professional discretion.

ETHICAL ASPECTS OF ECT

By the time of the GAP report on electroshock in 1947, numerous ethical issues had been identified. They included charges of abuse of professional and scientific authority and discretion ("promiscuous and indiscriminate use of electroshock therapy"), administration of the therapy by untrained psychiatrists, and lack of research and reporting about safety and efficacy of the treatment. Similar accusations years later led to the medical, legislative, and judicial standards established in the 1970s. The medical standards concentrated on the proper indications for and the appropriate techniques of administration of ECT. The legislative and judicial standards emphasized the rights of competent patients to an informed choice or refusal of ECT, and the rights of incompetent patients to have their interests protected through proper peer review of treatment recommendations and choices made by authorized representatives. Given that ECT, like other forms of invasive treatment, may have uncertain benefits and potentially serious risks, the rights of patients have been given much greater weight than in years past. The regulation of ECT use is an area that most professionals as well as the public agree is appropriate (Mills, 1978). The medical, legislative, and judicial standards of the 1970s have created the background for the ethical issues that have emerged in the 1980s.

The most significant ethical issue germane to ECT is informed consent. This reflects the recognition that when persons are in need of medical care, they normally have a right—legal and moral—to consent to or refuse a proposed treatment. Moral, legal, and psychological values underlie this practice. The moral principle of respect for persons implies respect for personal preference; the legal doctrine of informed consent supports self-determination; the psychological value of self-esteem is promoted by respect for personal preferences (Jonsen et al, 1986).

Despite the legal, ethical, and psychological justification for informed consent requirements, questions are frequently raised about its feasibility and practicality. Some clinicians tirelessly point out that medical patients in general and psychiatric patients in particular are often incompetent, sometimes lacking the ability to take in or process relevant information. Some patients who understand the issues are indifferent to or unable to make a voluntary choice. Clinicians who deal regularly with severely compromised patients are particularly critical of informed consent requirements, viewing them as at best required rituals, and at worst as obstructions to providing needed treatment.

Other clinicians and researchers believe that informed consent can, with concentrated effort and education of professionals and patients, be implemented and integrated into routine psychiatric practice (Lidz et al, 1984; Roth, 1986). Although further research is needed to determine the extent to which informed consent practices can be adapted to the nuances of clinical situations, empirical studies and clinical reports indicate the informed consent process can be improved. With respect to ECT, consensus exists that informed consent issues are especially important because so much confusion and controversy accompanies its use. Proponents of ECT emphasize that competent patients—voluntary and involuntary—have a right to treatment in general and a right to choose ECT in particular. To the extent that ECT offers a better or safer treatment option than other alternatives, such as medication or psychotherapy, it is especially important to make it available. Even opponents of ECT use acknowledge that voluntary patients have a right to choose or refuse ECT if they have been adequately informed of its alleged benefits and risks as well as its controversial status. The disagreements between proponents and opponents turn on *what* patients should be told, not *whether* they should be informed or have a right to choose.

Among those who endorse ECT as an appropriate form of treatment in certain cases, disagreements have arisen concerning the relationships among mental illness, incompetence, and irrationality. Although mental illness, incompetence, and irrationality are often found together, their precise connections to each other are not always clear. Mental illness occurs with varying degrees of severity, and even the severely mentally ill, such as seriously depressed persons, may be neither incompetent nor irrational. Other persons who are mentally ill may be both incompetent and irrational. By incompetent we mean that a person is unable to take in and assess information about his or her illness and need for treatment. By irrational we mean that a person is unable to appreciate and make reasonable choices. Both incompetence and irrationality are, however, elusive concepts. They defy precise definition; they occur in varying degrees; cultural, attitudinal, and other subjective factors influence our ideas of incompetence and irrationality. A recent debate in the literature of psychiatric ethics about mental illness, competence, and rationality illustrates the difficulties of applying these concepts to patients who are appropriate candidates for ECT treatment (Culver et al, 1980; Lesser, 1983; Sherlock, 1983; Taylor, 1983). Some psychiatrists believe that mentally ill but competent patients should be permitted to refuse ECT treatment even if their decision is irrational. Others agree that serious mental illness and irrationality are evidence that a person is incompetent and that such refusals should be overridden. Underlying the semantic dispute are different ethical orientations. Those who would override the choices of competent but irrational, mentally ill persons are disposed to paternalistic interventions. Those who would permit irrational refusal of treatment lean toward protection of patient preferences. In a clinical setting it is always difficult to determine the extent to which mental illness undermines capacity to make one's own decisions.

In a particularly thoughtful article, a British psychiatrist articulates the ethical issues that arise in practice when ECT is under consideration (Taylor, 1983). Dr. Taylor emphasizes the practical aspects of ethics in the giving and receiving of information and the nuances of the informed consent *process*. It is acknowledged that, in practice, assessment of competency is the most difficult part of the process. How one combines the subjectivity of the psychiatrist and the subjectivity of the patient to make an assessment of competency is extremely subtle. Perhaps that is why determinations of competency are a legal matter as well—and this despite the fact that there is little legal guidance about definitions of competency. The virtue of a legal proceeding to determine competency in contested or difficult cases is that it provides a forum for opposing views to be fully presented and defined. Yet, court determinations themselves are sometimes cumbersome, slow, and controversial. It is also possible, however, for psychiatrists, administrators, patients, attorneys, and families to utilize a legal forum quickly and efficiently to determine questions about competency to consent to ECT.

Perhaps the most disputed issue is whether involuntary patients should receive ECT. Some psychiatrists argue that no involuntary patients, even arguably competent ones, should be eligible for ECT because the environment is inherently coercive. Others believe that competent, involuntary patients should be free to choose or refuse medically indicated ECT. It is argued that administrative or legal procedures can protect against undue institutional or professional influence. The law generally permits the use of ECT with competent involuntary patients; this seems consistent with most ethical writings, which stress the rights of competent persons to make their own medical decisions. With respect to incompetent, involuntary patients the greatest risk of disregard of rights or even abusive practices exists. Incompetent patients are particularly vulnerable to exploitation because of their disability. Often such patients are abandoned by their families, disliked by staff, and stigmatized in the courts. Severely mentally ill patients are typically difficult to manage and control as well as often intractable to treatment. ECT provides a means of control and possible benefits, so it was and still is tempting to use, at least as a last resort. From an ethical perspective it is important that decisions made on behalf of incompetent, involuntary patients be scrutinized carefully. Public accountability for the decision, as well as protective procedures, are necessary to avoid the appearance and to insure against the reality of impropriety. The most vulnerable patients need the most protection from overzealous therapeutic efforts as well as unwarranted neglect.

Ethical concerns about ECT are likely to continue. At best, ECT is a form of treatment that arouses deep and passionate reactions among its proponents and opponents. Uncertainties about its reliability or duration of its therapeutic effect, uneasiness about using electricity to affect the brain, past occurrences or future potential for overuse and abuse, disputes about the appropriateness or effectiveness of legal restrictions, and doubts about adequate implementation of the informed consent process all contribute to a cloud of suspicion about ECT. To protect minimally the rights and interests of patients and to regulate properly professional discretion, legal regulation is desirable and necessary. To establish and maintain maximum standards of psychiatric practice, ethical self-criticism is essential. And to prevent overzealous as well as abusive practices, external vigilance and scrutiny must be maintained.

REFERENCES

American Psychiatric Association: Task Force Report 14: Electroconvulsive Therapy. Washington, DC, American Psychiatric Association, 1978

Bloch S, Chodoff P: Psychiatric Ethics. Oxford, Oxford University Press, 1984

Brakel SJ, Parry J, Weiner BA: The Mentally Disabled and the Law, third edition. Chicago, American Bar Foundation, 1985

Brandon S: The history of shock treatment, in Electroconvulsive Therapy: An Appraisal. Oxford, Oxford University Press, 1981

Breggin PR: Electro-Shock: Its Brain-Disabling Effects. New York, Springer, 1979

Culver CM, Gert B: Philosophy in Medicine. New York, Oxford University Press, 1982

Culver CM, Ferrell RB, Green RM: ECT and special problems of informed consent. Am J Psychiatry 1980; 137:5

Donaldson K: Insanity Inside Out. New York, Crown Publishers, 1976

Fink M: Convulsive Therapy: Theory and Practice. New York, Raven Press, 1979

Gap: Circular letters. Nov. 8, 1946, no. 9; and Jan. 22, 1947, no. 18.

Greenblatt M: Psychopolitics. New York, Grune & Stratton, 1978

In the Matter of Loretta Schuoler, Supreme Court, State of Washington, No. 5133-1, August 7, 1986

Jonsen AR, Siegler M, Winslade WJ: Clinical Ethics, second edition. New York, Macmillan, 1986

Lesser H: Consent, competency and ECT: a philosopher's comment. J Med Ethics 1983; 9:144-145

Lidz C, Meisel A, Zerubavel E, et al: Informed Consent. New York, Guilford Press, 1984

Mahler H, Co BT, Dinwiddie S: Studies in involuntary civil commitment and involuntary electroconvulsive therapy. J Nerv Ment Dis 1986; 174:97-105

Mills MJ, Avery D: The legal regulation of electroconvulsive therapy, in Mood Disorders: The World's Major Public Health Problem. Edited by Ayd FJ. Baltimore, Frank Ayd, 1978

NIH Consensus Development Conference: Electroconvulsive Therapy. Bethesda, MD, NIH and NIMH, 1985

Northern California Psychiatric Society, et al. v. City of Berkeley, California, Appellate Court, A026125, 1986

Parry B: Tragedy of legal impediments involved in obtaining ECT for patients unable to give informed consent (letter). Am J Psychiatry 1981; 138:1128-1129

Perr IN: Liability and electroshock therapy. J Forensic Sci 1980; 25:508-573

Roth L: Data on informed consent. Psychopharmacol Bull 1986; 22:494-495

Roth L, Lidz CW, Meisel A, et al: Competency to decide about treatment or research. Int J Law Psychiatry 1982; 5:29-50

Rothman D: ECT: The historical, social and professional sources of the controversy, in NIH Consensus Development Conference: Electroconvulsive Therapy. Bethesda, MD, NIH and NIMH, 1985

Senter NW, Winslade WJ, Liston EH, et al: Electroconvulsive therapy: the evolution of legal regulation. American Journal of Social Psychiatry Fall 1984; IV: 4

Sherlock R: Consent, competency and ECT: some critical suggestions. J Med Ethics 1983; 9:141-143

Slawson P, Guggenheim FG: Psychiatric malpractice: a review of the national loss experience. Am J Psychiatry 1984; 141:979-981

Taylor PJ: Consent, competency and ECT: a psychiatrist's view. J Med Ethics 1983; 9:146-151

Winslade WJ, Liston EH, Ross JW, et al: Medical, judicial, and statutory regulation of ECT in the United States. Am J Psychiatry 1984; 141:1349-1355

Wyatt v. Hardin, No. 3195-m, (M.D. Ala., Feb. 28, 1975), 1 MDLR 55

Afterword

by Robert M. Rose, M.D., and Harold Alan Pincus, M.D.

While, clearly, electroconvulsive therapy (ECT) remains a treatment surrounded by considerable public controversy, there are a number of consistent themes emphasized in this section around which, at least within the scientific and professional community, there is a great deal of consensus. At the same time, there are some areas where there is conflicting evidence and no clear conclusions can be drawn. Finally, there are a great many questions which have very little good empirical data available to provide answers, yet from which emerges firm agreement on one point: the need for further research on ECT.

A number of important issues have been emphasized in this section:

- The profession itself has provided little self-regulation of ECT. Along with unfavorable public perceptions of the procedure, this may have contributed to increased bureaucratic and judicial intrusion. There is a need for the profession to develop and enforce its own guidelines for training and practice regarding ECT, to ensure accountability and public confidence.
- It is essential that informed consent be regarded as a process—an integral component of the doctor/patient relationship—not a piece of paper to be signed by a patient. There should be much effort expended in educating patients (including, for example, the use of videotapes) about the procedure. Special concerns and procedures exist with regard to involuntary patients and patients who are not competent.
- There does exist an established body of knowledge regarding procedures for administering ECT in a way that provides the greatest safety and efficacy, minimizing potential side effects and risks. At the same time it is essential that facilities providing ECT be appropriately staffed and equipped. Moreover, psychiatrists providing ECT must have specific training in these procedures (in fact, all psychiatrists should), and their level of knowledge must be continually augmented and maintained through regular continuing medical education.
- There is a great deal of impressive evidence regarding the efficacy of ECT. This is most evident with regard to the treatment of depression, but there have also been recent data from controlled studies in mania. While ECT is not the first-line treatment in schizophrenia, and its overall utility for this disorder has not been fully resolved, it may be useful in certain specific instances. There are also anecdotal reports of ECT effectiveness in other mental disorders. Also, specific subgroups of mental disorders may be more responsive to ECT (for example, delusional depression).
- Importantly, there are variations in the effects of different techniques used in administering ECT. Unilateral nondominant ECT is generally as or nearly as effective, and produces less side effects, as bilateral ECT. In certain circumstances, however (for example, clinical urgency, mania), bilateral ECT may be more appropriate. Similarly, pulse stimuli are generally preferred over sine

wave stimuli. While general guidelines exist for the frequency and number of treatments, clearly more research is needed in this area.

- ECT does carry with it the potential for significant side effects. Acute confusional states are common, but are usually brief. Specific forms of memory deficits also are a concern, with varying degrees of length and significance. Furthermore, the assessment of memory deficits is confounded by difficulties in teasing out objective memory loss from patient perceptions or complaints of such loss from the effects of the illness itself. There is no substantial support for those who portray ECT, as currently administered, as permanently damaging to brain tissue.
- While various systemic changes are associated with ECT, cardiac effects are of greatest concern. These are most frequent in patients with pre-existing cardiac disease, and even in high risk patients these can generally be managed effectively.
- Importantly, with regard to most side effects, their frequency and severity generally vary with regard to specific stimulus parameters, electrode placement, and so on. Furthermore, the conclusions generally reflect group norms. The existence of subgroup and individual responses must also be considered.
- While the precise mechanisms by which ECT exerts its effects are not known, there is a wide array of theories which have been put forward. Most recently these have emphasized changes at the neurophysiological and neurochemical levels. While advances in the techniques of research in biological psychiatry and neuroscience have resulted in much progress in delineating the neurobiologic effects of ECT, complicating investigations in this area are the range of disorders in which ECT is effective as well as the range of cognitive and other central nervous system (CNS) effects of ECT. Also, recent evidence suggests that the relative role of the seizure itself, as compared to the stimulus used, is more complex than had been previously known.
- Finally, there is a great deal more research that needs to be done. Research on ECT must be brought further into the mainstream of psychiatric investigation. More sophisticated research is needed on the basic mechanisms by which ECT exerts its therapeutic and other effects. Studies are also needed to better identify characteristics of subgroups for whom the treatment is particularly beneficial or who are more likely to be subject to significant side effects. In addition, much more information is needed, based on carefully designed studies, to refine techniques to maximize the efficacy and minimize side effects, including such issues as the frequency and number of treatments, electrode placement, and such stimulus parameters as form and, particularly, intensity. Finally, we do not have enough good information about the role of maintenance ECT for prophylactic treatment of episodic disorders in patients who have had a good response to ECT for an acute condition.

As is evident from this review, ECT is clearly a powerful element in the therapeutic armamentarium of psychiatrists. Much like other treatments in psychiatry and, for that matter, in all of medicine, we are much more carefully specifying its role with regard to its indications and the manner in which it is administered; more clearly delineating the nature of its side effects; and we are building a more substantial information base derived from systematic empirical research. As noted earlier, however, we must also assure that this information is appropriately integrated into the education, training, and clinical practice of psychiatrists.

V

Cognitive Therapy

Section V

Cognitive Therapy
Foreword

by Aaron T. Beck, M.D., and A. John Rush, M.D.,
Section Editors

HISTORY

Precursors

The inclusion of a section on cognitive therapy in this distinguished series indicates that this approach to psychotherapy has come of age. From a historical vantage point, cognitive therapy shows the confluence of a variety of approaches to psychopathology. The theoretical underpinnings are derived from three main sources: 1) the phenomenological approach to psychology, 2) structural theory and depth psychology, and 3) cognitive psychology. The phenomenological approach to psychology emphasizes the view of the self and the personal world as central to the determination of behavior. This concept was originally formulated in Greek Stoic philosophy and in most recent times was evident in the writings of Adler (1936), Alexander (1950), Horney (1950), and Sullivan (1953).

The structural theory and depth psychology of Kant and Freud, particularly Freud's concept of the hierarchical structuring of cognition into primary and secondary processes, was the second major influence. The third sphere of influence stems from developments in contemporary cognitive psychology. George Kelly (1955) is generally recognized as being the first to describe the personality in terms of "personal constructs" and to define the role of beliefs in behavior change. The cognitive theories of emotion of Magda Arnold (1960) and Richard Lazarus (1984), which assigned primacy to cognition in emotional and behavioral change, also contributed to the theoretical structure of cognitive therapy.

Developmental History

Cognitive therapy dates back to the 1960s and stems, in part, from Beck's research on depression (Beck, 1963, 1964, 1967). Trained in psychoanalysis, Beck attempted to validate Freud's formulation of depression as having at its core "hostility turned on the self." To confirm his hypothesis, Beck made a systematic study of his depressed patients in traditional psychoanalysis. Instead of the expected finding of increased hostility in the thoughts and dreams, Beck observed a negative bias against the self. This finding was confirmed in a larger scale study in a hospital population. Continued clinical observations and experimental testing led to the development of the cognitive model of emotional disorders and a therapeutic system designed to reverse the systematic bias in information processing—cognitive therapy.

The rational–emotive therapy of Albert Ellis (1962) was a major influence in the development of cognitive therapy. Beck and Ellis, both, eschewed components of their analytic training and replaced passive listening with active, direct, face-to-face interviews.

The work of a number of contemporary behaviorists contributed to the development of cognitive therapy. Bandura's (1977) social learning theory concepts of expectancy of reinforcement, self and outcome efficacies, the interaction between person and environment, modeling, and vicarious learning helped to stimulate the shift in behavior therapy to the cognitive domain. Mahoney's (1974) emphasis on the cognitive control of behavior and his continuing theoretical contributions furthered the development of cognitive therapy. Along with cognitive therapy and Ellis's rational–emotive therapy, Meichenbaum's (1977) cognitive–behavioral modification is recognized as one of the three major cognitive–behavioral therapies.

RESEARCH

It is worthwhile to review research in the field of cognitive therapy since the first papers on cognitive theory and therapy were published (Beck, 1963, 1964). This research can be considered in terms of specific phases.

Tests of the Cognitive Model

The first phase revolved around the systematic testing of the cognitive model in both correlational and experimental studies (Beck, 1961). The investigations and investigators of the past 10 years are so numerous that only a representative few can be mentioned by name. Among these are Kuiper, Olinger, MacDonald, and Shaw (1985), supporting the concept of cognitive schemas; and the work by Wilkinson and Blackburn (1981) and Eaves and Rush (1984), demonstrating the negative bias of depressed patients in their view of themselves, their future, and their personal worth. The negative cognitive bias in the memory of depressed patients was amply demonstrated by Clark and Teasdale (1982). The specificity of cognitive distortions in depression has been supported by the studies by Krantz and Hammen (1979), Fennel and Campbell (1984), and Miller and Norman (1986).

The differentiation of depression and anxiety disorder on the basis of their "cognitive profiles" supported the specificity hypothesis. A review of the literature by Ernst (unpublished manuscript, 1987) showed that of 120 empirical studies designed to test the cognitive model of depression, specifically, the "negative cognitive triad" and "biased processing" hypotheses, approximately 90 percent supported this model.

Tests of Cognitive Therapy of Depression

The next major thrust was the development of the strategies and techniques of cognitive therapy preparatory to their testing in controlled clinical trials. Following the initial findings in Philadelphia (Rush et al, 1977), the efficacy of cognitive therapy as compared with antidepressant medication was validated in nine clinical trials. Most notable was the finding of superiority of cognitive therapy over drugs at one- or two-year follow-up in four studies (Kovacs et al, 1981; Simons et al, 1986; Blackburn et al, 1987; and Hollon et al, 1983).

The efficacy of cognitive therapy in groups was supported by Covi and his group in Baltimore (Roth and Covi, 1984; Covi et al, 1982), and by Beutler and his team in Tucson, working with the elderly (in press). Further success with the elderly depressed has been reported by Thompson and Gallagher (1984) and Gottlieb and Beck (1987).

Cognitive Therapy with Other Disorders

There have been numerous applications of cognitive therapy to other disorders. A few of the pioneers have been Salkovskis (Salkovskis and Warwick, 1985; Salkovskis, 1985) with obsessive-compulsives; Bradley and Gossop (1982) with drug addicts; Moorey (in press) with mentally handicapped; Wright and his team in Louisville (Wright and Beck, 1983), and J. Scott (personal communication, 1986) in Newcastle with inpatient depressives. A particularly effective area has been the application of cognitive concepts to marital therapy by Epstein and his group (Epstein et al, 1987).

CURRENT STATUS

The formation of systematic inpatient units centered around cognitive therapy has represented an "institutionalization" of cognitive therapy in Umea (Sweden), Oxford, Louisville, and San Diego. The First International Congress of Cognitive Therapy was held in Philadelphia in 1983, and the Second World Congress in 1986, in Umea.

Numerous units in cognitive therapy have sprung up in many centers where cognitive therapy research has been carried out. In the United States there are over 15 training centers for cognitive therapy. The largest research and training program is at the Center for Cognitive Therapy associated with the University of Pennsylvania in Philadelphia. Two journals devoted to cognitive therapy have appeared in the past 10 years—*Cognitive Therapy and Research* (founded by Mahoney, Meichenbaum, Goldfried, and Beck) and *Journal of Cognitive Psychotherapy* (founded by Dryden).

This section of this volume highlights some of the more recent work in cognitive therapy. In Chapter 24, Drs. Shaw and Segal introduce the reader to cognitive theory and its relationship to behavioral theory, as well as to cognitive psychology. In Chapter 25, Dr. Wright reviews the specifics of the cognitive model as it applies to depression, and describes the general approach of Beck's cognitive therapy to these disorders. Ruth Greenberg and Dr. Aaron T. Beck, in Chapter 26, further elaborate both theory and therapeutic methods that have recently been applied to and tested in patients with panic disorder. Further evidence for this expanded application comes from two recent studies of cognitive therapy with generalized anxiety disorder. Lindsay and associates (1987) found cognitive therapy to be superior to wait-list and anxiety management, and marginally superior to treatment with lorazepam. Durham and Turvey (in press) found cognitive therapy to be superior to behavior therapy in this patient group.

Chapter 27, by Drs. Trautman and Rotheram, suggests interesting new modifications of the model and specific techniques derived from their work with depressed adolescents. In Chapter 28, Drs. Covi and Primakoff review their clinical experience and relate empirical data on the use of cognitive therapy in a group format. Chapter 29, by Dr. Rush, proposes a cognitive model for identifying adherence obstacles to medication regimens in medically or psychiatrically ill patients, and illustrates its utility by case example. Finally, in Chapter 30, Dr. Hollon and Ms. Najavits provide a very thorough and most up-to-date review of the empirical studies of cognitive therapy in various psychiatric disorders.

In summary, while cognitive therapy has been most thoroughly explicated and evaluated in depressive disorders, the present field is rapidly expanding into modification and amplification of the theory and therapeutic techniques to an ever-widening group of disorders or set of clinical problems. These revisions have resulted in the development of new treatment manuals (Beck and Emery, 1985) for specific disorders, as well as new empirical studies of efficacy. It is this interaction of clinical experience with empirical science that fuels the careful, further development of this model and its related techniques. We believe that this section provides a clinically relevant overview of new advances in cognitive theory and therapy.

REFERENCES

Adler A: The neurotic's picture of the world. Int J Ind Psychol 2:3-10, 1936

Alexander F: Psychosomatic medicine: its principles and applications. New York, Norton, 1950

Arnold M: Emotion and Personality, vol. 1. New York, Columbia University Press, 1960

Bandura A: Social learning theory. Englewood Cliffs, NJ, Prentice Hall, 1977

Beck AT: A systematic investigation of depression. Compr Psychiatry 1961; 2:163-170

Beck AT: Thinking and depression, 1: idiosyncratic content and cognitive distortions. Arch Gen Psychiatry 1963; 9:324-333

Beck AT: Thinking and depression, 2: theory and therapy. Arch Gen Psychiatry 1964; 10:561-571

Beck AT: Depression: Clinical, Experimental and Theoretical Aspects. New York, Hoeber, 1967. (Reprinted as Depression: Causes and Treatment. Philadelphia, University of Pennsylvania Press, 1972)

Beck AT, Emery GE: Anxiety Disorders and Phobias: A Cognitive Perspective. New York, Basic Books, 1985

Beutler LE, Scogin F, Kirkish P, et al: Group cognitive therapy and alprazolam in the treatment of depression in older adults. J Consult Clin Psychol (in press)

Blackburn IM, Eunson KM, Bishop S: A two-year naturalistic follow-up of depressed patients treated with cognitive therapy, pharmacotherapy, and a combination of both. J Affective Disord 1987; 10:67-75

Bradley B, Gossop M: Differences in attitudes toward drug taking among drug addicts: implications for treatment. Drug Alcohol Depend 1982; 10:361-366

Clark DM, Teasdale JD: Diurnal variation in clinical depression and accessibility of memories of positive and negative experiences. J Abnorm Psychol 1982; 91:87-95

Covi L, Roth D, Lipman RS: Cognitive group psychotherapy of depression: the close-ended group. Am J Psychother 1982; 36:459-469

Durham R, Turvey A: Cognitive therapy versus behavior therapy in the treatment of chronic general anxiety: outcome at discharge and six-month follow-up. Behav Res Ther (in press)

Eaves G, Rush AJ: Cognitive patterns in symptomatic and remitted unipolar major depression. J Abnorm Psychol 1984; 93:31-40

Ellis A: Reason and emotion in psychotherapy. New York, Lyle Stuart, 1962

Epstein N, Pretzer J, Fleming B: The role of cognitive appraisal in self-report of marital communication. Behavior Therapy 1987; 18:51-69

Fennell MJ, Campbell EA: The cognitions questionnaire: specific thinking errors in depression. Br J Clin Psychol 1984; 23:81-92

Gottlieb G, Beck AT: Cognitive therapy and pharmacotherapy in geriatric depressants: a pilot randomized clinical trial. Paper presented at the 140th Annual Meeting of the American Psychiatric Association, Chicago, May 1987

Hollon SD, Evans MD, DeRubeis RJ: The cognitive–pharmacotherapy project: study design, outcome and clinical follow-up. Paper presented at the World Congress of Behavior Therapy, Washington, DC, December, 1983

Horney K: Neurosis and Human Growth: The Struggle Toward Self-Realization. New York, Norton, 1950

Kelly G: The Psychology of Personal Constructs. New York, Norton, 1955

Kovacs M, Rush AJ, Beck AJ, et al: Depressed outpatients treated with cognitive therapy or pharmacotherapy. Arch Gen Psychiatry 1981; 38:33-39

Kuiper NA, Olinger LJ, MacDonald MR, et al: Self-schema processing of depressed and nondepressed content: the affects of vulnerability to depression. Special Issue: Depression. Social Cognition 1985; 3:77-83

Lazarus R: On the primacy of cognition. Am Psychol 1984; 39:124-129

Lindsay WR, Gamsu CV, McLaughlin E, et al: A controlled trial of treatments for general anxiety. Br J Clin Psychol 1987; 26:315

Mahoney MJ: Cognition and Behavior Modification. Cambridge, MA, Ballinger, 1974

Meichenbaum D: Cognitive-Behavior Modification: An Integrative Approach. New York, Plenum, 1977

Miller IW, Norman WM: Persistence of depressive cognitions within a subgroup of depressed inpatients. Cognitive Therapy Research 1986; 10:211-224

Moorey S: Cognitive therapy in adults with learning difficulties, in Cognitive Therapy in Clinical Practice. Edited by Scott J, Williams JMG, Beck AT. London, Croom Helm (in press)

Roth D, Covi L: Cognitive group psychotherapy of depression: the open-ended group. Int J Group Psychother 1984; 34:67-82

Rush AJ, Beck AT, Kovacs M, et al: Comparative efficacy of cognitive therapy and imipramine in the treatment of depressed outpatients. Cognitive Therapy Research 1977; 1:17-37

Salkovskis PM: Obsessional-compulsive problems: a cognitive-behavioral analysis. Behav Res Ther 1985; 23:571-583

Salkovskis PM, Warwick HM: Cognitive therapy of obsessive-compulsive disorder: treating treatment failures. Behavioral Psychotherapy 1985; 13:243-255

Simons AD, Murphy GE, Levine JL, et al: Cognitive therapy and pharmacotherapy: sustained improvement over one year. Arch Gen Psychiatry 1986; 43:43-48

Sullivan HS: The Interpersonal Theory of Psychiatry. New York, Norton, 1953

Thompson LW, Gallagher D: Efficacy of psychotherapy in the treatment of late-life depression. Advances in Behavior Research Therapy 1984; 6:127-139

Wilkinson IM, Blackburn IM: Cognitive style in depressed and recovered patients. Br J Clin Psychol 1981; 20:283-292

Wright JH, Beck AT: Cognitive therapy of depression: theory and practice. Hosp Community Psychiatry 1983; 34:1119-1127

Chapter 24

Introduction to Cognitive Theory and Therapy

by Brian F. Shaw, Ph.D., and Zindel V. Segal, Ph.D.

A PARADIGM SHIFT IN PSYCHOTHERAPY

The importance of studying cognitive processes in human adaptation is now generally accepted. Yet, when viewed in its historical context, this development represents a significant shift (some would say revolution) over the past two decades, which witnessed the ascendancy of a cognitive mediation perspective over radical behavioral or drive-based models of psychopathology (Dember, 1974; Erwin, 1978; Lazarus et al, 1982). The proliferation of cognitive paradigms employed in the investigations of diverse clinical disorders such as schizophrenia (Cromwell, 1978; Mathysse et al, 1979), unipolar depression (Ingram, 1984), panic disorder (D.M. Clark, 1986), and social anxiety (Mathews and MacLeod, 1985) provides ample evidence of the incursion this perspective has made into territory once considered the domain of more traditional psychopathology research.

A confluence of developments in the early 1960s served to usher in this change of focus. Chief among these was the shift in behavioral psychology from a simplistic stimulus–response model, dominated by animal conditioning studies, to a framework that admitted the possibility of cognitive mediation (Wilson, 1978). Bandura's influential work (1969) legitimized the study of such intra-individual cognitive variables as expectancies, self-verbalizations, predictions, and other covert processes that had heretofore been excluded from accounts of human learning and behavior. A second important development was the surge of data from the neurosciences and computer sciences which began to focus psychology on issues such as the nature of perception and the mechanisms of memory. Loosely termed the information-processing perspective, this viewpoint emphasizes that humans are active and selective seekers, creators, and users of information. This perspective stands in contrast to nonmediational models that relied on historical and environmental variables to account for the control of behavior (Pribram, 1986; Turk and Salovey, 1985).

The existence of a cognitive-learning perspective, with its emphasis on an internal determinism of human action, was gradually recognized by the field of psychotherapy. Practitioners who had previously endorsed the external determinism of a purely behavioral perspective, a view that accepted only stimuli, responses, and contingencies, were now willing to consider the possibility that the modification of cognitions and dysfunctional information processing may be an important intervention in the treatment of maladaptive behavior (Mahoney, 1977). This model was articulated by Mahoney (1977) who outlined its four basic tenets: 1) The human organism responds primarily to cognitive representations of its environments rather than to those environments per se; 2) these cognitive representations are functionally related to the processes and parameters of learning; 3) most human learning is cognitively mediated; and 4) thoughts, feelings, and behaviors are causally interactive (pp. 7–8). The translation process through which these assertions were applied to the conceptualization and treatment of emotional disorders yielded a number of different schools or methods of cognitive–behavior therapy.

COGNITIVE THERAPY AND BEHAVIOR CHANGE

The cognitive reanalysis of such clinical phenomena as phobic avoidance, depression, lack of assertion, and poor anger control led to the development of novel treatment modalities that instructed clients in 'distancing' or 'decentering' from intense emotional experiences and then engaging in objective appraisal, in the use of coping skills, or in developing an active problem-solving set (see, for example, Wilson, 1978). While the comparative outcome between these relatively new procedures and the more traditional behavioral approaches is still an unresolved issue in the field (Beidel and Turner, 1986), this lack of knowledge has not prevented their adoption by increasing numbers of practitioners (Smith, 1982). Mahoney and Arnkoff (1978) pointed out that the commonalities among the different cognitive–behavioral schools are stronger than their procedural variations and that all approaches subscribe to three basic principles. These principles state that: 1) humans develop adaptive and maladaptive behavior patterns by way of cognitive processes (for example, selective attention, symbolic coding); 2) these cognitive processes are functionally activated by procedures that are generally isomorphic with those of the human learning laboratory; and 3) the resultant task of the therapist is that of a diagnostic-educator who assesses maladaptive processes and subsequently arranges learning experiences that will alter cognitions, and the behavior and affect patterns with which they correlate (p. 692).

An important point that at times is underemphasized in discussions about the role played by cognitive theory in the development of cognitive therapies, is the distinction between treatment procedures and theoretical processes. While a basic tenet of cognitive and social learning theories is the reliance upon cognitive mechanisms to explain the acquisition and maintenance of abnormal behavior (Bandura, 1969), recognition is also given to the fact that performance-based procedures are among the most powerful methods of producing behavior change. The use of homework assignments and behavioral tasks is an implicit part of cognitive therapy as practiced by Beck and colleagues (1979) and others. At first glance, this inclusion might seem to present a contradiction to those interested in heralding the claims of cognitive procedures, yet upon closer inspection this distinction is not really problematic. Social learning theory acknowledges that performance-based procedures offer a powerful means for modifying maladaptive behavior, but that all behavior change, in order for it to be enduring and generalizable to new settings, must modify the patient's belief that he or she can carry out the more adaptive response. Changes in the patient's cognitive construct of self-efficacy is what this process describes, and is considered to be the common point of action as well as the ultimate goal of most cognitive interventions (Bandura, 1969, 1977). Thus, directly produced behavior change is considered to be one of the most effective means of altering the cognitive mechanisms that mediate subsequent performance. Of course, as will be clear from the other chapters in this section, many of the interventions of cognitive therapy address the patient's maladaptive thinking. Ultimately, change in self-defeating cognitive patterns, including incorrectly appraising life events, jumping to conclusions, and reasoning on the basis of dysfunctional assumptions, is the goal of cognitive therapy. Our task now is to review the theoretical and empirical base for cognitive therapy of emotional disorders.

COGNITIVE MODELS OF EMOTIONAL DISORDERS

Understandably, most of the chapters in this section focus on two prevalent emotional disorders (unipolar major depression and panic disorder), as these areas have received the greatest attention from theorists and clinicians. Cognitive behavior therapists tend to address these emotional disorders in part because there are adequate theoretical models and experimental work to provide a foundation for such efforts. One of Ford and Urban's (1963) criteria for a system of psychotherapy is that the therapy is based on a "theory supported by a public and verified body of knowledge" (p. 18). Cognitive therapy, as will be seen, meets this criterion.

We agree that, "A therapist's primary purpose is not to establish principles of behavior, but rather to apply established principles to achieve behavioral change . . . therapists require some principles by which to proceed. Theoretical statements are needed to account for the manner in which unwanted behaviors arise and for the procedure whereby they can become changed. Without a systematic point of view, therapists are likely to become quite inefficient and on occasion perhaps even haphazard in seeking behavioral change in their patients" (Ford and Urban, 1963, p. 9). This chapter addresses the theoretical base concerning the relationship between cognitive changes and either depressive disorders or anxiety disorders. Other chapters in this section will deal with the actual procedures used to facilitate change in these variables.

Several cognitive models have been presented to account for the development and maintenance of the emotional disorders. As such, it may be confusing for the clinician to identify the salient features of each model and to determine the clinical constructs that stem from the various models. We plan to present a few prominent cognitive models of depression and anxiety, to define the central constructs used by cognitive therapists, and to review briefly the current experimental work in this field. Our goal is to provide a framework for the clinician to understand our conceptualization of psychopathology and therapeutic change. The reader should note that this chapter is a selective and not an exhaustive review.

Definition of Terms/Constructs

Many terms are used to describe the products, processes, and structure associated with psychopathology (Hollon and Kriss, 1984). By cognition, we refer to the verbal or pictoral events in a person's stream of consciousness. It will be apparent that terms such as cognitive therapy and cognitive assessment depend on knowledge of a particular type of self-referent thinking rather than on the more traditional evaluations of intelligence, memory functioning, the ability to think abstractly, and so on.

Cognitive therapists are most concerned with patients' automatic thoughts (other terms that refer to the same phenomenon include self-statements and internal dialogue), their attitudes (assumptions, beliefs), and the organization of their self-perceptions and of their perceptions of the world. Typically, the term cognitive is considered to reflect the content of the patient's thinking (that is, the actual words or pictures that come to mind), or the processes of their thinking (that is, the ways in which information from the world and from one's memories are managed). Several theorists have cautioned us that simply describing the content or processes of a person's ideation does not explain it (Meichenbaum and Butler, 1980; Arnkoff and Glass, 1982). "Adaptive living is not necessarily incompatible with holding a belief that diverges somewhat from reality or with saying negative things to oneself; the determinant of adaptation is the meaning or function of the belief or self-statement" (Arnkoff and Glass, 1982, p. 3).

Automatic thoughts (Beck, 1963) are a special type of cognition that occur in normal states, but are of particular clinical significance in emotional disorders. Automatic thoughts occur without deliberation (that is, they have an involuntary quality) and are characterized by a habitual and steretyped content, an unquestioned plausibility and an almost instantaneous accessibility (Beck et al, 1979). Given these qualities it is essential to recognize that automatic thoughts may not be easily elicited by a simple inquiry from the therapist. In many cases the patients must be trained to identify and report this ideation.

Cognitive therapists often try to alter their patients' beliefs, attitudes, and assumptions, three related constructs that refer to the individual's rules about themselves and others. This information is typically inferred from the patient's pattern of thinking and behavior. Beliefs are rigid and absolutistic; there are demands, commands, and musts that people endorse (for example, the belief that one should [must] have certain and perfect control over events in one's life [Ellis, 1979]). Attitudes that focus on the self can be seen as the rules that guide an individual's behavior evaluations and/or expectations (for example, you cannot be happy unless others respect you). Bandura (1977) introduced the concept of self-efficacy to characterize, in a general way, the types of beliefs and outcome expectations people have about their behavior. Self-efficacy is the belief that one has the personal resources to perform certain behaviors that will, in turn, lead to desirable outcome (for example, pain reduction, successful attempts to cope with phobic reactions). Assumptions typically involve a contingency about one's self-worth (Kuiper and Olinger, 1986).

The clinically relevant points about beliefs, attitudes, and assumptions are that a) they are unspoken (silent), abstract regulators of behavior; b) they are inferred from a set of automatic thoughts; and c) they may be maladaptive or dysfunctional in the sense that they disrupt the person's commonsense responses and produce painful emotional reactions. For example, if a person presents with several automatic thoughts concerned with having to be intimately involved with someone, it may be that in their interactions with others they place strong demands on others, are easily disappointed and hurt, and even minimize or demean friendly contacts. A vicious cycle is established in which individuals guided by their assumptions behave in a way that influences their perceptions. In this case the assumption might be, "If others don't express their love for me at all times then I'm worthless." This example illustrates a vulnerability to experience a lowered sense of worth contingent upon the reactions of others. Clearly, this assumption is dysfunctional given the unpredictability of others' responses and the person's inability to control such reactions. Such an orientation empowers external sources to determine the person's value rather than a more adaptive mode whereby the person draws on intrinsic values.

At an even greater level of abstraction, dysfunctional beliefs and attitudes are hypothesized to reflect knowledge structures or schema. Schema are cognitive structures consisting of the person's basic organization of personal and environmental information and are constructed from information gleaned from past experiences (Thorndyke and Hayes-Roth, 1979). What is represented is often the most meaningful and emotionally salient experiences in an individual's life, although clearly it is not limited to these events. Once activated, schema influence the processing of new experiences by way of selective attention and the reconstruction of past memories by way of selective recall. They determine which bits of new experience are important and promote efficient and coherent information processing (Markus, 1977; Turk and Speers, 1983). In the service of greater efficiency, schema give rise to cognitive distortions, a concept used to describe various biases in information processing.

Clinically, cognitive therapists are most interested in self-schema (Markus, 1977), an active organizer of personally relevant information. The schema construct, along with automatic thoughts and dysfunctional attitudes (including a lowered sense of self-efficacy), are prominent in the prevailing cognitive models of depression and anxiety. Self-schema that have been frequently activated are difficult to change. These structures assimilate information in such a way that it is unlikely that naturally occurring "corrective experiences" are detected (Segal, in press). For example, if one is sensitized to one's "unlovable" qualities, he or she may perceive others as rejecting or uncaring if they do not acknowledge him or her in all situations (this reaction is an example of a cognitive distortion, namely selective abstraction—focusing on a detail without considering other salient features of the experience). He or she may even interpret a positive comment as a reflection of the other person's pity rather than caring (an arbitrary inference—the process of drawing a conclusion in the absence of evidence or even when the evidence is contrary to the conclusion). Another type of cognitive distortion is overgeneralization, the pattern of drawing a general rule or conclusion on the basis of one fact. In this case, perhaps the person's spouse has separated and is no longer loving, with the result that the person concludes, "No one cares for me. I'll never be loved again." While cognitive distortions clearly occur in normal states and are by no means specific to only one psychopathological condition (Kruglanski and Ajzen, 1983; Nisbett and Ross, 1980), they are frequently observable in reports of depressed and anxious patients.

Two other important cognitive constructs employed by cognitive theorists are also readily observable in patient reports. *Expectations* refer to inferences about the outcomes of actions or about future events, while *causal attributions* refer to inferences regarding the causes of events, including behaviors (Hollon and Kriss, 1984). These constructs are important because they reflect two aspects of the self-fulfilling prophecy (Merton, 1948)—the notion that people behave in a manner consistent with their expectations, thereby altering the response of others and themselves and making reality match their preconceptions. Furthermore, once certain outcomes occur (particularly negative events such as a failure or a panic attack) the cause of the event is *attributed* to the expected factor ("I'm no good in math"; "My heart won't take it"). As a result, patients may be caught in the negative downward spiral of depression or the upward spiral of anxiety.

Cognitive Models of Depression

The two prominent cognitive models of depression are Seligman's reformulated, learned helplessness model (Abramson et al, 1978; Peterson and Seligman, 1985) and Beck's model (1967; Beck et al, 1979). The learned helplessness model was originally based on the observation that when humans expect that they cannot control events in their life they manifest certain changes consistent with depression (passivity, lowered aggression, loss of appetite, negative expectations). The attributional reformulation focused on the person's explanations for this uncontrollability. Abramson and colleagues (1978) proposed three dimensions to account for the individual's attributional style (internal versus external, stable versus unstable, and global versus specific). Depression was predicted to result from internal, stable, and global attributions for negative events, basically a propensity for self-blame. The individual's expectation that he or she cannot control the outcome of future events are exacerbated by his or her causal attributions. For example, "I'll never marry again because I'm not capable of love. I poison every relationship that I'm in." Notably, the person's explanatory style is viewed as a trait, and thus should show consistently across situations and may even serve as a vulnerability marker for some types of depressives (Peterson and Seligman, 1985).

Beck's (1967) model of depression places even greater emphasis on the individual's vulnerability to depression in the face of stressful life events. Beck and associates (1979) hypothesized that excessively rigid and dysfunctional assumptions about one's self-worth constitute a predisposition to depression. These dysfunctional attitudes were proposed to reflect negative self-schema that have formed as a result of earlier experiences, particularly the experiences of loss, deprivation, and death. Later, the spiral of depression begins when negative life events (specifically, perceived loss or losses) impinge on the dysfunctional attitudes, increasing the accessibility of negative self-schema. These self-schema ". . . become overly active in a depressive episode . . . organize those aspects of the person's experience that concern self-evaluation and relationships with other people . . . information about life situations or events that the individual perceives as real or potential subtractions from his personal domain" (Kovacs and Beck, 1978, p. 529). As the patient becomes depressed, negative automatic thoughts become increasingly evident. "The cognitive model postulates three specific concepts to explain the psychological substrate of depression: (1) the cognitive triad, (2) schema, and (3) cognitive errors (faulty information processing)" (Beck et al, 1979, p. 10). The patient's automatic thoughts fit within a negative cognitive triad: negatively biased views of the self, the world, and the future. The model gives a primacy to these cognitive changes as the central factors that maintain many depressions. The relative stability with which personal information is interpreted in a negative way and with which memories are recalled are seen as functionally related to the other symptomatic changes in depression. Furthermore, the cognitive distortions in depression promote an assimilation of information about the self from all sources into this negative structure. In other words, the activation of negative self-schema in response to life events leads to a potential domination of the person's thinking. The initial task of therapy is to decrease the accessibility of these negative self-schema.

Cognitive Models of Anxiety

The cognitive models of anxiety emphasize the person's expectations and appraisals of situation. Where the theme of depression is loss, anxiety disorders are seen from the perspective of extreme threat reactions. Beck and Emery (1985) posit that "anxiety disorders represent a malfunction of the system for activating and terminating a defensive response to a threat" (p. 22). Furthermore, in anxiety the central cognitions are unrealistic perceptions of danger following such events as illness and death, or catastrophising about the loss of control, or negative changes in a relationship (Clark and Beck, 1987).

As Watts and colleagues (1986) pointed out, however, a cognitive model that relies solely on expectancy is not likely to account for the complex cognitive changes associated with the anxiety disorders or their treatment. For this reason, cognitive therapists are also concerned with schema for feared objects or situations and with dysfunctional beliefs that may serve as vulnerability factors to anxiety states. The cognitive distortions associated with anxiety states were viewed by Beck (1976) as following Lazarus's (1966) stress model. Lazarus and Launier (1978) defined stress as "any event in which environmental or internal demands (or both) tax or exceed the adaptive resources of an individual" (p. 87). Lazarus (1966) proposed three processes in response to a stressor: primary appraisal, the initial impression of the situation; secondary appraisal on evaluation of the available resources, both internal and external, that will counter the stressor; and reappraisal, the re-evaluation of the stressor in the context of coping resources. Thus, the distortions associated with anxiety involve: a) overestimating the probability of the feared event; b) overestimating the severity of the feared event; c) underestimating coping resources (what you can do about it); and d) underestimating rescue factors (what other people can do to help you) (Beck, 1976).

A key aspect of cognitive models of anxiety concerns the "fear of fear": in other words, the patient's fear or dread of the symptoms of anxiety as differentiated from the actual stressor(s). Clark and Beck (1987) point out that ". . . the symptoms of anxiety are often perceived as a further source of threat leading to a series of vicious circles which tend to maintain or exacerbate anxiety reactions" (p. 142). In a broad-based analysis, Reiss and associates (1986) identified two component processes of the fear of fear. "Anxiety expectancy is primarily an associative learning process in which the individual has learned that a given stimulus arouses anxiety/fear. Anxiety sensitivity is an individual difference variable consisting of beliefs that the experience of anxiety/fear causes illness, embarrassment or additional anxiety" (pp. 1–2).

It is the emphasis on the patient's belief and interpretations that distinguishes the cognitive model. Several theorists have pointed to expectations and the recall of past experiences with the sensations of anxiety as critical variables in anxiety disorder. Van den Hout and Griez (1984), Beck and Emery (1985), and D.M. Clark (1986) all point to the "catastrophic misinterpretations of certain bodily sensations" as central to panic disorder, "examples of catastrophic misinterpretations would be a healthy individual perceiving palpitations as evidence of impending heart attack; perceiving a slight feeling of breathlessness as evidence of impending cessation of breathing and consequent death; or perceiving a shaky feeling as evidence of impending loss of control and insanity" (Clark, 1986, p. 462). Other anxiety disorders are characterized by differing ideational content. Thus, social phobia involves exaggerated concerns about the valuations of others, particularly being seen as weak and being rejected or abandoned by others (Clark and Beck, 1987). Simple phobias involve exaggerated perception of danger in specific situations (for example, going away from home, high places, or confined places) or specific objects (for example, snakes or cats). Generalized anxiety is often associated with a decreased sense of self-efficacy (Bandura, 1977) in dealing with life's threats (Rappee, 1985; Hibbert, 1984).

The person is judged to be vulnerable to anxiety disorders if he or she chronically accesses a view of the self as subject to "internal or external dangers over which his or her control is lacking." This pattern results in a focus on danger-oriented ("what if") rather than problem-oriented ("if I see x then I'll do y") thinking.

EXPERIMENTAL EVIDENCE FOR COGNITIVE CHANGE IN DEPRESSION AND ANXIETY

In this section we will summarize some of the main experimental findings related to cognitive models of depression and anxiety. Several extensive reviews of the current cognitive assessment measures related to these disorders are available (Segal and Shaw, 1987; Goldberg and Shaw, in press). In addition, the literature evaluating the adequacy of the cognitive models of depression has captured many of the extent controversies in the field (see Coyne and Gotlib, 1983; 1986; Segal and Shaw, 1986a, 1986b).

In general, depressed states are associated with thoughts of loss and failure, while anxiety states are associated with cognitions of future harm and danger (Harrel et al, 1981; Thorpe et al, 1983; D.M. Clark, 1986). Depression has received considerably more attention from experimental psychopathologists than has anxiety, probably because of the relative recency of anxiety models. Readers should recall, however, the significant overlap between depressive and anxiety states, estimated by some investigators to be as high as 60 percent (see Hamilton, 1981). For the most part, this overlap is ignored in studies using the Research Diagnostic Criteria (RDC) (Spitzer et al, 1978) because of exclusion clauses in this system. Thus, it may be that many of the cognitive changes reported in the following pages may not be specific to either disorder.

Depression

The literature on depression almost exclusively concerns unipolar, nonpsychotic, depressive disorders (major depression, intermittent depression, dysthymic disorder) and may in nonclinical samples (for example, students) involve transient mood states (Shaw, 1985). We will only report on studies that assessed a clinical sample. There are several reliable findings of cognitive change in depression. These changes include: a) an increase of negative automatic thoughts; b) negative expectancies for success; c) a negatively biased recall of self-referent information; d) an abnormally high level of dysfunctional attitudes; and e) following a failure experience, a bias toward internal, stable, and global attributions.

Findings that depression involves negative thinking and, particularly, negative automatic thought will surprise no one, but the importance of documenting these changes and determining whether they are state-dependent should not be overlooked. Several studies have documented an increase in negative automatic thoughts in depression (for example, Hollon et al, 1986; Dobson and Shaw, 1986) with a corresponding return to normal levels once the depression remits (see also Miller and Norman, 1986; Eaves and Rush, 1984). Negative expectancies for success and depression are clearly related. Studies have documented that depressed patients have lower expectancies of success in skill-related tasks compared with nondepressed individuals (for example, Norman et al, 1983; Lunghi, 1977). The notable point is that the depressed subjects' actual performance on many tasks does not differ from others, although clearly, when considering interpersonal skills, these negative expectations may be veridical. Following these tasks depressed subjects are more likely to describe themselves in negative terms and to recall the negative aspects of their performance (for example, Gotlib, 1983). Whether the biased recall evident in depression is also observable in other types of psychopathology remains unknown. As with automatic thoughts, cognitive changes are probably a function of the depressed state.

If we consider the role played by dysfunctional attitudes and biased attributional style we run into more controversy. While there are several methods to measure self-schema, one of the most widely used is actually a measure of attitudes, the Dysfunctional Attitude Scale (DAS) (Weissman, 1979). This instrument asks subjects to indicate their degree of agreement with statements describing contingencies between various outcomes and self-worth (for example, "My value as a person depends greatly on what others think of me"; "If I fail at work then I am a failure as a person"). The DAS quantifies a number of attitudes that have been shown to correlate significantly with depression (see Segal and Shaw, 1986a). The controversy emerges when investigators try to establish whether these evaluations of dysfunctional attitudes persist beyond the depressive episode. On balance, it appears that the majority of studies reveal that DAS scores return to normal once the episode remits (for example, Silverman et al, 1984). There is enough of a range of response, however, to suggest that, in some patients, elevated DAS scores in a nondepressed phase may be consistent with a vulnerability to future symptoms (Rush et al, 1986; Simons et al, 1986).

Similar data have been obtained with respect to the attributional bias in depression. Again, various scales and methods have been used to assess attributional style. Some studies have found that the depressive style of attributing negative or failure events to internal, stable, and global causes is predictive of future depressed symptoms (Eaves and Rush, 1984; Hollon et al, in press), but like so many other findings, this result is not conclusive (see Dobson and Shaw, 1986). One important study was that of Miller and colleagues (1982), who found that differences in attributional style varied according to whether the investigator used hypothetical events, stressful life events, or experimental tasks as stimuli. Peterson and associates (1985) summed up this area nicely with the comment ". . . there is a style of attributing bad events that is sometimes associated with depression and sometimes not. The determinants of this 'sometimes' correlation need to be established" (p. 168).

Anxiety

When we turn to anxiety, the experimental literature is interesting despite the fact that it is in an earlier stage of productivity. Clark and Beck (1987) identified four predictions to test the cognitive models. These are: 1) the thinking of anxious patients will be characterized by thoughts concerned with the perception of danger; 2) within individuals, anxiety ratings will correlate with the believability and frequency of thoughts concerned with danger; 3) the temporal occurrence of thoughts concerned with danger will be such that they *could* logically contribute to the initiation or maintained activation of the anxiety program; 4) experimental manipulations of the frequency and believability of thoughts concerned with the perception of danger will have systematic effects on patients' level of anxiety (p. 145).

Clark and Beck (1987) go on to discuss the literature as related to these predictions. The first prediction held across six studies, with most patients identifying danger-related automatic thoughts. One study (Butler and Mathews, 1983) found that anxious patients (and depressed patients with significant anxiety) overestimated the likelihood of future negative hypothetical events. Anxious patients appear to notice threatening situations more readily and so dwell on the danger inherent in these situations. This attention to threat in phobics was illustrated in a study by Watts and colleagues (1986). These researchers developed a task from cognitive psychology and showed that the performance of spider phobics was significantly affected by the presentation of words such as "creepy," "hairy," and "legs." One interesting study by Foa and McNally (1986) demonstrated differential sensitivity on the part of patients with obsessive-compulsive disorder for fear-related words (for example, dirt, germs) compared to neutral words. Using a dichotic listening task, a procedure in which subjects are presented with two simultaneous audio recordings and are asked to repeat the content of one recording, patients detected more fear-related words in the unattended channel. Following treatment, this sensitivity was significantly reduced.

The third and fourth predictions require more study. Some investigators (for example, Beck et al, 1974; Last and Blanchard, 1982) have shown that phobics and other anxious patients report danger related thoughts *before* their anxiety peaked, but more prospective work is needed before any conclusions can be reached.

FUTURE DIRECTIONS

From a Popperian standpoint (Popper, 1968), the emergence of a new approach to the study of psychopathology, as well as for modeling the process of behavior change in psychotherapy, is necessarily inadequate and often wrong in detail. The most important consideration, however, is that the model is a feasible one and that it can be progressively sharpened by recourse to experimental disconfirmation (Pribram, 1986). Research-based attempts to test this model's predictions have occupied an important role in this theory's development over the past 10 years, and in spite of critical disclaimers (Coyne and Gotlib, 1983), support for a number of its central assertions has been reported (Segal and Shaw, 1986b).

One of the continuing challenges for cognitive models of depression and anxiety lies in their integration with other models investigating the functioning of depressed or anxious patients, so that a more comprehensive understanding of these disorders can be attained. The development of such multifaceted models is seen as an alternative to the poor explanatory power of theories that aim to account for the complexity of depressive or anxiety phenomena in a single theoretical position (Hammen, 1985; Segal and Shaw, 1986a; Zubin and Steinhauer, 1981). One research direction that derives from such a focus examines the covariance of both biological (for example, dexamethasone suppression, rapid eye movement [REM] latency) and cognitive (for example, schematic processing, attributional style) markers in depression in an effort to map the interaction among these correlates of the disorder. Research of this type can have direct implications for causal theory building, as well as for designing more sensitive change measures for patients still in the episode. The simultaneous assessment of changes at both these levels of response would begin to answer the question of whether patients effectively treated with cognitive therapy show improvement on biological markers of the episode, and whether tricyclic treatment has an impact on cognitive distortions and other types of dysfunctional information processing. Demonstration of such interactive effects would serve to strengthen the view that, at least in unipolar depression, cognitive and pharmacological treatments work by altering different aspects of the same dysfunctional system and represent alternative points of entry into the system (Beck, 1984), rather than being seen as separate treatments of a single problem. This conceptualization is consistent with the view proposed by Akiskal and McKinney (1975), and may serve to discourage dichotomous thinking with respect to the findings of cognitive and pharmacotherapy outcome trials which are often taken as evidence of the superiority of one approach over the other.

An issue closely related to treatment is that of secondary prevention, the goal of which is to identify those individuals who, once out of the depressive episode, are at greatest risk for relapse. Such a focus shifts the emphasis away from speculation about initial causes, and attempts instead to understand the cognitive processes associated with relapse, regardless of what may have led into the index episode. Considering that estimates for risk of relapse are discouragingly high (Keller et al, 1983) and that this presents a danger for the development of a chronic course of the disorder, a focus on relapse seems warranted. One recent development that contributes to this discussion is the emergence of the 12- to 18-month follow-up data from a number of clinical trials in which cognitive therapy was compared to pharmacotherapy for depression. The data point to a differential relapse effect in favor of patients treated with cognitive therapy, suggesting that perhaps this treatment approach is modifying some aspect of the underlying causal mechanisms which drive the episode, while medication-based treatment is acting mainly in a symptom suppressive fashion and has less impact on causal factors (Hollon et al, in press). In addressing the issue of the apparent prophylaxis associated with cognitive treatment, Hollon and colleagues (in press) outlined a promising model for disentangling state and trait variables during and after the depressive episode, as well as for identifying the causally active mechanisms underlying it. The systematic adoption of this model in future studies examining the basic psychopathology of depression could yield important information regarding possible markers of vulnerability to the disorder.

This strategy would also augment our knowledge about the differences between patients who relapse and those who manage to stay well after treatment.

Shifting the focus away from the expansion of the cognitive model into new research areas and back to the viability of the model itself, it is becoming increasingly apparent that the consideration of life-stress variables by cognitive approaches to the study of depression and anxiety is a future priority. Model building within the cognitive–behavioral tradition would benefit greatly from a classification of the role that stress plays in precipitating the types of cognitive shifts that lead to dysphoria, depression, or anxiety. Such a strategy may serve to bolster the modest correlations obtained between measures of stressful life events and depression, for example, as well as redress the lack of attention that cognitive theories have paid to the ways in which cognitive and personality variables interact with stressful life events to produce depression. The work by Hammen (1985) is instructive in its adoption of a cognitive–environmental perspective in which contributions from these two sources of variance are both assessed and expected. By studying event and cognitive distortion interactions, Hammen (1985) was able to demonstrate that dysphoria followed the occurrence of a specific type of stressor in individuals belonging to one depressive subtype grouping and not another. This level of specificity is laudable, given that past research has shown the correlation between specific life events and depression in general to be quite low. Whether the predictions provided by such a differentiated model will be comparable to those afforded by more traditional predictors such as past history of depression or positive family history for affective disorder remains to be seen, and will probably be an important focus for future research in the area.

Two clinical developments related to both the practice and conceptualization of cognitive therapy are important to mention. The first of these relates to the identifiction of subtypes of depressed patients who present with a recognizable and unique cognitive organization around issues of either affiliation or achievement. Beck's (1967) original cognitive model of depression was amended to include this level of personality functioning, which is thought to be more stable and consistent than cognitive distortions or dysfunctional schemata. The two dominant personality modes, identified as sociotropy and autonomy, represent different characterological constellations and may be vulnerability subtypes that react to different stressors. This differentiation is congruent with the concerns described above and is also valuable clinically, since each personality subtype brings a different set of clinical concerns and issues to therapy. Sociotropes, for example, often have a strong orientation to be loved by others, or need to feel that someone else cares about them. Their entrance into therapy may be due to a rejection or loss of someone they love. Autonomous types, on the other hand, are concerned about being respected and feeling worthy through their accomplishments. Their entrance into therapy may be preceded by a failure to achieve in the work place or a business loss of some sort (Beck, 1983).

The second development relates to the practice of cognitive–behavioral therapy and is a conceptual framework for choosing interventions at choice points in the session. The description of core cognitive processes (Safran et al, 1986) is meant to serve as a guide for helping therapists choose which of the numerous thoughts accessed during the session are most likely to lead to the greatest clinical change. A number of principles were outlined. These include: 1) importance of self-referential thinking; as noted previously, the thoughts that relate to perceptions of the self may provide the best leads toward the understanding of cognitive processes that are more central to the patient; 2) using emotion to prime the accessibility of negative self-referent cognition (that is, monitoring the patient's mood during the session and introducing situations that are emotionally laden in order to facilitate the experiencing of negative automatic thoughts). Furthermore, advances in technical interventions such as the horizontal versus vertical exploration of cognitive content and the use of process versus content markers to understand in-session client responses are described (Safran et al, 1986). With continued refinement, these guidelines and others spawned by their usage may help to systematize and advance treatment of emotional disorders from a cognitive–behavioral perspective.

REFERENCES

Abramson LY, Seligman MEP, Teasdale JD: Learned helplessness in humans: critique and reformulation. Abnorm Psychol 1978; 87:49-74

Akiskal HS, McKinney WT: Overview of recent research in depression: integration of ten conceptual models into a comprehensive clinical frame. Arch Gen Psychiatry 1975; 32:285-305

Arnkoff DB, Glass CR: Clinical cognitive constructs: examination, evaluation, and elaboration, in Advances in Cognitive–Behavioral Research and Therapy, vol. 1. Edited by Kendall PC. New York, Academic Press, 1982

Bandura A: Principles of Behavior Modification. New York, Holt, Rinehart & Winston, 1969

Bandura A: Self-efficacy: toward a unifying theory of behavioral change. Psychol Rev 1977; 84:191-215

Beck AT: Depression: Clinical, Experimental and Theoretical Aspects. New York, Harper & Row, 1976

Beck AT: Thinking and depression: idiosyncratic content cognitive distortion. Arch Gen Psychiatry 1963; 9:324-333

Beck AT: Cognitive Therapy and the Emotional Disorders. New York, International Universities Press, 1976

Beck AT: Cognitive therapy of depression: new perspectives, in Treatment of Depression: Old Controversies and New Approaches. Edited by Clayton PJ, Barrett JE. 1983

Beck AT: Cognition and therapy. Arch Gen Psyciatry, 1984; 411:1112-1114

Beck AT, Emery G: Anxiety Disorders and Phobias. New York, Basic Books, 1985

Beck AT, Laude R, Bonhert M: Ideational components of anxiety neurosis. Arch Gen Psychiatry 1974; 31:319-325

Beck AT, Rush AJ, Shaw, et al: Cognitive therapy of depression. New York, Guilford, 1979

Beidel DC, Turner SM: A critique of the theoretical bases of cognitive behavioral theories and therapy. Clin Psychol Rev 1986; 6:177-197

Butler G, Mathews A: Cognitive processes in anxiety. Advances in Behaviour Research and Therapy 1983; 5:51-62

Clark DA: Cognitive–affective interaction: a test of the "specificity" and "generality" hypothesis. Cognitive Therapy and Research 1986; 10:607-623

Clark DM: A cognitive approach to panic. Behav Res Ther 1986; 24:461-470

Clark DM, Beck AT: Cognitive approaches, in Handbook of Anxiety Disorder. Edited by Last CG, Hersen M. New York, Pergamon, 1987

Coyne JC, Gotlib IH: The role of cognition in depression: a critical appraisal. Psychol Bull 1983; 94:472-505

Coyne JC, Gotlib IH: Studying the role of cognition in depression: well-trodden paths and cul-de-sacs. Cognitive Therapy and Research 1986; 10:695-705

Cromwell R: Attention and information processing: a foundation for understanding schizophrenia?, in The Nature of Schizophrenia: New Approaches to Research and Treatment. Edited by Wynne LC, Cromwell RL, Matthysse S. New York, Wiley, 1978

Dember WN: Motivation and the cognitive revolution. Am Psychol 1974; 29:161-168

Dobson KS, Shaw BF: Cognitive assessment of major depressive disorder. Cognitive Therapy and Research 1986; 10:13-29

Eaves G, Rush AJ: Cognitive patterns in symptomatic and remitted unipolar major depression. J Abnorm Pyshcol 1984; 93:31-40

Ellis A: The theory of rational-emotive therapy, in Theoretical and Empirical Foundations of Rational-emotive therapy. Edited by Ellis A, Whitley JM. Monterey, CA, Brooks/Cole, 1979

Erwin E: Behavior Therapy: Scientific, Philosophical, and Moral Foundations. Cambridge, Cambridge University Press, 1978

Foa EB, McNally RJ: Sensitivity to feared stimuli in obsessive-compulsives: 1986; a dichotic listing analysis. Cognitive Therapy and Research 1986; 10:477-486

Ford DH, Urban HB: Systems of Psychotherapy. New York, Wiley, 1963

Goldberg JO, Shaw BF: The measurement of cognition in psychopathology: clinical and research applications, in Handbook of Cognitive Therapy. Edited by Arkowitz H, Beutler LE. New York, Plenum (in press)

Gotlib IH: Perception and recall of interpersonal feedback: negative bias in depression. Cognitive Therapy and Research 1983; 5:399-412.

Hamilton M: Depression and anxiety: a clinical viewpoint, in Psychiatry in the 80's: Ideas, Research. Edited by Hamilton M, Bakker JB. London, Excerpta Medica, 1981

Hammen CL: Predicting depression: a cognitive–behavioral perspective, in Advances in Cognitive–Behavioral Research and Therapy, vol. 4. Edited by Kendall PC. Orlando, FL, Academic Press, 1985

Harrell T, Chambless D, Calhoun J: Correlational relationships between self-statements and affective states. Cognitive Therapy and Research 1981; 5:159-173

Hibbert GA: Ideational components of anxiety: their origin and content. Br J Psychiatry 1984; 144:618-624

Hollon SD, Bemis KM: Self-report and the assessment of cognitive functions, in Behavioral Assessment: A Practical Handbook (second edition.) Edited by Hersen M, Bellack AS. New York, Pergamon, 1981

Hollon SD, Kriss MR: Cognitive factors in clinical research and practice. Clin Psychol Rev 1984; 4:35-76

Hollon SD, Kendall PC, Lumry A: Specificity of depressotypic cognitions in clinical depression. J Abnorm Psychol 1986; 95:22-59

Hollon SD, Evans MD, DeRubeis RJ: Preventing relapse following treatment for depression: the cognitive-pharmacotherapy project, in Stress and Coping Across Development. Edited by Field T, McCabe P, Schneiderman N. Hillsdale, NJ, Lawrence Erlbaum (in press)

Ingram RE: Toward an information-processing analysis of depression. Cognitive Therapy and Research 1984; 8:443-477

Keller MB, Lavori PW, Lewis CE, et al: Predictors of relapse in major depressive disorder. JAMA 1983; 250:3299-3304

Kovacs M, Beck AT: Maladaptive cognitive structure in depression. Am J Psychiatry 1978; 135:525-533

Kruglanski AW, Ajzen I: Bias and error in human judgment. European Journal of Social Psychology 1983; 13:1-44

Kuiper NA, Olinger LJ: Dysfunctional attitudes and a self-worth contingency model of depression, in Advances in Cognitive-Behavioral Research and Therapy, vol. 5. Edited by Kendall PC. Orlando, FL, Academic Press, 1986

Last CG, Blanchard EB: Classification of phobic versus fearful non-phobic: procedural and theoretical issues. Behavioral Assessment 1982; 4:195-210

Lazarus RS: Psychological Stress and the Coping Process. New York, McGraw-Hill, 1966

Lazarus RS, Launier R: Stress-related transactions between person and environment, in Internal and External Determinants of Behavior. Edited by Pervin LA, Lewis M. New York, Plenum, 1978

Lazarus RS, Coyne JC, Folkman S: Cognition, emotion and motivation: the doctoring of Humpty-Dumpty, in Psychological Stress and Psychopathology. Edited by Neufeld RVJ. New York, McGraw-Hill, 1982

Lunghi ME: The stability of mood and social perception measure in a sample of depressed inpatients. Br J Psychiatry 1977; 130:598-604

Mahoney MJ: Reflections on the cognitive-learning trend in psychotherapy. Am Psychol 1977; 32:5-13

Mahoney MJ, Arnkoff DB: Cognitive and self control therapies, in Handbook of Psychotherapy and Behavior Change, second edition. Edited by Garfield SL, Bergin AE. New York, Wiley, 1978

Markus H: Self-schema and processing information about the self. J Pers Soc Psychol 1977; 35:63-78

Mathews A, MacLeod C: Selective processing of threat cues in anxiety states. Behav Res Ther 1985; 23:563-569

Matthysse S, Spring BJ, Sugarman J: Attention and Information Processing in Schizophrenia. New York, Pergamon, 1979

Meichenbaum D, Butler L: Egocentrism and evidence: making Piaget kosher, in Psychotherapy Process: Current Issues and Future Directions. Edited by Mahoney MJ. New York, Plenum, 1980

Merton RK: The self-fulfilling prophecy. Antioch Review 1948; 8:193-210

Miller IW, Norman WH: Persistence of depressive cognitions within a subgroup of depressed inpatients. Cognitive Therapy and Research 1986; 10:211-224

Miller IW, Klee SH, Norman WH: Depressed and nondepressed inpatients' cognitions of hypothetical events, experimental tasks and stressful life events. J Abnorm Psychol 1982; 91:78-81

Nisbett R, Ross L: Human Inference: Strategies and Shortcomings of Social Judgments. Englewood Cliffs, NJ, Prentice-Hall, 1980

Norman WH, Miller IW, Klee SH: Assessment of cognitive distortion in a clinically depressed population. Cognitive Therapy and Research 1983; 7:1333-1340

Peterson D, Seligman MEP: The learned helplessness model of depression: current status of theory and research, in Handbook of Depression: Treatment, Assessment and Research. Edited by Beckham EE, Leber WR. Homewood, IL, Dorsey, 1985

Peterson C, Villanova P, Raps CS: Depression and attributions: factors responsible for inconsistent results in the published literature. J Abnorm Psychol 1985; 94:165-168

Popper KR: The Logic of Scientific Discovery. New York, Harper & Row, 1968

Pribram KH: The cognitive revolution and mind/brain issues. Am Psychol 1986; 41:507-520

Rappee RM: (1985). Distinctions between panic disorder and generalized anxiety disorder: clinical presentation. Aust NZ J Psychiatry 1985; 19:227-232

Reiss S, Peterson RA, Gursky DM, et al: Anxiety sensitivity, anxiety frequency and the prediction of fearfulness. Behav Res Ther 1986; 24:1-8

Rush AJ, Weissenburger J, Eaves G: Do thinking patterns predict depressive symptoms? Cognitive Therapy and Research 1986; 10:225-236

Safran JD, Vallis TM, Segal ZV, et al: Assessment of core cognitive process in cognitive therapy. Cognitive Therapy and Research 1986; 10:509-526

Segal ZV: Appraisal of the self-schema construct in cognitive models of depression. Psychol Bull (in press)

Segal ZV, Shaw BF: Cognition in depression: a reappraisal of Coyne and Gotlib's critique. Cognitive Therapy and Research 1986a; 10:671-694

Segal ZV, Shaw BF: When cul-de-sacs are more mentality than reality: a rejoinder to Coyne and Gotlib. Cognitive Therapy and Research 1986b; 10:707-714

Segal ZV, Shaw BF: Cognitive assessment: issues and methods, in Handbook of Cognitive–Behavioral Therapies. Edited by Dobson KS. New York, Guilford, 1987

Shaw BF: Closing commentary: social cognition and depression. Social Cognition 1985; 3:135-144

Silverman JS, Silverman JA, Eardley DA: Do maladaptive attitudes cause depression? Arch Gen Psychiatry 1984; 41:28-30

Simons AD, Murphy GE, Levine JL, et al: Cognitive therapy and pharmacotherapy for depression. Arch Gen Psychiatry 1986; 43:43-48

Smith D: Trends in counseling and psychotherapy. Am Psychol 1982; 37:802-809

Spitzer RL, Endicott J, Robins E: Research diagnostic criteria: rationale and reliability. Arch Gen Psychiatry, 1978; 35:773-782

Thorndyke PW, Hayes-Roth B: The use of schemata in the acquisition and transfer of knowledge. Cognitive Psychology 1979; 11:82-106

Thorpe G, Barnes G, Hunter J, et al: Thoughts and feelings: correlations in two clinical and two nonclinical samples. Cognitive Therapy and Research 1983; 7, 565-574

Turk DC, Salovey P: Cognitive structures, cognitive processes, and cognitive behavior modification, I: client issues. Cognitive Therapy and Research 1985; 9:1-17

Turk DC, Speers MA: Cognitive schemata and cognitive processes in cognitive-behavioral intervention: going beyond the information given, in Advances in Cognitive-Behavioral Research and Therapy, vol. 2. Edited by Kendall PC. New York, Academic Press, 1983

Van den Hout MA, Griez E: Panic symptoms after inhalation of carbon dioxide. Br J Psychiatry 1984; 144:503-507

Watts FN, McKenna FP, Sharrock R, et al: Colour naming of phobia-related words. Br J Psychol 1986; 77:97-108

Weissman AN: The Dysfunctional Attitude Scale: A Validation Study. Unpublished doctoral dissertation. Philadelphia, University of Pennsylvania, 1979

Wilson GT: Cognitive behavior therapy: paradigm shift or passing phase, in Cognitive Behavior Therapy. Edited by Foreyt JP, Rathjen DP. New York, Plenum. 1978

Zubin J, Steinhauer S: How to break the logjam in schizophrenia: a look beyond genetics. J Nerv Ment Dis 1981; 169:477-492

Chapter 25

Cognitive Therapy of Depression

by Jesse H. Wright, M.D., Ph.D.

Distorted thinking is a widely recognized part of the depressive syndrome. Pathological guilt, low self-concept, hopelessness, and self-destructive thoughts are observed frequently in depressed patients, and such symptoms are usually included in systems for the diagnosis of depression (Wright and Beck, 1983, 1986). However, the etiological and therapeutic significance of cognitive distortion received little attention until about 25 years ago, when Beck (1963, 1964) first described his cognitive theory of depression. Beck and others (Beck et al, 1979; Rush and Beck, 1978; Rush, 1983) have subsequently developed a cognitive therapy of depression which has been tested extensively in controlled outcome studies.

Cognitive therapy of depression is based on the theory that cognitive distortion is one of the major factors in the development of depression, and that specific cognitive treatment techniques can reverse depressive symptomatology. Cognitive theory is reviewed in Chapter 24 of this volume. Cognitive therapy outcome studies are analyzed in Chapter 30. This chapter will describe practical applications of cognitive theory and research to the treatment of depression.

A COGNITIVE MODEL FOR DEPRESSION

It is often helpful to translate theoretical constructs and research findings into a working model for clinical practice. This can provide the therapist with a pragmatic guide for decision making within the complex milieu of psychotherapy. The use of such models should of course be tempered by an awareness of significant theoretical questions, conflicting data, and alternate approaches. Ingram (1984), Safran and colleagues (1986), and Shaw and Segal (in Chapter 24 of this volume) have recently reviewed such issues.

Figure 1 depicts a cognitive model for the treatment of depression. Information processing is given the central role in this elaboration of the classic stimulus–response model. Emotional arousal and behavior are seen as being dependent upon a cognitive appraisal of the significance of environmental information.

This point of view can be illustrated by contrasting the responses of different individuals to the same life stress. A depressed or depression-prone man whose wife threatens to leave him might interpret this event as follows: "I always knew this would happen; I've lost everything; my whole life is ruined." A nondepressed man who experienced the same stressful event might appraise it differently: "There's something obviously wrong with our marriage; she's really upset, but maybe we can work on it; what can I do?" Although both interpretations could cause significant emotional arousal, it is likely that the first individual would develop a higher level of sadness and anxiety.

The behavioral inclinations (cognitions about behavioral alternatives) of these individuals would probably also be quite different. The depressed man might

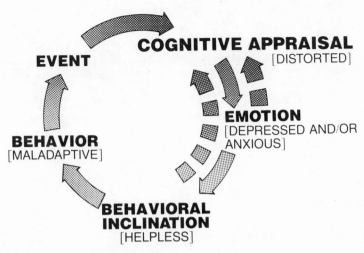

EVENT

COGNITIVE APPRAISAL
[DISTORTED]

EMOTION
[DEPRESSED AND/OR ANXIOUS]

BEHAVIOR
[MALADAPTIVE]

BEHAVIORAL INCLINATION
[HELPLESS]

Figure 1. A cognitive model for depression

think: "I should leave now and save her the trouble of getting rid of me"; or "I couldn't stand being alone; I'd be better off dead." The second individual might think of other possibilities such as changing his personal habits, having an in-depth talk with his wife, or starting marital counseling. It is likely that the depressed man, because of his negative constructions, will ultimately behave in a maladaptive way (for example, decreased communication, withdrawal, or even suicide), whereas the nondepressed individual would be more likely to behave in an adaptive manner.

This working model emphasizes the close relationship between cognitive distortion and depressive behavior. Distorted thinking can lead to depressive behavior such as lack of effort, poor motivation, and isolation from others. Depressed behavior then provides evidence that confirms and solidifies negative cognitions. A "vicious cycle" ensues in which negative cognitions and behavior continue to aggravate and reinforce one another. Therapeutic efforts are usually directed at both cognitive and behavioral pathology because positive changes in one area will favorably influence the other (Meichenbaum, 1977). For example, a depressed male patient with low self-esteem would probably try harder in his daily work if he were able to recognize previously ignored personal strengths. Alternatively, self-esteem could increase if he were able to improve work productivity through behavioral procedures.

Emotion is viewed as an important part of depression but not as the major feature of the disorder. Bower and others (Bower, 1981; Breslow et al, 1981; Greenberg and Safran, 1984; Mayer and Bower, 1985) have described the influ-ence of emotion on cognitive processing. It has been found that depressed mood can stimulate negative cognitive distortion, including selective recall of negative versus positive memories. Thus, modulation of affect through cognitive, behav-ioral, or other techniques would be expected to alter cognitive distortion and thereby influence treatment outcome.

The working model in Figure 1 does not describe other possible etiologies or treatment approaches to depression (for example, biological, interpersonal, or social). This model is intended to give general direction for cognitive interventions in the treatment of depression. However, it is assumed that depression is a "psychobiological final common pathway" syndrome (Akiskal and McKinney, 1975) and that a cognitive framework provides just one of the possible approaches to this disorder. Beck and others (Beck, 1985; Wright and Beck, 1983, 1986) have formulated integrative models that account for multiple etiological factors in depression. Integrated treatment approaches such as combined pharmacotherapy and cognitive therapy have also been described (Wright, 1987).

The major thrust of cognitive therapy is to identify and correct pathological information processing. Therefore, a thorough knowledge of basic cognitive processes in depression is required for proper selection and administration of treatment techniques. The main components of cognitive disorder in depression will be summarized briefly to provide a background for understanding cognitive therapy procedures.

COGNITIVE DISORDER IN DEPRESSION

Beck (1963, 1964) proposed that depressed individuals have negatively distorted thinking in three areas: self, world, and future (the "negative cognitive triad"). Subsequently, numerous research studies have documented distorted thinking in these three areas (Wright and Beck, 1983, 1986). Negative thinking about the future (hopelessness), has been shown to be more labile in depression than low self-esteem or distorted perceptions about the world (Wright, 1986a, 1986b; Dobson and Shaw, 1986). Hopelessness is a particularly important target for change because of its highly significant association with suicide (Minkoff et al, 1973; Beck et al, 1975; Fawcett et al, 1987).

Two main levels of cognitive distortion have been identified: negative automatic thinking, and disturbances of deeper, basic assumptions or schemata (Guidano and Liotti, 1983, 1985; Dobson and Shaw, 1986). Automatic thoughts are the cognitions that occur rapidly while a person is in a situation (Rush, 1983). These thoughts are usually not subjected to rational, systematic analysis. Patients may be subliminally aware of automatic thoughts. However, they do not realize the significance of these thoughts until questioning by the therapist brings them into full awareness. Negative automatic thoughts have been detected in normal individuals but are about twice as frequent in depressed patients as in control subjects (Harrell and Ryon, 1982). A detailed analysis of the content of automatic thinking usually reveals typical errors in logic such as selective abstraction, arbitrary inference, personalization, magnification or minimization, and absolutistic thinking (Beck et al, 1979; LeFebvre, 1981; Wright and Beck, 1983; Watkins and Rush, 1983).

It has been suggested that depression occurs when stressful life events stimulate the emergence of latent maladaptive schemata. These schemata are thought to be responsible for negative automatic thoughts and other distortions of information processing in depressed patients (Beck et al, 1979). Schemata are defined as basic rules for screening and coding environmental information (Wright and Beck, 1983). Bowlby (1985) has noted that these cognitive structures are generally adaptive because humans need coherent strategies for managing the enormous amount of information that is available to them.

Schemata can be maladaptive when they lead to the filtering out of relevant positive information or overattention to negative information. There has been considerable argument about the cause–effect relationship between schemata and depression (Silverman et al, 1984; Simons et al, 1984). Definitive prospective research on this issue has not been completed, but there seems to be little doubt that schemata and related attitudes are negatively biased during depression (Weissman, 1979; Simons et al, 1984; Silverman et al, 1984; Dobson and Shaw, 1986; Wright, 1986a, 1986b). Cognitive therapy is directed at changing maladaptive schemata in order to provide both acute symptom relief and protection against relapse (Beck et al, 1979; Hollon et al, 1983; Simons et al, 1986). It is thought that alteration in basic attitudes may explain a lower rate of relapse in patients treated with cognitive therapy as compared to pharmacotherapy (Simons et al, 1986).

Abramson and co-workers (1978) have offered another perspective on information processing in depression. They have suggested that depressed persons are likely to make attributions (causal explanations for environmental events) that are distorted in three dimensions: internal, global, and stable. For instance, a depressed student who received a poor grade might conclude that this was entirely due to his or her own personal failings, that the event has general significance, and that the circumstances will persist indefinitely. Conversely, a nondepressed student would be likely to make attributions in the opposite direction. Although most of the research concerning attributions has been done with college students, misattributions have also been identified in patients with major depression (Miller et al, 1982; Zimmerman et al, 1984; Wright, 1986a).

Distorted responses to feedback information have also been described in depressed patients (Loeb et al, 1964; Loeb et al, 1971; DeMonbreun and Craighead, 1977; Nelson and Craighead, 1977; Rizley, 1978). It has been found that depressed patients underestimate the amount of positive feedback they receive, while control subjects overestimate the number of times they receive positive feedback. Feedback distortion has been shown to be dependent on the amount of information presented. DeMonbreun and Craighead (1977) noted that depressed patients were most likely to make misjudgments about feedback when they received large amounts of data.

Research on learning and memory functioning in depression has consistently found significant differences between depressed and control subjects (Donnelly et al, 1972; Cutting, 1979; Breslow et al, 1980; Wright, 1985, 1986b). It has been shown that deficiencies are most pronounced for cognitive operations that require abstract thinking, deep levels of memory encoding, or considerable effort (Braff and Beck, 1974; Weingartner et al, 1981; Cohen et al, 1982; Wright, 1986b). Learning and memory functioning are usually slowed in depression (Glass et al, 1981; Wright, 1986b). However, Glass and co-workers (1981) have demonstrated that depressed patients can correct for some cognitive deficits by devoting more time to performing tasks.

Most of the emphasis in the development of cognitive therapy for depression has been on cognitive distortion. However, learning and memory impairment is also an important part of the information processing disturbance in depression. Impaired learning and memory functioning can limit the patient's ability to understand, remember, and effectively utilize information from many sources, including the immediate environment and the therapy process itself. Therapy procedures described in this chapter rely heavily on techniques that facilitate improved learning and memory functioning.

COGNITIVE THERAPY TECHNIQUES

Overview of Therapy Procedures

Cognitive therapy is a pragmatic, problem-oriented approach to depression. Duration of treatment is usually 12 to 20 sessions. Occasionally, mild cases can be treated with only a few sessions. At other times it may be necessary to extend the course of treatment. Reasons for continuing therapy beyond the short-term format can include chronic treatment-resistant depression, extensive character pathology in a depressed patient, and bipolar illness in which cognitive therapy is being used as an adjunct to lithium.

During the initial session a detailed history is taken, differential diagnosis is considered, and patient variables that could affect outcome are assessed (see Case Selection, below). This evaluation helps the therapist decide whether cognitive therapy, combined cognitive therapy and pharmacotherapy, or an alternate approach is indicated. Young and Beck (1982) have suggested six major goals for the early sessions of cognitive therapy: 1) define specific problems; 2) prioritize problems; 3) decrease hopelessness; 4) demonstrate relationship between cognition and emotion; 5) socialize patient into therapeutic milieu of cognitive therapy; and 6) stress importance of self-help homework assignments. Reaching these goals is dependent on the establishment of a good working relationship, the pre-eminent goal of early therapy sessions.

Middle therapy sessions are devoted primarily to eliciting and correcting negative automatic thoughts and cognitive errors. Behavioral assignments are given to test hypotheses generated in therapy sessions, collect "in vivo" cognitive data, and improve social skills. This work is continued throughout the therapy. In later sessions there is an added focus on deeper cognitive structures (schemata) and relapse prevention.

Case Selection

Unipolar major depression is the major indication for cognitive therapy. Substantial evidence has been collected that cognitive therapy is effective for outpatients with unipolar major depression (Wright and Beck, 1983, 1986; Chapter 30 in this volume). Bishop and associates (1986) have described the treatment of a psychotically depressed patient with cognitive therapy, but there has been no controlled research to support the use of cognitive therapy with patients who have major depression with psychotic features. Electroconvulsive therapy or pharmacotherapy with combined tricyclic antidepressants and antipsychotic drugs remain the treatments of choice for such patients.

The role of cognitive therapy in the treatment of melancholic depressed patients or those with a positive dexamethasone suppression test (DST) remains unresolved. Although Kovacs and colleagues (1981) and Blackburn and co-workers (1981) found no differences in the response of endogenous and nonendogenous patients to cognitive therapy, Rush (1983) has described a small series of patients with positive DSTs who did not respond to cognitive therapy alone. Hollon and associates (1983) found that 3-methoxy, 4 hydroxyphenylglycol (MHPG) levels did not predict outcome to either cognitive therapy or pharmacotherapy. As yet, there have been no outcome studies with hospitalized depressed patients in which cognitive therapy alone has been compared to pharmacotherapy.

Wright (1986b) studied cognitive functioning in nonpsychotic depressed inpatients who were treated with combined pharmacotherapy and cognitive psycho-therapy. Seriously depressed inpatients were able to participate fully in cognitive therapy. Patients with plasma nortriptyline concentrations below or above the "therapeutic window" (50–150 ng/ml) were as likely to respond to treatment as those within the desired range. Miller and colleagues (1985) have observed that chronic drug-resistant depressed inpatients responded well to combined cognitive therapy and pharmacotherapy. These studies provide some support that cognitive therapy can be used successfully in depressed inpatients. However, it is recommended that cognitive therapy usually not be used without medication in the treatment of hospitalized patients until further outcome research is completed. Indications for using cognitive therapy alone in depressed inpatients could include: pregnancy, medical illness that prevents use of antidepressants, drug intolerance, and patient objections to pharmacotherapy.

Cognitive therapy has been used adjunctively for patients with bipolar depression, but it is not considered a primary treatment for this disorder. There has only been a single case report describing the treatment of bipolar illness with cognitive therapy alone (Fuchs and Himmelhoch, 1980). Cochran (1982) studied the effect of using cognitive therapy with lithium in recently discharged patients who had bipolar disorder. Patients who received cognitive therapy were less likely to discontinue lithium against medical advice than those who were treated with lithium and standard aftercare procedures. It appeared that the collaborative and psychoeducational aspects of cognitive therapy improved treatment compliance. Thus, cognitive therapy may be indicated for supportive purposes in depressed patients who are being treated primarily with somatic approaches.

Akiskal (1982) has noted that many chronic or treatment-resistant depressed patients are given personality disorder diagnoses. He suggests that diagnosis of personality disorders be made with great caution in depressed patients because depression often causes personality traits to become more prominent. The diagnosis of a personality disorder may lower expectations and negatively influence treatment choices. The cognitive therapist usually concentrates on treatment of the depression, assuming that undesirable personality traits will fade as the depression improves. Yet, at times, severe personality disorders can coexist with depression. This can significantly hinder the treatment process (Rush and Giles, 1982). Patients with antisocial personality are particularly difficult to treat because of problems in developing the working relationship required for cognitive therapy. Borderline personality disorder is another condition that can limit the effectiveness of cognitive therapy (Pretzer, 1983).

Simons and co-workers (1985) observed that patients who had high scores on the Self-Control Schedule were more likely to respond to cognitive therapy than were those with low scores. Their work suggests that cognitive therapy may be more appropriate for depressed patients who believe that their personal efforts are important in the recovery process than for those who look only to external sources for help. The patient's level of intelligence and educational background are usually not major factors in selecting cognitive therapy as a treatment approach. A wide range of individuals can be treated if the material of therapy is adjusted to the intellectual level of the patient.

Therapy Format

Cognitive therapy uses a number of procedures designed to improve the efficiency of information processing in the depressed patient. Techniques used for this purpose include structuring, feedback, and learning reinforcement. Structuring of therapy begins with the setting of an agenda. Therapist and patient work together to come to mutual agreement on a list of problems or topics for the session. The agenda should contain significant problems that can be reasonably expected to yield to treatment efforts over a short-term period. Lumping of problems into broad categories is avoided because this reinforces the tendency of depressed persons to think in an absolutist and overgeneralized manner. Agenda setting can reduce hopelessness if problems are broken down into manageable pieces that can be understood and resolved.

A typical agenda for a therapy session with a depressed patient might contain the following items: 1) reactions to an argument with spouse; 2) coping with increased pressure at work; 3) review of homework from last session. Examples of agenda items that are likely to be too diffuse are: 1) my mother; 2) relationships with people; 3) the future. Although each of these latter areas may be of critical importance, a narrowing of focus would be suggested before the patient attempts to resolve global issues. Correction of cognitive distortions in a relatively small area can then be followed by generalization to the broader context.

Directive techniques are used to keep the patient on task and avoid digressions from the agenda. However, the agenda can change during the session if new information becomes available or if a different direction appears to be indicated. An example of an event that might require an agenda change would be the uncovering of an important underlying schema during the course of reviewing a homework assignment. The therapist also might suggest a change of topic if it appears that further exploration of a particular agenda item would be of limited value.

Feedback between patient and therapist is encouraged throughout the course of cognitive therapy. The therapist stops at frequent intervals to comment on his or her understanding of the progress of the session and to ask the patient to do the same. The therapist also asks for feedback on how he or she is being perceived. Is the therapist being understood? What would the patient like the therapist to do differently? Similarly, the therapist tries to give the patient an accurate picture of how the therapy is going, and at times suggestions are made for actions that might be helpful to the patient.

A considerable amount of attention is also devoted to procedures that enhance learning. The therapist is presented with a somewhat difficult situation: New learning is the goal of treatment, but deficits in learning and memory interfere with this process. Some of the typical procedures used to reinforce learning in cognitive therapy of depression include repetition, checking for understanding, note taking, reading assignments, and homework. An individualized assessment of each patient is used to provide data on the status of learning and memory functioning, and the types and degree of cognitive distortion. Learning-reinforcement techniques can then be selected which match the individual patient's level of cognitive functioning (Wright, 1985).

Note taking by both patient and therapist is strongly encouraged. The process of writing cognitions and then visualizing them helps to draw attention to important information discovered in the therapy session. Learning can be augmented further if these notes are reviewed between therapy sessions. Patients often report that they consult their therapy notes even after treatment has been completed. This helps them to retain the concepts learned in therapy and to use this information for long-term maintenance of rational thinking and self-esteem.

Typical reading assignments for depressed patients include the pamphlet *Coping with Depression* (Beck and Greenberg, 1974) and sections of the book *Feeling Good* (Burns, 1980). Assignments are reviewed carefully to check for understanding. Core concepts discussed in these readings are explained, clarified, and demonstrated in therapy sessions. The use of other types of homework assignments will be discussed later, in the section on cognitive and behavioral treatment techniques.

Therapeutic Relationship

Effective utilization of any of the cognitive or behavioral techniques is contingent upon the formation of a good therapeutic relationship. Therapist and patient work together as an investigative team. This has been termed "collaborative empiricism" (Beck et al, 1979). Automatic thoughts, dysfunctional schemata, and other cognitions are identified and set forth as hypotheses. Data are then collected to prove or disprove the hypotheses. This approach substitutes a spirit of inquiry for the self-blaming attitudes used by most depressed patients.

Kindness, understanding, and a confident attitude from the therapist help give the depressed patient hope that recovery is possible. Therapists who have an overly pessimistic world view or who are struggling with cognitive distortion and depression themselves may have difficulty using cognitive therapy with depressed patients. Such individuals may tend to identify with the patients' negative distortions and not see possibilities for change.

However, it should be noted that some of the patient's negative evaluations may be found to be accurate (Krantz, 1985). To illustrate, it could be found that a depressed woman with low self-esteem has actual deficits in social skills that impair her ability to work and maintain relationships. In this case, the therapist would not try to ignore or downplay deficits. Instead, he or she would begin to engage the patient in behavioral procedures that could help the patient develop more effective social skills.

Feedback between patient and therapist helps to avoid a regressive transference that would interfere with the "here and now" nature of this short-term therapy. Yet, when distortions do occur about the therapeutic relationship, material is provided for understanding disordered information processing in other interpersonal situations. Like the psychoanalyst, the cognitive therapist is interested in transference, but in this case the "transference" is the recurrence of habitual information processing errors within the context of a therapeutic relationship.

Cognitive Techniques

The technique used most commonly to uncover cognitive distortion is "guided discovery." Direct questions are asked which encourage inductive reasoning and help the patient to recognize automatic thoughts, cognitive errors, and other distorted cognitions. The choice of questions is influenced by factors such as:

status of learning and memory functioning; degree of cognitive distortion; stage of the therapy; strategy for change; new information derived from previous questions; and emotional arousal cues.

Direct questioning techniques can be illustrated with the example of Mr. A, a 44-year-old businessman who developed major depression after separating from his wife. During the course of an early treatment session, the discussion centered on one of the patient's main concerns—the effect of the marital separation on Mr. A's children:

> Mr. A: I'm worried about what my wife is saying to the children.
> Therapist: What worries do you have?
> Mr. A: Mainly that she'll make me sound like the bad guy.
> Therapist: In what way?
> Mr. A: I don't know. I guess she blames everything on me. (Patient's eyes turn down, and he struggles to hold back tears.)
> Therapist: I can see that this upsets you a great deal. What thoughts were running through your head just now?
> Mr. A: She's right. I was never at home. All I could think about was my job. It's really all my fault, and I wouldn't blame them if they never saw me again. (He cries freely.)
> Therapist: I can see why you would feel so badly when you think that way about yourself. Perhaps we could begin to take a look at how your thoughts influence your emotions.

The questioning of Mr. A demonstrates how emotional cues often indicate the presence of intense and highly relevant cognitions. The therapist correctly identified the "emotional shift" and in an empathic way helped the patient to identify negative automatic thoughts. Further questioning could be used to demonstrate the relationship of cognition to emotion, thus giving a highly personalized demonstration of the basic cognitive model. Questioning is generally most effective when it is directed toward clearly meaningful and emotionally charged situations or issues.

Several other procedures, including imagery and role play, can be used when direct questioning does not uncover suspected negative automatic thoughts and distorted beliefs. Imagery techniques can facilitate the recall of salient thoughts and emotions by having the patient temporarily suspend current concerns while focusing on reliving a significant scene from the recent past. The therapist usually asks several questions to help "set the scene." For example, Mrs. B, a depressed woman who became very upset at a church meeting, was asked to describe the circumstances of the meeting. "What did the room look like? What did you do when you first came into the room? Describe the people who were there." The patient was then asked to imagine that she was actually in the scene and to report her thoughts and feelings.

A portion of the dialogue between Mrs. B and the cognitive therapist went as follows:

> Therapist: Can you picture yourself in the room now?
> Mrs. B: Yes, I can see it very clearly.
> Therapist: Now, when did you begin to get upset?
> Mrs. B: It was when they started to talk about the new building fund drive.

Therapist: What was said?

Mrs. B: The chairman stood up and looked at each of us. I started to get upset right then.

Therapist: Try to imagine yourself back at the meeting at that exact moment. (Pause) What was going through your head?

Mrs. B: He knows I haven't tried as hard as I should. I never stick things out like others do. They're having trouble with this drive, and I haven't been pulling my share. I'll probably give up on this just like everything else.

Therapist: And how did you feel?

Mrs. B: Angry at myself and sad, just like I do now.

Role play is a related technique used to discover cognitions not readily accessible to direct questioning. In this procedure, the therapist and patient play out the roles of persons involved in a significant interpersonal situation. The role play is stopped at several intervals to review cognitions generated by the exercise. Roles may be switched to give the patient an improved perception of the thinking of the other individual. This procedure can be illustrated with the case of Mr. C, a young depressed man who had been unable to face the stress of job interviews. Mr. C was asked to role play himself at a job interview while the therapist played the prospective employer. The roles were then reversed so the patient could attempt to understand the thoughts and motivations of the employer. After identifying distorted cognitions, the role play was repeated so Mr. C could practice more adaptive cognitions and behavior in the job interview situation.

Cognitive techniques have been described as having two phases, eliciting and testing of cognitive distortion (Beck et al, 1979; Young and Beck, 1982). In practice, these two components of cognitive therapy usually occur simultaneously. Specific hypothesis-testing procedures are not required when the patient recognizes and changes cognitive distortion as a result of guided discovery. Simply bringing cognitive distortion to awareness is often enough to stimulate more rational patterns of thinking and behaving. However, other procedures can be employed when direct questioning does not provide sufficient evidence to change cognitive distortion (Beck et al, 1979; Wright and Beck, 1983). Several examples of these techniques will be described.

Thought recording is one of the standard techniques used in cognitive therapy of depression. It provides a method of both identifying and changing distorted cognitions. One of the commonly used forms for recording thoughts is the Daily Record of Dysfunctional Thoughts (Young and Beck, 1982). This instrument contains five columns (situation, negative automatic thoughts, emotional reaction, rational thoughts, and change in emotions after rational thoughts). The patient is asked to write down negative automatic thoughts that occur in real life situations, and to examine these thoughts in relationship to the situation that has stimulated them and the emotions that were induced. The rational thought column is used to record alternate thoughts about the situation. Cognitions are rated for degree of belief and emotions are rated for intensity on 0–100 scales. The numerical ratings encourage less absolutistic thinking by pointing out that thoughts and feelings have gradations. They also help the patient to recognize and measure change.

The use of the Daily Record of Dysfunctional Thoughts can be illustrated with the following example of a middle-aged physician who was being treated for depression:

1. *Situation:* I get a message to call an angry parent whose daughter isn't doing well.
2. *Automatic thoughts:* I must have done something wrong (100). I'm going to get sued (70). I won't know what to say (80). I'm such a pushover (80).
3. *Emotions:* anxiety (95), sadness (50), anger (30)
4. *Rational thoughts:* Wait a minute, I did everything that I should have done for her daughter (95). I was jumping to conclusions again (100). Even if there is something wrong, I can take care of it (95). If I stay calm and ask questions, I can manage the situation (90).
5. *Change in emotions:* anxiety (15), sadness (10), anger (15)

At times it is helpful to begin with only a portion of the Daily Record of Dysfunctional Thoughts. For example, two columns, situation and automatic thoughts, could be used early in therapy when the focus is on learning how to identify automatic thoughts. The rational thought column could then be employed later in therapy when the patient has had experience in correcting distorted thinking. Thought recording usually begins in therapy sessions and is continued as a homework assignment. Used in this manner, it extends the work of therapy into everyday life and also provides material for subsequent therapy sessions.

Two other techniques for testing the validity of cognitive distortions, examining the evidence and "in vivo" experiments, are illustrated in the treatment of a 30-year-old depressed woman, Mrs. D, who reported that she was having trouble at work and was sure that she was about to be fired. She described her situation as follows: "It's just too much for me; I'm not very smart; they all think I'm incompetent." She indicated that she saw this as proof of her general incapacities and was certain that she would continue to have problems in the future.

After a series of questions that gave a more detailed picture of the situation, the therapist asked Mrs. D to examine the evidence that her negative cognitions were valid. She was able to find some evidence that the automatic thoughts were accurate (for example, significant decline in work output, had been making more mistakes than usual, late to work on two occasions). However, when all available evidence was explored, Mrs. D found that there had also been inaccuracies in her automatic thoughts. She had worked for the company for nine years with job ratings consistently in the excellent category, had completed graduate work in her job area, and had received supportive comments from co-workers that she had been asked to do too much). It was discovered that Mrs. D had been assuming that her employer was displeased but had not discussed the situation with him. She was asked to consider an "in vivo" experiment in which she would talk with her employer about the job situation, gather information about her performance and any need for change, and bring this information back to therapy.

At the next therapy session, Mrs. D revealed that she had a productive talk with her employer. He had complimented her on being a highly valued employee. Although he voiced concern about the decline in her job performance, he noted that an increased volume of work seemed to be affecting many of his employees.

They agreed to make several changes in Mrs. D's workload, and suggestions were made for how she might organize her efforts more efficiently.

This case also illustrates the use of cognitive therapy techniques for reattribution. A review of the "in vivo" experiment helped to demonstrate to Mrs. D that she had made attributions about her work problems that were distorted in several dimensions. She had originally concluded that the situation was entirely her fault, had general significance for her life, and was predictive of future failures. Specific reattributions were formulated which included both internal and external causes for the work problems, avoided overgeneralization, and provided room for possible changes in the future.

As therapy progresses into the middle and late phases, the therapist begins to recognize recurring patterns of automatic thoughts and cognitive errors that reflect underlying schemata. The patient usually has greater difficulty identifying schemata than more superficial cognitive distortions (Young and Beck, 1982). An attempt is made to have the patient identify schemata by pointing out consistent patterns of cognitive distortion. However, at times the therapist may need to suggest that possible schemata are operative. Once the patient and therapist agree that a certain schema exists, its validity can be tested with standard cognitive therapy techniques described earlier.

It is often helpful to list the advantages and disadvantages of basic assumptions. This facilitates an understanding of the powerful effects of schemata on self-concept and personal efficacy. Alternative schemata can then be proposed. An example of therapeutic work with schemata can be found in the case of a 48-year-old heart transplant patient, Mr. E. This patient was seriously depressed and was also doing poorly in his rehabilitation program. He had started to smoke again, was not exercising, and had stopped following his prescribed diet. This behavior was related to two main cognitive factors: hopelessness about recovery and a significant underlying maladaptive schema.

Early treatment efforts with Mr. E had been directed at hopelessness, and significant improvement had resulted. Nonetheless, he still adamantly refused to change his dangerous habits. A breakthrough occurred when, during the course of a therapy session, the following schema was uncovered: "If someone tells me what to do, it means I'm stupid." This assumption had been generated during childhood and had been reinforced with military and work experiences. He had always rebelled when he was told how to behave. After listing advantages and disadvantages and then examining evidence for the validity of this assumption, Mr. E was able to see that the schema was quite detrimental and had been based on previous erroneous conclusions that did not apply in the current situation. There was no evidence that he was unintelligent; he was just sick. His medical team had good ideas that could benefit him. They recognized that many patients had problems with their habits. Instead of thinking that he was stupid, his doctors liked him and wanted to help him change so he could live longer. Mr. E stopped smoking and resumed rehabilitation efforts shortly after this schema was altered.

Guidano and Liotti (1983, 1985) have argued that schemata continually evolve and unfold throughout the life cycle. They note that life themes are constructed "day by day, year by year, based on events and experience and how the individual has interpreted and dealt with them" (Guidano and Liotti, 1985). Their constructivist orientation to cognitive therapy suggests that therapeutic work with basic self-constructs can often lead the patient beyond the original therapy goals of reducing symptoms of depression.

Not all patients need or desire to focus on deep personal exploration and growth. However, after synthesizing information from therapy, some patients who have largely recovered from the symptoms of depression wish to proceed further with identification and modification of schemata. For example, a young professional man, Mr. F, had only mild residual symptoms of depression after 16 sessions of treatment. He had identified several important schemata, one of which was, "If I try something, I must not fail."

During the course of therapy, Mr. F had discovered that this schema had almost led to his suicide. He did not love his wife and recognized that his marriage was over, but he could not consider divorce because his schema would not permit "failure." Suicide had appeared to be his only option. Mr. F's driven, perfectionistic behavior in all areas of his life was related to this schema formed in childhood. Revision of the schema helped Mr. F to accept both his strengths and his weaknesses. This subsequently led to less pressured behavior as he accepted a more realistic performance standard. However, he also realized that he needed new, more meaningful constructs to give him direction for the future.

Patients such as Mr. F can benefit from a shift late in therapy to the growth-directed forms of cognitive therapy recommended by Guidano and Liotti (1983, 1985), Mahoney (1985), and Frankl (1985). The reader is referred to recent writings by these authors for an elaboration of constructivist and existentially oriented cognitive therapy procedures. A detailed description of these techniques is beyond the scope of this chapter.

Behavioral Techniques

Behavioral procedures are used to reverse depressive behavior (for example, low effort, isolation, decreased activity), and to stimulate new patterns of thinking. Direct questioning about behavior is the most commonly used technique. Questioning helps to distinguish between actual behavioral problems and distorted reports about behavior. Most depressed patients initially describe their daily activities in a derogatory manner. For instance, a depressed 48-year-old man, Mr. G, reported, "I don't do anything after I go home, I just sit and vegetate." Detailed questioning revealed that this patient was less active than usual but typically was able to read the newspaper, do homework with his son for 20 to 30 minutes, and work in the garden for about an hour each night. Previously, he had been heavily involved in a number of activities, including tennis, running, and civic clubs.

Not uncommonly, behavioral change results from insights gained from direct questioning. After he was questioned about his behavior, Mr. G commented that, "I guess I dropped out of some things that mean a lot to me; it would be a good idea if I started exercising again." A daily activity record was then used with this patient to obtain a more systematic inventory of behavior. He was instructed to use this form to report his activities, hour by hour, throughout the week. Each activity was rated on 0–10 scales for both mastery and pleasure. Mr. G observed that there were differences in his ratings of various activities. Sitting alone reading the newspaper was rated 7 for mastery, but was given a pleasure rating of 3. Watching T.V. was rated 5 for mastery and 1 for pleasure, but attending a concert was rated 8 for mastery and 9 for pleasure. Data from this record was used to design a program for behavioral change. Patient and therapist agreed on scheduling several activities that would heighten the sense of both mastery and pleasure.

Graded task assignments are used to help patients reach major behavioral goals that may seem unattainable when first considered. Behaviors are broken down into small steps that have a good chance of being mastered if taken one at a time. Self-confidence, hopefulness, and adaptive behavior grow with the completion of each successive step. The use of graded task assignments with depressed patients can be illustrated with the case of Mrs. H, a 42-year-old depressed woman who had never worked outside the home and believed that she was incapable of doing so. She wanted to return to school to complete her degree, but believed that she was "too old" and "had forgotten everything." She was convinced that she would fail and that this would just make things worse. Despite these negative predictions, Mrs. H was willing to try a behavioral experiment to see if her predictions were wrong. The steps were as follows: 1) obtain college catalog; 2) select five courses of interest and rank them for degree of difficulty; 3) choose one of the less difficult courses; 4) obtain text for this course; 5) read first chapter of text; 6) rate self on level of mastery of the material and on level of interest; and 7) consider enrolling in this course if ratings in number 6 were satisfactory. These assignments were reviewed in therapy sessions so cognitive distortions and behavioral problems could be identified and worked through before moving on to the next step.

The use of cognitive–behavioral rehearsal was suggested earlier in the section on role play exercises. This technique involves practicing new behaviors and cognitions prior to using them in actual life situations. Other behavioral procedures include assertiveness training, modeling, and social skills training (Meichenbaum, 1977; Young and Beck, 1982). These techniques can be used to treat actual behavioral deficits or to reverse depressive behavior generated by cognitive distortion.

SUMMARY AND CONCLUSIONS

Arieti (1985) once observed that "cognition teaches us that the human being is 'homo symbolicus,' for which a small part becomes a symbol that stands for the whole." Cognitive therapy of depression is directed at uncovering repetitive patterns of distorted information processing that influence the depressed patient's mood and behavior. Treatment is usually short term, and the agenda for therapy sessions is circumscribed, but global improvement is possible when recurrent cognitive distortions are scrutinized and changed.

Studies of cognitive disorder in depression indicate that depressed patients have impaired learning and memory functioning, frequent cognitive distortions, maladaptive schemata, abnormal responses to feedback information, and misattributions to environmental events. Although depression is probably a "psychobiological final common pathway" disorder with many possible treatments, alteration of cognitive pathology appears to be one of the more important avenues for intervention. This chapter describes the basic cognitive model and commonly used treatment techniques. A growing research effort on the nature of cognitive disorder in depression will likely influence the further evolution of this treatment approach to depression.

REFERENCES

Abramson LY, Seligman MEP, Treasdale JD: Learned helplessness in humans: critique and reformulation. J Abnorm Psychol 1978; 87:49-74

Akiskal HS: Factors associated with incomplete recovery in primary depressive illness. J Clin Psychiatry 1982; 43:266-271

Akiskal HS, McKinney WT: Overview of recent research in depression: integration of ten conceptual models into a comprehensive clinical frame. Arch Gen Psychiatry 1975; 32:285-305

Arieti S: Cognition in psychoanalysis, in Cognition and Psychotherapy. Edited by Mahoney MJ, Freeman A. New York, Plenum, 1985

Beck AT: Thinking and depression, I: idiosyncratic content and cognitive distortions. Arch Gen Psychiatry 1963; 9:36-45

Beck AT: Thinking and depression, II: theory and therapy. Arch Gen Psychiatry 1964; 10:561-571

Beck AT: Cognitive therapy, behavior therapy, psychoanalysis, and pharmacotherapy: a cognitive continuum, in Cognition and Psychotherapy. Edited by Mahoney MJ, Freeman A. New York, Plenum, 1985

Beck AT, Greenberg RL: Coping with Depression. New York, Institute for Rational Living, 1974

Beck AT, Kovacs M, Weissman A: Hopelessness and suicidal behavior. JAMA 1975; 234:1146-1149

Beck AT, Rush AJ, Shaw BF, et al: Cognitive Therapy of Depression. New York, Guilford, 1979

Bishop S, Miller IW, Norman W, et al: Cognitive therapy of psychotic depression: a case report. Psychotherapy 1986; 23:167-173

Blackburn IM, Bishop S: Changes in cognition with pharmacotherapy and cognitive therapy. Br J Psychiatry 1983; 143:609-617

Blackburn IM, Bishop S, Glen AIM, et al: The efficacy of cognitive therapy in depression: a treatment using cognitive therapy and pharmacotherapy, each alone and in combination. Br J Psychiatry 1981; 139:181-189

Bower GH: Mood and memory. Am Psychol 1981; 36:129-148

Bowlby J: The role of childhood experience in cognitive disturbance, in Cognition and Psychotherapy. Edited by Mahoney MJ, Freeman A. New York, Plenum, 1985

Braff DL, Beck AT: Thinking disorder in depression. Arch Gen Psychiatry 1974; 32:456-459

Breslow R, Kocsis J, Belkin B: Memory deficits in depression: evidence utilizing the Wechsler Memory Scale. Percept Mot Skills 1980; 54:541-542

Breslow R, Kocsis J, Belkin B: Contribution of the depressive perspective to memory function in depression. Am J Psychiatry 1981; 138:227-230

Burns DD: Feeling Good. New York, Morrow and Company, Inc., 1980

Cochran SD: Effectiveness of cognitive therapy in preventing noncompliance with lithium regimens. Paper presented at the annual meeting of the American Psychological Association, Washington, DC, August 1982

Cohen RM, Weingartner H, Smallberg SA, et al: Effort and cognition in depression. Arch Gen Psychiatry 1982; 39:593-597

Cutting J: Memory in functional psychosis. J Neurol Neurosurg Psychiatry 1979; 42:1031-1037

DeMonbreun BG, Craighead WE: Distortion of perception and recall of positive and neutral feedback in depression. Cognitive Therapy and Research 1977; 1:311-329

Dobson KS, Shaw BF: Cognitive assessment with major depressive disorders. Cognitive Therapy and Research 1986; 10:13-29

Donnelly EF, Dent JK, Murphy DL: Comparison of temporal lobe epileptics and affective disorders on the Halstead–Reitan test battery. J Clin Psychol 1972; 28:61-62

Fawcett J, Scheftner W, Clark D, et al: Clinical predictors of suicide in patients with major affective disorders: a controlled prospective study. Am J Psychiatry 1987; 144:35-40

Frankl VE: Logos, paradox, and the search for meaning, in Cognition and Psychotherapy. Edited by Mahoney MJ, Freeman A. New York, Plenum, 1985

Fuchs CZ, Himmelhoch JM: Pseudomanic-depressive illness and cognitive–behavior therapy. J Nerv Ment Dis 1980; 168:382-384

Glass RM, Uhlenhuth EH, Hartel FW, et al: Cognitive dysfunction and imipramine in outpatient depressives. Arch Gen Psychiatry 1981; 38:1048-1051

Greenberg LS, Safran JD: Integrating affect and cognition: a perspective on the process of therapeutic change. Cognitive Therapy and Research 1984; 8:559-578

Guidano VF, Liotti G: Cognitive Processes and Emotional Disorders: A Structural Approach to Psychotherapy. New York, Guilford, 1983

Guidano VF, Liotti G: A constructivistic foundation for cognitive therapy, in Cognition and Psychotherapy. Edited by Mahoney MJ, Freeman A. New York, Plenum, 1985

Harrell TH, Ryon NB: Cognitive assessment of depression: clinical validation of the ATQ–30. Paper presented at the 16th annual meeting of the American Association of Behavior Therapy, Los Angeles,1982

Hollon SD, Kendall PC: Cognitive self-statements in depression: development of an automatic thought questionnaire. Cognitive Therapy and Research 1980; 4:383-395

Hollon SD, DeRubeis RJ, Evans MD: Final report of the cognitive–pharmacotherapy trial: outcome, prophylaxis, prognosis, process, and mechanism. Presented at the 17th annual meeting of the Association for the Advancement of Behavioral Therapy, Washington, DC, December 1983

Ingram RE: Toward an information-processing analysis of depression. Cognitive Therapy and Research 1984; 8:443-477

Kovacs M, Rush AJ, Beck AT, et al: Depressed outpatients treated with cognitive therapy or pharmacotherapy. Arch Gen Psychiatry 1981; 38:33-39

Krantz SE: When depressive cognitions reflect negative realities. Cognitive Therapy and Research 1985; 9:595-610

LeFebvre MF: Cognitive distortion and cognitive errors in depressed psychiatric and low back pain patients. J Consult Clin Psychol 1981; 49:517-525

Loeb A, Beck AT, Feshbach S, et al: Some effects of reward on the social perception and motivation of psychiatric patients varying in depression. Journal of Abnormal and Social Psychology 1964; 68:609-616

Loeb A, Beck AT, Diggory J: Differential effects of success and failure on depressed and nondepressed patients. J Nerv Ment Dis 1971; 152:106-114

Mahoney MJ: Psychotherapy and human change processes, in Cognition and Psychotherapy. Edited by Mahoney MJ, Freeman A. New York, Plenum, 1985

Mayer JD, Bower GH: Naturally occurring mood and learning: comment on Hasher, Rose, Zacks, Sanft, and Doren. J Exp Psychol 1985; 114:396-403

Meichenbaum D: Cognitive-Behavior Modification. New York, Plenum, 1977

Miller IW, Klee SH, Norman WH: Depressed and nondepressed inpatients' cognitions of hypothetical events, experimental tasks, and stressful life events. J Abnorm Psychol 1982; 91:78-81

Miller IW, Bishop SB, Norman WH, et al: Cognitive/behavioral therapy and pharmacotherapy with chronic, drug-refractory depressed inpatients: a note of optimism. Behavioral Psychotherapy 1985; 13:320-327

Minkoff K, Bergman E, Beck AT, et al: Hopelessness, depression, and attempted suicide. Am J Psychiatry 1973; 130:455-459

Nelson RE, Craighead WE: Selective recall of positive and negative feedback, self-control behaviors, and depression. J Abnorm Psychol 1977: 86:379-388

Pretzer JL: Borderline personality disorder: too complex for cognitive therapy? Presented at 91st annual meeting of the American Psychological Association, Anaheim, CA, August 1983

Rizley R: Depression and distortion in the attribution of causality. J Abnorm Psychol 1978; 87:32-48

Rush AJ: Cognitive therapy of depression: rationale, techniques, and efficacy. Psychiatr Clin North Am 1983; 6:105-127

Rush AJ, Beck AT: Cognitive therapy of depression and suicide. Am J Psychother 1978; 32:201-219

Rush AJ, Giles DE: Cognitive therapy: theory and research, in Short-Term Psychotherapies for Depression. Edited by Rush AJ. New York, Guilford, 1982

Rush AT, Beck AT, Kovacs M, et al: Comparison of the effects of cognitive therapy and pharmacotherapy on hopelessness and self-concept. Am J Psychiatry 1982; 139:862-866

Safran JD, Vallis TM, Segal ZV, et al: Assessment of core cognitive processes in cognitive therapy. Cognitive Therapy and Research 1986; 10:509-525

Silverman JS, Silverman JA, Eardley DA: Do maladaptive attitudes cause depression? Arch Gen Psychiatry 1984; 41:28-30

Simons AD, Garfield SL, Murphy GE: The process of change in cognitive therapy and pharmacotherapy of depression. Arch Gen Psychiatry 1984; 41:45-51

Simons AD, Lustman PJ, Wetzel RD, et al: Predicting response to cognitive therapy of depression: the role of learned resourcefulness. Cognitive Therapy and Research 1985; 9:79-89

Simons AD, Murphy GE, Levine JL, et al: Cognitive therapy and pharmacotherapy for depression. Arch Gen Psychiatry 1986; 43:43-48

Watkins JT, Rush AJ: Cognitive Response Test. Cognitive Therapy and Research 1983; 7:425-436

Weingartner H, Cohen RM, Murphy DL, et al: Cognitive processes in depression. Arch Gen Psychiatry 1981; 38:42-47

Weissman AN: The dysfunctional attitude scale: a validation study. Dissertation Abstracts International 1979; 40:1389-1390b

Wright JH: The cognitive paradigm for treatment of depression, in Psychiatry, vol 4. Edited by Pichot P, Berner P, Wolf R, et al. New York, Plenum, 1985

Wright JH: Cognitive research: implications for the psychotherapy of depression. Paper presented at the World Congress of Psychiatry Regional Symposium, Copenhagen, August 1986a

Wright JH: Nortriptyline effects on cognition in depression. Dissertation Abstracts International 1986b; 47:2667b

Wright JH: Cognitive therapy and medication as combined treatment, in Cognitive Therapy. Edited by Freeman A, Greenwood V. New York, Human Sciences Press, 1987

Wright JH, Beck AT: Cognitive therapy of depression: theory and practice. Hosp Community Psychiatry 1983; 34:1119-1127

Wright JH, Beck AT: Cognitive therapy, in Depression. Edited by Munich SS. Ernst Reinhardt Publishers, 1986

Young JE, Beck AT: Cognitive therapy: clinical applications, in Short-Term Psychotherapies for Depression. Edited by Rush AJ. New York, Guilford, 1982

Zimmerman M, Coryell W, Corenthal C: Attribution style, the dexamethasone suppression test, and the diagnosis of melancholia in depressed inpatients. J Abnorm Psychol 1984; 93:373-377

Chapter 26

Cognitive Therapy of Panic Disorder

by Aaron T. Beck, M.D., and Ruth L. Greenberg, Ph.D.

Distorted cognition is an obvious feature of panic attacks, yet one that is generally dismissed or neglected in the treatment of panic disorder. According to the *Diagnostic and Statistical Manual of Mental Disorders, Third Edition, Revised (DSM-III-R)* (American Psychiatric Association, 1987), the belief that one is dying, going crazy, or about to lose control of behavior is a defining characteristic of panic attacks. Reassurance, disconfirming medical tests, and positive "self-talk" often have only a limited effect in loosening the hold of these tenacious beliefs. Nevertheless, we have had considerable preliminary success in treating panic disorder with a program that focuses directly on the cognitive features.

The program attempts, through repeated demonstrations, to undermine the belief that the panic attack is a malignant foreboding of impending disaster. We have found that when it is effective, the program reduces anticipatory anxiety and facilitates the reversal of avoidant and dependent behavior. Further, these interventions provide an opportunity to teach the patient that thoughts and images, beliefs and assumptions, may play a role in panic as well as other disturbing emotional reactions, a principle that can then be applied to modifying dysfunctional reactions to background stressors.

COGNITIVE MODELS OF ANXIETY AND PANIC

Like cognitive therapy for depression, our approach to panic disorder is based on a cognitive model of emotional disorders (Beck, 1976; Beck et al, 1979). In this model, disturbing affect is associated with "automatic" thoughts and images which distort or exaggerate reality and arise from dysfunctional basic assumptions about the self and the environment. The automatic thoughts and images in anxiety reactions are characterized by themes of danger—threat to the individual's physical, social, or psychological well-being. The presence of such thoughts was demonstrated in studies by Beck and colleagues (1974), Beck and Rush (1975), Hibbert (1984), Mathews and Shaw (1977), and in a case study by Zane (1984).

The cognitive model of anxiety was developed further by Beck and Emery (1985). Here it was argued that the anxiety patient has a core belief in his vulnerability to internal and environmental dangers. When this belief has been activated, perhaps by life stress, he begins to attend selectively to potential sources of harm. Perceiving risk, he tends both to exaggerate the degree of harm it portends and to underestimate his own capacity to cope with or ward off that harm. The perception of extreme danger sets off an "alarm system," at the center of which are primal responses of organisms to threat, all of which may have had adaptive value at some time in the evolution of our long-suffering species. Thus, the individual experiences an inclination to faint, freeze, flee, or fight. Unhappily, these responses tend to increase the sense of threat: As the public speaker "freezes," focusing ever more intently on cues from the audience that seem to signal disgrace, he or she perceives growing internal disability as an additional danger. Cognition, affect, and somatic sensations tend to reinforce one another, creating a vicious cycle which maintains anxiety.

In the case of panic disorder, physical sensations generally constitute the salient source of danger. Terrifying panic attacks, marked by strong somatic symptoms, leave the patient feeling vulnerable to further episodes, which he or she misinterprets as threats to survival, sanity, or social acceptability. Vigilant regarding possible recurrence of symptoms, the patient may react with alarm to any change in somatic state. Frightening thoughts and images generate additional somatic symptoms, and spiraling anxiety tends to reinforce the idea that catastrophe is imminent. A desire to escape, seek help, or act aggressively may overwhelm the patient, yet the impulse may itself be perceived as threatening, as it signifies weakness and abnormality.

Panic patients tend to generate symptom "equations" which encapsulate the frightening misinterpretations of symptoms and sensations. Thus, palpitations may mean heart attack; racing pulse, a stroke. A sense of unreality, or difficulty concentrating on a task, suggest insanity or loss of control over behavior. Slight blurring of vision may produce automatic thoughts such as, "I am going blind," and disturbing images of future incapacity.

In addition, such patients hold fallacious assumptions about anxiety and panic. The assumptions tend to center on themes of *vulnerability* ("Since I had a panic attack in this situation before, I'm likely to have one again"), *escalation* ("If I have a little anxiety, it will get worse until it goes all the way; I'm only safe if I have no symptoms at all"), and *copelessness* ("I'm completely helpless when I have the attack. I need a companion to get help").

Finally, a body of rules may develop that tend to maintain dysfunctional behavior: "It's best to avoid thinking about stressful problems that make me nervous"; "It's best to avoid being alone"; "It's best to stay busy at all times lest I experience frightening feelings and thoughts."

Although they may not be aware of this factor initially, panic patients often react with anxiety to a variety of life situations. The cognitive model suggests that here, too, as in their reactions to somatic sensations, they are exaggerating danger. Further, their appraisals reflect the operation of basic assumptions about themselves and their environment. For example, the homemaker who frequently has thoughts such as, "What if I don't finish cleaning the house?" may perceive a half-swept kitchen as a significant threat to her security; she may hold the assumption, "I will only be cared for if my performance is perfect." The stress generated by such assumptions helps to predispose this woman to the stronger anxiety symptoms characteristic of the panic attack. At the same time, her need to appear perfect undermines her ability to tolerate symptoms: "What if I have an attack during the party?"

Similarly, a young agoraphobic woman responds anxiously to a variety of interpersonal contacts. She holds the assumption, "I'm unloved and unloveable—a social misfit." Panic symptoms produce the thought, "I'm going to die alone." They signify that she is "different," likely to perish without achieving others' love and regard. In some cases, such as these two, we have discerned connections between the meaning given to panic symptoms and broader issues.

Sensations other than those related to anxiety may also trigger panic. Unpleasant emotions, such as anger or sadness, may themselves be frightening to the patient who feels incapable of coping with them; the effort to elude such disturbing experiences may maintain or generate arousal, which is then given a catastrophic interpretation. When in a vulnerable "mode" (Beck and Emery, 1985), the patient may even interpret as threatening a variety of purely physical changes: a sharp intake of breath as she emerges onto a frigid wintry street; faint feelings in a hot, stuffy room or after skipping meals; slight dizziness produced by fluorescent lights or by driving past vertical posts of a guardrail on a curving highway exit ramp. The sensations are accompanied by thoughts such as, "My heart can't take this," "I won't be able to catch my breath," "I'll lose control and drive my car off the road," "If I don't get help, something terrible will happen."

In a cognitive conceptualization, then, the panic attack occurs when physical symptoms and sensations, which may or may not themselves be related to anxiety, are given catastrophic interpretations and take on exaggerated, negative meaning for the individual. The panic patient may also be reacting to other life circumstances with distorted appraisals of potential harm.

COGNITIVE–BEHAVIORAL TREATMENT: PRINCIPLES AND MAJOR TECHNIQUES

Our treatment program is based on the observation that disturbing affect and dysfunctional behavior often resolve when related thoughts and assumptions are identified and subjected to rigorous reality-testing. Patients are trained to recognize and monitor their "automatic" thoughts and images, then assess their validity objectively. Although therapists draw on logic, general information, and other tools to help patients "test" their thoughts, we have found that the most effective tests often involve active "experiments" in which patients themselves gather data and evaluate them. In treating panic disorder, the key experiments lead the patient toward the conclusion that symptoms may be produced by simple mechanisms that are neither dangerous nor highly abnormal, and not entirely out of their control.

In the initial session, the therapist attempts to help the patient identify specific fears, and, if possible, the idiosyncratic meaning of symptoms. In order to accomplish this, we elicit as precise a description as possible of a typical panic attack. In what situation did symptoms occur? What did you notice first—then what? Exactly what sensations, what emotions, what thoughts, what images? What did you think was the worst thing that could happen, and how strongly did you believe it might? What did you do to try to cope with the symptoms? What does it mean to you when this happens? And how dangerous do you think the attack was, *right now?*

The therapist responds to this account with "capsule summaries" (Beck et al, 1979) that underscore the presence of danger-laden thoughts and images and the interplay among cognition, sensation, emotion, and behavior. The patient is then asked to consider the possibility that exaggerated thoughts exacerbate symptoms. At this point, patients are often relieved that some sense can be made of their painful, bewildering, and heretofore rather lonely experience, and they are receptive to information that tends to "normalize" anxiety—to place it in the context of the body's normal repertoire of responses to threat. If there is a discrepancy between the patient's estimates of danger from the panic attack during the attack and during the therapy session, that datum is used as evidence that thoughts about panic are distorted under certain circumstances. As "homework," the patient is asked to monitor and record panic-related sensations, emotions, thoughts, and images, and the situations in which they occur.

When enough data have been gathered to permit the identification of the patient's "symptom equations," an attempt is made to test their validitiy by replicating key symptoms in the office. When symptoms are reproduced by simple means, they tend to lose their mystery, and patients find alternative "equations" more credible. A method that succeeds with many patients is to ask them to "overbreathe"—breathe rapidly and deeply—for a two-minute period. Patients are then asked to close their eyes and briefly introspect, to report what they are experiencing (sensations, emotions, thoughts, images), and to estimate the degree to which the effects of overbreathing resemble those of a panic attack.

If, as often happens, the patient reports at least some similarity, she is asked to try to recall whether there is anything "special" about her breathing during the attack (for example, gulping air, breathing through the mouth). Together, therapist and patient explore the possibility that hyperventilation may account for numbness, tingling, dizziness, and other sensations. She is "re-educated" about anxiety as the therapist explains the effects of "blowing off" carbon dioxide through overbreathing, and the operation of a "vicious cycle" in which symptoms lead to fear, which leads to more symptoms and more fear. The patient is then taught "control breathing," a pattern of breathing slowly and regularly, through the nose, which controls hyperventilation if initiated early in an attack. The overbreathing demonstration and the control breathing technique are drawn from the work of Clark and colleagues (1985) and Salkovskis and co-workers (1986).

The essential goal of the overbreathing demonstration and other "replication experiments" is to correct the erroneous "symptom equations." We find it valuable to make this correction in writing, so that the patient can remind herself, during an attack, of the factual explanation of symptoms. Thus, if the initial equation reads, "Heart racing = heart attack," the new equation might read, "Heart racing = normal, harmless reaction of the body to perception of danger, related to hyperventilation." A self-instruction may follow: "Slow your breathing, remember symptoms do not last long." Such instructions prepare the patient to cope with symptoms, and erode the belief that they are entirely uncontrollable.

Replication of symptoms can take many forms. The therapist may ask the patient to rate the severity of symptoms before and after he is asked to bring into his mind the frightening image that has occurred to him during an attack, or an image of himself having an attack or walking in a shopping mall. If body discomfort has increased, the patient is asked to reflect on that observation, and again is led to reattribute symptoms to benign processes. Specialized interventions may be required to simulate particular symptoms. Salkovskis (personal communication, 1987) notes that chest pain can be produced by filling the lungs with air, then trying to breathe even more deeply; intercostal muscles will be strained, and may even be sensitive to the touch. Having the patient run stairs, jog in place, rise suddenly from a horizontal position, closely monitor his body state, or drink coffee may also produce characteristic sensations. To simulate visual effects, Greenberg (1987) used printed grid designs that produce optical illusions such as blurring and movement. The designs were adapted from Grafton (1976).

On occasion, we have taken advantage of the phenomenon of "relaxation-induced anxiety" (Heide and Borkovec, 1984) to replicate symptoms. We attempt to induce deep muscle relaxation in the standard fashion, but embrace any resulting *increase* in anxiety as an opportunity for cognitive restructuring (for example, "You are misinterpreting normal, 'floaty' feelings that ocurr in a relaxed state"). It is worth noting that, in a small number of patients, medical problems may limit the types of replication experiments that are advisable.

In these initial sessions, we also review the circumstances surrounding the first panic attack. We consider both distal factors, such as concurrent life stress and emotional tension, and proximal factors, such as weather, illness, use of "recreational" drugs, exertion, and fatigue. Again, the technique helps to develop a noncatastrophic interpretation of symptoms.

The search for alternative explanations for symptoms also involves examining the patient's daily life for sources of stress. Although many patients vigorously deny that any life problem they may have is sufficient to cause such distressing symptoms, logging attacks not infrequently makes them aware of environmental precipitants. Diaries also help to clarify internal triggers, such as effects of exercise, excitement, or ingestion of alcohol; menstrual symptoms; or frightening images (Clark, personal communication, 1985). As the treatment continues, we encourage patients to notice and record not only panic symptoms, but other changes in their levels of emotional distress, along with related "automatic thoughts" and images.

Because patients sometimes think a "Pandora's box" of overwhelming, unendurable pain will be opened if they attend to their feelings, we try to deepen affective experience in the sessions. We emphasize that even very difficult problems are often susceptible to some solution, and that even great emotional pain can be tolerated. Indeed, simply surviving such a session can be viewed as evidence that disconfirms frightening expectations. When other life problems are identified, we apply appropriate problem-solving or cognitive-restructuring techniques.

RELATED PROBLEMS AND TECHNIQUES

Fear of Loss of Control

In many cases, the patient's key belief is that during a panic attack he will "lose control" and act foolishly or aggressively. Some patients picture themselves running frantically through the streets, accosting strangers and begging for help. Such patients need to learn that although their physical symptoms, emotions, or thoughts appear to be "out of control," it is unlikely their behavior will be. They are asked to examine relevant evidence: "What have you done in the past that was 'out of control'?" These patients may respond to simple experiments, such as giving themselves a command during the next attack ("Raise your arm"; "Walk four steps to the right"), and observing whether they follow it.

When patients believe they must rigidly control their thoughts for fear of going insane and "doing something weird," we experiment by having them deliberately abandon control or think "mad" thoughts, and observe the effects. Particular "loss of control" experiments depend on patients' specific fears and therapists' ingenuity.

We also explore what the patient perceives as the consequences of "acting foolish" or expressing anger. Often the patient believes that behaving in less than a perfectly controlled manner is a sign of intolerable weakness or inadequacy, and would seriously imperil others' regard. To help test these beliefs, our therapists have been known to leap unexpectedly onto office chairs and implore mall security guards for help (during occasional *in vivo* sessions). To date, no patient has lost regard for us because of our foolish behavior. It may be appropriate to have the patient ask for help or express anger, and observe others' responses.

Fear of Being Trapped

Here the patient generally believes that she will be in a situation where it will either be impossible to escape the disastrous effects of panic, or she will have to commit an egregious public error to do so, such as leaving the classroom during a test or the boardroom during a presentation. Again, behavioral options and their perceived consequences must be explored. Patients may gain a sense of control simply by planning in advance what they will do in the event of intolerable anxiety: exit briefly, take a few sips of water, pinch themselves, remind themselves the speech has limited importance. Some of the strategies are never actually employed: the sense of having options seems to alleviate anxiety.

Diversion (Distraction)

Diverting attention away from symptoms and frightening thoughts can be a surprisingly powerful way to cope with anxiety, and one that many patients have discovered on their own. We encourage moderate use of this technique to increase the sense of mastery or control. In fact, we enhance these skills by teaching patients to focus on the sights, sounds, smells, and textures in their immediate environment, or by suggesting they carry small puzzles, take walks, or chat with fellow passengers when panicky (also see Newman, 1985). Conversely, we might have the patient focus on the sensations rather than on frightening thoughts. However, the most important use of these techniques is to demonstrate the role of frightening cognitions and cast doubt on the likelihood of impending catastrophe: "If you were having a heart attack or becoming insane, do you think you could slow it down by looking at a poster of a Gauguin beach scene?" Diversion seems to be most effective if demonstrated in the session when the patient is feeling anxious.

Fear of Unending Anxiety

In spontaneous images that occur during the attack, panic patients sometimes see themselves experiencing anxiety or emotional pain that never comes to an end. We ask such patients to time periods of acute distress; generally they conclude that episodes are time-limited.

Modifying Appraisal of Risk

Gradually, patients acquire the idea that when anxious or panicky, they tend to overestimate potential harm and underestimate safety factors. We train them to recalculate the probability of harm by attending to factual "evidence," and to look actively for the neglected safety factors. For example, patients learn, through repeated observations, that a little anxiety does not necessarily signal a full-blown attack. We also teach patients to reappraise danger from external sources. A patient who avoided shopping in malls feared her child might be kidnapped there; she estimated the probability of kidnapping at 50 percent. As a "homework" assignment, the patient was asked to telephone her local police department for relevant statistics; she discovered there had never been a kidnapping in the district! The search for safety factors similarly comprises both internal and external domains: the patient's demonstrated capacity to cope, the body's self-regulatory mechanisms, the likelihood strangers will think badly of them for getting lost. We emphasize resources available to any adult, rather than the false safety provided by dependent relationships or proximity to home.

Fear of Ultimate Consequences: Death, Rejection, Isolation

Our energetic beginning thrust is designed to reduce the immediate fear of death or social disgrace by affecting the perceived probability of harm. At a later stage, we explore the ultimate feared consequences. When the problem is fear of death, we carefully elicit the patient's concept of death. One patient pictured himself lying in a coffin, with his senses intact, aware of separation from loved ones. A young woman believed death meant the loss of God's grace—punishment for wrongdoing. For some, the real fear is of dying without leaving a mark, earning respect, completing a project. Fears of rejection or isolation prompt an examination of existing social relationships that aims at defining solvable problems.

Modifying Images

A woman who had developed a panic disorder following a severe reaction to penicillin experienced, during attacks, a vivid image of herself lying in bed in the hospital with an oxygen mask over her face, as she had during the drug reaction. A second woman, agoraphobic after betrayal by her lover, pictured herself fainting in the street, regarded with disdain by indifferent passers-by.

Such images respond to various restructuring techniques. Repeated inductions of the drug-reaction image taught the patient to distinguish between the anxiety-producing fantasy and the reality of sitting safely in the physician's office. The agoraphobic woman was asked to carry her image further, and visualized a caring stranger helping her to safety. Patients may also be trained to substitute a pleasant image for the frightening one.

Reversing Avoidant Behavior

Once the patient has learned to reappraise symptoms and has a grasp of coping techniques, we instigate a program of exposure to feared situations. The patient's manual by Mathews and co-authors (1981) has been a valuable adjunct to this procedure. Exposure exercises are viewed as additional opportunities to test assumptions about anxiety symptoms and about the self and the environment, as well as to practice anxiety management skills.

Avoidance may be subtle in nonphobic panic disorders. For this reason, we inquire of patients who have improved, "Are there circumstances under which you would still be alarmed by symptoms?" We have found in this way that patients were avoiding taking antibiotics, visiting their family, or exercising strenuously, and exposure tasks were contrived.

On occasion, when patients are "stuck," we accompany them into phobic situations.

Experiencing Panic

Although we train patients in coping skills at an intermediate stage of treatment, eventually we encourage patients to experience attacks without using anxiety management techniques. When earlier interventions have worn down the fearful ideation, the patient is usually ready to conduct this more elegant test of catastrophic expectations. As preparation for this phase, we make use of the language and writing of Weekes (1978). This step is crucial for patients who overcontrol anxiety, becoming preoccupied with using techniques to ward off attacks.

Modifying Rules and Assumptions

As therapy progresses, we draw on the accumulating store of data regarding the patient's emotional and behavioral reactions to formulate hypotheses regarding underlying rules and assumptions. If the patient agrees that the hypotheses fit the data, we then examine the validity and usefulness of the assumptions and rules. In treating panic, we might address the assumption, "I can solve the problem by staying close to others," or weigh the costs and benefits of the rule, "Wait until I'm calm before trying anything new." Basic assumptions about the self and the environment are also formulated: "I am completely and solely responsible for my family's well-being"; "I should be able to prevent anything bad from happening"; "A strong man is essential to my survival—and I'm not good enough to get one." Like those uncovered in the treatment of depression, these assumptions are modified in the manner described by Beck and colleagues (1979).

Case Example

The case of Ann illustrates a number of the principles outlined above.

Status at Intake

A 31-year-old elementary school teacher entered treatment with panic attacks two or three times a day. She frequently experienced anxiety and a rapid heart rate, which she feared were symptomatic of a life-threatening heart condition. Other symptoms—blurred vision, palpitations, dizziness, sweating, paresthesias, shaking—also occurred during the attacks. Because of the attacks she stopped working, driving her car, or staying at home alone. She became increasingly dependent on her husband, frequently checked her pulse, and was preoccupied with worries about her physical condition. Panic symptoms typically came "out of the blue" and disappeared within 30 minutes.

During a previous period of frequent panic attacks, Ann (not her real name) had consulted several cardiologists and was prescribed a variety of cardiac medications, which had produced little improvement. In fact, Ann attributed some of her more troubling symptoms to the medications. She had mitral valve prolapse and frequent migraine headaches.

Family Background and Precipitating Stresses

Circumstances that involved her family of origin were clear precipitants of the patient's problems. The obedient oldest child of fanatically religious parents, Ann had carried much of the responsibility for managing the household and her six siblings, including a disruptive, delinquent brother. While her mother worked a night shift, Ann would often be beaten by her authoritarian father.

Over time, tension had developed between Ann and her brother, who as an adult was troubled by joblessness and drug abuse. Despite the disturbing facts of his life, the patient felt her mother was partial to the brother and acted coldly and capriciously toward Ann. Eventually, the brother was arrested on burglary charges. In an emotional scene that followed the incident, Ann expressed anger at her brother's behavior, and her mother responded by defending him and angrily withdrawing from Ann. Almost immediately, Ann experienced panic symptoms, and a generalized anxiety state also began to develop.

Sessions 1–7

In her first sessions, Ann complained of a variety of symptoms that frightened her and reported automatic thoughts such as, "What if my heart beats faster while I'm driving the car?" When driving into the city that week, she had had severe anxiety accompanied by the thought, "What if I have to get home and have to wait to get my car out of a parking lot?" In both cases she pictured an incapacitating medical emergency.

She also identified fears of performing inadequately at work. She was able quickly to discern a pattern of expecting the worst of her own performance and of others' reactions, and she could see that these expectations had generally not been confirmed by subsequent events. Ann also realized that she constantly felt compelled to hurry.

In the third session, Ann agreed to try to overbreathe for two minutes. She had a strong physical and emotional reaction to the procedure—indeed, tearfulness interrupted the overbreathing. She described her experience as follows: "My heart is pounding. I feel very dizzy, lightheaded, spaced out, unreal. I don't feel particularly anxious. I'm a little afraid. It's a little scary. My palms are sweaty. My mouth feels dry. I'm a little shaky. I feel like I can't catch my breath . . . I did have a thought about my heart. I hope it doesn't beat very fast. I did feel that I feel safe here."

Thus, the procedure did evoke Ann's fear of having a potentially dangerous heart condition; the automatic thoughts also suggest an implicit appraisal of how perilous the symptoms might be, given particular circumstances. Ann concluded that it was plausible that overbreathing might be contributing to her symptoms and that regulating her breathing might help her.

At the following session, Ann had observed that when anxious she had been holding her breath. Breathing slowly and regularly had helped. Further, she had applied the idea of conscious pacing to other activities, and noted with satisfaction that the tactic had worked very well. Pacing herself had made it obvious that she would need to stand up to her principal, who had been extracting hours of uncompensated service from her each week.

Here some basic assumptions were elicited: "I'm not such a hot person because I don't want to do what's expected of me. You are supposed to do without getting back." For homework, Ann recorded her activities for a week to see whether it was *possible* comfortably to add responsibilities to her current schedule. By her next session, the "evidence" had convinced Ann that no time was available for additional work—and that turning down the principal had nothing to do with whether she was a "hot person," but merely with assessment of priorities.

In the fourth session, guided imagery was used to reduce Ann's fear of public places from which escape would be difficult. Ann pictured herself shopping in a large department store, her car blocks away in a huge garage. In her initial image, she saw herself gasping for breath, desperate to reach her car, finally collapsing for lack of medical attention. Asked to form an alternate image, she pictured herself managing symptoms on her own until they passed, aware that a rescue team would likely be summoned in the event of a true emergency.

Simultaneously, Ann was trained in testing danger-laden automatic thoughts regarding her health ("What if my blood pressure is high?" "If the anxiety keeps up, my heart won't be able to take it") and her work performance ("I can't do it!" "What if something went wrong?"). By the sixth session, she was able to respond on her own to such thoughts. Ann was feeling better during the day, "churning" at night.

During the following week, Ann became frightened by symptoms that started when she drank wine. At the root of this may have been a church prohibition against drinking. Ann appeared to have interpreted signs of anxiety about breaking the prohibition as manifestations of a dangerous reaction to the alcohol itself. However, she had coped with a rapid heartbeat that awakened her that night by breathing slowly and reminding herself that such symptoms always passed. She was pleased to have achieved some control over her symptoms and her fears.

Sessions 8–12

Concerns about Ann's family began to move into the foreground at about session seven. She expressed fear that her helpless, troubled brother would become her responsibility as her parents aged, if the parents failed to correct his behavior. The assumption, "If others aren't doing the job, I am responsible," seemed to be at work. In retrospect, it had also been operating at school. The assumption accounted in part for her anger at her mother—"I have to assume this burden because you refuse to." Ann recalled that she had long been angry at her mother for abandoning her responsibilities: "Why didn't you protect me from Dad?"

Two related assumptions could soon be articulated: "If I don't take care of things, and do it properly, a catastrophe will happen," but at the same time, "There's more to taking care of things than I can handle." Visiting her family, which she had been avoiding since the beginning of her illness, Ann caught automatic thoughts such as, "Something bad will happen. I have to fix it." The assumptions could be traced readily to childhood, when she had been expected to manage potentially dangerous situations that were beyond her level of competence. A memory surfaced of having aborted a sister's suicide attempt while her mother sewed.

During this period of therapy, Ann was helped to reassess the probability that she or her parents *could* set her brother straight. She began to see that she was quite able to succeed at any *reasonable* goal she set for herself, although she would likely have to give up trying to change her brother: "I see I can't control some things."

Fear and anger about the mother were also addressed: "I might deserve her mistreatment." An alternative hypothesis was proposed to account for the mother's behavior. Far from disapproving of Ann, the mother might feel she must apologize to the successful sibling for the unsuccessful one.

Ann was encouraged to "gather data" related to this hypothesis by speaking assertively to her mother, assisted by in-session role plays and "cognitive rehearsals," and found the mother more accepting than she had imagined. Later, Ann said she had learned to "be more bold," and to try to express feelings and solve problems in a timely manner.

In later sessions, earlier lessons were reinforced. A short episode of "spaceyness" made Ann recall the period of florid symptoms and fear it would recur. She also was distraught that anger at her parents meant she was not fulfilling the commandment to "honor" them. In both cases, she learned that "all or nothing thinking" was at fault: Some anxiety did not inevitably foretell severe anxiety, and angry behavior was not a sign of total disrespect.

SUMMARY

Through a course of cognitive–behavioral treatment, Ann overcame helplessness in regard both to physical symptoms and a daunting family problem, which had triggered a drastic and generalized loss of self-confidence. Anxiety at work and church provided an initial domain for developing skills in thought-testing and anxiety management, which she was later able to apply to the resonant, core issues evoked by family conflict.

Questions of family structure were explored within a cognitive framework that involved hypothesis formulation and data collection; coaching in assertive behavior facilitated the process. Responsibility and "control" proved to be dominant themes, with the patient seeking control in areas where success was unlikely, while shrinking from action that might have proved beneficial.

Empirical Status

Although efforts to test the effectiveness of this treatment program are still at a preliminary stage, a number of studies do support the cognitive model of anxiety disorders. Studies by Mathews and MacLeod (1985) and MacLeod and colleagues (1986) demonstrated that patients with generalized anxiety attend selectively to cues related to threat. Mathews and MacLeod (1986) obtained similar results; this study suggests, in addition, that selective processing occurs at a preconscious level. In a study by Butler and Mathews (1983), anxious patients were more likely than controls to interpret ambiguous scenarios as threatening; patients also rated the "subjective cost" of the events higher than controls.

Further, selective attention and selective memory effects have been demonstrated in relation to phobic populations. Agoraphobic and social phobic subjects studied by Burgess and colleagues (1981) showed greater recognition of fear-related words than controls when a dichotic-listening paradigm was employed. Nunn and co-workers (1984) found that agoraphobic subjects had enhanced recall for danger-related material. Agoraphobic women with driving phobias, studied by Williams and Rappaport (1983), had more fearful thoughts, more thoughts about their body states and their anxiety level, and fewer diversionary thoughts than controls while driving along a prescribed route.

Nonphobic panic patients interviewed by Hibbert (1984) reported thoughts and images associated with physical, psychological, and social disaster. These patients insisted that their expectations of extreme physical harm were a reaction to body sensations. Finally, Greenberg (1987) found that panic patients and normal subjects reacted differently to procedures designed to alter body sensations: panic subjects had fewer positive responses to a two-minute period of overbreathing and more negative responses to a series of disturbing visual patterns.

In relation to therapy, we can report that an initial cohort of 23 patients (19 with panic disorders and 4 with agoraphobia with panic attacks), treated according to the program outlined above at the Center for Cognitive Therapy, did show marked improvement. Frequency of panic attacks reduced significantly over the course of treatment and were completely remitted at termination (mean = 22 sessions). The effect was maintained throughout the 3–12 month follow-up period (Beck and Sokol-Kessler, 1986).

Our clinical experience suggests that the cognitive strategies can provide relatively rapid relief from potentially disabling symptoms, while establishing a practical and conceptual framework for work with related difficulties. The "replication experiments" permit us to expose patients to fearful stimuli while remaining in our own offices, a clear advantage both for patients whose attacks do not occur in particular situations and for many phobic patients, who seem more willing to enter feared settings after their "reeducation." These procedures are, of course, particularly appropriate for patients who have reacted adversely to medications or who are unwilling to use them, and for patients who have not benefited from other treatments. We see the cognitive method as an integrative approach that unites diverse elements in a coherent program of relearning and behavior change.

REFERENCES

American Psychiatric Association: Diagnostic and Statistical Manual of Mental Disorders, third edition, revised. Washington, DC, American Psychiatric Association, 1987

Beck AT: Cognitive Therapy and the Emotional Disorders. New York, International Universities Press, 1976

Beck AT, Emery G: Anxiety Disorders and Phobias: A Cognitive Perspective. New York, Basic Books, 1985

Beck AT, Rush AJ: A cognitive model of anxiety formation and anxiety resolution, in Stress and Anxiety, vol. II. Edited by Sarason ID, Spielburger CD. Washington, DC, Hemisphere Publishing, 1975

Beck AT, Laude R, Bohnert M: Ideational components of anxiety neurosis. Arch Gen Psychiatry 1974; 31:319-325

Beck AT, Rush AJ, Shaw BF, et al: Cognitive Therapy of Depression. New York, Guilford, 1979

Beck AT, Sokol-Kessler L: Cognitive therapy of panic disorder. Poster presentation at the meeting of the Association for Advancement of Behavior Therapy, October, 1986

Burgess IS, Jones LM, Robertson SA, et al: The degree of control exerted by phobic and nonphobic verbal stimuli over the recognition behaviour of phobic and nonphobic subjects. Behav Res Ther 1981; 19:233-243

Butler G, Mathews A: Cognitive processes in anxiety. Advances in Behavior Research Therapy 5:51-62, 1983

Clark DM, Salkovskis PM, Chalkley A: Respiratory control as a treatment for panic attacks. J Behav Ther Exp Psychiatry 1985; 16:23-30

Grafton CB: Optical Designs in Motion with Moire Overlays. New York, Dover, 1976

Greenberg RL: Cognitive components of panic disorder. Doctoral dissertation, University of Pennsylvania, 1987

Heide FJ, Borkovec TD: Relaxation-induced anxiety: mechanisms and theoretical implications. Behav Res Ther 1984; 11:1-12

Hibbert GA; Ideational components of anxiety: their origin and content. Br J Psychiatry 1984; 144:618-624

MacLeod C, Mathews A, Tata P: Attentional bias in emotional disorders. J Abnorm Psychol 1986; 95:15-20

Mathews A, Shaw P: Cognitions related to anxiety: a pilot study of treatment. Behav Res Ther 1977; 15:503-505

Mathews A, Gelder MG, Johnston DW: Agoraphobia: Nature and Treatment. New York, Guilford, 1981

Mathews A, MacLeod C: Selective processing of threat cues in anxiety states. Behav Res Ther 1985; 23:563-569

Mathews A, MacLeod C: Discrimination of threat cues without awareness in anxiety states. J Abnorm Psychol 1986; 95:131-138

Newman F: Fighting Fear. New York, MacMillan, 1985

Nunn JD, Stevenson RJ, Whalan G: Selective memory effects in agoraphobic patients. Br J Clin Psychol 1984; 23:195-201

Salkovskis PM, Jones DRO, Clark DM: Respiratory control in the treament of panic attacks: replication and extension with concurrent measurement of behaviour and pCO$_2$. Br J Psychiatry 1986; 148:526-532

Weekes C: Simple, effective treatment of agoraphobia. Am J Psychother 1978; 32:357-369

Williams SL, Rappaport A: Cognitive treatment in the natural environment for agoraphobics. Behav Ther 1983; 14:299-313

Zane MD: psychoanalysis and contextual analysis of phobias. J Am Acad Psychoanal 1984; 12: 553-568

Chapter 27

Cognitive Behavior Therapy with Children and Adolescents

by Paul D. Trautman, M.D., and
Mary Jane Rotheram-Borus, Ph.D.

This chapter presents a model of cognitive–behavioral intervention, with depressed children and adolescents, that focuses on coping skills. This program evolved from clinical work with suicidal and suicide-attempting adolescents. It includes training families and children in interpersonal problem solving; ways of talking to oneself; identifying, controlling, and expressing feelings; and practicing behavioral skills. The components of this model are not new. The integration emerges from clinical experience, which indicates that focusing only on dysfunctional thinking patterns is insufficient for changing behavior and feelings in children and adolescents.

THERAPEUTIC MODEL

There are four differences between the basic assumptions of cognitive therapy with adults and those we employ.

1. *The therapist aims to increase idealistically positive thoughts, perceptions, feelings, and actions.* People like good feelings, want positive events to recur, and will act to receive rewards from others (Skinner, 1953). Beck and colleagues (1979, p. 299) carefully distinguish positive thinking from realistic thinking and encourage patients to be realistic. However, in reviewing the literature on negative attributions and depression, Layne (1983) concludes that nondepressed persons are unrealistically positive in their expectations and attributions. Our therapeutic goal is to increase idealistically positive feelings, thoughts, and experiences (Stuart, 1980), even though they may be initially unrealistic. That is, we want people to act "as if" their lives were happy and good, even if life is not so good at present. This approach emphasizes the strengths and accomplishments of the child and the family, however small, and might be called "success therapy." The therapist helps families to identify and experience positive feelings, thoughts, and behaviors within and outside the session. Family strengths and the loving bonds among family members are emphasized, while negative perceptions and feelings are relabeled in a positive context.

There is theoretical support for this strategy. Depression has been conceptualized as a response to the loss of social rewards that were formerly present (Skinner, 1953), to the diminished effectiveness of social rewards (Ferster, 1966;

Preparation of this chapter was supported in part by grants from the William T. Grant Foundation and the Administration for Children, Youth and Families (HD6638). We wish to acknowledge the help of Jeffrey Young, PhD, in adapting the cognitive therapy model to an adolescent population. We also wish to acknowledge the support of the Leon Lowenstein Foundation, Inc.

Costello, 1981), to the failure to obtain rewards because of poor social skills, to the reward of inappropriate behavior (for example, attention for crying), or to punishment of coping behaviors (Lewinsohn and Shaw, 1969). Depressed children and adults have a negative view of themselves, the world, and the future (Beck et al, 1979).

Emphasis on success and positive events addresses the family's thinking style, not by modifying thinking, but by forcing the family to engage in behavior incompatible with negativistic thinking (Vailhinger, 1924; James, 1948). By encouraging positive behaviors incompatible with depression, we employ the principle of reciprocal inhibition (Wolpe, 1958). By asking the family to act in an idealistically positive manner, the therapist is also attempting to implement a positive self-fulfilling prophecy. Believing one is effective can lead to positive behavioral change (Bandura, 1977, 1978).

A family's thinking style shapes not only its perception of problems, but also its expectations of therapeutic outcome (Heine and Trosman, 1973; Overall and Aronson, 1963). Idealistic positivism helps both patient and therapist to develop the belief that change is possible. Patients and families expect change to occur quickly in therapy and will drop out without early assurance that this will occur (Bent et al, 1975; Strupp, 1978; Haley, 1977; Stuart, 1980; Nichols and Beck, 1960). Successful therapeutic outcome is also dependent on the therapist's positive regard for the patient and positive expectations about outcome (Parloff et al, 1979; Heine and Trosman, 1973; Heller and Goldstein, 1961). By structuring a pleasant first meeting, outlining a treatment plan and goals, and planning pleasant activities between sessions, therapist and patient will establish rapport and positive expectations.

2. *Cognition, behavior, and affect are interactive* (Murray and Jacobson, 1971; Izard and Schwartz, 1986). We do not attempt to change the child's thinking style and hope for a generalization to behavior and feelings, but rather to teach a new habit of processing feelings, thoughts, and actions in problem situations. We assume that stresses during periods of developmental crisis act as precipitants for depressive symptoms in children who lack the competence to resolve developmental challenges successfully (Waters and Sroufe, 1983; Cicchetti and Schneider-Rosen, 1986).

Behaviors are easier to observe and monitor than thoughts. We first build behavioral success and later examine the child's thoughts and beliefs about problem situations. Younger patients must be taught to label and to gauge the intensity of feelings *before* considering associated automatic thoughts.

We train children and families to increase social competence in solving daily problems (Phillips, 1985). Depressed children and adults expect life to bring negative events, and see these events as their own fault (internal), unchanging (stable), and pervasive (global) (Seligman et al, 1984; Kaslow et al, unpublished manuscript; Kaslow et al, 1984). They also lack the ability to generate solutions to interpersonal problems (Sacco and Graves, 1984) and to evaluate the cost and effectiveness of various solutions (Levenson, 1974; Rotheram and Trautman, 1986). These deficits are addressed by developing social competence.

Strategies for effective social interaction, and their requisite cognitive, behavioral, and emotional skills, are outlined in Table 1 (Rotheram, 1980). Each skill outlined must be acquired by adolescents and their families in order to deal effectively with day-to-day life problems. The social adjustment of children and

Table 1. Model for social interaction process with associated prerequisite cognitive, behavioral, and emotional responses for effective interpersonal style*

Model of Strategy for Social Interactions	Adaptive Skills		
	Cognitive	Behavioral	Emotional
1. Problem orientation	1. Social inferential ability	1. Social inferential ability	1. Self-monitoring of internal discomfort
2. Negative emotional response	2. Labeling of negative emotion (e.g., anxiety, depression, excitement) and assessing intensity of response	2. Ability to control behavioral response	2. Labeling of negative emotion (e.g., anxiety, depression, excitement) and assessing intensity of response
3. Cope with negative emotional response	3. Identify covert self-punishment, catastrophic thinking; intervene with coping self-talk, self-reinforcement	3. Control of nonverbal responses, use of time out	3. Relax physiologically
4. Problem solve (a) clarify goal (b) generate alternatives (c) evaluate and select alternative	4. (a) state one goal in one sentence (b) divergent thinking (c) social inferential ability to assess realistic consequences of behavior	4. (a) direct requests, refusals, (b) behavioral repertoire to implement any alternative	4. Assessment and ability to control new emotional states that arise

Table 1. Model for social interaction process with associated prerequisite cognitive, behavioral, and emotional responses for effective interpersonal style* *(continued)*

Model of Strategy for Social Interactions	Adaptive Skills		
	Cognitive	Behavioral	Emotional
5. Respond behaviorally	5. Belief you have right to be assertive, self-esteem in ability to respond	5. Verbal skill (disclosures, I statements, requests, refusals), nonverbal skills (eye contact, voice tone, latency level, facial expression)	5. Relaxation techniques
6. Evaluate	6. Self-reinforce, goal set	6. Request feedback from environment	6. Monitor and assess internal state

*Reprinted with permission from Rotheram MJ: Social skills training with elementary school and high school students, in Social Skills throughout the Lifespan. Edited by Rathjen D, Foreyt J. New York, Pergamon Books Ltd., 1980 adolescents has been shown to be related to each of the components of this model, although the components have not been fully evaluated in depressed children. For example, the acquisition of social inferential ability (that is, the ability to empathize) is related to altrustic behavior (Hartup, 1970; Rothenberg, 1970) peer popularity, and cognitive problem-solving ability in children (Sobol, 1974) and adolescents (Platt and Spivack, 1972). Early findings on the relationship of social inferential ability to adjustment were unclear (Schantz, 1975), until the interaction of cognitive and behavioral skills was examined (Barrett and Yarrow, 1977; Dodge et al, 1987). Social inferential ability apparently influences prosocial behavior only if the child already has the ability to act assertively. In other words, understanding how others felt made a difference only for those who could act upon that understanding. Similarly, studies which focused on children's social (Oden and Asher, 1977; Rucker and Vincenzo, 1970) or cognitive skills (McChure, 1975) found that initial gains were not maintained. However, when a process of thinking, feeling, and acting assertively is taught, gains are maintained at follow-up (Rotheram et al, 1982; Robin, 1981; Sarason and Sarason, 1981). All these studies were conducted in nonclinical samples.

Few data support the integration of cognitive and behavioral skills in clinical populations of children (Shaffer, 1984), but the recommendation for such integration is consistently made, especially with reference to depressed children and adolescents (Emery et al, 1983; Di Giuseppi, 1981). Outcome studies of behavioral interventions with depressed children (single case studies) support the use of behavioral interventions (Matson, 1982; Frame et al, 1982; Calpin and Kornblith, 1978; Calpin and Cinciprini, 1978; Matson et al, 1980), but the authors give no indication of generalized improvement beyond the treatment setting or of elimination of the depressive disorder.

Two studies have examined the relative efficacy of cognitive and behavioral interventions with children. Coats and Reynolds (unpublished manuscript) found that a combination of cognitive and behavioral skills training exceeded a wait list control in decreasing adolescents' depression. In a study of depressed fifth and sixth graders, Butler and colleagues (1980) found that children who were trained to role-play problem-solving solutions were less depressed and better adjusted in the classroom than children who were taught cognitive restructuring or who received attention control or no treatment. No follow-up data were provided. These studies suggest the importance of developmental differences to the design of treatment interventions. Since fifth and sixth graders are very concrete in their cognitive abilities, it might be expected that the concrete behavioral role-playing techniques would be more effective than cognitive restructuring; whereas, in adolescents, cognitive techniques might be equally effective. The integration of cognitive and behavioral components may be superior to either component, and needs to be tested.

3. *Therapy with children and adolescents must include the family and others from the child's network.* Cognitive therapy is usually conducted as individual therapy, although group work has also been described (see Chapter 28 in this volume). Beck and co-workers (1979) have pointed out the advantages of utilizing others in therapy with adult patients, especially for severely depressed individuals and those with interpersonal difficulties. We believe cognitive therapy with children and adolescents must include members of the child's interpersonal network, especially his or her family.

Children's thoughts and behavior patterns evolve in a social context and are influenced by that context (Bandura, 1977). Mothers (but not fathers) and their children appear to share depressive feelings and attributional style for negative events (Seligman and Peterson, 1986). Outcome studies of therapy consistently show that parental participation (and especially fathers' participation) contributes to successful outcome (Rutter, 1972; Shaffer, 1984; Reisinger et al, 1976; Strain et al, 1981; D'Angelo and Walsh, 1967; Gluck et al, 1964). Outcome of behavioral parent-training programs is enhanced by focusing on parental isolation, depression, and marital difficulties (Greist et al, 1979).

There are problems in the families of depressed and suicidal children which are not based on cognitive distortions. For example, a foreign-born mother and her Americanized daughter may quarrel about dating and "hanging out" after school. This conflict is not based on cognitive distortion. It needs to be relabelled as the natural consequence of immigration and acculturation. By relabelling, the family may employ its coping skills to resolve specific conflicts in a broader context. Parent and child can acknowledge that they simply have different life experiences and roles, and can profit from one another's experience.

4. *Problems must be examined in the context of development.* Children and adolescents are faced with new developmental challenges as their biological, psychological, social, and cognitive resources shift throughout childhood (Erikson, 1948). Families also evolve through developmental phases (Combrink-Graham, 1985). Developmental changes affect the behavioral, cognitive, and affective expression of depressive symptoms, and the nature of the unresolved parent–child difficulties.

Very young children respond to pain and frustration with anger but without a sense of hopelessness, while children six to nine begin to evince shame, guilt, low self-esteem, excessive self-criticism, and masochistic behavior (Carlson and Garber, 1986; Izard and Schwartz, 1986). Depressive symptoms of middle childhood are reflected in social isolation, behavior problems at school, and separation anxiety. In adolescence depression may be reflected in drug and alcohol abuse, eating disorders, and antisocial behavior as well as the typical vegetative, cognitive, and psychological symptoms of adulthood (Chambers et al, 1985). These shifts in emotions reflect changes in children's cognitive capacity to process their world.

Kendall (1981) argues that children lack thinking skills, rather than have defective thinking styles. Therefore, interventions with children should be aimed at skill building, not just remediation. Research with nondepressed children has demonstrated the importance of different cognitive skills at different ages. Behavioral adjustment of children in middle childhood is more related to the ability to generate alternative problem solutions, whereas in adolescents the ability to evaluate the costs and benefits of alternatives (means–ends thinking) is more salient (Spivack et al, 1976).

The problems of depressed children also depend on the family's developmental stage. From middle childhood on, parents are freer to pursue activities and interests outside the home and are less focused on family intimacy issues. In adolescence, their children assume increasing responsibilities outside of the family and focus more and more attention on peer relationships (Peterson and Hamburg, 1986). These shifts provide a developmental context for family problems. For example, a mother who focuses solely on her family may experience great benefits while her children are young. As the children grow older and the mother fails to expand her interests and relationships, overwhelming parent–adolescent conflicts may emerge. The therapist must recognize and assess the congruence or compatibility of the family members' developmental tasks.

OVERVIEW OF TREATMENT STRATEGY

These assumptions lead us to develop a cognitive–behavioral intervention program that has four main components: 1) identification of child and family problems and strengths and a focus on idealistic positivism; 2) labeling and assessing feelings; 3) interpersonal problem solving; and 4) altering dysfunctional thoughts and attributional styles. Table 2 outlines the stages of therapy in a hypothetical 15-session treatment program. The therapist need not carry on for 15 sessions, nor limit himself or herself to 15 sessions. We sometimes find it useful to alternate family and individual adolescent sessions, and sometimes conduct family sessions only. This depends on the types of problems presented and the teen's preference. Without disrupting a confidential relationship, one can use information gathered in the individual session in the family session, and vice versa.

Therapist's role. Cognitive–behavioral therapists have generally ignored the therapeutic process and relationship in outlining their treatment techniques (Rotheram, 1982). A "supershrink" for children (Ricks, 1974; Kolvin et al, 1981) and adults (Slaney, 1978) has been characterized as active, assertive, directive, explanatory, responsive, and one who supports autonomy, emphasizes skills training, utilizes outside resources (for example, tutors), and structures the treatment. With children, the therapist's age, sex, race, religion, experience, and theoretical orientation make little difference (Parloff et al, 1979), nor is there an interaction between diagnosis and therapeutic outcome (Shaffer, 1984).

In addition to emulating the "supershrink," the cognitive–behavior therapist should:

1. *Think strategically.* Therapy is a problem-solving activity. If one intervention is not effective, try another. There are many routes to reach the same goal. For example, after identifying a cognitive distortion, a therapist may have the patient: 1) set her wrist watch alarm and self-reward for every three-minute period in which she did not engage in the distortion; 2) say, "Stop," each time the thought occurs; 3) read alternative, useful thoughts from a 3×5 index card hourly; 4) join in a contest with a friend to practice disputing dysfunctional thoughts; or 5) make a contract that each time the dysfunctional thoughts occur, the patient will ask mother for a compliment—"What do you like about me?" Each strategy attempts to change the existing reward contingencies for the dysfunctional thought. The possible strategies are endless.

2. *Be positive.* The therapeutic relationship is a model of the relationship the therapist hopes the family will reestablish. This is one in which positive interactions occur repeatedly, while negative interchanges are seen as temporary and serve as cues for identifying and resolving problems. It is more effective to focus on an adolescent's strengths than on his or her deficits (Liberman et al, 1973). For example, instead of saying, "You are a bum! Get off your duff and study," a parent could be taught to say, "You obviously have high potential and I would like to see you reach your potential. What can we do to help you study more effectively?" The therapist should develop skills in finding the positives in an

apparently negative situation. For example, if the adolescent says he or she didn't do the homework assignment, he or she is directed to write or discuss the homework in the session, and the therapist finds a way to compliment the patient; for example, "No wonder you didn't write your homework. You were so busy practicing that conversation we rehearsed there was no time left. Good going!"

3. *Be a model of what you are trying to change in the child or family.* The interactions between therapist and family should serve as examples of the style which one hopes will develop outside the session. The therapist may disclose positive events in her or his life, mention solutions she or he has found to daily problems, and demonstrate coping self-instructional talk (for example, "Kristie, I felt terrible after our last session. I said to myself, 'What a lousy therapist! You argued with your patient and there was no reason for that.' Then I remembered, 'Everybody makes mistakes. You can talk to Kristie next time and we can work things out.' That made me feel better. How did you feel about our last session?"). The family will copy the therapist's social skills for better or worse.

4. *Establish clear roles.* The therapist a) defines the problem so that the strengths of the family are highlighted and the existing reward contingencies of the problem are clear; b) teaches problem solving and interpersonal skills; c) provides positive and negative feedback to the family; d) develops a positive relationship with the family; and e) models interpersonal skills. The patient or family is asked a) to fully disclose their problems, thoughts, and feelings; b) to want to change one or more of these problems; c) to attend sessions; d) to share responsibility for problem resolution with the therapist; e) to provide positive and negative feedback to the therapist; and f) not to engage in suicidal behavior.

5. *Be concrete.* A discrete problem lends itself to concrete intervention strategies. Ask for specific examples: for example, "What do you mean Jerry never listens to you? When was the last time he didn't listen? What did you say? What did he do?" The therapist uses cues, such as tokens and flash cards, to punctuate the intervention. For example, the family can hand one another poker chips each time they give or receive compliments. Specific, simple homework assignments carry the learning program outside the therapist's office.

Step 1: Assessment and Positivity

There are two goals in assessing the family: to obtain information on the individual's biological, psychological, and social resources and deficits, and to clarify family communication patterns. These goals are implemented in an atmosphere which helps the family to identify and acknowledge its positive attributes.

Interviewing the adolescent first conveys a message that the therapist is interested in *the adolescent's point of view.* What are his or her beliefs about self, the world (particularly the family), and the future? The parents' view of the child's and family's problems and their goals for treatment are reviewed next. The therapist asks, "Why do you bring your child now? What do you want me to do?" Since the child's problems have not developed in a vacuum, it is important to review systematically the parents' difficulties, particularly depression, alcohol and drug abuse, and the marital relationship. The parents may have identified their child as having a problem, but is he or she the one, or the only one, who needs treatment? Our bias is clearly that adolescent problems exist in a family context, and that change will occur most quickly if the entire family is involved.

Table 2. Stages of Therapy

Session	Skill	Context	Task	Homework
1,2 family	Positivity: self-reward, reinforce others; identify problems	Chief complaint, recent and past history, precipitating events	5 self positives; 5 family rewards; build family problem hierarchy	Chart successes with low level problems
3 family	Interpersonal problem solving (IPS): recognize problems, set goals	Problem list; parent–child communication	Starting with easy problems, resolve problems	Chart problem situations; monitor feelings; caring days
4,5 teen	IPS: generate alternative behaviors and thoughts	Parent–child communication	Build teen problem list	Chart problems, set goals, generate alternatives
6 family	IPS: evaluate consequences	Check-up: parent–child communication; start peer relations	Assess consistency of evaluations of family interactions; adult view of peer relations	Chart problems; generate alternatives to problems
7,8 teen	IPS: evaluate consequences	Peer relations	Teen's view of peer relations; teacher and peer perceptions; male/female relations	Chart problems; evaluate means–ends– consequences of actions

Table 2. Stages of Therapy (*continued*)

Session	Skill	Context	Task	Homework
9 family	IPS: integration of steps	Parent–parent communication	Present problem situation for family to solve	Chart problems, goals, alternatives, consequences
10,11,12 teen	Attributions: beliefs, self-talk	Problem list: peers, parents, new situations	Build dysfunctional beliefs list; practice self-talk; role-play self-talk in problem situations	Chart situations, dysfunctional beliefs, self-talk, success
13,14 family	Attributions: self-talk	Problem list; set future goals	Identify parents' dysfunctional beliefs; role-play problem sequence from identification to resolution	Chart problems, successes, self-talk
15 family	Summary and evaluation; future goals	Review goals; set future goals	Review successes; discuss future problems and how to solve problems	List all past successes

Discrepancies between the adolescent's and parents' reports inevitably arise and may be resolved by reinterviewing the adolescent; for example, "Your parents mentioned you stay in your room all evening and have a 'Do not disturb' sign on your door. Tell me more about that." A joint interview with parents and teen is also useful for clarifying discrepancies, but riskier because another quarrel or parental lecture may ensue. The therapist simply states, "You've all given me a lot of important information but there are some different points of view that we'll begin to discuss next time. An important part of cognitive therapy is communication, and that begins with being able to understand the other's point of view, even if you don't agree with it. We'll be working on this together."

The quality of parent–child and parent–parent relations may be observed during a joint interview. Where do people sit, who talks for whom, and who cuts whom off? We have used family tasks to assess family social interaction (for example, families were asked to decide how to spend $200 on a weekend together), and found that families of adolescent suicide attempters exchanged few positive rewards, made nonspecific plans, and either allowed one child to wield undue power, or allowed the children no input whatsoever (Rotheram, unpublished manuscript).

In the initial interview, the therapist begins to build a positive therapeutic relationship and asks family members to start identifying positive things about themselves; for example, "Tell me three good things about yourself and three good things about your family." Any effort to answer this question receives praise. If the adolescent cannot think of anything, we prompt him or her by giving compliments. The same strategy is true for the parents, who are often stumped when asked to say three positive things about their child. The family might be given a first homework assignment of repeating these attributes at home, or thinking of a new one each day. The therapist should actively model positivity by giving compliments in this and every session—"I like your shirt." "This information you're giving me is terrific! Really helpful!" This aspect of treatment is fun, and most sessions include a good deal of joking.

Step Two: Developing a List of Problems and Strengths

The written problem list should include problems big and small, identified by the adolescent, parents, siblings, teachers, therapist, and any other available informants. The adolescent need not agree with all the problems on the list; these can be labeled as to source. The list of strengths includes positives mentioned by adolescent or parent, and things 'ruled out' during the course of interview. Table 3 presents a sample problem/strengths list. Give a copy of the list to the family to take home and hang up in a place accessible to all, or give each a copy.

The problem list is often an eye opener for adolescents, who tend to see themselves as having one big, amorphous problem, rather than a few, often small, discrete ones. The list is useful, too, for the therapist because one problem may stand out as needing immediate attention or as being quickly solvable, which will bring early success to the therapy.

While the initial problem list is somewhat general (for example, "depressed all the time"), the therapist will help clarify the frequency, intensity, circumstances, and response of others to each problem situation. Transforming global attributions into specific, concrete, and modifiable states is one of the most

Table 3. A Problem List

Name: Bill D. Age: 14	
Problems	Strengths/positives
1. depressed all the time	1. pretty smart
2. sometimes think of killing myself	2. have two good friends
3. no girlfriend	3. sister o.k.
4. parents: "They'd dance on my grave"	4. dad brought me for help when I said I was suicidal
5. father has heart condition	5. Mom working part time
6. father unemployed	6. Bill wants to talk
7. maternal grandmother: "We all hate her"; prefers granddaughters; rich but cheap	7. parents concerned and interested in family therapy
8. had a fight in school yesterday	8. no really terrible teachers this year
9. worried about school	
10. Bill doesn't want to attend any family sessions	
11. headaches every other day	

powerful aspects of a behavioral approach. Negative global perceptions are addressed through cognitive–behavioral technology. See further discussion under steps 3 and 4.

In conducting the initial interview, the therapist does not want to reinforce the family's problems and dysfunctional beliefs and moods by an overly detailed examination of every symptom. A list of strengths emphasizes from the beginning that the adolescent is successful in many areas even if he or she is reluctant to say so. The list promotes a sense of well-being and at the same time clarifies for therapist and family what is and is not a problem. Adolescents (and, often, their parents) are not very good at organizing problems and putting them into perspective and will readily conclude, "Oh God! I didn't know I had so many problems. The doctor thinks I'm crazy. It's hopeless." Instead, we want the adolescent to leave the office feeling better about himself ("At least I'm passing three subjects. And I can talk to Aunt Lila when Mom won't listen") and better about the therapist ("She's not bad, for a shrink. Maybe she can help me"). The therapist promotes the belief that the teen's problems are not insurmountable, that the therapist will take *action* to help him or her feel better. By the end of therapy the adolescent will have acquired skills for solving his or her own problems. Early therapeutic contact emphasizes the collaborative relationship and the greater experience of the "teacher–therapist."

Step 3: Identifying Feelings—The Feeling Thermometer (SUDS):

Adolescents, particularly younger adolescents, have difficulty identifying their feelings and automatic thoughts. When asked why they took an overdose, for example, many adolescents reply, "I don't know." This reply generally reflects not a lack of cooperation, but a real confusion about feelings and motives at the time of the overdose, difficulty verbalizing these feelings and motives, and the cognitive complexity of expressing multiple, sometimes contradictory, ideas and feelings.

We teach our patients how to identify feelings, measure their intensity, and clarify contradictions, using the "feeling thermometer" or "Subjective Units of Distress Scale" (SUDS) (Wolpe, 1958). The feeling thermometer is simply a scale marked 0 to 100, on which 100 represents the most uncomfortable feeling one can remember, and 0 represents one's most comfortable memory, a time free of trouble. For each feeling, the situational context is identified as graphically as possible. In addition, the feeling's physical context should also be identified; for example, "How did your body feel in that situation? Where do you get tense?" An example of a feeling thermometer is given in Table 4.

Examples at the extreme ends of the scale are readily identified, but adolescents have difficulty filling in the middle range; that is, situations which were somewhat upsetting, but not the worst. The purpose of the scale is to identify feelings and recognize their strength vis-à-vis other life problems. Each teen's SUDS scale is subjective and unique to the individual. A situation which may be a "20" for one person may be an "80" for another. Also, each teen has a

Table 4. SUDS (Feeling Thermometer)

Name: Paula G. Age: 15		
(worst)	100	when my father hit me for staying out late
	90	
	87	when mom and dad fight (headache, tired)
	80	Ray quit me for another girl
	72	Ray's new girlfriend said nasty things, we almost fought
	70	
	60	math final exam (stomach queasy)
	55	Mom nagging me about the dishes and my room
	50	
	40	math tests
	39	getting up in front of class to give a speech (hands shake)
(not bad, can	30	
can handle it)	20	
	18	returning spoiled milk to the grocery
	10	
	1	the second time I saw Johnnie; summer camp
(best)	0	the first time I saw Johnnie from 'Menudo' (a rock group)

unique threshold for problem intervention; that is, situations which fall below 30 or 40 on the scale may require no intervention. It is important to discuss low-SUDS situations, however, as examples of successful coping and problem solving. The goal of therapy will be to use alternative thoughts and behaviors to reduce SUDS to less than the teen's threshold. Most of a 45-minute session will typically be required to develop a feeling thermometer. The adolescent takes home a copy. A homework assignment might be to add other problem situations to the SUDS scale, or to monitor SUDS as new situations arise during the week. "SUDS" should become part of the child and family's everyday vocabulary.

Step 4: Identifying Automatic Thoughts, Goals, Alternative Thoughts, and Alternative Behaviors

We use the thought and action sheet to examine problem situations recorded on the feeling thermometer and new problem situations which arise during the course of therapy. This sheet is derived from Beck's Dysfunctional Thought Record (Beck et al, 1979). Problem solving is conducted by breaking each problem situation into components in a systematic fashion: describe the problem and its associated feelings; identify automatic thoughts; list goals for the situation (what would be a good outcome?); generate, evaluate, and test alternative thoughts and behaviors; and, finally, reassess the situation: Have the goals been met? If not, test second-choice alternatives.

A sample thought and action sheet is shown in Table 5. The problem is described briefly, and its associated feelings and their strength (SUDS) measured in relation to other situations on the feeling thermometer. A good homework assignment is to have the adolescent or family rate the SUDS of three problem-feeling situations over the course of the next week.

Next, identify the automatic thoughts that occurred in the problem situation. Automatic thoughts are negative, extreme, and "all or nothing" in quality; for example, "I'll never pass this course," "I hate my mother," "I'm a terrible daughter," "I'm a failure," and so forth. Younger adolescents have difficulty identifying such thoughts, and often need to be given examples at first. One might say, "Another girl I know thought, 'I'll never get another boyfriend now. All my friends will hate me.' Did you think something like that?" Often alternative thoughts and behaviors are mixed in with automatic thoughts when the adolescent is first learning. For example, "I'll punch that guy out" is an alternative thought/behavior (albeit not a very adaptive one!) and should be written in the alternative section and discussed later.

Next, the therapist inquires about goals. Ideally, how would the adolescent or family like the problem situation to be resolved? For example, is the teen's goal: a) simply to feel less angry, b) to never argue with Mom again, c) to argue less often, or d) to have Mom acknowledge how you feel, even if she doesn't let you do everything you want? Adolescents are often surprisingly modest and reasonable in their goals, and the solution may be obvious and simple.

Alternative thoughts and behaviors are the means to achieving goals. Alternative thoughts modify the extremes of automatic thoughts, and are more reasonable and rational; they take a middle ground; for example, "I got an F on this exam, but I really didn't study very much, and I had a cold that day. Failing one test doesn't mean you fail the whole course." Alternative behaviors are actions one can take to change a situation; for example, asking for extra help

Table 5. Thought and Action Sheet

Name: Jim R.   Age: 17   Date: 5/1/86

Event: Playing guitar in the basement with Rob and Eddie. Trying to make up a new song. They're just messing around, not serious. Drank some beer.

Feelings/emotions (rate strength 0–100): disappointed (60), discouraged (50), tired (82), depressed (75)

Automatic thoughts: I can't talk to them; I'm dead; I don't feel like doing anything anymore

Behaviors (what happened next?): Told them I wanted to watch football so I wouldn't have to hang out with them anymore; they left; want to sleep.

Goals (desired outcomes): Make up a new tune; practice with Rob and Eddie; tell them what I want to do; talk to them, just an easy conversation

Alternative thoughts: When Eddie doesn't talk, it's harder for me to talk; beer makes me feel worse; when things don't work out the way I want them to, I often feel tired; I made up a song last week, it was pretty good

Alternative behaviors: Tell them I never want to see them again; tell them off; tell them I want to really practice for an hour, then we can hang out someplace; find some new guys to play with; quit guitar

Costs and benefits (advantages/disadvantages): They're the best friends I've got!; they might not listen; a new bass player would improve the band—Rob's not very good and not motivated

Plan of action, final outcome: Practice again on Wednesday night; played my new tune, Eddie's a great drummer; only a little depressed (40), not tired at all, Eddie still doesn't talk much

---

from the teacher, changing teachers, or changing schools. Because alternative behaviors are more readily generated than alternative thoughts, we tend to discuss interpersonal problem-solving, assertiveness skills, and behavioral rehearsal, *before* self-attributions in our work with young people. First the adolescent does something new, then she learns to talk to herself about the achievement (or failure).

The ability to generate many alternative thoughts and behaviors is an important prerequisite of problem solving. The therapist must be careful to accept any and all alternatives, regardless of their feasibility or quality, and should insist that family members do the same. Have one member write them all down, ask for more, and make suggestions of your own (for example, "Yes, you could say to youself, 'I hate that guy!'; and you could kick your teacher in the shin. Think of some more things. What about a lawsuit for educational malpractice? Or a nice long vacation in Tahiti?"). Suggested alternatives should be acceptable to the family, but not necessarily possible. Generating alternatives is fun, as therapist and family think of wacky things to do, think, or say.

Alternative thoughts and behaviors have their advantages and disadvantages, which may be evaluated in a variety of ways; for example, by developing a list of pros and cons; role-playing; or by gathering information. A hierarchy of alternative behaviors can be developed and tried sequentially. For example, a 16-year-old boy felt depressed and suicidal after a drinking companion threw his radio into the park lake. We developed a list of solutions to be tried, starting with the easiest and working up to the most complicated: 1) ask him to replace the radio; 2) ask mutual friends to speak to him; 3) call his father; 4) ask my father to speak to his father; 5) go to small claims court. Over a period of two or three weeks we rehearsed conversations for each alternative, discussed his experiences in implementing them, and developed many alternative thoughts, including, "Who cares about a lowlife who hangs out in the park?" and "When I have a problem there are steps I can take to solve it." This approach has the advantage of supporting the adolescent as he or she tests out new skills learned during the session.

Step 5: Changing Behaviors and Cognitions: Evaluating Consequences and Self-Attributions

Interpersonal problem solving is developed in both individual and family sessions. When the adolescent identifies a problem which is interpersonal in nature, we ask for detailed information (what did she say, what did you say?), discuss the patient's goals in the situation, and then rehearse or role-play the situation in the session. We teach the adolescent how to be appropriately assertive and how to handle negativity from others (Rotheram, 1980). In the family sessions, we ask family members to restate what another member has said before replying, to give positive statements to one another, and to plan family activities.

We teach family members to use coping self-instructional thought to alter negative self-attributions. For example, when mother and daughter argue, the daughter may think, "I'm a bad daughter"; "We'll never stop arguing"; and I'm also a lousy friend, a poor student, and lazy" (internal, stable, and global attributions). One must not assume that attributions will automatically change as behavior changes; we have frequently observed, for example, that a mother and daughter will continue to say, "We never talk to each other," after successfully completing three five-minute conversations given as a homework assignment.

Coping, self-instructional thought may take the form of flashcards (for example, "Give yourself a compliment"; "If you start to get angry, take three deep breaths and say, 'I can handle this if I take it easy'") or a list of instructions for crisis situations. One of us treated a girl who was terrified that her former stepfather, who had just been released from jail, would try to break into the house, beat her mother, and steal their money. Although the mother was not particularly worried, they prepared a list of things to do if he came when the girl was home alone: Stay calm, repeat, "I can handle this"; don't unlock the door; call the neighbor; call the police; go down the fire escape. While most of this list consists of behaviors, it functioned as coping self-instruction since she carried it wherever she went and reviewed it many times daily, with relief of anxiety. Coping, self-instructional thought increases the adolescent's personal efficacy; that is, it teaches the teen that he or she can make good things happen and stop bad things from happening, or at least modify the impact of negative events.

THE STYLE OF COGNITIVE THERAPY WITH CHILDREN AND ADOLESCENTS

Cognitive therapy with children and adolescents is fast-paced, with much give and take between adolescent, parents, and therapist. Silences are avoided—if the patient will not or cannot talk, the therapist keeps the conversation going. We make jokes and do some gentle teasing. We avoid intense displays of negative emotion—tears and so forth. Understanding how the adolescent feels and letting him express himself are fine, but "getting out feelings," as the jargon goes, is not in itself therapeutic. Identifying the dysfunctional behaviors and thoughts that promote those feelings is the therapeutic measure.

Homework assignments are an integral part of cognitive therapy with adolescents. Assignments force the family to actively participate in their own treatment program. They can take many forms: For example, writing components of the thought and action sheet; gathering information to support or refute automatic thoughts; or testing out new skills learned during the session. Family homework assignments include giving one another compliments, "caring days" (that is, family members take turns being taken care of and indulged; Mother's Day need not happen just once a year), and mother–daughter activities.

The following case example illustrates the content of a treatment session in which dysfunctional attributions are addressed.

Tony is an 11-year-old who was brought in by his mother because of suicidal threats. He had recently begun to refuse to attend school, and teachers had noted a fall-off in classroom attention and in the quality of his work. When asked what problems he was currently having, he listed two:

1. I can't get along with my mother; she's always yelling at me.
2. I'm stupid, or I think I'm stupid.

Tony went on to describe depressive hallucinations—a man's voice inside his head ("Maybe it's my conscience") which sometimes spoke roughly, saying, "Go ahead and kill yourself," and sometimes in a falsely 'nice' way, saying "So what if one person likes you. That don't mean nothing."

Here we see the absolute quality of automatic thoughts (she *always* yells; I *am* stupid) and one example of irrationality which Beck has called 'disqualifying the positive' (even if one person likes me, nobody likes me). We also see the beginning of an alternative thought ("or I think I'm stupid"). The therapist used this material to *collect evidence* and *generate alternative thoughts*.

Therapist: Tony, you said one of your problems is you're stupid.
Patient: Yes, I am.
T: (T does not attempt to refute this.) When you think, "I am stupid," how do you feel?
P: Bad. And sad.
T: Uh huh. And what's your SUDS when you feel like that?
P: 100.
T: Wow. The worst. (Siding with the patient) I guess my SUDS would be 100, too, if I believed I was stupid. (Labeling the thought) "I'm stupid" is an automatic thought. It's negative and absolute. Let's talk about it and see if we can figure out if it's true.
P: It is true.

T: Well, you may be right. But I don't know you very well yet so I'm just not sure. Let's gather some facts about it.

P: What kind of facts?

T: Well, you said, "I'm stupid, or I think I'm stupid." What made you say that?

P: The social worker told me it's not that I *am* stupid but that I think I am.

T: Well, which is it?

P: I'm not sure.

T: Good, then we'll try to figure it out together. (Getting specific) Now think of a situation that made you think, "I'm stupid."

P: When me and my mom argued yesterday because I forgot to take out the garbage.

T: Good. (Siding with the patient first) Now, I suppose there are things your mother does that make you angry?

P: Yeah, she yells at me all the time, for nothing.

T: (Taking the other's point of view) And what's one thing that you do that makes her angry?

P: If I forget things she tells me to do.

T: And then what happens?

P: She screams at me. She calls me stupid.

T: (Therapist does *not* empathize with this. The boy feels bad enough. Don't stress the negative.) Gotcha. Now, what about others. Does anyone else call you stupid? What about teachers?

P: They think I am.

T: They do? Well, has any teacher said so recently?

P: No.

T: And do any of your teachers think you're smart?

P: Well . . . (Shows therapist a "poem" which describes his deep unhappiness and yearning for father, who is in jail. A teacher has written a long note in the margin.)

T: (Positivity) Your poetry teacher wrote that this is beautifully written, that she wants you to write more, and says you may grow up to be a writer like she is. I suppose you were pleased by these comments?

P: Yes.

T: (Compliments) Well you should be. I agree it's beautifully written. Now one other thing. While I was talking to the social worker, you were playing with G.I. Joe. Were you thinking, "I'm stupid"?

P: No, I wasn't thinking about it.

T: (Summary, feedback) Fine. So now we have some facts. I'll summarize them and you tell me if I've got them correctly. You think, "I'm stupid," when you and your mom argue. But you don't think this all the time. Your mom says, "You're stupid," when she gets mad. No teacher has said this, but it's possible some think it; we just don't know. One teacher thinks you write well. And so do I. Did I get the facts right?

P: Yes.

T: So now let's make up an alternative thought that takes the facts into account. One might be, "When my mom and I argue I feel stupid. But I don't think that way all the time. And I'm a good writer."

P: But I'm only in the sixth grade!

T: (Turning a possible refutation into a positive) An excellent addition! Thank you. We should say, "I'm a good writer for a sixth grader." Is that right?

P: Yeah!

T: Great. Now you say the whole thing. (He does so.) You got it! Now what's your SUDS?

P: Maybe 65?

T: Good. Sixty-five is better than 100. We'll put your alternative thought on a 3×5 card and you keep it. And five times each day I want you to pull the card out of your pocket and read it, say, when you eat and when you go to the bathroom. Can you do it?

P: Yep.

T: You did good work today.

This boy's comments about his mother's angry criticism make it clear that cognitive–behavior therapy with the child alone would be insufficient. The mother was herself quite depressed and needed help in developing a more positive, effective parenting style.

SPECIAL POPULATION: SUICIDE ATTEMPTERS

While the principles outlined above are applicable to a variety of adolescent and family problems, the suicidal and suicide-attempting adolescent presents some unique problems for the cognitive therapist. First, it is very often the case that neither the adolescent nor the parents are motivated for treatment (Trautman, 1986a, 1986b). The family comes to the hospital for emergency care and goes away with a psychiatric follow-up appointment for which it did not ask. Suicidal crises (and parental anxiety) often defuse as quickly as they blow up. The families of adolescent suicide attempters are highly dysfunctional; chronic marital and parent–child conflict are common (Trautman and Shaffer, 1984). The therapist must be very active in identifying the immediate precipitants of the crisis and the longer-standing conflicts and problems, and must point out that the adolescent attempter is at very high risk for further attempts. New and better ways must be found to solve family problems or a suicidal crisis will recur.

In our experience, it is more critical to motivate the parents for treatment than the adolescent, since much can be accomplished around family communication and problem solving without the adolescent's participation. On the other hand, if the parents are unmotivated but the adolescent agrees to attend, they overtly or covertly will sabotage the treatment. Parents will feel they are being criticized and their authority undermined. The adolescent is unable to solve family problems on his or her own.

When the parents cannot be engaged, it is better for the therapist to restate their decision in a positive light and discharge them, offering future help. For example, "I feel good that Judy isn't suicidal now although my experience tells me that there's a high probability her problems will recur and that she's at risk for hurting herself again. You know your family better than I, and you have to do what you think is best. If problems do come up again, will one of you call me? I'll be glad to try to help." Of course, an adolescent can be hospitalized without parental consent if a physician believes she or he may be a danger to self or others.

Second, we ask the adolescent to make a commitment to no further suicide attempts, and to promise to tell us if he or she again thinks about suicide. This commitment, which includes steps the adolescent will take and individuals he or she will turn to should suicidal feelings recur, is written as a contract and sealed with a handshake (Rotheram, 1987). The adolescent who cannot make such a commitment needs to be hospitalized. With this commitment and parental cooperation to remove pills and weapons and to remain with the adolescent 24 hours a day (at least initially), the psychiatrist can feel confident about releasing the patient for outpatient care. Such contracts are equally useful in an inpatient setting. A psychotic adolescent (for example, one hearing voices telling him to kill himself) cannot be expected to comply with such a contract. This is an absolute indication for hospitalization.

The suicide attempt should become the first problem on the patient's problem list. Beck's "reasons for living and dying" technique (Beck et al, 1979) is useful at the beginning of treatment with adolescents. If the patient has difficulty thinking of reasons for living, we suggest reasons so that the first list is at least as long as the second. If the patient is unable to generate or endorse reasons for living, the clinician should consider hospitalization.

Similarly, we find it useful to explore in some detail the adolescent's several and often contradictory motives for making the suicide attempt. These might include wanting to die, not wanting to die, hurting oneself, hurting Dad, sleeping for awhile to forget all the problems, getting out of the house, seeing who will visit in the hospital, and letting a girlfriend know how much she is loved. Preparing such a list teaches a useful cognitive lesson: That it is possible (and not crazy) to have goals which contradict one another. The next therapeutic step is to weigh the pros and cons of each motive, and then to choose actions and thoughts that are in the adolescent's best interest.

Because both the adolescent and family are prone to stop talking about the attempt after a week or two, it is important for the therapist to keep bringing it up. One can remind the teen that a new problem situation sounds like the one that led to the suicide attempt. Did it make him or her feel suicidal? If not, why not? What were the thoughts that led him or her to reach some other problem solution? Ask him to convince you and his parents that he's not going to take an overdose the next time his parents yell at him for coming in late. Occasionally parents can be overly vigilant, fearing a suicide plan behind every request to go out or to be alone. What are the parents' automatic thoughts, and can they generate rational alternatives? It is helpful to make a plan about how family members can reassure one another at home, and to practice this plan as a homework assignment. For example, the adolescent might agree to say every day before supper, "I'm feeling okay today" or "I started to have some suicidal thoughts so I telephoned the doctor," and parents might say, "You looked a little down to me before and I started to get my automatic thoughts, so I thought I better ask if you're okay."

SUMMARY AND CONCLUSIONS

In this chapter we have tried to illustrate the ways in which we have adapted cognitive and behavioral theories and therapies to the treatment of depressed and suicide-attempting adolescents. We believe that a lack of skills as well as dysfunctional thoughts and behaviors promote and maintain adolescent problems. Cognitive–behavior therapy with adolescents is active, concrete, and didactic. The adolescent and his or her family are guided through explicitly stated and rationally planned steps which teach intrapsychic and interpersonal problem-solving skills. This treatment is unlike traditional psychotherapies in that positivity within the family is actively taught, while unhappy feeling-states receive minimum attention. The therapist uses herself or himself actively to model positivity, problem-solving, and coping self-instructional thought. The treatment may be distinguished from cognitive therapy with adults in that cognition is approached from a developmental standpoint; behavior change is emphasized before change in self-attributions; and thoughts, feelings, and actions are considered to be interactive and inseparable. We have also tried to show that cognitive–behavior therapy with adolescents and their families is engaging and fun for both patients and therapist.

REFERENCES

Bandura A: Social Learning Theory. Englewood Cliffs, NJ, Prentice-Hall, 1977

Bandura A: The self system in reciprocal determinism. Am Psychol 1978; 33:344-358

Barrett DE, Yarrow MR: Prosocial behavior, social inferential ability and assertiveness in children. Child Dev 1977; 48:475-481

Beck AT, Rush AJ, Shaw BF, et al: Cognitive Therapy of Depression. New York, Guilford Press, 1979

Bent RJ, Putnam DG, Kiesler DJ, et al: Expectancies and characteristics of outpatient clients applying for services at a community mental health facility. J Consult Clin Psychol 1975; 43:280

Butler L, Miezitis S, Friedman R, et al: The effect of two school-based intervention programs on depressive symptoms in pre-adolescents. American Educational Research Journal 1980; 17:111-119

Calpin J. Cinciprini P: A multiple baseline analysis of social skills training in children. Paper presented at Midwestern Association for Behavioral Analysis, Chicago, 1978

Calpin J, Kornblith S: Training of aggressive children in conflict resolution skills. Paper presented at the meeting of the Association for the Advancement of Behavior Therapy, Chicago, 1978

Carlson G, Garber J: Developmental issues in the classification of depression in children, in Depression in Young People: Developmental and Clinical Perspectives. Edited by Rutter M, Izard C, Read P. New York, Guilford Press, 1986

Chambers WJ, Puig-Antich J, Hirsch M, et al: Assessment of affective disorders in children and adolescents by semi-structured interview. Arch Gen Psychiatry 1985; 42:696-702

Cicchetti D, Schneider-Rosen K: An organizational approach to childhood depression, in Depression in Young People: Developmental and Clinical Perspectives. Edited by Rutter M, Izard C, Read P. New York, Guilford Press, 1986

Combrinck-Graham L: A developmental model for family systems. Fam Process 1985; 24:139-150

Costello CG: Childhood depression, in Behavioral Assessment of Childhood Disorders. Edited by Mash EJ, Terdal L. New York, Guilford Press, 1981

D'Angelo RY, Walsh JF: An evaluation of various therapy approaches with lower socio-economic group children. J Psychol 1967; 67:59-64

DiGiuseppe RA: Cognitive therapy with children, in New Directions in Cognitive Therapy. Edited by Emery G, Hollon S, Bedrosian R. New York, Guilford Press, 1981

Dodge KA, Pettit GS, McClaskey CL, et al: Social competence in children. Monograph of the Society for Research in Child Development 1987; 51:1-81

Emery G, Bedrosian R, Garber J: Cognitive therapy, in Affective Disorders in Childhood and Adolescence—An Update. Edited by Cantwell DP. Jamaica, NY, Spectrum Publications, 1983

Erickson E: Identity, Youth and Crisis. New York, WW Norton, 1948

Ferster C: Animal behavior and mental illness. Psychological Record 1966; 16:345-356

Frame D, Matson J, Sonis W, et al: Behavioral treatment of depression in a prepubertal child. J Behav Ther Exp Psychiatry 1982; 13:239-243

Gluck MR, Tanner MM, Sullivan DF, et al: Follow-up evaluation of child guidance cases. Behav Res Ther 1964; 2:131-134

Greist J, Klein M, Eischen R, et al: Running as a treatment for depression. Compr Psychiatry 1979; 20:41-54

Haley J: Problem-Solving Therapy. San Francisco, Jossey-Bass, 1977

Hartup WW: Peer interaction and social organization, in Carmichael's Manual of Child Psychology, vol 2. Edited by Mussen P. New York, John Wiley, 1970

Heine RW, Trosman H: Initial expectations of the doctor–patient interaction as a factor in continuance in psychotherapy. Psychiatry 1973; 23:275-278

Heller K, Goldstein AP: Client dependency and therapist expectancy as relationship-maintaining variables in psychotherapy. J Consult Clin Psychol 1961; 25:371-375

Izard C, Schwartz C: Patterns of emotion in depression, in Depression in Young People: Developmental and Clinical Perspectives. Edited by Rutter M, Izard C, Read P. New York, Guilford Press, 1986

James W: Essays in Pragmatism. New York, Hafner Publishing, 1948

Kaslow NJ, Rehm LP, Siegel AW: Social and cognitive correlates of depression in children. J Abnorm Child Psychol 1984; 12:605-620

Kendall PC: Cognitive–behavioral interventions with children, in Advances in Clinical Behavior Psychology. Edited by Lahey BB, Kazdin AE. New York, Plenum Press, 1981

Kolvin I, Garside RE, Nicol A, et al: Help Starts Here: The Maladjusted Child in the Ordinary School. London, Tavistock, 1981

Layne C: Painful truths about depressives cognitions. Journal of Clinical Psychology 1983; 39:848-854

Levenson M: Cognitive correlates of suicidal risk, in Psychological Assessment of Suicidal Risk. Edited by Neuringer C. Springfield, IL, Charles C. Thomas, 1974

Lewinsohn P, Shaw D: Feedback about interpersonal behavior as an agent of behavior change: a case study in the treatment of depression. Psychother Psychosom 1969; 17:82-88

Liberman M, Yalom I, Miles M: Encounter Groups: First Facts. New York, Basic Books, 1973

Matson JL: The treatment of behavioral characteristics of depression in the mentally retarded. Behavior Therapy 1982; 13:209-218

Matson J, Esvelt-Dawson K, Andrasik M, et al: Observation and generalization effects of social skills training with emotionally disturbed chlidren. Behavior Therapy 1980; 11:522-531

McChure LF: Social problem-solving training and assessment: an experimental intervention in an elementary school setting. Unpublished dissertation, University of Connecticut, Storrs, 1975

Murray EJ, Jacobson LI: The nature of learning in traditional and behavioral psychotherapy, in Handbook of Psychotherapy and Behavior Change. Edited by Bergin AE, Garfield SL. New York, John Wiley, 1971

Nichols RC, Beck KW: Factors in psychotherapy change. Journal of Consulting Psychology 1960; 24:388-399

Oden S, Asher SR: Coaching children in social skills for friendship making. Child Dev 1977; 48:495-506

Overall P, Aronson H: Expectations of psychotherapy in patients of lower socioeconomic class. Am J Orthopsychiatry 1963; 33:421-430

Parloff MB, Waskow IE, Wolfe BE: Research on therapist variables in relation to process and outcome, in Handbook of Psychotherapy and Behavior Change: An Empirical Analysis, second edition. Edited by Garfield SL, Bergin AE. New York, John Wiley, 1979

Peterson A, Hamburg B: Adolescence: a developmental approach to problems and psychopathology. Behavior Therapy 1986; 17:480-499

Phillips E: Social skills: history and prospect, in Handbook of Social Skills Training and Research. Edited by L'Abate L, Milan MA. New York, John Wiley, 1985

Platt JJ, Spivack G: Problem-solving thinking of psychiatric patients. J Consult Clin Psychol 1972; 39:148-151

Reisinger JJ, Frangia G, Hoffman EH: Toddler management training: generalization and marital status. J Behav Ther Exp Psychiatry 1976; 7:335-340

Ricks DF: Supershrink: methods of a therapist judged successful on the basis of adult outcomes of adolescent patients, in Life History Research in Psychopathology, vol 3. Edited by Ricks DF, Thomas A, Roff M. Minneapolis, University of Minnesota Press, 1974

Robin AL: A controlled evaluation of problem-solving communication training with parent–adolescent conflict. Behavior Therapy 1981; 12:593-609

Rothenberg B: Children's social sensitivity and the relationship to interpersonal competence, interpersonal comfort, and intellectual level. Developmental Psychology 1970; 2:335-350

Rotheram MJ: Social skills training with elementary school and high school students, in Social Skills throughout the Lifespan, edited by Rathjen D, Foreyt J. New York, Pergamon Press, 1980

Rotheram MJ: Variations in children's assertiveness due to trainer assertion level. Journal of Community Psychology 1982; 10:228-236

Rotheram MJ: Evaluation of imminent danger for suicide among youth. Am J Orthopsychiatry 1987; 57:102-110

Rotheram MJ, Trautman PD: Assessment of cognitive and behavioral deficits among adolescent suicide attempters. Paper presented at the annual meeting of the American Academy of Child Psychiatry, Los Angeles, October 1986

Rotheram MJ, Armstrong M, Booraem C: Assertiveness training with elementary school children. Am J Community Psychol 1982; 10:567-582

Rucker CH, Vincenzo FM: Maintaining social acceptance gains made by mentally retarded children. Exceptional Children 1970; 36:679-680

Rutter M: Critical notice. J Child Psychol Psychiatry 1972; 13:219-222

Sacco WP, Graves D: Childhood depression, interpersonal problem-solving and self-ratings of performance. Journal of Clinical Child Psychology 1984; 13:10-15

Sarason IG, Sarason BR: Teaching cognitive and social skills to high school students. J Consult Clin Psychol 1981; 49:908-918

Schantz CV: The development of social cognition, in Review of Child Development Research. Edited by Hetherington EV. Chicago, University of Chicago Press, 1975

Seligman M, Peterson C: A learned helplessness perspective on childhood depression: theory and research, in Depression in Young People: Developmental and Clinical Perspectives. Edited by Rutter M, Izard C, Read P. New York, Guilford Press, 1986

Seligman ME, Kaslow N, Alloy LB, et al: Attributional style and depressive symptoms among children. J Abnorm Psychol 93:235-238, 1984

Shaffer D: Notes on psychotherapy research among children and adolescents. J Am Acad Child Psychiatry 1984; 23:552-561

Skinner BF: Science and Human Behavior. New York, Free Press, 1953

Slaney RB: Therapist and client perceptions of alternative roles for the facilitative conditions. J Consult Clin Psychol 1978; 46:1146-1147

Sobol DE: The effects of psychosocial awareness classes on self-esteem, behavior, and academic achievement in the elementary grades. Dissertation Abstracts International, 271a, 1974

Spivack G, Platt J, Shure M: The Problem-Solving Approach to Adjustment. San Francisco, Jossey-Bass, 1976

Strain PS, Young CC, Horowitz J: An examination of child and family demographic variables related to generalized behavior change during oppositional child training. Behav Modif 1981; 5:12-26

Strupp H: Psychotherapy research and practice: an overview, in Handbook of Psychotherapy and Behavior Change: An Empirical Analysis, second edition. Edited by Garfield SL, Bergin AE. New York, John Wiley, 1978

Stuart R: Helping Couples Change: A Social Learning Approach to Marital Therapy. New York, Guilford Press, 1980

Trautman PD: Coping with refusal of treatment and dropouts among adolescent suicide attempters. Paper presented at the 63rd annual meeting of the American Orthopsychiatric Association, Chicago, IL, 1986a

Trautman PD: Specific treatment modalities for adolescent suicide attempters. Paper to the Secretary's Task Force on Youth Suicide, Oakland, California, 1986b

Trautman PD, Shaffer D: Treatment of child and adolescent suicide attempters, in Suicide in the Young. Edited by Sudak HS, Ford AB, Rushforth NB. Boston, John Wright PSG, 1984

Vailhinger H: The Philosophy of As-If. Translated by Ogden CK. New York, Scribners, 1924

Waters E, Sroufe LA: Competence as a developmental construct. Developmental Review 1983; 3:79-97

Wolpe J: Reciprocal Inhibition Therapy. Palo Alto, Stanford University Press, 1958

Chapter 28

Cognitive Group Therapy

by Lino Covi, M.D., and Laura Primakoff, Ph.D.

HISTORICAL BACKGROUND

Cognitive therapy in its many variations and "schools" is most commonly provided in an individual or dyadic format. However, one of the earliest cognitive therapies, rational-emotive therapy (RET), was introduced simultaneously as both an individual and a group therapy (Wessler, 1983). Originally conceptualized in 1955, the RET approach has a strong didactic emphasis, and most typically employs open-ended, time-unlimited treatment in small groups of 8 to 13 members (Ellis, 1982).

Another pioneering cognitive theory is described in G.A. Kelly's (1955) *Psychology of Personal Constructs*. Kelly suggested group therapy as an important clinical application of his approach, but did not generate formally developed group techniques. However, Neimeyer and colleagues (1985) has recently integrated Kelly's framework with A.T. Beck's cognitive therapy for depression (Beck et al, 1979). It remained for Beck and his colleagues (1979) to fully develop well defined individual and group cognitive techniques.

Several authors have provided clinical descriptions of cognitive group therapy for depression (Covi et al, 1982; Eidelson, 1985; Hollon and Evans, 1983; Hollon and Shaw, 1979; Roth and Covi, 1984). There have also been several controlled treatment-outcome studies demonstrating the efficacy of cognitive–behavioral group therapy for depression (Covi and Lipman, in press; Gioe, 1975; Rush and Watkins, 1981; Shaffer et al, 1981; Shaw, 1977; Taylor and Marshall, 1977).

CLOSE-ENDED COGNITIVE GROUP THERAPY FOR DEPRESSION

Covi and his associates developed the close-ended, cognitive group therapy for depression that is presented in this chapter (Covi et al, 1982). The treatment protocol is derived in part from Shaw's (1977) pioneering group study and from Hollon and Shaw's (1979) elaboration of cognitive group clinical techniques. The protocol has been employed in a preliminary treatment outcome study (Covi and Lipman, 1987) and has been revised for use in our currently ongoing treatment-outcome study comparing cognitive group therapy to imipramine to the combined treatments.

A close-ended group is one in which all group members start and finish treatment at the same time. The treatment is of a predetermined length. Close-ended, time-limited cognitive groups usually range from 8–15 sessions in length. Sessions are 1½ to 2 hours in duration. Groups typically have a membership of four to eight patients with one or two co-therapists.

Group Composition

HOMOGENEITY. The traditional clinical expectation has been that depressed patients, as a result of their need for intensive support, as well as their "self-absorption, unrelieved pessimism, desire for immediate symptom relief, and rejection of others' suggestions" (Hollon and Shaw, 1979, p. 329), would be poor candidates for group treatment, both in terms of their own individual clinical improvement, as well as their negative impact on therapeutic group processes.

Yalom (1970) suggests, however, that the problems associated with depressed patients' suitability for group psychotherapy may be more applicable to depressed patients' participation in a heterogeneous group rather than in homogeneously depressed groups. Hollon and Shaw (1979) concur with Yalom's recommendation of homogeneity. They found that the high degree of structure and the active cognitive restructuring process in cognitive group therapy are effective antidotes to the "contagious negative, affective slide" that can occur in traditional psychotherapy groups in which depressed patients' painful renditions of reality are uncritically accepted and "absorbed" by fellow group members.

It has been our clinical experience that the homogeneous composition of cognitive groups produces unique benefits for depressed patients. It has been observed that in initial group sessions it often comes as a powerful revelation for patients to encounter individuals who are experiencing virtually identical affective, motivational, cognitive, and behavioral depressive symptomatology as themselves. As the group endures, patients' experiences of identifying with and having compassion for other group members appears to have a softening effect on their excessively harsh attitudes toward themselves.

PATIENT SELECTION CRITERIA. Close-ended, time-limited cognitive group therapy for depression is most directly applicable to patients with primary depressive symptomatology. Hollon and Shaw (1979) contend that for the most part those problems addressed by individual cognitive therapy can also be treated in group cognitive therapy. In general, however, the traditional diagnostic contraindications are relevant; that is, patients presenting with acute psychotic symptoms, schizoaffective disorder, organic brain syndromes, those who are acutely suicidal, homocidal, or withdrawn, severe substance abusers, and borderline and antisocial personality disorders (Rush, 1984; Woods and Melnick, 1979). With regard to severely suicidal or withdrawn patients, Hollon and Shaw (1979) suggest that if supplemental individual sessions can be made available, it may be possible for such patients to benefit from group treatment.

Conducting Cognitive Group Therapy

PREPARATORY INDIVIDUAL SESSIONS. Two individual sessions are conducted prior to the beginning of the first group session (Covi et al, 1982). The major purpose of these preparatory sessions is to begin teaching patients about the theoretical and therapeutic rationale of cognitive therapy. An important secondary purpose is to establish initial rapport with the group therapist and to provide the patient with some individual attention.

There is an initial determination of the patient's past experiences with psychotherapy and/or pharmacotherapy, as well as his or her expectations of cognitive group therapy. The therapist may then clarify how cognitive therapy differs from previous therapy experiences. Patients develop a target symptom list, and the cognitive model of depression is illustrated by helping the patient to recall and discuss concrete examples of mood changes being associated with specific cognitions. Self-help assignments are developed involving activity scheduling and the self-monitoring of moods. The patient is also taught how to rate the degree of mastery and pleasure experienced in relation to daily activities. The sessions end with a request for feedback regarding, in particular, any untoward reactions to the therapist or to the cognitive model, as well as any concerns about the group sessions. When appropriate, the therapist provides realistic feedback regarding the patient's reactions.

A third individual session is held subsequent to the first two group sessions. The primary purpose of this session is to elicit any particularly problematic reactions to the group or to the cognitive approach to depression. The therapist attempts to either help the patient solve any actual problems or to help the patient correct any distorted thoughts that may be occurring. An additional purpose of the session is to strengthen the collaborative therapeutic alliance.

STRUCTURE OF GROUP SESSIONS. The initial group session has several unique items on the group agenda. The therapists begin by establishing some basic ground rules. First and foremost is the issue of confidentiality. The suggested guideline is that group members are free to discuss their own problems outside of the group, but are encouraged not to reveal the identity of any of their fellow group members. The emphasis on confidentiality helps to foster a sense of trust and willingness to disclose delicate and often shame-producing material.

The structure of the group in terms of agenda setting is explained. At each group session, there is a predetermined group agenda, as well as individual agenda items chosen by each group member for that session. One of the standard group agenda items is a go-around in which each group member has the opportunity to discuss the week's events and any significant changes in symptomatology. Quite frequently, because of time constraints, the therapists will have to limit the number of individual agenda items which can be the focus of discussion. It is emphasized, however, that every effort is made over the course of treatment to provide each group member with an equal amount of group time, although this is not always possible in any given session.

The next item on the initial session's agenda is used to illustrate: 1) the relationship between an external situation, moods, and cognitions, and 2) how the same external event can precipitate a variety of emotional and cognitive reactions. Group members are asked to report what their moods and thoughts were in anticipation of the group session. Patients are often quite amazed that they share such similar apprehensions, as well as excitement and optimism. This exercise fosters group cohesiveness, as well as being illustrative of cognitive principles.

The next agenda item is members' descriptions of what has brought them for treatment and the target problems that they intend to address during the course of treatment. It is stressed that group members should reveal as much or as little as they feel comfortable disclosing. The remaining portion of the initial session includes a review of the self-help assignments from the second individual session, the assigning of new self-help work, patient feedback, and a summary of the current session.

In general, group agendas for subsequent group sessions are similar in structure to individual cognitive therapy agendas as suggested by Beck and his associates (Beck et al, 1979). The following items are always included on the group agenda:

1. individual patient agenda items
2. patients' reactions to the previous session
3. significant shifts in clinical status as revealed by Beck Depression Inventory (BDI) scores
4. patients' self-reported clinical status and significant events during week
5. therapists' review of previous sessions' self-help assignments
6. any new cognitive theory or technique
7. discussion of selected individual agenda items
8. new self-help assignments
9. summary of session
10. patients' reactions to the current session

The Group Course and its Phases

As in individual cognitive therapy, the nature of group sessions changes as the group progresses. The initial sessions are quite didactic in nature. A major goal of the first phase of treatment (individual sessions 1–3, and group sessions 1–3) is for patients to understand the cognitive model of depression. Patient agenda items are used to demonstrate cognitive concepts and methods. Homework assignments are behaviorally oriented in order to provide symptom reduction and mood improvement as quickly as possible. The behavioral assignments also serve a cognitive restructuring function by providing patients with contradictory evidence to their negative predictions and selective focus on negative memories regarding the daily events in their lives.

The second phase of treatment (group sessions 4–7) involves the formal introduction of cognitive restructuring techniques. Thus, in time-limited groups, the first half of the group is spent learning techniques for challenging distorted, negative automatic thoughts. Once patients' moods have improved sufficiently through learning the thought correction techniques, the third phase (group sessions 8–15) is begun. At this point, patients are better able to tackle questioning their basic depressogenic assumptions. Usually, intensive work over multiple sessions is required to weaken any one of these fundamental beliefs. The final portion of the third phase involves termination issues. Often, patients are anxious about relapses of depressive symptomatology and coping independently without the structure and support of the group. Since relapse is a realistic concern, this phase of treatment includes a relapse prevention component. The relapse prevention consists of patients' identification of the specific cognitive and behavioral skills learned which have been most effective in addressing their initial target problems, as well as any significant new targets that have emerged during the course of treatment. This assessment provides clarification as to remaining risk factors for future depressive episodes. The final homework assignment in the protocol requests that patients identify precise posttherapy goals. They are then asked to generate the necessary cognitive and behavioral strategies required to work toward their goals and to minimize their vulnerability to future depressions. At termination, group members have at their disposal the entire armamentarium of self-help forms, bibliotherapy references, their own completed homework, and all written didactic materials provided during the course of treatment.

The length of time that patients need to work on the skills presented in each phase of treatment varies from patient to patient and is related to patients' differential ability to learn and utilize the various techniques. Those patients who are most severely depressed may remain in the behavioral self-help assignment phase for most of the treatment. Others are able to master challenging their automatic thoughts, but may not succeed in identifying or changing their underlying depressogenic assumptions.

It is important, as will be discussed later in the chapter, for the therapists to be alert to any negative comparisons that patients may be making vis-à-vis their own progress in relation to the other patients in the group.

Clinical Management Issues

TARGET PROBLEM-ORIENTED VERSUS PROCESS-ORIENTED GROUPS. Cognitive group therapy has a highly structured and problem-focused format. The therapeutic stance is educative; the therapists have a specific body of cognitive theory and technique to teach group members. Within this didactic context, the emphasis is on individual agendas, rather than on the interaction among group members. Because of the clinical demands intrinsic to cognitive groups with depressed patients, therapists most often focus their efforts on patients' separate clinical concerns. Thus, close-ended cognitive group therapy has been practiced as essentially individual therapy carried out *in* a group. Treatment strategies have been virtually identical to individual cognitive therapy protocols. However, because of depressed persons' vulnerability to construing interpersonal events in negative and distorted ways, it is important to give group members a chance to express their reactions to the group interaction. The feedback solicited at the beginning and end of each session is a structured opportunity for patients to report any upsetting reactions that they may have had to the group process. Hollon and Shaw (1979) encourage therapists to make didactic use of any negative automatic thoughts that may be triggered by the group interaction. They suggest that such thoughts may be vividly illustrative of distorted cognitive processes, and can be subjected to cognitive disputation by the group. They provide examples such as, "I am taking up too much of the group's time; I don't have anything to offer; I don't fit in" (Hollon and Shaw, 1979, p. 336).

The following is a clinical example of the therapeutic benefit derived from a negative, distorted reaction to group process:

> A female group member told the group that 15 years prior to treatment she had given up an illegitimate child for adoption. This was the first time she had disclosed this information to anyone other than her current husband. Since the adoption, she had condemned herself mercilessly; that is, "I am a *bad* (totally irresponsible and selfish) mother." Upon returning to the group session following her disclosure, she felt extremely guilty and depressed at having revealed this information. She had spent the entire week ruminating that "I am selfish for having burdened the group with this. I have upset them and made them uncomfortable coming to the group. They now know what a sinful person I am."

The therapists and the group members were able to provide realistic feedback which allowed her to question the validity of these ideas.

NEGATIVE SELF-COMPARISONS. In a group format, patients experience a constant "barrage" of therapists' and other patients' remarks and actions. There is the resultant increased likelihood of negative social comparisons being triggered. Typical automatic thoughts that can emerge are: "Other group members seem so much more intelligent (less depressed) than I; I've been working at this for weeks longer than G., yet he's catching on much faster than I am; He's doing this much better than me, I never do anything right" (Hollon and Shaw, 1979, pp. 331, 333).

Because patients cannot always be the focus of the therapists' efforts, they can easily engage in silent rumination involving these negative comparisons. However, the alert group therapist makes a point of attending to any potential rumination and inquires of the patient as to the content of the thinking. The patient can then test the validity of the thoughts, both in the group session and in homework outside of the group.

Self-denigrating comparisons with other patients may appear to be a weakness of the group format. However, to the contrary, the skillful evocation and correction of negative social cognitions is a unique benefit of cognitive group therapy. This type of interpersonal material might never be activated in individual treatment.

PATIENTS AS CO-THERAPISTS. In the initial phase of group treatment, the therapists have major responsibility for helping patients correct their distorted thinking. However, as the group progresses, the responsibility shifts from the therapist to the other group members. An analogous shift takes place with regard to patients becoming increasingly active in generating their own self-help assignments.

The high degree of identification and compassion between group members which can exist in homogeneously depressed groups facilitates patients working with each other in the role of co-therapist. The social cognition (Pietromonaco and Markus, 1985), as well as clinical literatures (Hollon and Shaw, 1979), have noted depressives' ability to think about others in significantly more objective and flexible terms than they do about themselves. Hollon and Shaw (1979) describe the "universal" cognitive distortions that patients discover they share in a homogeneous group. They emphasize the value for patients in being able to recognize the cognitive distortions of others, and thereby learn better to realistically evaluate their own "idiosyncratic cognitive sets."

Acting as co-therapist gives patients additional practice in identifying and disputing depressive thinking. In addition, the co-therapist role provides them with "experiential" disputation of such dysfunctional beliefs as, "I can't give anything to others; I am a burden to others; I cannot think rationally" (Eidelson, 1985). Such beliefs are experientially disconfirmed by the actual experience of offering emotional support and helping to correct the depressive thinking of their fellow group members.

A unique opportunity that exists in cognitive group therapy is "group collaboration" (Sank and Shaffer, 1984). This is the collaborative process in which the patients–co-therapists challenge their fellow group members' self-rejecting ideas, or brainstorm solutions to seemingly insoluble problems. The therapeutic benefit of such group collaboration is that it becomes increasingly difficult for patients to totally discount the bombardment of contradictory data to which they are being exposed. Thus, cognitive group therapy, in contrast to the dyadic format, offers multiple sources of therapeutic change in the form of four to eight additional patient–co-therapists.

TIME MANAGEMENT—USE OF COMMON THEMES. As is evident from the previous listing of group agenda items, the group agendas are quite demanding in terms of the quantity of material to be covered. As Eidelson (1985) has pointed out, much of the skill involved in conducting cognitive group therapy is the ability to intervene as efficiently as possible within the time constraints, without compromising clinical quality or sensitivity. There are a number of strategies that cognitive group therapists employ in order to consolidate the therapeutic material.

Although an effort is made to cover all patients' agendas, it has been the authors' clinical experience that it is often unrealistic to address all individual agendas and to also maintain high clinical quality. It has been more therapeutic to focus on three, or at the most, four individual agenda items and to work on those in depth. Patients whose agendas are not being directly addressed can actively participate in the session as co-therapists. An attempt is made to work on those individual agendas which have the most in common with other group members' agendas.

The selection of agenda items is based on a variety of factors. Clinical considerations are first and foremost. The agenda of any patient who is in crisis or has had a particularly distressing week is definitely addressed. Second, if a patient's agenda will effectively demonstrate the cognitive theory or technique which is being presented during that session, it may be chosen as an agenda item. A third frequent selection criterion is overlapping content among patients' agendas. One such agenda can then be used efficiently as illustrative of the common theme among agendas. Finally, a self-help assignment which reveals a lack of understanding of either cognitive theory or methods might be chosen for didactic purposes as an agenda item.

A distinct advantage of homogeneous groups is that they are more likely to contain group members with shared cognitive distortions and depressogenic assumptions. Within any homogeneously depressed group, there often exists a continuum of dysfunctional beliefs that are held with varying degrees of rigidity and extremity; for example, the degree to which patients believe that without love they are worthless or that life's problems are too difficult to endure.

A clinical example serves to illustrate the therapeutic impact of working on a shared cognitive theme.

> In one of the close-ended cognitive therapy groups for depression, most of the group members shared the belief that they required the love and approval of significant others, in particular, their spouses, in order to be "worthwhile." However, one group member who had been divorced and living alone for a number of years struggled throughout the duration of the group to control overwhelming suicidal urges. Her desire to die was based on the idea that life was literally not worth living without a male partner. The dichotomous nature of her thinking—that is, "husband versus death"—was identified and persistently challenged. Suggestions were made as to alternative types of relationships other than conjugal, as well as other sources of life satisfaction and meaning. When the group progressed to the phase of working on basic assumptions, the following group theme/continuum was

identified and challenged: "I *must* have love: 1) in order to be happy; 2) in order to be worthwhile; and 3) in order to survive." The intensive and repetitive therapeutic work done with the suicidal group member appeared to jolt several group members into a clearer recognition than might have occurred otherwise of their own more moderate, but self-defeating and unrealistic notions of self-worth being contingent on love from others.

ROLE OF THE THERAPIST AND CO-THERAPIST. It is considered advisable to employ co-therapy teams because of the wealth of in-session, as well as written material, that is generated in cognitive group therapy. The "primary therapist" conducts the preparatory individual sessions and has thereby established some initial rapport with group members, and has a working knowledge of their respective target problems (Covi et al, 1982). The primary therapist assumes responsibility for actively directing the sessions by selecting the individual agenda items, presenting the didactic material, helping patients to question the validity of their thinking, summarizing important points, and eliciting patients' feedback.

The co-therapist has a complementary and supportive role; for example, noting any significant changes in symptomatology as reflected in the BDI scores, offering illustrative examples of homework assignments, suggesting additional techniques, disputations, and clarifications. With a co-therapy team, the primary therapist can actively intervene with the targeted patient while the co-therapist closely observes the ongoing reactions of the other group members. As mentioned previously, it is especially important in a homogeneously depressed group for the co-therapist to be alert to group members who may slip into negative ruminative states. Attempts are made to encourage group members to be in an active teaching or learning role during as much of the session as possible.

Other Close-Ended Therapies for Depression

Most cognitive–behavioral group treatments for depression employ a close-ended format and have a strong psychoeducational emphasis. The Self-Control Therapy program for depression was developed by Fuchs and Rehm (1977) on the basis of Rehm's self-control model of depression (Rehm, 1977). Rehm identified six self-control dysfunctions that are implicated in the development of depression: 1) excessive monitoring of negative events; 2) attention to immediate versus delayed consequences of behavior; 3) stringent standards of self-evaluation; 4) inaccurate attributions of causality; 5) insufficient self-reward; and 6) excessive self-punishment. The group treatment consists of 6 to 12 sessions which are 90 to 120 minutes in duration. Over the course of treatment, in-session didactic material and homework exercises systematically address each of the six hypothesized dysfunctions (O'Hara and Rehm, 1983). The self-control treatment package has been tested in five outcome studies (O'Hara and Rehm, 1983).

Coping with Depression (CWD), developed by Lewinsohn and colleagues (1985), is an explicit psychoeducational approach. The treatment is based on a social learning theory of depression; that is, emotional disorders are considered to be learned responses that affect and are affected by individuals' interactions with the environment. Treatment goals are implemented through multimodal techniques aimed at increasing positively reinforcing interactions between the depressed person and the environment and at decreasing negative, punishing interactions. Twelve two-hour sessions are held over an eight-week period, with two follow-up "reunions" at one and six months posttreatment. The group is conducted in the form of an academic class with formal lectures, homework assignments, a textbook, and "student" workbooks. An instructor's manual provides specific lecture and agenda materials for the group therapists. Effectiveness of the CWD course has been demonstrated in three outcome studies (Teri and Lewinsohn, 1985).

Problem Solving Training (PST) has been developed by Nezu (1986) on the basis of the observation that depressed individuals evince interpersonal problem-solving deficits. The first five sessions are didactic and include practice of the five stages of PST; that is, problem definition, generation of alternatives, decision making, solution implementation, and verification. The remaining three sessions are devoted to applied integration of the problem-solving model and practice of its different components. Homework is assigned at each session. A controlled outcome study with depressed patients demonstrated the effectiveness of PST as compared to: 1) a nondirective treatment group and 2) a wait-list control group (Nezu, 1986).

Multimodal therapy is a cognitively oriented individual and group technique developed by A. Lazarus (1982). Multimodal group treatment includes depressed patients in diagnostically heterogeneous groups of 4 to 10 members which meet for 20 weekly sessions of 90 to 120 minutes. The two initial sessions focus on an assessment of the individual members' BASIC I.D. Modality Profiles; that is, problem areas in seven critical modalities—behavior, affect, sensation, imagery, cognition, interpersonal, and biological. Thereafter, therapy is directed toward the elimination of specific excesses and deficits in each member's profile using a variety of group techniques. At times, therapists and individual group members interact much as they would in an individual session—"therapy *in* the group"—while at other times, group interaction is active—"therapy *by* the group" (Lazarus, 1981).

Neimeyer and colleagues (1985) have developed a group therapy for depression which integrates G.A. Kelly's (1955) cognitive model and Beck and colleagues (1979) cognitive therapy. Sank and Shaffer (1984) have formulated a time-limited group therapy for a mixed depressed and anxious population based on a modification of Beck and colleagues' (1979) cognitive therapy.

Zeiss and associates (1979) have attempted to elucidate the critical components that the recent cognitive–behavioral treatments for depression may have in common. They hypothesized the following four dimensions: 1) the presentation of a therapeutic rationale that encourages patients to believe that they can exercise self-control over their behavior, including their depression, 2) skills training consistent with the self-control rationale so that patients experience increased self-efficacy in their daily lives; 3) emphasis on skills practice outside of therapy; and 4) attribution of improvement in mood to patients' skill acquisition, rather than to therapists' interventions.

CLOSE-ENDED, COGNITIVE GROUP APPROACHES WITH OTHER CLINICAL DISORDERS

The purpose of the following summary is to provide a selected listing of the use of close-ended, cognitively oriented groups with a variety of clinical disorders. Reference will be made to treatment manuals or protocols, as well as to experimental and treatment outcome studies in which cognitive treatment takes place within a group context. As Rose and co-workers (1985) have pointed out, many reports of the use of the group format are contained in the experimental literature on cognitive–behavioral therapy. In these studies, the targeted treatment is carried out *within* a group context. However, little mention may be made of the group format per se; group therapy frequently appears to have been employed in such studies for practical rather than for theoretical or therapeutic reasons.

Within the loosely defined context of cognitive group approaches, a spectrum of treatment methods have been used, including stress inoculation training, rational-emotive therapy, cognitive restructuring, self-instructional training, self-statement modification, and rational restructuring. Detailed descriptions of these techniques are beyond the scope of this chapter. However, treatment manuals and protocols are either referenced or are often available from cited authors.

Stress inoculation training (Meichenbaum, 1977) teaches coping skills for managing a variety of stress-induced disorders. Meichenbaum and Cameron (1983) delineate three phases of training: 1) conceptualization: a conceptual model of stress is introduced and a treatment plan is formulated; 2) skills acquisition and rehearsal: training in self-monitoring of stress-engendering thoughts, images, feelings, and behaviors, self-instructional training in generating coping self-statements, and training in problem-solving and coping skills; 3) application and follow through: modeling and rehearsal of coping skills and graded in vivo behavioral assignments.

Two major reference texts (Meichenbaum and Jaremko, 1983; Turk et al, 1983) describe in detail the application of stress inoculation procedures to a host of stressors. *Stress Reduction and Prevention* (Meichenbaum and Jaremko, 1983) includes descriptions of training methods with regard to burn patients, psychophysiological disorders (chronic headache, bronchial asthma), rape victims, social anxiety, and adolescent anger problems. *Pain and Behavioral Medicine* (Turk et al, 1983) focuses attention primarily on stress inoculation applications to the treatment of chronic pain as well as a review of behavioral medicine applications; for example, essential hypertension, obesity, Type-A coronary-prone behavior, and irritable bowel syndrome.

A particularly well developed application of stress inoculation training is R.W. Novaco's treatment for *anger management* (Novaco, 1978; 1985). Hazaleus and Deffenbacher (1986) demonstrated the effectiveness of a modified version of Novaco's stress inoculation for anger management.

Cognitive group approaches have been applied to the treatment of a variety of *anxiety disorders*, including social phobia (Butler et al, 1984; Emmelkamp et al, 1985; Kanter and Goldfried, 1979); heterosexual dating anxiety (Glass et al, 1976; Jaremko, 1983); and public speaking anxiety (Jaremko, 1980; Lent et al, 1981). Cognitive approaches to assertiveness training with socially anxious patients have also been evaluated (Jacobs and Cochran, 1982; Linehan et al, 1979; Wolfe and Fodor, 1977). Finally, Jasin (1983) has described a cognitive–behavioral group treatment for agoraphobics. Jasin's protocol is largely based on Chambless and Goldstein's (1980) work with agoraphobia, but she also incorporates Beck and colleagues' (1979) cognitive restructuring and Meichenbaum's (1977) self-instructional training. Several controlled treatment-outcome studies have evaluated cognitive group protocols for agoraphobia (Emmelkamp et al, 1982; Marchione et al, in press; Mavissakalian et al, 1983).

Eating disorders have been successfully treated with cognitive–behavioral group therapy. A cognitive–behavioral group format has been employed in a number of controlled outcome studies in the treatment of bulimia nervosa (see Garner et al, in press; Wilson, 1986, for detailed reviews). K.D. Brownell has developed a cognitive–behavioral group approach to treating obese patients (Brownell and Foreyt, 1985) and has written a detailed self-help manual for the lay public (Brownell, 1985). Collins and associates (1986) have evaluated the effectiveness of a group cognitive–behavioral approach to the treatment of obesity.

The foremost approach to working with *addictive disorders* is G.A. Marlatt's relapse prevention (RP) program (Marlatt and Gordon, 1985). The reference text *Relapse Prevention* describes the wide array of cognitive and behavioral procedures that are delivered in both an individualized and a group format. RP strategies fall into three categories: 1) skill training strategies, which include cognitive and behavioral coping skills to manage high-risk situations; 2) cognitive reframing procedures, and 3) lifestyle intervention strategies; for example, relaxation and exercise. Detailed reviews of RP application and outcome studies in relation to specific addictive disorders (that is, alcoholism, smoking, and obesity) are included in the text.

Cognitive–behavioral group methods have been applied to a variety of disorders affecting *adolescents*. Grossman and Freet (1987) have described cognitive group therapy with hospitalized adolescents with problems ranging from attention deficit disorders to impulsive or aggressive behavior problems to psychotic disorders. Reynolds and Coats (1986) demonstrated the effectiveness of cognitive–behavioral group therapy with depressed adolescents. E.L. Feindler has developed a stress-inoculation approach to adolescent anger problems (Feindler and Fremouw, 1983) and has demonstrated its effectiveness with adolescent inpatients (Feindler et al, 1986) and junior high school delinquents (Feindler et al, 1984).

Several cognitive–behavioral group approaches have been developed and evaluated with the *depressed elderly*. Two clinical research teams (Steuer et al, 1984; Steuer and Hammen, 1983; Yost et al, 1986) have created cognitive group treatments based on Beck and colleagues' (1979) methods. Steuer and co-workers (1984) demonstrated the effectiveness of their cognitive treatment in a controlled outcome study. Steinmetz and associates (1985) have applied Lewinsohn and colleagues' (1985) psycho-educational approach to the treatment of subclinical depression in older adults. The program is largely behavioral, but a cognitive component is included.

OPEN-ENDED GROUP THERAPY FOR DEPRESSION AND RELATED DISORDERS

Covi and his associates developed the open-ended cognitive group therapy presented in this chapter (Roth and Covi, 1984). The open-ended, time-unlimited group is a flexible but more intensive version of the close-ended format (Covi et al, 1982). The objectives and procedures in the two formats are extremely similar. However, differences exist in terms of patient selection criteria, preparatory "role induction" procedures, and the sequence of techniques and phases of treatment.

Patient Selection Criteria

Some of the best candidates for inclusion in open-ended groups are depressed patients who have completed a course of close-ended treatment. Many patients who enter close-ended cognitive group therapy in a major depressive episode show marked improvement or complete remission of symptoms at termination. However, a certain percentage of patients fail to improve sufficiently. Others are remitted from their major depressive syndrome, but continue to exhibit symptoms that may be part of a chronic dysthymia, a generalized anxiety disorder, or a personality disorder coexisting with the major depression. While true nonresponders may be more appropriately referred to other therapeutic modalities, those individuals who have experienced some benefit from the time-limited group may be helped significantly from participation in an open-ended cognitive group.

Previously untreated major depression can also be helped by an open-ended cognitive group. A fairly rapid response to treatment is expected in these cases. A lack of symptom amelioration in the depressive syndrome within five or six weeks of treatment may indicate a need for reevaluation of the treatment plan; for example, the institution of adjunctive pharmacological treatment or other disposition. Anxiety disorders, as well as borderline, avoidant, dependent, compulsive, and passive-aggressive personality disorders, can be successfully treated in an open-ended cognitive group. In general, the open-ended format is definitely indicated for patients across the diagnostic spectrum for whom social anxiety and isolation are central features of their disorder.

Preparatory Role Induction

This crucial phase of cognitive therapy needs to be individually tailored to new members of an open-ended group. Those patients who have had previous courses of individual or close-ended group cognitive therapy may only require a minimal orientation in a single individual session with the group therapist. However, patients with no prior cognitive therapy experience, and who are experiencing moderate to severe distress, usually require four to eight individual preparatory sessions in order to understand the cognitive model and methods and to gain adequate symptom relief (Roth and Covi, 1984). Veteran group members play a critical role in the "socialization" process into the open-ended group. At a new member's initial group session, current members review their respective progress to date. At times, such reviews constitute powerful "testimonials" to the efficacy of cognitive therapy.

Variation of Group Techniques and Phases

The structure of the close-ended group dictates a particular didactic sequence of cognitive techniques. However, because of the heterogeneous membership and fluid entry of new members into an open-ended group, flexibility of sequence and type of techniques utilized are indispensable. For example, an entering dysthymic patient may be able to begin working immediately on depressogenic assumptions, rather than requiring weeks of basic behavioral assignments. Anxious patients may benefit from techniques such as decatastrophizing, cognitive rehearsal of anxiety-provoking events, and in vivo exposure to feared situations. Patients with personality disorders often require intensive work on erroneous beliefs regarding interpersonal relationships.

The unlimited time dimension of the open-ended group has several important clinical benefits. Because of the luxury of time, therapists can help patients to intensively challenge deeply entrenched dysfunctional assumptions. In addition, therapy *by* the group is much more possible and likely to take place. Over the course of treatment, because of the availability of time, relationships among group members can flourish. An atmosphere of trust can more easily be engendered. The interpersonal consequence of such trust is patients' willingness to engage in more intimate self-disclosure, as well as to offer and receive constructive, straightforward feedback.

Within the context of more stable and intimate relationships in the group, dysfunctional interpersonal rules are more likely to be "acted out" between group members. This provides a unique opportunity for the group therapists to focus patients' attention on the reciprocal relationship between personal rules and the interpersonal behaviors associated with the rules. Interactions in the group can thus be utilized to identify and correct long-standing, dysfunctional social cognitions, as well as self-defeating interpersonal behaviors that unwittingly invite unwanted response from others (see Kiesler, 1986; Safran, 1984, for discussion of integration of cognitive and interpersonal models).

Case Illustration

Norma, a 30-year-old, divorced data analyst and mother of two, was self-referred to our clinic. She met the criteria for major depression and avoidant personality disorder.

Norma recalled a depressed, isolated childhood and adolescence. She reported three prior episodes of suicidal depression, each of which had been precipitated by marital and extramarital relationship conflicts. Her mother had committed suicide by drug overdose after years of severe depression and alcohol abuse. Norma described her father as "stern and cold." Her sister had been chronically depressed and alcoholic; her brother was described as "aloof" with no obvious depressive symptomatology.

After several individual cognitive therapy sessions, Norma remained fairly apprehensive about participating in a group, but was willing to join the open-ended group that we conducted. She formulated the following target problems: guilt for being "uncaring," feeling overwhelmed by life's tasks, afraid to allow herself enjoyment, feeling rejected when not appreciated, unassertive, socially withdrawn, unable to cope with emergencies, and use of avoidance as her main approach to life.

Norma's social contact was narrowly restricted to her two children and a male cohabitant, Michael, with whom she had been living for the past five years. The first target problems addressed were her social withdrawal and telephone phobia. She neither made phone calls nor answered the phone. The initial behavioral assignments involved making a prescribed number of phone calls and saying "hello" to a prescribed number of people on a daily basis. Over several months' time, she felt sufficiently confident to be willing to ask people to lunch. Her strong resistance to each assignment revealed to her some immobilizing dysfunctional beliefs; that is, "If I am rejected, then I am worthless; I am responsible for others' happiness; If I don't give others whatever they expect or demand, then I am selfish *and* they will reject me."

Norma's moderate success at making positive contact with people, at "surviving" several negative encounters, and at being assertive by making and refusing a number of requests, provided her with preliminary evidence that countered her depressive rules.

What emerged from Norma's increasing social activity was her greater enjoyment of other people and her intensified estrangement from Michael. However, whenever she would consider asking him to move out, she would be flooded with the following thoughts: "I don't deserve to be happy; I must not hurt him; I should love someone who loves me; I will fall apart without him; having fun (with new friends) is bad."

Norma struggled for several sessions with her increasing ambivalence about Michael. We then encouraged the other group members to help her to question the validity of her thinking. An older, divorced female group member, Rhonda, was particularly forceful and articulate in her questioning. Rhonda had a strong, expansive, and charming personality, and men were constantly pursuing her. As a result, Rhonda had developed a very self-protective and aggressive style with men.

Rhonda asked Norma why she should not enjoy an active social life separate from Michael, if he was not satisfying to her? Why was it selfish to ask him to leave if the relationship had become that painful? She pointed out that Michael was an adult; he could survive rejection. Was Norma obligated to remain with him for the rest of her life because he had "tolerated" her depressions?

Week after week Rhonda would persist in this confrontative style of questioning. The other significant feedback was from two male group members who repeatedly disconfirmed Norma's negative self-concept and negative predictions regarding rejection by men. They provided her with their own perceptions, as well as objective evidence, that she was strong, attractive, interesting, and likeable, versus her conviction of being weak, a "chronic depressive," boring, and "no fun to be with."

A crucial turning point in Norma's cognitive change process was telling Michael that she wanted him to leave. None of her negative predictions were borne out. He was neither angry, rejecting, nor overwhelmingly distressed. In fact, his passivity and inability to communicate was a significant aspect of her dissatisfaction with the relationship. He told her that he wanted to stay and that he cared for her, but that he would leave if she really wanted him to. Norma was able to stand her ground, and he moved out.

Since that time, Norma has worked hard at remaining socially active and not slipping into her previous social isolation. Additional cognitive and interpersonal difficulties have emerged, and she has continued her attempts to resolve them with the help of the group.

Other Open-Ended Techniques

As mentioned previously, the first cognitive group therapy approach to be developed was rational-emotive therapy (RET), which was typically practiced in small, open-ended groups. Wessler (1983) points out that classical RET, principally directed at modifying basic irrational beliefs, has traditionally been provided in an individual format, whereas group RET is more "comprehensive," and almost indistinguishable from cognitive–behavioral approaches such as Beck and colleagues' (1979). RET groups are usually diagnostically heterogeneous, but may be homogeneous with regard to target problems such as loneliness, smoking cessation, or sexual dysfunctions.

Comparative Efficacy of Various Cognitive Formats

The selection of individual, close-ended group, or open-ended group cognitive therapy for a given patient should be guided by clinical judgment; that is, diagnosis and current severity of psychosocial stress. However, some data exist on the comparative efficacy of individual versus group cognitive therapy with depressed patients. Rush and Watkins (1981) have compared individual and group cognitive therapy in well matched samples, and found a significant advantage for the individual format. However, the mean of the posttreatment BDI scores of depressed patients completing the cognitive group protocol in the Covi and Lipman (1987) controlled outcome study is comparable to the mean of the posttreatment scores of Rush and Watkins's (1981) individual therapy completers, and significantly lower than that of their group therapy completers (see Table 1). The greater effectiveness of cognitive group therapy in the Covi and Lipman study may be partially a function of the treatment being delivered in a clinical research setting that is highly group-oriented.

Comparative Efficacy of Cognitive Group Therapy and Other Group Approaches

Several well designed outcome studies have compared cognitive group therapy to other group therapy approaches for depression. Shaw (1977) compared a cognitive–behavioral group therapy for depression, based on Beck and colleagues' (1979) cognitive treatment, to Lewinsohn's (1974) behavioral treatment for depression. Results of the study indicated that cognitive–behavioral therapy was the more effective treatment. Neimeyer and co-workers (1983) compared a cognitive group therapy, similar to that employed by Shaw (1977), to a group approach based on Klerman and associates' (1984) Interpersonal Psychotherapy of Depression (IPD). They found significantly greater improvement with cognitive therapy. Covi and Lipman (1987) compared close-ended, cognitive group treatment alone (the treatment protocol described earlier in the current chapter); to cognitive group with imipramine; to a traditional, nondirective, interpersonal group without medication. Randomized samples of depressive patients participated in the study. Both the cognitive group alone and the cognitive group with imipramine were superior in effectiveness to the traditional group.

The above-cited studies compared cognitive group treatment to traditional approaches in diagnostically homogeneous groups of depressed subjects. Depressed individuals are generally considered to be poor responders to tradi-

Table 1. A Comparison of BDI Scores for Completers of Group and Individual CBT

	Covi, Lipman		Rush, Watkins	
	Group		Group	Individual
Pre mean	26.2		29.2	29.5
s.d.	5.5		6.2	7.8
		versus		
Post mean	9.7		16.2*	8.6
s.d.	8.1		12.8**	6.7
N	23		23	8

*9.7 versus 16.2:
 t = 2.10; df = 22; p ≤ .05
**8.1 versus 12.8:
 F = 2.50; df = 22; p ≤ .05

tional, psychodynamically oriented group therapy in diagnostically homogeneous groups. It would be informative to compare cognitive and traditional approaches with depressed subjects treated in diagnostically heterogeneous groups. The effectiveness of cognitive group therapy for depression has not as yet been studied in diagnostically heterogeneous groups. Our clinical experience suggests that the close-ended format may be therapeutically limited with a diagnostically heterogeneous membership, but that the open-ended format may be quite effective.

CONCLUSIONS

In the past decade, cognitively oriented group approaches have been applied and, in many cases, demonstrated to be effective across an impressive range of clinical disorders. Frequently, cognitive group treatment appears to be delivered essentially as individual therapy carried out in a group, primarily for time and cost efficiency reasons. However, especially in the open-ended format, the group *qua* group and group members' participation has been considered to be an explicit and integral part of treatment.

The current chapter has suggested that cognitive group therapy provides a unique opportunity for cognitive restructuring in terms of the activation and correction of dysfunctional social cognitions. The interpersonal dimensions of cognitive group therapy have only begun to be explored by cognitive clinicians, theorists, and researchers. We would agree with Rose and colleagues' (1985) call for future outcome research on cognitive group therapy, including measures of group process variables' contribution to treatment outcome.

Whether cognitive group treatment is differentially effective from other group treatments or from the individual cognitive format remains to be specified. Our clinical experience, as well as the preliminary outcome data summarized herein, suggests promise in the efficacy of cognitive group treatments.

REFERENCES

Beck AT, Rush AJ, Shaw BF, et al: Cognitive Therapy of Depression. New York, Guilford Press, 1979

Brownell KD: The LEARN Program for Weight Control. Philadelphia, University of Pennsylvania Press, 1985

Brownell KD, Foreyt JP: A clinical approach to the treatment of the obese patient, in Clinical Handbook of Psychological Disorders. Edited by Barlow DH. New York, Guilford Press, 1985

Butler G, Cullington A, Manby M, et al: Exposure and anxiety management in the treatment of social phobia. J Consult Clin Psychol 1984; 52:642-650

Chambless DL, Goldstein AJ: The treatment of agoraphobia, in Handbook of Behavioral Interventions. Edited by Goldstein A, Foa E. New York, Wiley, 1980

Collins RL, Rothblum ED, Wilson GT: The comparative efficacy of cognitive and behavioral approaches to the treatment of obesity. Cognitive Therapy Research 1986; 10:299-318

Covi L, Lipman R: Cognitive behavioral group psychotherapy combined with imipramine in major depression. Psychopharmacol Bull 1987; 23:173-176

Covi L, Roth D, Lipman RS: Cognitive group psychotherapy of depression: the close-ended group. Am J Psychother 1982; 36:459-469

Eidelson JI: Cognitive group therapy for depression: "why and what." International Journal of Mental Health 1985; 13:54-66

Ellis A: Rational-emotive group therapy, in Basic Approaches to Group Therapy and Group Counseling, third edition. Edited by Gazda GM. Springfield IL, Charles C Thomas, 1982

Emmelkamp PMG, Mersch PP: Cognition and exposure in vivo in the treatment of agoraphobia: short-term and delayed effects. Cognitive Therapy Research 1982; 6:77-88

Emmelkamp PMG, Mersch PP, Vissia E, et al: Social phobia: a comparative evaluation of cognitive and behavioral interventions. Behav Res Ther 1985; 23:365-369

Feindler EL, Fremouw WJ: Stress inoculation training for adolescent anger problems, in Stress Reduction and Prevention. Edited by Meichenbaum D, Jaremko ME. New York, Plenum Press, 1983

Feindler EL, Marriott SA, Iwata M: Group anger control training for junior high school delinquents. Cognitive Therapy Research 1984; 8:299-311

Feindler EL, Ecton RB, Kingsley D, et al: Group anger control training for institutionalized male adolescents. Behavior Therapy 1986; 17:109-123

Fuchs CZ, Rehm LP: A self-control behavior therapy program for depression. J Consult Clin Psychol 1977; 45:206-215

Garner DM, Fairburn C, David R: Cognitive–behavioral treatment of bulimia nervosa: a critical appraisal. Behav Mod (in press)

Gioe VJ: Cognitive modification and positive group experience as a treatment for depression. Doctoral dissertation. Philadelphia, Temple University, 1975

Glass CR, Gottman JM, Shmurak S: Response acquisition and cognitive self-statement modification approaches to dating-skills training. Journal of Counseling Psychology 1976; 23:520-526

Grossman RW, Freet B: A cognitive approach to group therapy with hospitalized adolescents, in Cognitive Therapy—Applications in Psychiatric and Medical Settings. Edited by Freeman A, Greenwood VB. New York, Human Sciences Press, 1987

Hazaleus SL, Deffenbacher JL: Relaxation and cognitive treatments of anger. J Consult Clin Psychol 1986; 54:222-226

Hollon SD, Evans MD: Cognitive therapy for depression in a group format, in Cognitive Therapy for Couples and Groups. Edited by Freeman A. New York, Plenum Press, 1983

Hollon SD, Shaw BF: Group cognitive therapy for depressed patients, in Cognitive Therapy for Depression. Edited by Beck AT, Rush AJ, Shaw BF, et al. New York, Guilford Press, 1979

Jacobs MK, Cochran SD: The effects of cognitive restructuring on assertive behavior. Cognitive Therapy Research 1982; 6:63-76

Jaremko ME: The use of stress inoculation training in the reduction of public speaking anxiety. J Consult Clin Psychol 1980; 36:735-738

Jaremko ME: Stress inoculation training in the reduction of public speaking anxiety, in Stress Reduction and Prevention. Edited by Meichenbaum D, Jaremko ME. New York, Plenum Press, 1983

Jasin S: Cognitive–behavioral treatment of agoraphobia in groups, in Cognitive Therapy with Couples and Groups. Edited by Freeman A. New York, Plenum Press, 1983

Kanter NJ, Goldfried MF: Relative effectiveness of rational restructuring and self-control desensitization in the reduction of interpersonal anxiety. Behavior Therapy 1979; 10:472-490

Kelly GA: The Psychology of Personal Constructs. New York, Norton, 1955

Kiesler DJ: Interpersonal methods of diagnosis and treatment, in Psychiatry, vol. 1. Edited by Cavenar JO. Philadelphia, J.B. Lippincott, 1986

Klerman GL, Weissman MM, Rounsaville BJ, et al: Interpersonal Psychotherapy of Depression. New York, Basic Books, 1984

Lazarus AA: The Practice of Multimodal Therapy. New York, McGraw-Hill, 1981

Lazarus AA: Multimodal group therapy, in Basic Approaches to Group Therapy and Group Counseling, third edition. Edited by Gazda GM. Springfield IL, Charles C Thomas, 1982

Lent RW, Russell RK, Zamostny KP: Comparison of cue-controlled desensitization, rational restructuring, and a credible placebo in the treatment of speech anxiety. J Consult Clin Psychol 1981; 49:608-610

Lewinsohn PM: A behavioral approach to depression, in The Psychology of Depression: Contemporary Theory and Research. Edited by Friedman RJ, Katz MM. New York, Wiley, 1974

Lewinsohn PM, Steinmetz JL, Antonuccio D, et al: Group therapy for depression: the coping with depression course. International Journal of Mental Health 1985; 13:8-33

Linehan MM, Goldfried MR, Goldfried AP: Assertion therapy: skill training or cognitive restructuring. Behavior Therapy 1979; 10:372-388

Marchione KE, Michelson L, Greenwald M, et al: Cognitive–behavioral treatments of agoraphobia: tri-partite outcome of cognitive therapy, relaxation training and exposure. Behav Res Ther (in press)

Marlatt GA, Gordon JR: Relapse Prevention. New York, Guilford Press, 1985

Mavissakalian M, Michelson L, Greenwald D, et al: Cognitive–behavioral treatment of agoraphobia: paradoxical intention vs. self-statement training. Behav Res Ther 1983; 21:75-86

Meichenbaum D: Cognitive–Behavior Modification: An Integrative Approach. New York, Plenum Press, 1977

Meichenbaum D, Cameron R: Stress inoculation training: toward a general paradigm for training coping skills, in Stress Reduction and Prevention. Edited by Meichenbaum D, Jaremko ME. New York, Plenum Press, 1983

Meichenbaum D, Jaremko ME (Eds): Stress Reduction and Prevention. New York, Plenum Press, 1983

Neimeyer RA, Twentyman CT, Prezant D: A comparison of cognitive and interpersonal group therapies for depression: some preliminary findings. Paper presented at the annual meeting of the American Psychopathological Association, New York, March 1983

Neimeyer R, Heath A, Strauss, J: Personal reconstruction during group cognitive therapy for depression, in Anticipating Personal Construct Theory. Edited by Epting FR, Landfield AW. Lincoln, University of Nebraska Press, 1985

Nezu AM: Efficacy of a social problem-solving therapy approach for unipolar depression. J Consult Clin Psychol 1986; 54:196-202

Novaco RW: Anger and coping with stress, in Cognitive Behavior Therapy. Edited by Foreyt JP, Rathjen DP. New York, Plenum Press, 1978

Novaco RW: Anger and its therapeutic regulation, in Anger and Hostility and Cardiovascular Disorders. Edited by Chesney M, Rosenham R. New York, Hemisphere, 1985

O'Hara MW, Rehm LP: Self-control group therapy of depression, in Cognitive Therapy with Couples and Groups. Edited by Freeman A. New York, Plenum Press, 1983

Pietromonaco P, Markus H: The nature of negative thoughts in depression. J Pers Soc Psychol 1985; 48:799-807

Rehm LP: A self-control model of depression. Behavior Therapy 1977; 8:787-804

Reynolds WM, Coats KI: A comparison of cognitive–behavioral therapy and relaxation training for the treatment of depression in adolescents. J Consult Clin Psychol 1986; 54:653-660

Rose SD, Tolman S, Tallent S: Group process in cognitive–behavioral therapy. Behavior Therapist 1985; 8:71-75

Roth D, Covi L: Cognitive group psychotreatment of depression: the open-ended group. Int J Group Psychother 1984; 34:67-82

Rush AJ: Cognitive therapy, in Psychiatry Update, The American Psychiatric Association Annual Review, vol. III. Edited by Grinspoon L. Washington DC, American Psychiatric Press, 1984

Rush AJ, Watkins JT: Group versus individual cognitive therapy: a pilot study. Cognitive Therapy Research 1981; 5:95-103

Safran J: Some implications of Sullivan's interpersonal theory for cognitive therapy, in Cognitive Psychotherapies: Recent Developments in Theory, Research, and Practice. Edited by Reda MA, Mahoney MJ. Cambridge MA, Ballinger, 1984

Sank LI, Shaffer CS: A Therapist's Manual for Cognitive Behavior Therapy in Groups. New York, Plenum Press, 1984

Shaffer CS, Shapiro J, Sank LI, et al: Positive changes in depression, anxiety, and assertion following individual and group cognitive behavior therapy intervention. Cognitive Therapy Research 1981; 5:149-157

Shaw BF: A comparison of cognitive therapy and behavior therapy in the treatment of depression. J Consult Clin Psychol 1977; 45:543-551

Steinmetz JL, Thompson LW, Breckenridge JN, et al: Behavioral group therapy with the elderly: a psychoeducational approach, in Handbook of Behavioral Group Therapy. Edited by Upper D, Ross S. New York, Plenum Press, 1985

Steuer JL, Hammen CL: Cognitive–behavioral group therapy for the depressed elderly: issues and adaptations. Cognitive Therapy Research 1983; 7:285-296

Steuer JL, Mintz J, Hammen CL, et al: Cognitive–behavioral and psychodynamic group psychotherapy in treatment of geriatric depression. J Consult Clin Psychol 1984; 52:180-189

Taylor F, Marshall W: Experimental analysis of a cognitive–behavioral therapy for depression. Cognitive Therapy Research 1977; 1:59-72

Teri L, Lewinsohn PM: Group intervention for unipolar depression. Behavior Therapist 1985; 8:109-123

Turk DC, Meichenbaum D, Genest M: Pain and Behavioral Medicine. New York, Guilford Press, 1983

Wessler RL: Rational–emotive therapy in groups, in Cognitive Therapy with Couples and Groups. Edited by Freeman A. New York, Plenum Press, 1983

Wilson GT: Cognitive–behavioral and pharmacological therapies for bulimia, in Handbook of Eating Disorders. Edited by Brownell KD, Foreyt JP. New York, Basic Books, 1986

Wolfe JL, Fodor IG: Modifying assertive behavior in women: a comparison of three approaches. Behavior Therapy 1977; 8:567-574

Woods M, Melnick J: A review of group therapy selection criteria. Small Group Behavior 1979; 10:155-175

Yalom ID: The Theory and Practice of Group Psychotherapy. New York, Basic Books, 1970

Yost EB, Butler LE, Corbishley MA, et al: Group Cognitive Therapy—A Treatment Approach for Depressed Older Adults. New York, Plenum Press, 1986

Zeiss AM, Lewinsohn PM, Muñoz RF: Non-specific improvement effects in depression using interpersonal, cognitive, and pleasant events focused treatments. J Consult Clin Psychol 1979; 47:427

Chapter 29

Cognitive Approaches to Adherence

by A. John Rush, M.D.

Problems in adherence or compliance (these terms are used interchangeably) constitute a major dilemma for practitioners. There is only a 20 to 30 percent probability that a patient will follow a medication prescription 4 times a day for 10 consecutive days (Sackett and Haynes, 1976). It is likely that prescriptions over greater lengths of time will attain even lower rates of compliance. Numerous studies suggest that several factors affect the likelihood of adherence to medication prescriptions (for example, the patient's perceived seriousness of the illness, clinic administrative factors, side effects, dosage frequency, and so on). While we, as clinicians, often know what has to be done (which medications to prescribe, what behaviors to change), our ability to develop adherence in patients remains limited.

Cognitive psychotherapeutic strategies have been developed and tested in both depression and other conditions. This chapter provides a model for understanding and modifying adherence, derived mainly from clinical experience with cognitive techniques. The model allows for identification of specific obstacles to adherence, and suggests strategies to improve compliance with treatment recommendations. As these suggestions are derivations from clinical work, they may or may not be valid. Research to evaluate the efficacy, validity, and generalizability of these notions is needed.

ADHERENCE OBSTACLES

Various factors affect the probability of patients adhering to treatment recommendations (see Figure 1). Behavioral changes that: 1) are short-lived; 2) result in immediate positive gains; 3) are compatible with current beliefs within the immediate social system; 4) have general acceptance among professionals (that is, are "backed" by recognized authorities); and 5) which the patient has already become rather convinced are needed, can be accomplished most easily.

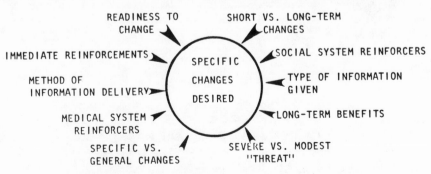

Figure 1. Factors that influence adherence

However, as clinicians, we often recommend behaviors that *do not* meet all of these criteria. Our suggestions often require long-term implementation that may include short-term discomfort (for example, maintenance medication), as well as extensive, long-lasting revisions in one's lifestyle. Both the culture and the patient's immediate social system may provide uneven, inconsistent, or negative reinforcement for such changes. In addition, both the type of information and the manner in which it is delivered to patients will critically influence whether patients will revise their behavior. For example, media advertising used to induce Americans to complete the 1980 census form consisted of a large group of people singing about being counted. Those who naturally distrust the government would not find being counted something to sing about.

Environmental Events

Figure 2 subdivides various potential contributants to high or low adherence. As patients enter the treatment system, a wide variety of events will likely occur. They interact with the physician, who renders a diagnosis and treatment plan, as well as the secretaries, nurses, physicians' assistants, laboratory technicians, and other patients.

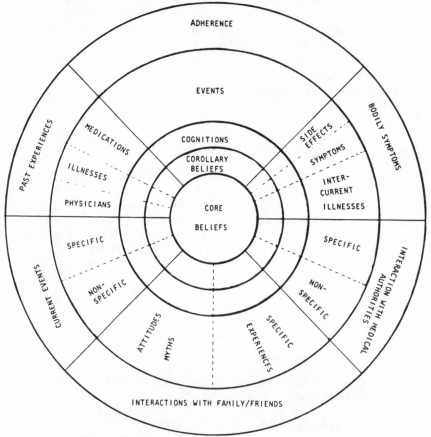

Figure 2. Adherence/events/cognitions/beliefs

This experience often results in recall of prior experiences with physicians, illnesses, hospitals, medication side effects, and so forth, which are conceptualized in different ways (for example, "medication makes me sick"; "doctors never tell me the whole truth"; "medical treatment is always impersonal"; and so on). These conceptualizations often importantly influence compliance. If treatments have failed, patients are less motivated to adhere to new treatments. If new treatments are not fully comprehended, the patient may use this view ("It's too complicated for me") to be nonadherent. Sometimes the disorder itself may impede proper adherence. For example, when depressed patients are presented with a treatment plan, their negative thinking biases may lead them to attend selectively to evidence of treatment dangers or possible lack of efficacy, which reduces adherence. Medical staff interactions (nonspecific factors) may also reduce adherence. An abrupt nurse, an impatient physician, or a belligerent clerk may dissuade ambivalent or nervous patients from attending a clinic or from taking prescribed medication. Some patients feel more comfortable with a friendly, less "professional" style of staff interaction, while others may tend to doubt the validity of information from a more casual staff.

Furthermore, during both diagnostic and treatment phases, patients focus on symptoms (both somatic and psychological). This heightened awareness of symptoms of the disorder may lead to an invalid inference about continued medication side effects ("the medication is making me sleepy") when the symptom is part of the disorder itself. Symptoms of an unrelated, intercurrent illness may be mistaken for medication side effects and, therefore, become the ground for treatment discontinuation. Alternatively, such symptoms may become cues for the idea that "The medication isn't working and, therefore, it should be stopped." In addition, patients often begin to search for more information about their illness, its treatment, and the dangers involved in both. Family and friends (particularly those who have suffered from the same illness) are often consulted. These outside opinions by important others are often given great weight by patients, as these other individuals have *actually* had the illness. Their reports, even if 10 to 20 years out of date, are taken as gospel. The family becomes the source of *specific* ideas about a particular illness or treatment, as well as a repository of *general* attitudes toward health, illness, physicians, and so on, which may either improve or inhibit adherence. Other culturally recognized "authorities" are often sought out or discovered by concerned patients (for example, books, newspapers articles, technical journal reports, television and radio reports) which may modify adherence, depending on how patients conceptualize this information. For example, news reports of physicians receiving kickbacks from laboratories may lead patients to question the need for, or even refuse, specific tests. Conversely, reports of new medications might lead patients to insist on treatment with these compounds when standard medications are preferable.

Thoughts and Beliefs

These events (bodily symptoms, news reports, statements by the treating physician or medical team members, family attitudes, or past experience with illnesses and treatment) are not objectively weighed by patients. A full, balanced account of the disorder, its treatment, and the dangers associated with each, is rarely available to patients and often only partially available to physicians at any given time. For example, many patients consult the *Physician's Desk Reference (PDR)*, which lists all Food and Drug Administration (FDA) approved prescription medications in this country. The *PDR*, however, often fails to distinguish *common* from *rare* and *serious* from *minor* side effects. It does not enumerate the consequences of the illness if it goes untreated, nor does it report drug interactions. Patients and families are usually unaware of the selective nature of the information in this publication and other sources.

In addition, patients themselves bias the information available based on previous experiences, which may modify adherence. A close examination of these thoughts in a particular patient often reveals stereotypical patterns that are surprisingly independent of the actual information or experiences encountered. For example, patients will overgeneralize or selectively attend to specific information or misconceptualize previous personal experiences or those of others close to them. A patient might believe that since an uncle died of heart disease while exercising, that exercising is bad for one's health. Alternatively, if a previous physician found "nothing wrong" after many tests, the patient may erroneously view all tests as useless.

How does such biased thinking arise? Biased access to information and specific experiences by important others are only two sources of bias. The *underlying disorder* (for example, depression or anxiety) may result in biased thinking. As noted in Chapter 25 of this volume, depressed patients may focus on information that reinforces their feelings of hopelessness. For example, when told that the average depression will have a 70 to 80 percent chance of complete response to antidepressant medication, such patients often think, "I'm in the other 20 to 30 percent," thereby discounting a very optimistic prognosis. Patient's current mood can also bias information. Anxious patients may overly emphasize the dangers of treatment or of the illness itself.

Basic beliefs or attitudes constitute a very important source of bias. Many patients would prefer to "deny" that they are ill or that they require treatment. This attitude ("I can't get sick") influences the amount and nature of information taken in, and it biases what patients admit to themselves about their illness or treatment. This denial may be particularly striking in patients whose health-reducing behavior (for example, smoking) have become habits. They know intellectually that smoking is dangerous, but they do not emotionally allow this information to affect current behavior. We hypothesize that a set of underlying beliefs influences the way in which specific information (such as smoking is dangerous) is managed so as to leave smoking behavior unaffected.

Symptoms themselves may become stimuli that are biased to fit preformed beliefs. For example, a headache may lead one person to immediately call for help or take a pill, while another may respond by trying to figure out what's irritating him or her. A patient who is distrustful of medication may ascribe the headache to the pill. Others who believe in medication may think the headache results from too little medication. Patients are likely to *selectively attend* to particular aspects of their experiences, to *magnify* selected portions of available information, to *generalize* from unique experiences, or to *personalize* the experiences of others. Consider, for example, the patient who leaves the clinic abruptly because the medical chart has been misplaced, thinking, "They don't know what they're doing here." This notion becomes the basis for justifying treatment dropout. This patient focused on a situational detail taken out of context, while ignoring more salient features. Conceptualization of the treatment process rests on a single incident, which was *selectively attended* to (Beck, 1976; Rush and Beck, 1978). Consider the patient who discontinues taking penicillin to treat pneumonia because the coughing has stopped. Here the patient has *arbitrarily inferred* that coughing is equated with pneumonia, while ignoring continued weakness, fever, and chest pain.

Cognitive theorists (Beck, 1976; Meichenbaum, 1977; Ellis, 1962) suggest that a series of silent assumptions or beliefs underlie and form the basis for specific thoughts. These beliefs and assumptions can be inferred from stereotypical thinking or behavioral patterns. A heirarchy of beliefs may be apparent. Corollary beliefs are those that can be easily inferred from stereotypical behavioral or thought patterns. While patients are often unaware of these notions, they are more easily changed with logic or brief targeted experiences. Core beliefs (general notions) can be inferred from a series of corollary beliefs. These core beliefs are not within the patients' awareness. They remain unquestioned and are not easily changed. They may even be vehemently denied by patients until recurrent experiences begin to *show* them that such beliefs exist. In fact, they are often reinforced by patients' repeated conceptualizations of specific current events. Implicit in this cognitive model is the notion that behavior influences specific beliefs and vice versa. Thus, significant behavioral change may result in modification of at least corollary, if not core, beliefs.

Figure 3 illustrates the ways in which thoughts, corollary beliefs, and core beliefs may interrelate. The patient, an anxious 45-year-old hypertensive executive, basically believed that no medication is best, all medication is dangerous, and that being sick is a sign of moral weakness. He claimed to be conscientious about his treatment, his work, and his role in the family. However, his blood pressure had been labile. He recorded a variety of thoughts, three of which were illustrated. He awoke one day and felt quite good—no headaches, fatigue, or stomach discomfort, and thought of not taking his medication as he was asymptomatic. At another time, while actually taking the medication, he felt anxious and attributed the anxiety to the medication. Thus, the presence *and* absence of symptoms were both cues for nonadherance. He also reported another thought about his aunt getting "hooked" or dependent on medicine while viewing a television program on hypertension. Corollary beliefs were inferred from this thinking pattern. He readily admitted to the first two beliefs: taking medicine is a crutch and that it causes problems. He less readily endorsed the idea that not taking medicine meant that he was not sick. Core beliefs were inferred from

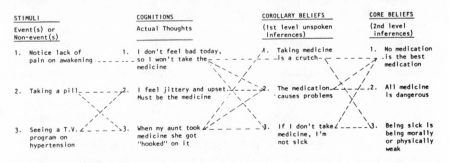

Figure 3. Cognitions and beliefs

the corollary beliefs. While he could see how these core beliefs logically followed from his stereotypical thinking pattern and corollary beliefs, he initially denied that he believed these notions.

Assuming that thoughts and beliefs affect adherence, how can clinicians modify them? Will patients change their attitudes simply with logical discussion? Not likely! Educational or informational methods alone have not been overwhelmingly powerful in modifying behaviors that contribute to illness. This model would suggest why this is so. Core beliefs are rarely changed by simple information. Rather, core beliefs dictate ways in which information is distorted to reinforce specific beliefs. The hypertensive patient just described used both the presence *and* absence of symptoms as cues for thinking about or actually failing to adhere to the prescribed medication. How can the clinician increase adherence in the face of such core beliefs?

SUGGESTIONS FROM PSYCHOTHERAPY FOR IMPROVING ADHERENCE

Psychotherapy research and experience provide some clues for solving this dilemma of how to persuade patients to adhere to appropriate regimens. Psychotherapy aims at changing behavior and reducing maladaptive emotional and behavioral responses while increasing adaptive ones. Psychotherapies differ in their approaches to persuading patients to undertake these changes. Patients frequently know what is appropriate, but somehow are unable or unwilling to undertake the needed changes, or are unable to maintain them. For example, obese patients know they should eat less, but do not.

Garfield (1980) has suggested common features of various psychotherapies. The *therapeutic relationship* provides a medium for problem identification and resolution. Such a relationship helps patients disclose thoughts, beliefs, and events that preclude or assist in compliance. Thus, specific obstacles to adherence become the target of friendly, yet professional, inquiry.

Most therapies provide a *cognitive map* or *rationale* for understanding problems. By analogy, nonadhering patients should be provided with a model of factors that affect adherence. This model should assist in objective discussion, inquiry, and problem solving. The model allows patients to evaluate behaviors, thoughts, and feelings associated with nonadherence.

Therapists provide *reassurance* to encourage new behaviors, and at times *catharsis* will clear the way for behavioral change. For example, the hypertensive patient described previously finally expressed his overwhelming fear of having a stroke (that is, his core belief was "I will end up just like my father" who also had high blood pressure, suffered a stroke, and died at age 57). In retrospect, his fear was in part displaced onto medication, doctors, and so on, and appeared to influence adherence. Somehow, the patient could pretend that his fate would differ from his father's if he did not take the medication.

Psychotherapy research further indicates that *specific techniques*, particularly behavioral ones, are effective in modifying specific behaviors (for example, phobias). However, more generalized behavioral changes (such as agoraphobia) may demand both cognitive, attitudinal, or behavioral change methods. Strupp and Bloxom (1973), Rush and Watkins (1980), and others have noted that improved adherence to psychotherapy results if *resistances* or *obstacles* to continued treatment are identified and discussed *before* they actually occur. With regard to adherence, the practitioner would be well advised to ask patients to anticipate or imagine what might happen that could reduce adherence. For example, patients should be asked to concretely imagine the steps involved in taking medication each day. Where will it occur? Who will be involved? Would a schedule change, an unexpected demand, running out of or misplacing the medication, or the presence of others from whom the patient wishes to conceal medication taking derail the plan? Would any specific symptoms, side effects, or intercurrent illnesses preclude adherence? Would symptomatic remission, opinions of other family members, or any other stimulus to attitude change modify adherence? By concretely anticipating various elements that may alter adherence (Figure 2), both patient and practitioner can adapt the treatment regimen to the individual. In addition, a detailed focus on adherence obstacles provides patients with a metamessage (indirect suggestion) that adherence is important enough to be planned for and discussed in detail.

Furthermore, the few psychotherapy studies available suggest that a supportive, collaborating immediate social system (for example, spouse, children, friends) will improve adherence. For example, Brownell and colleagues (1978) reported that greater weight reduction occurred in men using behavioral methods when spouses were willing to assist and were engaged by the therapist, in contrast to lesser weight loss in men whose spouses were unwilling to collaborate. Clinical experience suggests that marital or family relationships characterized by dissent may lead the spouse to undermine the patient's desire to adhere. Conversely, a collaborative relationship may increase adherence *if* the patient wants to adhere. Thus, the immediate social system may be an ally or an enemy of adherence.

To reduce the chances of misinterpretation and to enlist the spouse, it is recommended that another family member, usually the spouse, is *always* apprised of the problem or disorder to be treated, the treatment plan, and the expected effects, dangers, side effects, and so on. This education is best conducted as the treatment is initiated. The practitioner should speak directly to the spouse or family with the patient present. The spouse should be encouraged to raise questions, concerns, and misgivings which are answered directly by the clinician. As noted above, families often demonstrate a common general set of beliefs about treatment. These beliefs should be elicited, and if unfounded and biased, they should be corrected with specific information, not simply with general reassurances.

While the above suggestions are general guidelines, some specific suggestions can be gleaned from psychotherapy experience as well. Medical professionals too often use elaborate scientific explanations to motivate patients or to allay fears. This approach has a particular shortcoming, in that we may fail to elicit the patient's particular concern. For example, patients ask general questions about side effects, which we answer with a soliloquy on side effects ranging from A to Z, without first asking what specific side effects concern them. For example, patients may be especially concerned about becoming addicted to the medicine, though they are hesitant to ask this question directly without assistance from the practitioner. Thus, clinicians should withhold long explanations until they have more specific ideas about what the particular patient's concerns are. These concerns are easily elicited by dialogue with a series of questions. They are not easily revealed with premature, detailed explanations by clinicians.

Logic and scientific information often help patients to understand and get a much needed perspective on the illness and its treatment. However, corollary attitudes and core beliefs are not so easily changed by simplified science. In addition, patients may mislead the clinician about a concern by apparently seeking particular information (for example, "Is depression psychological or biological?" or "How does this drug lower my blood pressure?"). Such inquiries may only be of superficial emotional importance. While concrete and specific responses are appropriate to such questions, the practitioner is best advised, again, to use questions first to probe for what are often more meaningful personal concerns underlying patients' apparently "scientific inquiries." The first question, "Is depression psychological or biological?" often conceals the question, "Is there anything I or my family can do in addition to taking medication that will help?" The latter question about hypertensive mechanisms of action may overlie concerns about the probability of a stroke or heart attack. Probes in the form of 1) questions; 2) comments about how the patient appears emotionally (for example, "You sound like you are concerned with more than simply how the medication works"); 3) requests for specificity (for example, "Tell me more about what you have learned concerning hypertension"); or 4) inquiries about family attitudes (for example, "What does your wife think about your panic attacks?") often uncover key concerns that, if answered can lead to greater adherence.

Efficacy in adherence counseling can be increased by setting an agenda with the patient for each session. Patients are often tempted to divert discussion, obliquely express concerns, forget what was said, and so on. A proposed outline for the adherence interview is presented in the next section of this chapter. Each session should be verbally summarized, first by the patient, and then supplemented by the clinician. A written plan or set of instructions adds force to the conclusions reached, and it helps patients to play back and discuss the session with spouse or family.

Psychotherapy research also suggests that homework assignments may facilitate both behavioral and attitudinal changes and, by analogy, improve adherence. There is an art to developing and using such assignments. The key is to understand adherence induction as a stepwise, reiterative, trial-and-error process, in which first one obstacle and then another is identified and reduced or removed. Homework tasks can facilitate this reiterative process.

Simple environmental changes can be accomplished by directing patients to change some aspect of their daily life to increase adherence (for example, putting a reminder on the bathroom mirror that says, "Good morning, it's time to floss"). Reinforcer scheduling can be easily instituted by simple instructions (such as, "Take your pill at breakfast when the family is there and ask them to remind you"). A behavioral assignment may elicit thoughts or attitudes that patients are initially unaware of, or it may change those attitudes in the direction of increasing compliance. For example, a patient who believes that taking medication is morally weak might be asked to tactfully inquire of several others, whom they consider morally strong, whether they take medication of any type, in order to test out this belief. Alternatively, a careful record of thoughts at the time of medication ingestion or when patients "forget" often reveals ideas about medicine, illnesses, or life and death that are only on the edge of the patient's awareness. Attitude balancing is often a target of homework assignments. For example, after patients have read about the side effects in the *PDR*, readings about the effects of the untreated illness may be suggested to balance this information.

Finally, recent research in psychotherapy is beginning to focus on the types of information or experience most likely to influence specific sorts of people. Advertisers, marketing, and sales persons are quite aware that certain kinds of people are receptive to certain kinds of information that is delivered in specific ways. Some of us are inspired to believe in and, therefore, behave differently when, presented with an emotional or personal appeal. Others might be more receptive to a cold, hard look at the balance of facts—the "pros and cons" argument method. The practitioner who hopes to increase adherence might directly ask patients, "What kinds of information (or what can I or others tell you or show you that) would make it easier for you to accept and participate in your treatment?" Surprisingly, patients often know precisely what we should tell them! In addition, they are quite familiar with the types of information that have led them to make important decisions in the past—decisions that have changed their lifestyle, such as choosing an occupation, a spouse, or a place to live. By determining how they went about making these decisions, the clinician may have clues as to how to influence adherence.

THE ADHERENCE INTERVIEW

Most interactions with patients in treatment can affect compliance. If adherence improvement is a primary goal of an interview, some plan as to how to proceed is needed. In most clinical settings, the interview must be brief. However, the relationship to the clinician is often very powerful—particularly if the illness or symptoms are of significant meaning to the patient. Thus, the clinician's behavior in this interview importantly affects behavior because the context and the relationship magnifies the importance and effect of what the practitioner will do in treatment.

A rationale for treatment and changes in treatment regimen should be provided. In addition, given the pervasive difficulties with adherence, the practitioner should assume that specific obstacles to adherence always exist. The interviewer should inquire specifically about these anticipated obstacles and about possible solutions to them even before they are encountered. By directly inquiring about obstacles and solutions, clinicians prepare patients for a problem-solving approach.

How then should the interview proceed? Medication recall is the first step. It is preferable not to tell patients what they have been prescribed, but rather ask how they have been taking the medication. Some patients retort, "Well, you should know. After all, you prescribed it." The response to this should be, "I do not know how you have taken it. I simply know how I prescribed it. Everyone is individual when it comes to following prescriptions." Specifically, ask patients to recall, on a day-to-day basis, for the previous seven days, when, where, and how they took the medication, which usually takes about three to four minutes. This is facilitated by using some sort of weekly calendar or schedule. A check mark is placed at the appropriate time of each day when the patient is able to adhere to the prescribed schedule. A dash is placed in those spaces indicating when the patient failed to comply.

Next, ask the patient to describe what factors (events, ideas, information, and so on) assisted in adhering to the prescription. Here patients may recount a heightened awareness of the disorder by the presence of symptoms, by media information (from such sources as television, radio, or newspaper), or they may need assistance in recalling to take the medication from important others. This series of adherence-improving factors allows the clinician to gauge what kinds of information, or stimuli, are more likely to be of value when addressing those times of poor adherence.

Next, ask the patient to recall what factors impaired adherence by describing specifically what happened on each of the occasions when they failed to take the medication as prescribed. Where were they? Did the idea of taking medication come to mind? Was it dismissed or did the patient simply never consider the idea at all? What might have happened that would have modified the probability of taking the medication? When did they become aware of their failure to adhere? How often does this occur? Is there any pattern to those times when adherence failure occurs?

Next, the patient is shown a diagram (Figure 4), and is asked to rate the percentage that each of the factors shown in the diagram reduced adherence from 100 percent. This pie-shaped diagram displays the most common reasons for reduced adherence, including such elements as new medical information, recent interactions with other medical authorities, forgetting, schedule changes, the awareness or lack of symptoms, the awareness or lack of side effects, intercurrent illnesses, and interaction with important others and with the news media.

Next, patients are asked to detail how each of the two most likely weighted factors reduced adherence. For example, what was it that was said by the important other that led them to refrain from taking the medication? What specifically did they read in the newspaper that led them to be a bit more skeptical about taking medication and actually "forget" on several occasions? What was it about going on vacation that led them to decide not to take the medication? By inquiring how each of these elements contributed to adherence, one begins to uncover the underlying attitudes or beliefs that the patient has about medication, illness, and treatment.

As patients describe these factors, pay close attention to the patient's nonverbal behavior. Is the patient less than enthusiastic or even bored when talking about what sorts of things led him or her to "forget"? When the patient speaks about the spouse reminding him or her about the medication, is this related in a sarcastic tone of voice? Does the person feel "nagged" when reminded? Is the patient ashamed of failing to adhere? Is the patient "playing around with the medication," or does the patient regard the treatment as a serious and important aspect of life?

This nonverbal behavior allows the clinician to develop some hypotheses about attitudes and motivations. Then "feedback" can be provided to the patient by saying something such as, "You don't seem to be particularly concerned about failing to take your medication for a week. Are you really unconcerned, or perhaps do you feel that when you experience no symptoms, medication is not indicated?" As patients explain their underlying motivations, listen carefully for the attitudes about treatment, illness, and, specifically, the medication.

Sometimes, patients are able to conceal their underlying attitudes or beliefs. In this case, ask them to recall specifically what went through their minds on

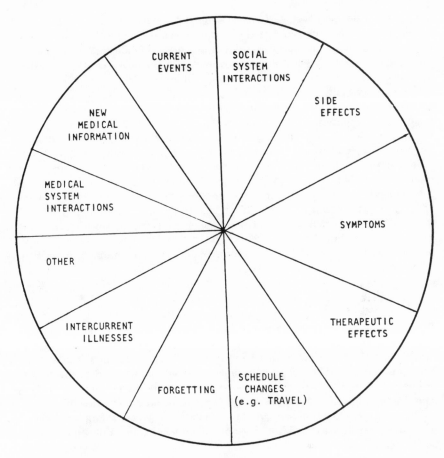

Figure 4. Clinician's guide: adherence-modifying factors.

each occasion when they failed to take the medication. As illustrated by the case example, these thoughts are often stereotypical and betray underlying attitudes. By recalling each time of forgetting in the past week, visualizing, and repeating aloud the thinking and feeling process that occurred at each occasion, patients become aware of their thoughts about the medication and illness.

Once these attitudes are identified, the basis for such beliefs is inquired about. The clinician might ask, "How did you come to believe that when there are no symptoms, the blood pressure medication is not indicated? Just because the medicine did not remove all of your headaches after just a few days, you somehow believe that this is evidence that the medicine is going to be ineffective in the future. I'm not sure how you came to understand this." Alternatively, phrases such as the following might be used, "It appears that you think, from time to time, that the medication may be doing you some harm. What sorts of things do you think it might be doing to you? What do you believe it could do to you that has not yet happened that might be dangerous or detrimental to you?"

Once patients explain and clarify the basis for their attitudes, one or two attitudinal or behavioral targets are chosen for planned intervention strategies. For example, if patients simply fail to recall to take the medication and had no thoughts about it, some sort of reminder technique is indicated, or some sort of cueing to high-frequency behavior is helpful. A calendar, alarm wristwatch, a pairing with morning coffee, and so on, will help develop the habit of recall and subsequent adherence.

Conversely, if patients have counteradherence attitudes as inferred from the recurrent, stereotypical thinking, these attitudes need to be tested and corrected when appropriate. Sometimes the clinician need only supply simple information (for example, "You know this antidepressant medication is not addicting, although it does elevate your mood"); however, sometimes specific attitude change techniques are needed (see the case example that follows).

If homework is used, its rationale must be explained to patients. Finally, patients are then asked to review the session by 1) *repeating* the high points, 2) *recording* what they plan to do, and 3) *rehearsing* or imagining how they are going to actually carry out the assignments. The interviewer provides interpersonal reinforcement for successful understanding of the interview and plans to improve adherence.

CASE EXAMPLE

The following case vignette illustrates how to identify factors that may reduce compliance. Selected portions of the adherence interview are presented. Medication recall forms the basis for identifying specific times of nonadherence. Thoughts and related beliefs surrounding specific adherence events were elicited or inferred. In some cases, dialogue is sufficient to modify thoughts and beliefs contributing to poor adherence. In other instances, specific homework assignments are created to modify antiadherence notions. This case example illustrates how unrelated life stressors interact with core beliefs and contribute to nonadherence.

Case Example: "To hell with it."

This 32-year-old nurse, single, a white female suffering from hypertension, had been taking hydrodiurnal once per day and alpha-methyl-dopa twice per day for the past four years. She was asymptomatic regardless of whether she took the medication. Her father had a history of hypertension and stroke. She had generally adhered to a low salt diet, even before her hypertension was diagnosed. The medications caused no side effects. She reported a belief that the medication was important, and denied that medication taking was a sign of weakness.

Medication recall revealed that she "forgot" her evening doses the preceding Tuesday and Thursday. Further questioning revealed that she actually had remembered, but thought, "Ah, to hell with it" at the time she actually "forgot," and went to bed without taking the medication.

T: Is this missing one or two doses per week typical?
P: Yes.
T: Do you usually think, "to hell with it," when you don't take your medication?
P: Yes.

T: Tell me what happened on Tuesday when you thought, "to hell with it," and "forgot."

P: My work was piling up. I was behind in my homework as well. I just felt pressured everywhere.

T: How were you feeling?

P: Frustrated. Like getting away from it all.

T: (Thinking that life stressors contributed to reduced adherence) How do you usually manage things when they pile up?

P: What do you mean?

T: Well, if you have too many things to do, what do you do?

P: I try my best.

T: What if your best isn't good enough to handle everything?

P: Well, I . . . I don't know.

T: Do you say "to hell with it," to some of the demands, or try to get help, or schedule what's important and delay the rest?

P: Well, not as clearly as you're saying it, but I must do something like that.

T: I don't think you do. I think you do what you said, which is to continue trying to do everything, get frustrated, and then whisper quietly, "to hell with it" by not taking your medication. Are the days that you don't take the medicine typically stressful as compared to others?

P: I think so.

(Here the patient might be asked to keep a daily record of "stressors" and medication ingestion to test whether stress or frustration inversely covaries with adherence).

T: (Believing the nonadherence pattern is an expression of frustration) Let's try to see if you can learn to manage these stressors differently. I mean, learn how to schedule, plan, say no, set priorities, and if needed, say "to hell with it," so that other people can hear you. If you can better manage stressors, then we'd predict you'd be adhering 100 percent to the prescribed medication. I want you to record your medication taking for the next week and to record the number of times you think something like, "to hell with it," and when you say it out loud. If you can learn to say it so that it actually helps reduce stressors and demands, then you won't have to say it by not taking the medication.

This case illustrates several important points. This patient appeared to have no medication-related reasons for nonadherence. Her father had suffered from a tragic, but not infrequent consequence of hypertension, namely, a stroke. She was quite cognizant of why medication was important and of the potential consequences of noncompliance. She had no side effects. In spite of these several factors contributing to adherence, she intermittently would rebel. Why?

A behavioral analysis revealed that she often thought "to hell with it" when she failed to take the medication. An accumulation of frustrations were reported on days of noncompliance. We hypothesized that she was the kind of person who too often says "yes" to demands that she or others make on her. This pattern would intermittently lead to feelings of frustration and overburden. Even if this were her usual pattern, formal psychotherapy was not needed.

The problem was reframed to provide her with a choice. She would either say "no" at work or "no" to her medication. The therapist might have explored further whether she expected significant negative consequences if she had said "no" at work, and whether they appeared to exceed the negative consequences she expected from saying "no" to her medication. However, in this case, the therapist judged that her father's stroke offered a dramatic reminder of what nonadherence might entail. If she continued to have difficulty with adherence, however, further exploration of this choice would have been indicated.

The therapist helped the patient to link "to hell with it" and nonadherence to the idea that she should speak up at work, say "no," and plan to reduce her frustrations. Thus, the impulse to nonadhere became a cue for reflection, planning, and stress management. The therapist also suggested a recording system for the following several weeks. The patient was to monitor the precipitating thoughts and subsequent medication taking. This strategy was chosen to help her attend to the link reported between frustration and medication nonadherence. An increased awareness of this link would result, hopefully, in increased compliance since she *wanted* to take the medication. Until now, she had failed to realize how frustration led to potentially self-destructive behavior.

If she were to have repeated difficulty with adherence, and reported continued "demands," the therapist might consider several options: 1) explore whether she actually believed medication taking was another demand; 2) determine whether she perceived situations as more demanding than they actually were; and 3) practice saying "yes" by doing things that she preferred (including taking the medication), rather than putting her wishes last.

CLINICIAN OBSTACLES TO IMPROVING ADHERENCE

Thus far, we have focused on patient obstacles to adherence. However, several factors within clinicians themselves may impair their capacity to deal with adherence. First, practitioners are particularly reluctant to follow an interview plan. Failure to follow a plan contributes to great inefficiency in patient interaction. Secondly, practitioners are uncomfortable with the specific nature of the interview methods and tend to use explanations, to avoid questions, and to rely too heavily on "scientific" rationales. The practitioner has become convinced of the prescription by a complex set of mental manipulations and reflections of which most patients are only dimly aware. Thus, when the diagnosis is arrived at, this is the first inkling to patients that there is, in fact, something wrong. Patients may have a lot of antipathy toward the diagnosis itself and initially are likely to misunderstand its meaning. Thus, without having been given time to consider the diagnosis and to understand the basis for it, patients are then asked to participate in a strange new treatment, which often entails ingestion of unknown and potentially dangerous substances that they are to undertake based on "faith."

A careful, detailed explanation of the disorder, the treatment plan, its potential dangers and specific requirements, as well as expected therapeutic benefits, should ensue. Again, an explanation is best conducted within the context of a dialogue between the practitioner and patient, in which a series of questions are posed by the practitioner to elicit patients' concerns.

Once the practitioner has decided upon a treatment course and the patient understands the rationale for it, it is wise to elicit "feedback" from patients— what sorts of ideas and feelings now occur to patients about themselves and their future life?

Another obstacle to adherence counseling appears to be a difficulty practitioners have in "creating" techniques. The idea of putting a reminder on the bathroom mirror for patients who need to take both A.M. and P.M. medication is a simple one, but one which many practitioners rarely consider. The easiest way to develop creative suggestions is to obtain a detailed description of the patient's day-to-day living, to "see" the world as the patient does. By going through the motions in imagination with the patient, the practitioner can often come up with several ideas individually tailored to the patient to assist in compliance.

Some practitioners have difficulty with adherence counseling because of their frustration with illogical behavior. It is wise to recall that many, if not most behaviors, are guided by both logical and irrational considerations. Practitioners need not become experts in unconscious motivations and neurotic conflicts. Rather, a compassionate understanding of the kinds of anxiety, fear, and confusion that many patients experience can help practitioners to empathize with and understand how this patient's behavior can fly in the face of "scientific" evidence.

Often, nonpsychiatric practitioners are fearful that specific questions and inquiry about the patient's attitudes, concerns, as well as their corollary and core beliefs is, in fact, conducting psychotherapy. They are afraid of uncovering a variety of factors in the patient's emotional life that they feel unable to deal with. This fear can be reduced by being aware that the target behaviors here have to do with adherence rather than with the patient's general joys and miseries. There are a few patients who require psychotherapy in order to obtain reasonable adherence. Patients, however, often confuse specific inquiries about their attitudes toward medication with general inquiries about their emotional life. The interviewer is best advised to focus the patient specifically on ideas, attitudes, and behaviors that impair or increase adherence.

Finally, perhaps the most difficult aspect of adherence counseling is that it significantly changes the content, nature, and method of interaction with patients. While medical practitioners begin to feel comfortable once a diagnosis is made and a prescription is written, patients begin to become anxious and confused. It is at this point, once the practitioner has solved his or her part of the "problem," that the search for specific compliance obstacles should begin. Thus, adherence counseling begins as soon as the diagnosis has been made and treatment has been selected.

Some reassurance can be gleaned by the would-be adherence counselor from the fact that a reiterative process is required (often over the course of several interviews) to help patients adapt to taking specific medication and to modify lifestyle and attitudes to facilitate adherence.

CONCLUSION

A model has been described here that clinicians can use to identify various factors that increase or decrease adherence. The scheme has a cognitive theoretical base. However, one need not be a cognitive psychotherapist to use this approach. If the target behavior is specified (for example, taking medication, exercising, and so on), then the ideas that surround the behavior can be easily gleaned by recall of specific times when the patient undertook or failed to perform the behavior. These thoughts form a pattern and are often based upon a number of beliefs (corollary beliefs), and, in turn, these corollary beliefs are based upon more core beliefs.

Many patients will not require extensive cognitive restructuring or revision of these corollary beliefs, particularly if the required change in behavior is short term, easily suited to the patient's lifestyle, and has an associated immediate reinforcement (for example, reduction of symptoms, improvement in looks, social system approval). For behavioral changes that are major revisions in lifestyle, contrary to the social system's beliefs, inconvenient, or not immediately reinforcing, the clinician may be required to elicit, confront, and attempt modification of specific corollary or core beliefs that obstruct these more substantive, long-lasting behavioral changes.

The obstacles to adherence immediately available to the patient include life events, information from medical authorities, beliefs and information within the patient's immediate social system and the culture as a whole, an awareness of symptoms, side effects and other bodily complaints, as well as environmental changes (for example, vacations, travel, and the like). The process of setting priorities upon these factors is a reiterative one in which the practitioner attempts to judge which factors contribute most profoundly to reduced compliance. The adherence interview provides a method for isolating and evaluating each factor and its cognitive concomitants. A careful assessment of these factors allows the clinician to select one or two specific techniques (such as recording side effects, cueing to high frequency behaviors, and so on) in a "trial" to modify adherence. The results of such interventions must be monitored carefully, and revision in these techniques might be required. Finally, several obstacles to effective adherence counseling in practitioners (for example, preference for explanations versus questions, failure to follow an interview format, and fear of "probing" too deeply into the attitudes of patients) have been reviewed.

Future work in this area might focus on elucidating the types of information that are most effective in changing behaviors and attitudes for specific types of individuals. In addition, careful comparative outcome studies to evaluate various adherence changing techniques in well defined populations should be conducted to evaluate the actual efficacy of specific strategies.

REFERENCES

Beck AT: Cognitive Therapy and Emotional Disorders. New York, International Universities Press, 1976

Brownell K, Heckerman CL, Westlake RJ, et al: The effect of couples training and partner cooperativeness in the behavioral treatment of obesity. Beh Res Ther 1978; 16:323-333

Ellis A: Reason and Emotion in Psychotherapy. New York, Lyle Stuart, 1962

Garfield S: Psychotherapy: An Eclectic Approach. New York, Wiley, 1980

Meichenbaum D: Cognitive–Behavioral Modification. Morristown, NJ, Plenum Press 1977

Rush AJ, Beck AT: Cognitive therapy of depression and suicide. Am J Psychother 1978; 32:201-219

Rush AJ, Watkins JT: Cognitive therapy with psychologically naive depressed outpatients, in Cognitive Therapy Casebook. Edited by Emery G, Hollon S, Bedrosian R. New York, Guilford Press, 1980

Sackett DL, Haynes RB: Compliance with Therapeutic Regimens. Baltimore, John Hopkins University Press, 1976

Strupp HH, Bloxom AL: Preparing lower-class patients for group psychotherapy: development and evaluation of a role-induction film. J Consult Clin Psychol 1973; 41:373-384

Chapter 30

Review of Empirical Studies on Cognitive Therapy

by Steven D. Hollon, Ph.D., and Lisa Najavits, B.A.

This chapter will focus on the empirical literature evaluating the efficacy of cognitive therapy. As will be seen, the bulk of the controlled empirical work to date has involved the treatment of depression, but work with other problem disorders is starting to emerge. Similarly, although the discussion will largely center on Beck's cognitive therapy (abbreviated throughout as CB, since it is, in fact, an integration of cognitive and behavior change principles [Beck et al, 1979]), some attention will be paid to its cognitive and cognitive–behavioral "first cousins," including rational-emotive therapy (RET), systematic rational restructuring (SRR), self-instructional training (SIT), and stress inoculation training (STI), among others.

A MODEL OF THE CHANGE PROCESS

Figure 1 (adapted from earlier theoretical work by Hollon and colleagues in an unpublished manuscript, Hollon et al, 1981, and first published in Hollon and Kriss, 1984) represents a model of the change process that will serve as a working

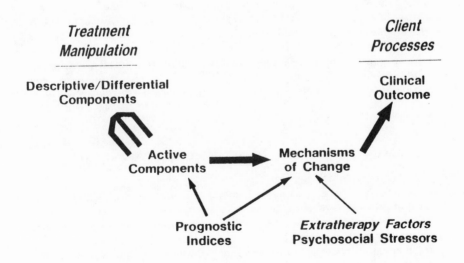

Figure 1. A model for the psychotherapy change process. Reprinted with permission from Hollon SD, Kriss MR: Cognitive factors in clinical research and practice. Clinical Psychology Review 1984; 4:35-76. Copyright 1984, Pergamon Journals, Ltd.

guide for the sections to follow. The uppermost nodes on the far left, "differ-ential treatments," and the far right, "clinical outcome," jointly define the mini-mal conditions for a controlled outcome study. Our primary emphasis will be on controlled trials that have compared cognitive therapy, or a closely related intervention, to one or more relevant alternative interventions (or no treatment). Clinical outcome can also be variously defined (Hollon, 1981). For our present purpose, we will be primarily concerned with initial response, and with the maintenance of that response after treatment termination.

As the number of trials evaluating cognitive therapy multiply, it becomes increasingly important to specify both the fidelity with which cognitive therapy was operationalized (whether the specified treatment was actually carried out) and the quality with which it was executed (how competently it was imple-mented). These twin aspects of treatment execution are represented by the term descriptive/differential components in Figure 1. Clearly, some of the variability in treatment outcome to be found in the empirical literature may be the conse-quence of variability across studies in treatment execution. Efforts to specify the active ingredients of change essentially attempt to identify that subset of differ-ential/descriptive components actually responsible for observed change. In essence, the search for active ingredients involves the search for what makes a therapy effective.

Active mechanisms are viewed as the mediators of change. When an inter-vention produces an effect, there must be some processes within the patient engaged by the therapy's active components which produce that change. As we have noted elsewhere (Hollon et al, 1987), efforts to identify causal mediators are remarkably complex. Few, if any, of the currently available studies have done more than evaluate some rather crude initial models, but these efforts deserve mention.

Finally, we will evaluate the literature pertaining to differential indicants for treatment; those variables that predict when a particular kind of patient would be better (or more poorly) served by receiving cognitive therapy than some other alternative intervention. This also turns out to be a more complex issue to resolve than it might first seem, since addressing it adequately requires all of the logical constraints needed to draw a solid differential treatment efficacy inference, plus large sample sizes and careful attention to the measurement of preexistent indi-vidual differences (Hollon, in press). Few existing studies meet all of these requirements.

COGNITIVE THERAPY AND ITS VARIATIONS

Cognitive therapy, as developed by Beck and colleagues (Beck, 1963, 1967, 1970, 1976; Beck et al, 1979) is, despite its name, an integrated set of cognitive and behavioral procedures designed to reduce aversive affective states and mal-adaptive behaviors by means of altering what a patient believes and how he or she processes information. The basic tenets underlying the approach and its central therapeutic strategies have been outlined elsewhere in this volume (see, for example, Chapters 24 and 25). In essence, cognitive therapy is presumed to rely most heavily on a process of empirical hypothesis testing to produce change in beliefs. Patients are encouraged to engage in behaviors that explicitly test the validity of their beliefs. Thus, cognitive therapy is an integration of cognitive and behavior change strategies.

Other types of cognitive or cognitive–behavioral interventions exist. Perhaps best know is Ellis's rational–emotive therapy (RET) (Ellis, 1962). RET shares many of its basic working principles with cognitive therapy, although it tends to emphasize a particular philosophy of life, stoicism, not explicitly promulgated by cognitive therapy (Ellis, 1973, 1980). Procedurally, RET probably relies most heavily on persuasion and reasoning to produce changes in patients' beliefs (Hollon and Beck, 1986). Thus, it seems fair to suggest that while cognitive therapy most emphasizes empirical hypothesis testing as its primary vehicle to change, RET relies most heavily on appeals to rationality. Systematic rational restructuring (SRR), (Goldfried et al, 1974), closely related to RET, also appears to rely largely on rationality to produce cognitive change. It is probably fair to say that SRR represents, in great measure, the efforts of university based researchers to develop a structured version of RET for use in controlled treatment trials. While RET is clearly the more widely utilized approach clinically, its very complexity and flexibility have tended to make it somewhat more difficult to execute competently in analogue studies, than has SRR.

Meichenbaum and colleagues have developed two related cognitive–behavioral interventions which rely, in large part, on repetition as their primary means of producing changes in cognition. The first, self-instructional training (SIT) (Meichenbaum, 1974, 1977), seeks to introduce appropriate mediational processes by having the patient first practice stating aloud, then rehearse covertly, the cognitions that the therapist believes would be more adaptive. This approach has found its greatest utility in work with impulsive children, for whom appropriate cognitive mediators appear to be absent (Kendall and Braswell, 1985). Whether it will prove as useful in work with adult populations, for whom existing maladaptive beliefs already exist, remains an open question.

The second approach, stress inoculation training (STI) (Meichenbaum, 1975), represents a combination of a skills training application phase, typically composed of a mixture of rationality and repetition-based efforts to change beliefs, with an opportunity for later application practice. This approach has been particularly prominent in efforts to deal with maladaptive habit problems such as chronic anger (Novaco, 1976) or substance abuse (Marlatt and Gordon, 1985), and with chronic pain and behavioral medicine (Turk et al, 1983).

Finally, there exist a variety of other more or less cognitive–behavioral approaches that have received less empirical attention. These include problem-solving therapy (D'Zurilla, 1986; D'Zurilla and Goldfried, 1971), self-control therapies (Kanfer, 1971a, 1971b; Rehm, 1977), self-control desensitization (Goldfried, 1971), covert conditioning (Cautela, 1966, 1967), and covert modeling (Kazdin, 1976), among others. While all have their place, they will not be the primary focus of this review. Our attention will primarily be centered on Beckian cognitive therapy, which has been tested primarily with depressed populations; and secondarily on the other major cognitive and cognitive–behavioral approaches, which have tended to be evaluated on other nondepressive problem types; for example, RET and SRR on anxiety and assertion, SIT on childhold impulse control disorders, and STI on habit disorders and chronic pain.

COGNITIVE THERAPY FOR DEPRESSION

Treatment Outcome

Few areas have received as much attention as the treatment of depression with cognitive therapy. As recently as the mid-1970s, Liberman (1975) concluded that most investigations of psychotherapy for depression did not meet acceptable scientific standards. Since that time, a wealth of well controlled studies have been added to the literature. Given that the various pharmacological and somatic interventions are already so well established in the treatment of depression (Klein and Davis, 1969; Morris and Beck, 1974), it would seem incumbent on proponents of approaches such as cognitive therapy to demonstrate some additional advantage; either superior acute response, specific subpopulation by treatment interactions, greater stability of response following treatment termination, or the like. Since the major finding emerging from this literature suggests a strong advantage for cognitive therapy over tricyclic pharmacotherapy with regard to treatment stability, we will review acute response versus the prevention of relapse/recurrence separately.

ACUTE RESPONSE.   Although the data are not wholly unambiguous, it would appear that cognitive therapy is an effective treatment for depression (see Hollon, 1981; Hollon and Beck, 1986; Jarrett and Rush, 1985, for expanded reviews).

Several studies have contrasted cognitive therapy with various minimal or no-treatment controls, typically in the form of an assessment-only wait list. All of the published trials have found cognitive therapy superior to no treatment (Bourque and Doucet, 1984; Comas-Diaz, 1981; Larcombe and Wilson, 1984; McNamara and Horan, 1986; Pecheur and Edwards, 1984; Shaw, 1977; Taylor and Marshall, 1977; Thompson and Gallagher, 1984; Wilson et al, 1983). Three additional unpublished doctoral dissertations evinced similar findings (Carrington, 1979; Magers, 1978; Morris, 1975). The only two studies failing to find differences favoring cognitive therapy were also unpublished doctoral dissertations (Besyner, 1979; Munoz, 1977). These studies are not above critique. Shaw's (1977) design utilized only a single therapist and a college student population (albeit one seeking treatment for depression). Several studies (Bourque and Doucet, 1984; McNamara and Horan, 1986; Taylor and Marshall, 1977) utilized brief treatments in analogue populations. Several other studies utilized specific samples which, while important special populations in their own right, were not representative of clinical depressives in general, including depression in Puerto Rican women (Comas-Diaz, 1981), geriatric populations (Thompson and Gallagher, 1984), persons with multiple sclerosis (Larcombe and Wilson, 1984), and the devoutly religious (Pecheur and Edwards, 1984). Put differently, none of these studies represented the ideal design for testing the proposition that cognitive therapy is superior to no treatment for a bona fide sample of clinical depressives.

In general, these studies come in one of three types; early analogue studies with fully realized cognitive therapy and minimal treatment controls (Shaw, 1977), later component analyses directed at dismantling CB (McNamara and Horan, 1986), and later clinical studies with fully realized CB and control conditions in special clinical populations, for whom the efficacy of the tricyclics have not been firmly established (Thompson and Gallagher, 1984). Given the existence of a known standard, the tricyclic antidepressants, such strategies are understandable. Despite the absence of any such ideal design, the available evidence is nearly wholly supportive of the conclusion that cognitive therapy is superior to no treatment.

Only four studies have contrasted cognitive therapy with the somewhat more informative attention-placebo or pill-placebo comparisons. Shaw (1977) found cognitive therapy superior to a nonspecific attention–placebo control condition in a sample of depressed college students requesting treatment at a university counseling center. Besyner (1979), in an unpublished doctoral dissertation, also found cognitive therapy superior to a nonspecific therapy in a sample of symptomatic community volunteers. Conversely, McDonald (1978) found no differences between cognitive therapy plus day care versus day care alone. The fourth trial may prove to be the most informative. In the NIMH Treatment of Depression Collaborative Research Program (TDCRP) (Elkin et al, 1985, 1986), carefully diagnosed primary and secondary depressed nonbipolar outpatients were randomly assigned to 16 weeks of cognitive therapy, interpersonal psychotherapy, imipramine pharmacotherapy plus clinical management, or pill-placebo plus clinical management (the attention-placebo/pill-placebo condition). Although the final report of the TDCRP is not yet available, it appears that cognitive therapy did not prove significantly superior to the attention/pill-placebo control. While it is the case that the pill-placebo condition represented a rather stringent control (it did involve the expectation of improvement from the "medication" and 20 to 30 minutes of weekly contact with an experienced psychiatrist offering support and encouragement), such a finding does not provide much support for the specific efficacy of cognitive therapy.

If this finding holds through the final report of the TDCRP, it may force a reevaluation of cognitive therapy's perceived efficacy. On the other hand, the TDCRP required off-site training and supervision of therapists recruited into the CB condition, a situation that may have undermined the adequacy with which CB was executed. All therapists did pass a preestablished competency criteria prior to participating in the study, with judgments made by experts in cognitive therapy, but only monthly consultations were provided on actual study cases. This schedule certainly provided less intensive ongoing case supervision than did other comparable studies involving cognitive therapy. It is quite likely that cognitive therapy, as practiced in the project, differed to a greater extent from what its practitioners were used to practicing than did the other modalities, a state of affairs that would place that modality at a relative disadvantage once the intensity of supervision was reduced. Clearly, we must await the full report of the TDCRP before its findings can be adequately evaluated. At this point, too few studies have been conducted to adequately determine whether cognitive therapy outperforms a nonspecific treatment control.

Cognitive therapy has typically fared well in comparison to other presumably active approaches. Several studies have indicated that cognitive therapy might be superior to essentially dynamic interventions; two unpublished dissertations (Carrington, 1979; Morris, 1975) and two published trials with clinical populations (Covi et al, in press; Steuer et al, 1984). Nonetheless, with the exception of the trial by Steuer and colleagues, in which indications favoring CB were limited to a single self-report measure, it is not clear that the psychodynamic interventions were powerfully executed by personnel capable of ensuring their representativeness. Thompson and Gallagher (1984) found no differences between

CB and a dynamic-eclectic approach in their geriatric population, while in the recently completed NIMH collaborative treatment trial (Elkin et al, 1985), interpersonal psychotherapy (IPT) (Klerman et al, 1984), derived from Sullivanian dynamic-eclectic principles, proved superior to placebo more often than did cognitive therapy (albeit not significantly superior to cognitive therapy in direct comparisons).

Comparisons to more purely behavioral interventions have been surprisingly few. Rude (1986) found CB comparable to assertion training in an unassertive depressed population. Both Shaw (1977) and Taylor and Marshall (1977) found that the combination of cognitive and behavioral procedures specified by cognitive therapy (see Beck et al, 1979) was superior to a more purely Lewinsohnian behavior therapy (Marshall and Taylor noted that the same result held when comparing the combination to the purely cognitive component). McNamara and Horan (1986) reported that the purely cognitive component of CB carried the basic weight of change, but also noted several factors that may have worked against the efficacy of their purely behavioral component. An unpublished dissertation by Besyner (1979) similarly favored cognitive therapy over the purely behavioral component, while a second unpublished dissertation by McDonald (1978) found no advantage when cognitive therapy was added to behavioral day care. While cognitive therapy, executed as an integration of cognitive and behavioral components, appears to be at least as effective, if not more effective than behavior therapy alone (or the purely cognitive component alone), the research speaking to this issue is surprisingly sparse and largely analogue in nature.

By far, the majority of the fully clinically representative trials involving cognitive therapy have contrasted the approach with tricyclic pharmacotherapy in the treatment of outpatient depressives. Given that such medications have been so clearly established as being effective change agents for depressed populations (most estimates suggest that approximately 70 percent of all primary nonbipolar outpatients can be expected to respond to antidepressant medications within one to two months of treatment initiation (Klein and Davis, 1969; Morris and Beck, 1974), it is clear that most investigators have pursued a strategy of evaluating cognitive therapy against a known standard.

The first such trial, conducted by Rush and colleagues (1977), suggested that cognitive therapy was not only comparable to tricyclic pharmacotherapy (imipramine) but superior to it, both in terms of acute symptom reduction and the minimization of attrition. However, that superiority emerged only once medication started being withdrawn two weeks before the end of the trial. This suggests that Rush and colleagues may have confounded acute response with relapse prevention. Consistent with this interpretation, subsequent studies have typically suggested comparability between cognitive therapy and tricyclic pharmacotherapy (for example, the psychiatric outpatient sample from Blackburn et al, 1981; Hollon et al, unpublished manuscript; Murphy et al, 1984). Only the general practice sample in Blackburn and colleagues (1981) also evinced a pattern of superiority for cognitive therapy over tricyclic pharmacotherapy, and that in the context of a response rate to pharmacotherapy so low (14 percent) as to call into question the adequacy with which that intervention was implemented. The single poorest outing for cognitive therapy vis-à-vis tricyclic pharmacotherapy came in the National Institute of Mental Health TDCRP (Elkin et al, 1986). Although not differing significantly from tricyclic pharmacotherapy by the end of the 16-week active treatment period, response to cognitive therapy was slower to develop and not as clearly discriminable from placebo as for tricyclic pharmacotherapy. Nonetheless, the issue of the adequacy of ongoing supervision previously discussed (and its potentially differential relevance for cognitive therapy) precludes any strong interpretation of those findings. Overall, there appears to be fairly compelling evidence that cognitive therapy alone is roughly comparable to tricyclic pharmacotherapy with regard to acute symptom reduction.

It remains unclear whether combined cognitive therapy and tricyclic pharmacotherapy is superior to cognitive therapy alone. Two trials have suggested such a superiority (the psychiatric outpatient sample in Blackburn et al, 1981; Hollon et al, unpublished manuscript), while four others have found no differences (Beck et al, 1985; the general practice sample in Blackburn et al, 1981; Covi et al, in press; Murphy et al, 1984). Where differences have been found, they have typically not been overwhelming in magnitude. There is somewhat more evidence to suggest that adding cognitive therapy to tricyclic pharmacotherapy is superior to pharmacotherapy alone, as four trials have demonstrated this superiority (both general practice and psychiatric outpatient samples in Blackburn et al, 1981; Hollon et al, 1986; Teasdale et al, 1984), while only one trial has indicated no advantage (Murphy et al, 1984). Clearly, there is no contraindication to combining the two approaches (unless one considers the risk of providing a potentially lethal medication to seriously suicidal depressed patients), with some indications of advantage over cognitive therapy alone and somewhat stronger indications of advantage over pharmacotherapy alone.

Overall, it is probably fair to conclude that cognitive therapy is an effective agent in the acute treatment of depression, although the available evidence derives from a series of designs that are not as solid as one might desire. The bulk of the studies utilizing no treatment or attention placebo controls are less than fully clinically representative in nature (Shaw, 1977; Taylor and Marshall, 1977; Wilson et al, 1983) or focused on narrowly defined populations (Comas-Diaz, 1981; Thompson and Gallagher, 1984). The single fully clinically representative trial using a pill-placebo control, the NIMH collaborative (Elkin et al, 1986), was not particularly supportive of cognitive therapy's efficacy, but may itself have reflected inadequate ongoing supervision for newly trained cognitive therapists, difficulties associated with off-site training, or other factors. Comparisons with other psychotherapeutic approaches have typically been supportive of at least comparable efficacy if not outright superiority, but were not themselves always ideal examples of powerful implementations of those alternative therapies. The most fully clinically representative trials, those contrasting cognitive therapy with tricyclic pharmacotherapy, rarely utilized control conditions (Rush et al, 1977; Blackburn et al, 1981; Hollon et al, unpublished manuscript; Murphy et al, 1984). Since the typical outcome emerging was one of general comparability, there remains the lingering concern that this literature has not so much documented comparability as failed to reject the null hypothesis. Nonetheless, given the comparability of the findings across studies, the magnitudes of the samples involved, the care that went into the execution of the pharmacotherapy conditions, and the comparability of the results produced by those pharmacological conditions relative to the best published indications, it seems very unlikely that this literature has failed to detect any "true" superiority for pharmacotherapy over cognitive therapy. The fairest conclusion would appear to be that cognitive therapy is an effective intervention for depressed outpatients, probably comparable to tricyclic pharmacotherapy alone in terms of acute response, and superior in combination with pharmacotherapy to either modality alone.

PREVENTION OF RELAPSE/RECURRENCE. If the available evidence suggests comparability between cognitive therapy and the current standard of treatment, tricyclic pharmacotherapy, with regard to acute response, there are strong indications of superiority for CB in preventing relapse or recurrence following treatment termination. Of the five studies that have followed successfully treated patients over treatment-free posttreatment intervals (typically ranging from one to two years), four have found cognitive therapy during the acute treatment phase (either alone or in combination with tricyclic pharmacotherapy) superior to medication without subsequent maintenance (Blackburn et al, 1986; Evans et al, 1985; Maldonado and Vila, 1986; Simons et al, 1986). In three of the four instances (Maldonado and Vila, 1986, used a much shorter follow-up period and a different analytic strategy), relapse rates in cognitive therapy, calculated as time to first relapse in life-table analyses, were only about one-half of what they were in tricyclic pharmacotherapy. The fifth trial, by Kovacs and colleagues (1981) (a follow-up to the earlier trial by Rush and associates) found only a nonsignificant trend favoring cognitive therapy, but overall relapse rates were roughly comparable to those in the other three studies. Recalling that the earlier trial by Rush and colleagues confounded response and relapse by withdrawing medications before the end of active treatment, thus overestimating end of treatment differences favoring cognitive therapy over pharmacotherapy, it seems likely that relapse in the report by Kovacs and colleagues systematically underestimated differences favoring cognitive therapy, by counting early relapses in the drug-treated cell as treatment nonresponders.

Overall, there appears to be strong convergent evidence that cognitive therapy provides greater protection against posttreatment relapse/recurrence than does tricyclic pharmacotherapy. Relapse rates appear to be in excess of 60 percent in pharmacotherapy without maintenance versus rates of approximately 30 percent in cognitive therapy. The higher rate in tricyclic pharmacotherapy is not simply an artifact of medication withdrawal, as indicated by the fact that relapse rates following the termination of combined cognitive-pharmacotherapy are typically no worse than for cognitive therapy alone (Evans et al 1985). Clearly, something very powerful is provided by cognitive therapy that survives the termination of treatment.

Pragmatically, of course, one could simply continue tricyclic pharmacotherapy for a period longer than is needed to bring about symptom remission. In the study by Evans and associates (1985), continuing medications for one year following symptomatic remission produced relapse/recurrence rates as low as those produced by having provided cognitive therapy during the acute phase (an extensive medication continuation literature exists indicating that pharmacotherapy should be extended across the expected length of the untreated episode; see, for example Glen et al, 1984; Prien et al, 1984). Whether cognitive therapy simply prevents *relapse* (the return of symptoms associated with the index episode) or provides a more comprehensive prophylaxis against *recurrence* (the onset of wholly new episodes) remains to be determined. Such studies will require even more extended follow-up periods than the one-year (Kovacs et al, 1981; Simons et al, 1986) and two-year designs (Blackburn et al, 1986; Evans et al, 1985) that have been utilized to date, since the average length of time between episodes appears to be about three years (Beck, 1967). Clearly, relapse and recurrence are somewhat distinct phenomena (Hollon, 1986; Prien and Caffey, 1977); indications of differential impact on each would have profound practical and theoretical implications. It remains unclear as to how cognitive therapy exerts its preventive effect, although early indications suggest that it may do so by virtue of altering the propensity of euthymic former patients to interpret negative life events as being the consequence of major flaws in their own abilities or character (Evans et al, 1985). Clearly, cognitive therapy's ability to prevent posttreatment relapse is the single most exciting (and robust) finding to emerge from this literature, one which will surely attract subsequent intensive investigation and influence clinical practice in this area. Providing booster sessions after the termination of acute sessions provided no additional prophylaxis in the only published trial to date to attempt such a manipulation (Baker and Wilson, 1985).

Prediction of Response

It is important to distinguish between prognostic indicators, variables which predict how different patients will fair in a given therapy, and prescriptive indicators, variables that indicate that a given type of patient will respond better to one type of therapy than another (Hollon, in press). Only the latter are actually useful in the selection of treatment for a given patient. In general, the prognostic factors predicting success in cognitive therapy are quite similar to those predicting success in imipramine tricyclic pharmacotherapy (see Bielski and Friedel, 1976, for a review). In general, patients who are older, female, unemployed, nonendogenous, neurotic, and/or chronically depressed tend to be less likely to respond to cognitive therapy than are other patients not evincing these characteristics. This does not mean that such patients are not suitable candidates for cognitive therapy (such a determination would require data speaking to how such patients would fare in the available alternative interventions), simply that other types of patients are more likely to respond to CB than they are.

Full prescriptive indicators are, to date, surprisingly few. Simons and co-workers (1985) found that patients high on pretreatment self-control did better in cognitive therapy than in pharmacotherapy. The endogenous/nonendogenous dichotomy has typically *not* proven predictive of differential response to cognitive therapy versus tricyclic pharmacotherapy (Blackburn et al, 1981; Hollon, 1986; Kovacs et al, 1981). This is surprising and not at all the case for other types of psychotherapy vis-à-vis pharmacotherapy (Prusoff et al, 1980). Few other prescriptive indicators are now known. Whether such indicants exist and have not yet been discovered, or whether they simply do not exist, remains undetermined at this time.

Active Ingredients and the Quality of Execution

While the efficacy of cognitive therapy appears to be reasonably well established, major questions remain as to how it exerts its influence. Presumably, it is the training in identifying and modifying one's own beliefs and information-processing strategies that carries the bulk of change (Beck et al, 1979). In particular, some have argued that it is the process of empirical hypothesis testing which is the most powerful change agent within the larger package that comprises cognitive therapy (Hollon and Beck, 1979; Hollon and Garber, 1981; Hollon and Garber, in press). To date, only a handful of studies have attempted to address these and similar issues. Teasdale and Fennell (1982) have found that efforts to change beliefs have a greater impact on symptomatic change than efforts to gather more information about beliefs. Jarrett and Nelson (1984) have found either self-monitoring plus logical analysis or self-monitoring plus empirical hypothesis testing to be superior to cognitive self-monitoring alone. Zettle and Hayes (1985) have similarly attempted to evaluate various components of cognitive therapy, finding them additive rather than interactive. Finally, Bourque and Doucet (1984) reported that a purely cognitive component of CB, completion of a dysfunctional thoughts record, equalled the full cognitive–behavioral integration advocated by Beck and colleagues (1979), but only after a two-month follow-up period.

Closely related is the desire to both describe and monitor the nature and quality of what goes on in cognitive therapy. Several instruments have recently been developed to do precisely that. These include the Collaborative Study Psychotherapy Rating Scale (CSPRS) (Evans et al, 1983; Hollon et al, 1984), a "fidelity" measure, and the Cognitive Therapy Scale (CTS) (Young and Beck, unpublished manuscript), a "quality" measure. Such instruments should make possible the ascertainment of whether cognitive therapy was executed in fact (fidelity) and with an appropriate level of competence (quality) in a given study relative to other studies. Further, correlational studies based on such instruments may help identify which components of the larger treatment package actually carried the bulk of observed change. For example, in the larger project by Hollon and co-workers (1986), the quality of modality-specific cognitive components and the quality of nonspecific relationship aspects jointly predicted acute response (Persons and Burns, 1985, reported a similar finding with regard to within-session mood changes), while only the quality of modality-specific cognitive components predicted prevention of relapse/recurrence. Clearly, the identification of active treatment ingredients and the growing capacity to specify and measure those behaviors associated with cognitive therapy represent important areas of future research activity.

Mechanisms of Change

Closely tied to the concern over which aspects of the treatment package account for its clinical efficacy is the issue of which mechanisms within the client are mobilized to mediate clinical change. In this regard, theory is easily specified. Cognitive therapy is presumed to operate by virtue of producing change in existing beliefs and information-processing strategies, which in turn produce reductions in overt symptomatology. In fact, efforts to evaluate mediational models are exceedingly complex and inferential errors quite easily made (Hollon et al, 1987).

In an early study based on Rush and colleagues' (1977) sample, Rush and co-workers (1981) found that for patients in cognitive therapy (but not pharmacotherapy), changes in patients' beliefs about themselves and their futures preceded changes in vegetative symptoms. Similarly, Rush and associates (1982) found greater change in measured hopelessness midway through therapy in cognitive therapy than in pharmacotherapy. Simons and colleagues (1984), however, found no differential change in either surface automatic thoughts or underlying differential attitudes between cognitive therapy and tricyclic pharmacotherapy. DeRubeis and colleagues, in an unpublished manuscript, similarly found no evidence for differential change in ongoing, surface ruminations, but did find that thinking propensities (for example, attributional styles) changed differentially in cognitive therapy relative to pharmacotherapy. Blackburn and Bishop (1983) also found evidence of greater change in cognitive content and process following cognitive therapy (either with or without medication) than in pharmacotherapy alone. Clearly, more work needs to be done in this regard, but the early studies suggest at least some initial support for cognitive mediational models.

Conclusion

It would appear that Beck's cognitive therapy is an effective intervention for depression, at least comparable to any other major alternative in the treatment of the acute episode, and perhaps superior to any other in terms of preventing subsequent relapse once treatment is terminated. It is important to note that these conclusions apply most clearly to primary, outpatient, nonpsychotic, nonbipolar depressives; virtually no controlled work has yet been done with secondary, inpatient, psychotic, or bipolar depressed populations. Within those populations that have been studied, surprisingly few indications of differential prescriptors have been documented. In this regard it is noteworthy that endogenicity does not appear to be a contraindication to cognitive therapy relative to pharmacotherapy. Studies of active ingredients and mediating mechanisms are few and, to date, rather primitive, but the initial findings emerging have not been at variance with the major hypotheses. Instruments capable of describing and evaluating the adequacy of treatment execution should both facilitate such research and help explain variance in outcomes across the empirical literature. On the whole, it would appear that cognitive therapy is a useful addition to the clinician's armamentarium. In particular, its capacity to reduce risk for relapse is a truly exciting dimension.

COGNITIVE AND COGNITIVE–BEHAVIORAL INTERVENTIONS FOR OTHER DISORDERS

The exposition to follow will be noticeably briefer and less detailed than the preceding discussion of cognitive therapy for depression. In part, this reflects our own interests, but it also reflects a subtle aspect of the empirical outcome literature. While cognitive therapy is far from the only type of cognitive–behavioral intervention that has been put forward, it has been, arguably, the most fully explored in the context of fully clinically representative trials. Curiously, virtually all of those trials have focused on clinical depression as the disorder of choice. In the section to follow, we draw heavily from a recent review of cognitive–behavioral interventions (Hollon and Beck, 1986), organizing our review around intervention strategies within discrete disorders.

Anxiety Disorder

SPECIFIC FEARS AND PHOBIAS. The bulk of the trials in this literature have been analogue in nature. In general, any of several cognitive or cognitive–behavioral interventions appear to be effective interventions for test anxiety. This statement appears to hold for systematic rational restructuring (Crowley et al, 1986; Goldfried et al, 1978; Wise and Haynes, 1983), self-instructional training (Holroyd, 1976; Meichenbaum, 1972), and, in more modest studies, stress inoculation training (Deffenbacher and Hahnloser, 1981; Hussian and Lawrence, 1978).

The literature with regard to speech anxiety is somewhat more modest. Various cognitive and cognitive–behavioral interventions were typically, but not invariably, superior to attention placebos or wait list controls. For example, Karst and Trexler (1970), Trexler and Karst (1972), and Thorpe and colleagues (1976) found RET superior, while Straatmeyer and Watkins (1974) did not. Gross and Fremouw (1982) found SRR superior to controls, but Lent and colleagues (1981) did not. Cradock and colleagues (1978), Glogower and colleagues (1978), Meichenbaum and colleagues (1971), and Weissberg (1977) similarly found SIT superior to controls, but Fremouw and Zitter (1978) did not. Nonetheless, these approaches have rarely outperformed more purely behavioral interventions, doing so in only two studies (Cradock et al, 1978; Glogower et al, 1978) and failing to do so in six others (Fremouw and Zitter, 1978; Gross and Fremouw, 1982; Hayes and Marshall, 1984; Lent et al, 1981; Meichenbaum et al, 1971; Weissberg, 1977).

These interventions have fared well in the treatment of social anxiety, typically proving superior to minimal treatment controls (SRR) Kanter and Goldfried, 1979; Shahar and Merbaum, 1981) and SIT (Glass et al, 1976; Elder et al, 1981), although RET did less well or no better than comparison conditions (DiLoreto, 1971; Emmelkamp et al, 1985). In the only trial to use Beck's cognitive therapy in this population (in this instance, combined with simulated exposure), Heimberg and colleagues (1986) found that approach superior to an educational supportive control condition. Cognitive–behavioral interventions typically performed as well as, but no better than, more purely behavioral interventions in the treatment of other specific phobias such as SRR (D'Zurilla et al, 1973; Wein et al, 1975) and SIT (Denny et al, 1977; Kanfer et al, 1975; Girodo and Roehl, 1978; Ladouceur, 1983). In Biran and Wilson (1981), the most fully clinically representative of all of these trials, a mixture of SIT and SRR was decidedly inferior to direct exposure.

GENERALIZED ANXIETY DISORDER. In the first relevant study in the area of generalized anxiety disorders, Woodward and Jones (1980) reported finding that a combined self-statement replacement plus desensitization was superior to either condition alone in a fully clinical population. Nonetheless, a careful reading of their published report makes it difficult to discern the empirical justification for this conclusion. A more recent project by Barlow and co-workers (1984), in which a combination of Beck's cognitive therapy and Meichenbaum's stress inoculation training was compared to a wait list control, indicated a strong advantage for the cognitive–behavioral intervention. Clearly, more work needs to be done, but this latter study is promising in light of the generally poor treatment response in this population.

OBSESSIVE-COMPULSIVE DISORDERS. In the only existent trial with an obsessive-compulsive population, again with a fully clinical sample, Emmelkamp and associates (1980) found little added advantage when cognitive restructuring was added to in vivo exposure.

AGORAPHOBIA. The bulk of the work in this area has involved fully clinical populations. In general, various cognitive or cognitive–behavioral interventions have typically failed to match more purely behavioral interventions in the treatment of agoraphobia (Emmelkamp et al, 1978, 1985, 1982). In two more studies, the addition of a cognitive component to behavior therapy did not enhance efficacy over the purely behavioral component alone (Emmelkamp and Mersch, 1982; Williams and Rappoport, 1983). In a sixth study, Mavissakalian and colleagues (1983) found that adding self-instructional training to in vivo exposure was less effective than adding paradoxical intent to in vivo exposure. The existing data are clearly not supportive of the utility of cognitive approaches in the treatment of agoraphobia. The question that emerges from this literature is whether cognitive approaches have been powerfully implemented in these trials. The research groups involved have generally been behaviorally oriented, and the cognitive approaches utilized have typically been treated largely as alternative control conditions rather than treatments of interest in their own right.

SUMMARY. In general, there appears to be a disparity between the utility of cognitive and cognitive–behavior interventions as evaluated in analogue trials, versus their utility for more representative clinical problems in more fully clinical populations. In general, analogue studies involving specific phobias typically produced evidence of superior efficacy relative to minimal treatment controls (but not more purely behavioral interventions), while studies involving bona fide clinical populations rarely found the cognitive and cognitive–behavioral combinations even comparable to the more purely behavioral approaches.

Assertion Problems

In general, the various cognitive and cognitive–behavioral approaches have fared well in the treatment of assertion problems. This statement appears to hold for RET (Alden et al, 1978; Carmody, 1978; Wolfe and Fodor, 1977), SRR (Derry and Stone, 1979; Hammen et al, 1980; Linehan et al, 1979), and SIT (Kazdin and Mascitelli, 1982; Kaplan, 1982; Safran et al, 1980; Thorpe, 1975). In general, these approaches have proven superior to various control conditions and at least equivalent to more purely behavioral interventions.

Anger and Aggression

Few controlled studies exist in this area but, to the extent that they do, the results typically have been promising. Forman (1980) and Camp and colleagues (1977) have both produced studies pointing to some efficacy for SIT-like approaches. Novaco (1976) and Schlicter and Horan (1981) have both demonstrated the utility of a stress inoculation approach in controlling chronic anger arousal. While the data are sparse, these two respective programs look quite promising.

Schizophrenia

At this time, there are no convincing data that cognitive or cognitive–behavioral interventions are at all effective in the treatment of schizophrenia. An early promising analogue by Meichenbaum and Cameron (1973) involving SIT failed an effort at replication by Margolis and Shemberg (1976). This is not to say that various cognitive and cognitive–behavioral approaches may not prove to be useful adjuncts to antipsychotic medication in dealing with the demoralization, depression, and anxiety that often accompany schizophrenia, but there is no reason to think that it is in any way a substitute for antipsychotic medications in terms of controlling the core thought disturbance.

Behavioral Medicine

Several studies have suggested the utility of any of the various cognitive approaches to the modification and control of headaches (Holroyd and Andrasik, 1978; Holroyd et al, 1977; Lake et al, 1979). Similarly, studies of analogue pain situations have found evidence of efficacy for cognitive interventions (Horan et al, 1977; Klepac et al, 1981). One study (Bradley et al, 1985) suggested that a combination of thermal biofeedback and cognitive–behavioral group therapy was superior to supportive group therapy and a no-treatment control in terms of reducing the pain associated with rheumatoid arthritis. Thurman (1985) found that a blend of RET and STI (with or without assertion training) was significantly more effective in reducing Type A behavior patterns and hostility, factors implicated in a variety of chronic health problems. In a particularly well executed study, Turner (1982) found a stress inoculation approach comparable to relaxation training, with both superior to wait list, in the treatment of chronic back pain. Finally, Kendall and colleagues (1979) found a stress inoculation condition superior to traditional patient education in preparing patients to cope with the stress of cardiac catheterization. The interested reader is directed to a recent monograph by Turk and associates (1983) for a thorough review of the role of cognitive and cognitive–behavioral approaches within the domain of behavioral medicine.

Marital Distress

Although an area of burgeoning interest, there has been, as yet, little controlled empirical work testing the utility of cognitive approaches to marital distress. Margolin and Weiss (1978) found the addition of rational restructuring to behavioral marital therapy superior to that latter condition alone, while Huber and Milstein (1985) found RET superior to a wait list control. Everaerd and Dekker (1985) found RET comparable to a standard Masters and Johnson sex therapy in terms of improving troubled sexual functioning, but superior in terms of reducing overall marital distress. Munjack and co-workers (1984) found RET superior to a wait list control in terms of reducing sexual dysfunction within marital dyads. Epstein and colleagues (1982) found an approach based on Beck's cognitive therapy superior to communication skills training. However, Baucom (1981) and Emmelkamp and associates (1984) found little advantage for the addition of a cognitive component styled after RET to more purely behavioral approaches. Beach and O'Leary (1986) found behavioral marital therapy superior to Beck's cognitive therapy in terms of reducing marital distress, although both were superior to a wait list control in terms of reducing depression. Clearly, more work needs to be conducted, paying careful attention to underlying theory and careful treatment implementation before any firm conclusions can be drawn.

Obesity and Eating Disorders

Surprisingly little work has been done in the area of eating disorders. Dunkel and Glaros (1978) found SIT superior to a more purely behavioral approach in the treatment of obesity. On the other hand, Wilson and colleagues (1986) found a cognitive intervention modeled after the purely cognitive component of Beck's cognitive therapy to be less effective than the same approach combined with exposure and response prevention in a bulimic sample, an advantage sustained through a one-year posttreatment follow-up. In addition to representing a worthwhile initial trial in an important population, this study appears to conform to the basic dictum that approaches which combine (and, especially, integrate) cognitive and behavioral components tend to prove more effective than either single modality alone (Bandura, 1977; Hollon and Beck, 1986). However, another major ongoing trial (Freeman et al, 1985) in which individual Beckian cognitive therapy (executed as the integration of cognitive and behavioral components) is being contrasted with both individual behavior therapy and a supportive-educational group therapy, may confound this basic principle. Early results suggest that the purely behavioral component may be at least comparable to the cognitive–behavioral integration in terms of reducing bulimic symptoms (but not associated depression). Little systematic work has yet been published in the area of anorexia, although a superb clinical-theoretical piece has been generated (Garner and Bemis, 1982) and important work is in progress.

Addictive Disorders

Despite the considerable interest in recent years in the role of cognitive factors in maintaining addictive processes (for example, Brownell et al, 1986; Marlatt and Gordon, 1985), there have been surprisingly few direct efforts to evaluate the contribution of cognitive interventions, at least as distinct from the more generic behavioral and behavioral self-control approaches. One study has looked at the utility of Beck's cognitive intervention in the treatment of heroin addicts, finding either cognitive therapy or supportive psychotherapy (each in combination with paraprofessional drug counseling) superior to that of drug counseling alone in terms of reducing subjective distress and drug usage (Woody et al, 1984). These treatment differences were largely confined to clients with more severe initial problems, suggesting that the formal therapies were most necessary for the more severely afflicted. Given the increasing theoretical prominence accorded cognitive factors in the maintenance of treatment gains, we anticipate accelerated controlled empirical work in this domain over the next decade.

Childhood Disorders

Along with the treatment of depression via Beck's cognitive therapy, no other set of disorders has been as fully and successfully explored as self-instructional training for impulsive children. Across a variety of studies (Arnold and Forehand, 1978; Kendall and Braswell, 1982; Kendall and Finch, 1978; Kendall and Wilcox, 1980; Kendall and Zupan, 1981; Meichenbaum and Goodman, 1971; Nelson and Birkimer, 1978; Parrish and Erickson, 1981), self-instructional training combined with modeling and response cost contingencies has proven superior to a variety of control conditions and alternative interventions. Nonetheless, important questions remain regarding the clinical representativeness of the changes observed (improvement is typically found on test tasks but is more equivocal on measures of impulsivity, attention, memory, and behavior) and the generalizability of those changes across situation and time (Abikoff, 1985; Gresham, 1985; Hollon and Beck, 1986; Whalen et al, 1985). Similarly, it is not clear whether these procedures will prove to be an effective alternative to medications and/or behavioral contingency management for working with seriously attention deficit disordered children (see, however, Hinshaw et al, 1984, for an exception).

CONCLUSIONS

The various cognitive and cognitive–behavioral interventions appear to have fulfilled some, but not all, of their original promise. The following conclusions can probably be drawn:

1. Beck's cognitive therapy for depression appears to be as effective as any other alternative intervention in the treatment of acute episodes, and more effective than other alternatives in terms of preventing posttreatment relapse. Little is yet known about inpatient, psychotic, or bipolar populations. Indicators of differential response are few. Work is underway to identify the active components leading to change and the mechanisms mediating that change but, to date, that work is not sufficiently well developed to be conclusive.
2. The utility of the cognitive–behavioral interventions for the various anxiety-based disorders remains an open question. The various interventions have fared better in analogue trials than in fully clinical samples. In those latter samples, the more generic cognitive and cognitive–behavioral interventions have not fared as well as the more purely behavioral interventions. Whether this state of affairs reflects the limited efficacy of rationality and repetition-based cognitive approaches, a more general inefficacy for all of the cognitive approaches, or some inadequacy in the execution of those interventions in these trials remains to be determined. To date, Beck's cognitive therapy, based on empirical hypothesis testing, has only begun to be tested in these populations, but initial indications are promising.
3. Interesting preliminary findings have emerged in some areas (for example, assertion training, anger control, behavioral medicine, marital distress, obesity and eating disorders, and addictive disorders) that merit further exploration. There appears to be little role for these interventions in the treatment of schizophrenia.
4. Meichenbaum's self-instructional training appears to be effective in modifying impulsive behavior patterns in children, although the generalizability and full clinical significance of these changes remain unclear.

Whether any one version of the cognitive–behavioral interventions is truly superior to any or all of the others remains to be determined. What is striking is the extent to which specific types of cognitive–behavioral interventions have been targeted to specific disorders (for example, Beck's cognitive therapy for depression, Meichenbaum's self-instructional training for childhood impulsivity, stress inoculation training in pain disorders, and so on). The approach relying most purely on rationality, RET, has perhaps the least carefully documented empirical support, although that state of affairs may be the result of its earlier clinical acceptance, leading, paradoxically, to a preponderance of earlier, less adequately executed clinical trials. The other approach relying largely on rationality, SRR, has held up somewhat better in somewhat better executed clinical trials, albeit trials that were mostly analogue in nature. Repetition-based approaches, SIT and STI, each have performed well in some populations, most notably childhood disorders for SIT and behavioral medicine for STI, although results are far less conclusive with other disorders in adults. Beck's cognitive therapy, with its emphasis on empirical hypothesis testing, has clearly performed well with respect to depression, but remains largely untested in other disorders. Clearly, more work is needed to explore how cognitive therapy exerts its influence in the treatment of depression, just as more work needs to be done in which fully clinically representative interventions are delivered to fully clinical populations in areas other than depression.

REFERENCES

Abikoff H: Efficacy of cognitive training interventions in hyperactive children: a critical review. Clinical Psychiatry Review 1985; 5:479-512

Alden L, Safran J, Weideman R: A comparison of cognitive and skills training strategies in the treatment of unassertive clients. Behavior Therapy 1978; 9:843-846

Arnold SC, Forehand R: A comparison of cognitive training and response cost procedures in modifying cognitive styles of impulsive children. Cognitive Therapy Research 1978; 2:183-188

Baker AL, Wilson PH: Cognitive–behavioral therapy for depression: the effects of booster sessions on relapse. Behavior Therapy 1985; 16:335-344

Bandura A: Self-efficacy: toward a unifying theory of behavioral change. Psychol Bull 1977; 84:191-215

Barlow DH, Cohen AS, Waddell MT, et al: Panic and generalized anxiety disorders: nature and treatment. Behavior Therapy 1984; 15:431-449

Baucom DH: Cognitive Behavioral Strategies in the Treatment of Marital Discord. Paper presented at the annual convention of the Association for the Advancement of Behavior Therapy, Toronto, November 1981

Beach SRH, O'Leary KD: The treatment of depression occurring in the context of marital discord. Behavior Therapy 1986; 17:43-49

Beck AT: Thinking and depression, I: idiosyncratic content and cognitive distortions. Arch Gen Psychiatry 1963; 9:324-333

Beck AT: Depression: Clinical, Experimental, and Theoretical Aspects. New York, Hoeber, 1967

Beck AT: Cognitive therapy: nature and relation to behavior therapy. Behavior Therapy 1970; 1:184-200

Beck AT: Cognitive Therapy and the Emotional Disorders. New York, International Universities Press, 1976

Beck AT, Hollon SD, Young J, et al: Combined cognitive–pharmacotherapy versus cognitive therapy in the treatment of depressed outpatients. Arch Gen Psychiatry 1985; 42:142-148

Beck AT, Rush AJ, Shaw BF, et al: Cognitive Therapy of Depression: A Treatment Manual. New York, Guilford Press, 1979

Besyner JK: The comparative efficacy of cognitive and behavioral treatments of depression: a multiassessment approach. Dissertation Abstracts International 1979; 39:4568-B

Bielski RJ, Friedel RD: Prediction of tricyclic antidepressant response: a critical review. Arch Gen Psychiatry 1976; 33:1479-1489

Biran M, Wilson GT: Treatment of phobic disorders using cognitive and exposure methods: a self-efficacy analysis. J Consult Clin Psychol 1981; 49:886-899

Blackburn IM, Bishop S: Changes in cognition with pharmacotherapy and cognitive therapy. Br J Psychiatry 1983; 143:609

Blackburn IM, Bishop S, Glen AIM, et al: The efficacy of cognitive therapy in depression: a treatment trial using cognitive therapy and pharmacotherapy, each alone and in combination. Br J Psychiatry 1981; 139:181-189

Blackburn IM, Eunson KM, Bishop S: A two-year naturalistic follow-up of depressed patients treated with cognitive therapy, pharmacotherapy and a combination of both. J Affective Disord 1986; 10:67-75

Bourque P, Doucet R: The reduction of the intensity of depression using Beck cognitive therapy. Revue de Modification du Comportement 1984; 14:105-111

Bradley LA, Turner RA, Young LD, et al: Effects of cognitive–behavioral therapy on pain behavior of rheumatoid arthritis (RA) patients: preliminary outcomes. Scandinavian Journal of Behavior Therapy 1985; 14:51-64

Brownell KD, Marlatt GA, Lichtenstein E, et al: Understanding and preventing relapse. Am Psychol 1986; 41:765-782

Camp BW, Blom GE, Hebert F, et al: "Think aloud": a program for developing self-control in young aggressive boys. J Abnorm Child Psychol 1977; 5:157-169

Carrington CH: A comparison of cognitive and analytically oriented brief treatment approaches to depression in black women. Dissertation Abstracts International 1979; 40:2829-B

Carmody TP: Rational-emotive, self-instructional, and behavioral assertion training: facilitating maintenance. Cognitive Therapy Research 1978; 2:241-254

Cautela JR: Treatment of compulsive behavior by covert sensitization. Psychological Record 1966; 16:33-41

Cautela JR: Covert sensitization. Psychol Rep 1967; 20:459-468

Comas-Diaz L: Effects of cognitive and behavioral group treatment on the depressive symptomatology of Puerto Rican women. J Consult Clin Psychol 1981; 49:627

Covi L, Lipman RS, Roth D, et al: Cognitive group psychotherapy in depression: a pilot study. Am J Psychiatry (in press)

Cradock C, Cotler S, Jason LA: Primary prevention: immunization of children for speech anxiety. Cognitive Therapy Research 1978; 2:389-396

Crowley C, Crowley D, Clodfelter C: Effects of a self-coping cognitive treatment of test anxiety. Journal of Counseling Psychology 1986; 33:84-86

Deffenbacher JL, Hahnloser RM: Cognitive and relaxation coping skills in stress inoculation. Cognitive Therapy Research 1981; 5:211-216

Denny D, Sullivan B, Thirty M: Participant modeling and self-verbalization training in the reduction of spider fears. J Behav Ther Exp Psychiatry 1977; 8:247-253

Derry PA, Stone GL: Effects of cognitive-adjunct treatments on assertiveness. Cognitive Therapy Research 1979; 3:213-222

DiLoreto AO: Comparative Psychotherapy. Chicago, Aldine-Atherton, 1971

Dunkel LD, Glaros AG: Comparison of self-instructional and stimulus control treatments for obesity. Cognitive Therapy Research 1978; 2:75-78

D'Zurilla TJ: Problem-Solving Therapy: A Social Competence Approach to Clinical Intervention. New York, Springer, 1986

D'Zurilla TJ, Goldfried MR: Problem solving and behavior modification. J Abnorm Psychol 1971; 78:107-126

D'Zurilla TJ, Wilson GT, Nelson R: A preliminary study of the effectiveness of graduated prolonged exposure in the treatment of irrational fear. Behavior Therapy 1973; 4:672-685

Elder JP, Edelstein BA, Fremouw WJ: Client by treatment interactions in response acquisition and cognitive restructuring approaches. Cognitive Therapy Research 1981; 5:203-210

Elkin I, Parloff MB, Hadley SW, et al: NIMH Treatment of Depression Collaborative Research Program, Arch Gen Psychiatry 1985; 42:305-316

Elkin I, Shea MT, Watkins J, et al: NIMH Treatment of Depression Collaborative Research Program: major outcome findings. Paper presented at the annual meeting of the American Psychiatric Association, Washington, DC, May 1986

Ellis A: Reason and Emotion in Psychotherapy. New York, Stuart, 1962

Ellis A: Are cognitive behavior therapy and rational therapy synonymous? Rational Living 1973; 8:8-11

Ellis A: Rational-emotive therapy and cognitive behavior therapy: similarities and differences. Cognitive Therapy Research 1980; 4:325-340

Emmelkamp PMG, Mersch PP: Cognition and exposure in vivo in the treatment of agoraphobia: short-term and delayed effects. Cognitive Therapy Research 1982; 6:77-90

Emmelkamp PMG, Kuipers ACM, Eggeraat JB: Cognitive modification versus prolonged exposure in vivo: a comparison with agoraphobics as subjects. Behav Res Ther 1978; 16:33-42

Emmelkamp PMG, van der Helm M, van Zanten BL, et al: Treatment of obsessive-compulsive patients: the contribution of self-training to the effectiveness of exposure. Behav Res Ther 1980; 18:61-66

Emmelkamp PMG, van der Helm M, MacGillavry D, et al: Marital therapy with clinically distressed couples: a comparative evaluation of system-theoretic, contingency constructing and communication skills approaches, in Marital Therapy and Interaction. Edited by Halweg K, Jacobson N. New York, Guilford Press, 1984

Emmelkamp PMG, Mersch PP, Vissia E, et al: Social phobia: a comparative evaluation of cognitive and behavioral interventions. Behav Res Ther 1985; 23:365-369

Emmelkamp PMG, Brilman E, Kuiper H, et al: The treatment of agoraphobia: a comparison of self-instructional training, rational emotive therapy and exposure in vivo. Behav Modif 1986; 10:37-53

Epstein N, Pretzer SL, Fleming B: Cognitive therapy and communication training: comparisons of effects with distressed couples. Paper presented at the annual meeting of the Association for the Advancement of Behavior Therapy, Los Angeles, November 1982

Evans MD, Hollon SD, DeRubeis RJ, et al: Development of a system for rating psychotherapies for depression. Paper presented at the annual meeting of the Society for Psychotherapy Research, Sheffield, England, July 1983

Evans MD, Hollon SD, DeRubeis RD, et al: Accounting for Relapse in a Treatment Outcome Study of Depression. Paper presented at the annual meeting of the Association for the Advancement of Behavior Therapy, Houston, November 1985

Everaerd W, Dekker J: Treatment of male sexual dysfunction: Sex therapy compared with systematic desensitization and rational emotive therapy. Behav Res Ther 1985; 23:13-25

Forman SA: A comparison of cognitive training and response cost procedures in modifying aggressive behavior of elementary school children. Behavior Therapy 1980; 11:594-600

Freeman C, Sinclair F, Turnbull J, et al: Psychotherapy for bulimia: a controlled study. J Psychiatr Res 1985; 19:473-478

Fremouw WJ, Zitter RE: A comparison of skills training and cognitive restructuring-relaxation for the treatment of speech anxiety. Behavior Therapy 1978; 9:248-259

Garner DM, Bemis KM: A cognitive-behavioral approach to anorexia nervosa. Cognitive Therapy Research 1982; 6:123-150

Girodo M, Roehl J: Cognitive preparation and coping self-talk: anxiety management during the stress of flying. J Consult Clin Psychol 1978; 46:978-989

Glass CR, Gottman JM, Shmurak SH: Response acquisition and cognitive self-statement modification approaches to dating skills training. Journal of Counseling Psychology 1976; 23:520-526

Glen AIM, Johnson AL, Shepherd M: Continuation therapy with lithium and amitriptyline in unipolar depressive illness: a randomized, double-blind controlled trial. Psychol Med 1984; 14:37-50

Glogower FD, Fremouw WJ, McCroskey JC: A component analysis of cognitive restructuring. Cognitive Therapy Research 1978; 2:209-224

Goldfried MR: Systematic desensitization as training in self-control. J Consult Clin Psychol 1971; 37:228-234

Goldfried MR, DeCanteceo ET, Weinberg L: Systematic rational restructuring as a self-control technique. Behavior Therapy 1974; 5:247-254

Goldfried MR, Linehan MM, Smith JL: Reduction of test anxiety through cognitive restructuring. J Consult Clin Psychol 1978; 46:32-39

Gresham FM: Utility of cognitive-behavioral procedures for social skills training: a critical review. J Abnorm Child Psychol 1985; 13:411-423

Gross RT, Fremouw WJ: Cognitive restructuring and progressive relaxation for treatment of empirical subtypes of speech-anxious subjects. Cognitive Therapy Research 1982; 6:429-436

Hammen CL, Jacobs M, Mayol A, et al: Dysfunctional cognitions and the effectiveness of skills and cognitive–behavioral assertion training. J Consult Clin Psychol 1980; 48:685-695

Hayes BJ, Marshall WL: Generalization of treatment effects in training public speakers. Behav Res Ther 1984; 22:519-533

Heimberg RG, Becker RE, Kennedy CR, et al: Treatment of social phobia with cognitive–behavior therapy versus education and support: posttest and follow-up. Paper presented at the annual meeting of the Association for the Advancement of Behavior Therapy, Chicago, November, 1986

Hinshaw SP, Henker B, Whalen CK: Self-control in hyperactive boys in anger-inducing situations: effects of cognitive–behavioral training and of methylphenidate. J Abnorm Child Psychol 1984; 12:55-77

Hollon SD: Comparisons and combinations with alternative approaches, in Behavior Therapy for Depression: Present Status and Future Directions. Edited by Rehm LP. New York, Academic Press, 1981

Hollon SD: Deconfounding cognitive vulnerability from symptom suppression: what we can learn from differential risk following treatment of depression. Paper presented at the annual meeting of the Association for the Advancement of Behavior Therapy, Chicago, November 1986

Hollon SD: Predicting outcome vs. differential response: matching clients to treatments, in Matching Clients to Treatments: A Critical Review. Edited by Pickens R. Rockville, MD, National Institute on Drug Abuse (in press)

Hollon SD, Beck AT: Cognitive therapy for depression, in Cognitive–Behavioral Interventions: Theory, Research and Procedures. Edited by Kendall PC, Hollon SD. New York, Academic Press, 1979

Hollon SD, Beck AT: Cognitive and cognitive–behavioral interventions, in Handbook of Psychotherapy and Behavior Change: An Empirical Analysis, third edition. Edited by Garfield, SL, Bergin AE. New York, Wiley, 1986

Hollon SD, Garber J: A cognitive-expectancy theory of therapy for helplessness and depression, in Human Helplessness: Theory and Applications. Edited by Garber J, Seligmen MEP. New York, Academic Press, 1980

Hollon SD, Garber J: Cognitive therapy: a social-cognitive perspective, in Social-personal Inferences in Clinical Psychology. Edited by Abramson LY. New York, Guilford Press (in press)

Hollon SD, Kriss MR: Cognitive factors in clinical research and practice. Clinical Psychology Review 1984; 4:35-76

Hollon SD, DeRubeis RJ, Evans MD: Toward a theory of therapy for depression: concepts and questions. Paper presented at the annual meeting of the American Psychological Association, Los Angeles, August 1981.

Hollon SD, Evans MD, Elkin I, et al: System for rating therapies for depression. Paper presented at the annual meeting of the American Psychiatric Association, Los Angeles, May 1984

Hollon SD, Garvey MJ, Evans MD, et al: Biological processes as predictors of response and mediators of change in cognitive therapy versus tricyclic pharmacotherapy of depression. Paper presented at the annual meeting of the Association for the Advancement of Behavior Therapy, Chicago, November 1986

Hollon SD, DeRubeis RJ, Evans MD: Causal mediation of change in treatment for depression: discriminating between nonspecificity and noncausality. Psychol Bull 1987; 102:139-149

Holroyd KA: Cognition and desensitization in the group treatment of test anxiety. J Consult Clin Psychol 1976; 44:991-1001

Holroyd KA, Andrasik F: Coping and the self-control of chronic tension headache. J Consult Clin Psychol 1978; 46:1036-1045

Holroyd KA, Andrasik F, Westbrook T: Cognitive control of tension headache. Cognitive Therapy Research 1977; 1:121-134

Horan JJ, Hackett G, Buchanan JD, et al: Coping with pain: a component analysis of stress inoculation. Cognitive Therapy Research 1977; 1:211-222

Huber CH, Milstein B: Cognitive restructuring and a collaborative set in couples work. American Journal of Family Therapy 1985; 13:17-26

Hussian RA, Lawrence PS: The reduction of test, state, and trait anxiety by test-specific and generalized stress inoculation training. Cognitive Therapy Research 1978; 2:25-38

Jarrett RB, Nelson RO: Mechanisms of change in cognitive–behavioral therapy in relation to depressives' dysfunctional thoughts. Paper presented at the annual meeting of the Association for the Advancement of Behavior Therapy, Philadelphia, November 1984

Jarrett RB, Rush AJ: Psychotherapeutic approaches for depression, in Psychiatry, vol. 1. Edited by Cavenar JO. Philadelphia, JB Lippincott, 1985

Kanfer FH: Self-regulation: research, issues and speculations, in Behavior Modification in Clinical Psychology. Edited by Neuringer C, Michael JL. New York, Appleton-Century-Crofts, 1971a

Kanfer FH: The maintenance of behavior by self-generated stimuli and reinforcement, in The Psychology of Private Events: Perspective on Covert Response Systems. Edited by Jacobs A, Sachs LB. New York, Academic Press, 1971b

Kanfer FH, Karoly P, Newman A: Reduction of children's fear of the dark by competence-related and situational threat-related verbal cues. J Consult Clin Psychol 1975; 43:251-258

Kanter NJ, Goldfried MR: Relative effectiveness of rational restructuring and self-control desensitization in the reduction of interpersonal anxiety. Behavior Therapy 1979; 10:472-490

Kaplan DA: Behavioral, cognitive and behavioral–cognitive approaches to group assertion training therapy. Cognitive Therapy Research 1982; 6:301-314

Karst TO, Trexler LD: An initial study using fixed role and rational-emotive therapies in treating public speaking anxiety. J Consult Clin Psychol 1970; 34:360-366

Kazdin AE: Assessment of imagery during covert modeling of assertive behavior. J Behav Ther Exp Psychiatry 1976; 7:213-219

Kazdin AE, Mascitelli S: Behavioral rehearsal, self-instructions, and homework practiced in developing assertiveness. Behavior Therapy 1982; 13:346-360

Kendall PC, Braswell L: Cognitive–behavioral self-control therapy for children: a components analysis. J Consult Clin Psychol 1982; 50:672-689

Kendall PC, Braswell L: Cognitive–behavioral modification with impulsive children. New York, Guilford Press, 1985

Kendall PC, Finch AJ: A cognitive–behavioral treatment for impulsivity: a group comparison study. J Consult Clin Psychol 1978; 46:110-118

Kendall PC, Wilcox LE: Cognitive–behavioral treatment for impulsivity: concrete versus conceptual training in non-self-controlled problem children. J Consult Clin Psychol 1980; 48:80-91

Kendall PC, Zupan BA: Individual versus group application of cognitive–behavioral self-control procedure with children. Behavior Therapy 1981; 12:344-359

Kendall PC, Williams L, Pechacek TF, et al: Cognitive–behavioral and patient education interventions in cardiac catheterization procedures. J Consult Clin Psychol 1979; 47:49-58

Klein DF, Davis JM: Diagnosis and Drug Treatment of Psychiatric Disorders. Baltimore, Williams & Wilkins, 1969

Klepac RK, Hauge G, Dowling J, et al: Direct and generalized effects of three components of stress inoculation for increased pain tolerance. Behavior Therapy 1981; 12:417-424

Klerman GL, Weissman MM, Rounsaville BJ, et al: Interpersonal Psychotherapy of Depression. New York, Basic Books, 1984

Kovacs M, Rush AJ, Beck AT, et al: Depressed outpatients treated with cognitive therapy or pharmacotherapy: a one-year follow-up. Arch Gen Psychiatry 1981; 38:33-39

Ladouceur R: Participant modeling with or without cognitive treatment for phobias. J Consult Clin Psychol 1983; 51:942-944

Lake A, Rainey J, Papsdorf JD: Biofeedback and rational-emotive therapy in the management of migraine headache. J Appl Behav Anal 1979; 12:127-140

Larcombe NA, Wilson PH: An evaluation of cognitive–behavioral therapy for depression in patients with multiple sclerosis. Br J Psychiatry 1984; 145:366-371

Lent RW, Russell RK, Zamostny KP: Comparison of cue-controlled desensitization, rational restructuring, and a credible placebo in the treatment of speech anxiety. J Consult Clin Psychol 1981; 49:608-610

Liberman M: Survey and Evaluation of the Literature on Verbal Psychotherapy of Depressive Disorders. Rockville, MD, Clinical Research Branch, National Institute of Mental Health, 1975

Linehan MM, Goldfried MR, Goldfried AP: Assertion therapy: skill training or cognitive restructuring. Behavior Therapy 1979; 10:372-388

Magers BD: Cognitive–behavioral short-term group therapy with depressed women. Dissertation Abstracts International 1978; 38:4468-B

Margolin G, Weiss RL: A comparative evaluation of therapeutic components associated with behavioral marital treatment. J Consult Clin Psychol 1978; 46:1476-1486

Margolis RB, Shemberg KM: Cognitive self-instruction in process and reactive schizophrenics: a failure to replicate. Behavior Therapy 1976; 7:668-671

Marlatt GA, Gordon JR (Eds): Relapse Prevention. New York, Guilford Press, 1985

Mavissakalian M, Michelson L, Greenwald D, et al: Cognitive–behavioral treatment of agoraphobia: paradoxical intention vs self-statement training. Behav Res Ther 1983; 21:75-86

McDonald AC: A cognitive/behavioral treatment for depression with Veterans Administration outpatients. Dissertation Abstracts International 1978; 39:2944-B

McNamara K, Horan JJ: Experimental construct validity in the evaluation of cognitive and behavioral treatments for depression. Journal of Counseling Psychology 1986; 33:23-30

Meichenbaum D: Cognitive modification of test-anxious college students. J Consult Clin Psychol 1972; 39:370-380

Meichenbaum D: Cognitive Behavior Modification. Morristown NJ, General Learning Press, 1974

Meichenbaum D: A self-instructional approach to stress management: a proposal for stress inoculation training, in Stress and Anxiety, vol. 2. Edited by Sarason I, Spielberger CD. New York, Wiley, 1975

Meichenbaum D: Cognitive–Behavior Modification. New York, Plenum, 1977

Meichenbaum D, Cameron R: Training schizophrenics to talk to themselves: a means of developing attentional controls. Behavior Therapy 1973; 4:515-534

Meichenbaum D, Goodman J: Training impulsive children to talk to themselves: a means of developing self-control. J Abnorm Psychol 1971; 77:115-126

Meichenbaum D, Gilmore JB, Fedoravicius A: Group insight vs group desensitization in treating speech anxiety. J Consult Clin Psychol 1971; 36:410-421

Morris JB, Beck AT: The efficiency of anti-depressant drugs: a review of research (1958-1972). Arch Gen Psychiatry 1974; 30:667-674

Morris NE: A group self-instruction method for the treatment of depressed outpatients. Ottawa, Ontario, National Library of Canada. Canadian Thesis Division, No. 35272, 1975

Munjack DJ, Schlaks A, Sanchez VC, et al: Rational-emotive therapy in the treatment of erectile failure: an initial study. J Sex Marital Ther 1984; 10:170

Munoz RF: A cognitive approach to the assessment and treatment of depression. Doctoral dissertation. Eugene, OR, University of Oregon, 1977

Murphy GE, Simons AD, Wetzel RD, et al: Cognitive therapy and pharmacotherapy, singly and together, in the treatment of depression. Arch Gen Psychiatry 1984; 41:33-41

Nelson WJ Jr, Birkimer JC: Role of self-instruction and self-reinforcement in the modification of impulsivity. J Consult Clin Psychol 1978; 46:183

Novaco RW: Treatment of chronic anger through cognitive and relaxation controls. J Consult Clin Psychol 1976; 44:681

Parrish JM, Erickson MT: A comparison of cognitive strategies in modifying the cognitive style of impulsive third grade children. Cognitive Therapy Research 1981; 5:71-84

Pecheur DR, Edwards KJ: A comparison of secular and religious versions of cognitive therapy with depressed Christian college students. Journal of Psychology and Theology 1984; 12:45-54

Persons JB, Burns DD: Mechanisms of action of cognitive therapy: the relative contributions of technical and interpersonal interventions. Cognitive Therapy Research 1985; 9:539-551

Prien RF, Caffey EM: Long-term maintenance drug therapy in recurrent affective illness: current status and issues. Diseases of the Nervous System 1977; 164:981-992

Prien RF, Kupfer DJ, Mansky PA et al: Drug therapy in the prevention of recurrences in unipolar and bipolar affective disorders. Arch Gen Psychiatry 1984; 41:1096-1104

Prusoff BA, Weissman MM, Klerman GL, et al: Research diagnostic criteria as predictors of differential response to psychotherapy and drug treatment. Arch Gen Psychiatry 1980; 37:796-803

Rehm LP: A self-control model of depression. Behavior Therapy 1977; 8:787-804

Rehm LP, Fuchs CZ, Roth DM, et al: A comparison of self-control and assertion skills treatments of depression. Behavior Therapy 1979; 10:429-442

Rehm LP, Kaslow NJ, Rabin AS, et al: Prediction of outcome in a behavior therapy program for depression. Paper presented at the annual meeting of the American Psychological Association, Los Angeles, August, 1981a

Rehm LP, Kornblith SJ, O'Hara MW, et al: An evaluation of major components in a self-control behavior therapy program for depression. Behav Modif 1981b; 5:459-490

Roth D, Bielski R, Jones M, et al: A comparison of self-control therapy and combined self-control therapy and antidepressant medication in the treatment of depression. Behavior Therapy 1982; 13:133-144

Rude SS: Relative benefits of assertion or cognitive self-control treatment as a function of proficiency in each domain. J Consult Clin Psychol 1986; 54:390-394

Rush AJ, Beck AT, Kovacs M, et al: Comparative efficacy of cognitive therapy and pharmacotherapy in the treatment of depressed outpatients. Cognitive Therapy Research 1977; 1:17-38

Rush AJ, Kovacs M, Beck AT, et al: Differential effects of cognitive therapy and pharmacotherapy in depressive symptoms. J Affective Disord 1981; 3:221-229

Rush AJ, Beck AT, Kovacs M, et al: Comparison of the effects of cognitive therapy on hopelessness and self-concept. Am J Psychiatry 1982; 139:862-866

Safran JD, Alden LE, Davidson PO: Client anxiety level as a moderator variable in assertion training. Cognitive Therapy Research 1980, 4:189-200

Schlichter KJ, Horan JJ: Effects of stress inoculation on the anger and aggression management skills of institutionalized juvenile delinquents. Cognitive Therapy Research 1981; 5:359-366

Shahar A, Merbaum M: The interaction between subject characteristics and self-control procedures in the treatment of interpersonal anxiety. Cognitive Therapy Research 1981; 5:221-224

Shaw BF: Comparison of cognitive therapy and behavior therapy in the treatment of depression. J Consult Clin Psychol 1977; 45:543-551

Simons AD, Garfield SL, Murphy GE: The process of change in cognitive therapy and pharmacotherapy for depression. Arch Gen Psychiatry 1984; 41:45-51

Simons AD, Lustman PJ, Wetzel RD, et al: Predicting response to cognitive therapy of depression: the role of learned resourcefulness. Cognitive Therapy Research 1985; 9:79-89

Simons AD, Murphy GE, Levine JE, et al: Cognitive therapy and pharmacotherapy for depression: sustained improvement over one year. Arch Gen Psychiatry 1986; 43:43-49

Steuer JL, Mintz J, Hammen CL, et al: Cognitive–behavioral and psychodynamic group psychotherapy in treatment of geriatric depression. J Consult Clin Psychol 1984; 52:180-189

Straatmeyer AJ, Watkins JT: Rational emotive therapy and the reduction of speech anxiety. Rational Living 1974; 9:33-37

Taylor FG, Marshall WL: Experimental analysis of a cognitive–behavioral therapy for depression. Cognitive Therapy Research 1977; 1:59-72

Teasdale JD, Fennell MJV: Immediate effects on depression of cognitive therapy interventions. Cognitive Therapy Research 1982; 6:343

Teasdale JD, Fennell MJV, Hibbert GA, et al: Cognitive therapy for major depressive disorder in primary care. Br J Psychiatry 1984; 144:400-406

Thompson LW, Gallagher D: Efficacy of psychotherapy in the treatment of late-life depression. Advances in Behavior Research Therapy 1984; 6:127

Thorpe GL: Desensitization, behavior rehearsal, self-instructional training and placebo effects on assertive-refusal behavior. European Journal of Behavioral Analysis and Modification 1975; 1:30-44

Thorpe GL, Amatu HI, Blakey RS, et al: Contribution of overt instructional rehearsal and specific insight to the effectiveness of self-instructional training. Behavior Therapy 1976; 7:504

Thurman CW: Effectiveness of cognitive–behavioral treatments in reducing type A behavior among university faculty. Journal of Consulting Psychology 1985; 32:74-83

Trexler LD, Karst TO: Rational emotive therapy, placebo and no treatment effects on public speaking anxiety. J Abnorm Psychol 1972; 79:60-67

Turk DC, Meichenbaum D, Genest M: Pain and Behavioral Medicine: A Cognitive–Behavioral Perspective. New York, Plenum, 1983

Turner JA: Comparison of group progressive-relaxation training and cognitive–behavioral group therapy for chronic low back pain. J Consult Clin Psychol 1982; 50:757-765

Wein KS, Nelson RO, Odom JV: The relative contribution of reattribution and verbal extinction to the effectiveness of cognitive restructuring. Behavior Therapy 1975; 6:459-474

Weissberg M: A comparison of direct and vicarious treatments of speech anxiety: desensitization, desensitization with coping imagery, and cognitive modification. Behavior Therapy 1977; 8:606-620

Whalen CK, Henker B, Hinshaw SP: Cognitive–behavioral therapies for hyperactive children: premises, problems, and prospects. J Abnorm Child Psychol 1985; 13:391-410

Williams SL, Rappoport A: Cognitive treatment in the natural environment for agoraphobics. Behavior Therapy 1983; 14:299-313

Wilson PH, Goldin JC, Charbonneau-Powis M: Comparative effects of behavioral and cognitive treatments of depression. Cognitive Therapy Research 1983; 7:111

Wilson TG, Rossiter E, Kleifield EI, et al: Cognitive–behavioral treatment of bulimia nervosa: a controlled evauation. Behav Res Ther 1986; 24:277-288

Wise EH, Haynes SN: Cognitive treatment of test anxiety: rational restructuring versus attentional training. Cognitive Therapy Research 1983; 7:69-78

Wolfe JL, Fodor IG: Modifying assertive behavior in women: a comparison of three approaches. Behavior Therapy 1977; 8:567-574

Woodward R, Jones RB: Cognitive restructuring treatment: a controlled trial with anxious patients. Behav Res Ther 1980; 18:401-407

Woody GE, McLellan AT, Luborsky L, et al: Severity of psychiatric symptoms as a predictor of benefits from psychotherapy: the Veterans Administration–Pennsylvania State Study. Am J Psychiatry 1984; 141:1172-1177

Zettle RD, Hayes SC: Cognitive therapy of depression: behavioral analysis of component and process issues. Affective Disorders Network Bulletin 2, March 1985

Afterword

by A. John Rush, M.D., and Aaron T. Beck, M.D.

Given the numerous advances in cognitive therapy detailed in the preceding chapters, the psychiatric practitioner may be confronted with several questions about this approach: How does cognitive therapy relate to psychodynamic theory and therapy? Can cognitive techniques be utilized in the context of a more psychodynamically oriented approach to therapy? Must the therapy be time-limited? Can this approach successfully be combined with medication treatment? What are common obstacles or problems encountered in learning cognitive therapy? How can one learn cognitive therapy?

As noted in the Foreword and in Chapter 24, as well as in other writings (Beck et al, 1979), cognitive therapy is compatible with ego psychoanalytic approaches. While both focus on "information processing" as a key determinant of behavioral and emotional response patterns, there is a fundamental paradigmatic shift implied in the cognitive approach. Namely, one's representation of reality or "phenomenal field" constitutes the key target of change for the cognitive therapist. The underlying motivational need for such a representation is not sought by the cognitive practitioner. Rather, it is assumed that both the pathological state itself and one's previous day-to-day experiences—especially, but not exclusively, in early life—create the basis for such a representation. It is a change in that representation, fostered by both discussions with the therapist and, most importantly, as facilitated by repeated homework assignments, that is deemed essential for a therapeutic effect. Some patients may, and others may not, develop a detailed knowledge or insight into the original sources of such a representation. In this sense, symptom reduction becomes an essential first target of cognitive therapy, with historically based insight taking on a somewhat secondary importance. In this respect, cognitive therapy is more akin to behavioral notions that change in behavior or thinking may precede, yet foster, such insight, rather than insight being viewed as a necessary antecedent of behavioral or cognitive change.

Some writings (Rush, 1980; Altshuler and Rush, 1984) have attempted to relate psychodynamic constructs and cognitive concepts. While the clarification of these relationships is yet unfolding, it is of clinical interest that that "therapeutic opportunities and targets" may be rather similar for cognitive and psychoanalytic practitioners (Altshuler and Rush, 1984). Conversely, the specific methods or techniques to facilitate therapeutic changes do more sharply distinguish these two approaches. Cognitive therapy, for example, involves a rather active, directed, yet collaborative therapist role. The initial objective of treatment is the elicitation of automatic thoughts, which may be viewed as "preconscious" from a dynamic perspective. It is for this reason that strong general therapeutic skills are essential for the would-be cognitive therapist. As most clinicians know, if these automatic thoughts are to be carefully elicited and confronted, a breach of the therapeutic alliance is likely (Rush, 1985; Chapter 29 of this volume). This poses a special problem, as noted by Trautman and Rotheram (in Chapter 27) in adolescents, or in those with significant Axis II problems (Beck et al, 1979). For those patients for whom the development of the therapeutic alliance is a painstaking, time-demanding exercise, the usual brief time limit suggested for cognitive therapy may have to be modified (Rush, 1985; Chapter 29 of this volume). Thus, while the fixed time limit can provide encouragement for some patients who do not have significant personality difficulties, it can have a negative therapeutic effect for those with more severe problems in relationship formation and trust (Rush and Shaw, 1983; Chapter 29 of this volume).

Alternatively, clinical experience would suggest (though no formal empirical studies are available) that selected cognitive techniques can be blended into a more psychodynamically oriented approach to therapy. Such a blending requires two key elements: 1) patients' willingness to modify their thinking and behavior to discover (gain "insight into") the consequences of their routine and modified response patterns, and 2) the therapist's ability/willingness to direct, motivate, and support the patient's attempts to explore alternative patterns of response. Since cognitive techniques are rather prescriptive—although based on a clear understanding of the patient's current view of the world—the therapist, whether cognitive or psychodynamic, must exercise both tact and judgment in initiating specific cognitive techniques, as described by Wright, Beck and Greenberg, Rush, and Trautman and Rotheram in the preceding chapters.

Turning to common obstacles or difficulties encountered by would-be cognitive therapists, one can divide these problems into two groups. The first group consists of problems encountered by less experienced, though eager, therapists. For these young practitioners, cognitive therapy appears to be so simply prescriptive that one need only follow the recipe manual, and an elegant souffle is sure to follow. Because descriptions of techniques appear to be clear, one need only emulate that which is written—with little regard for modification and titration based upon the individual patient's position or participation. These therapists often learn and cling to just a few techniques with which they approach all patients (for example, the Triple Column Technique [see Chapter 25]), or they bombard a single patient with too many directives/techniques in hopes of beating the time limit established by the proscribed treatment. Further, the emotional impact of these techniques—which is often substantial—is often not fully appreciated by inexperienced therapists. In some instances, patients feel overwhelmed and, as a consequence, withdraw from treatment.

Conversely, the experienced psychodynamically oriented practitioner will encounter rather different problems in attempting to learn cognitive therapeutic methods. The role of the therapist as a facilitator, guide, questioner, or collaborator often is felt as too active, intrusive, or insensitive. One assumes that the patient will ultimately move (with indirect and very gentle encouragement) to a desire to change. Thus, the use of what appears to be provocative techniques leads to a sense of discomfort and a tendency to retreat on the part of many such clinicians. Secondly, the cognitive model often appears to be too simplistic. Some of these clinicians will explore the deeper, unconscious "motivation" of patients. While such explorations may be especially enlightening for the therapist, they must be willing to forego this adventure in hopes of more immediate symptom reduction. That is, symptom reduction and collaborative correction of distorted thinking and dysfunctional person–environment interactions must become more important than a full historical reconstruction of the hidden motivations for pathological behavior. When the psychodynamically experienced practitioner is confronted with this choice, the response is often to be very tentative in the necessary role change. The cognitive therapist must be able to be both somewhat directive or probing, while maintaining an empathetic understanding of the patient. That is, special skill in both empathetic and directive roles is needed.

To date, there is no evidence at all that suggests a negative interaction between cognitive therapy and medication to control symptoms of a particular disorder. Alternatively, compliance with medication is not as easily obtained as might be thought (see Chapter 29). In addition, for some patients the combination treatment may not offer any advantage over either treatment alone (Beck et al, 1985), yet for others such a combination treatment may be especially useful (Blackburn et al, 1981). Now the challenge of the field is to identify and separate such patients. As noted in Chapters 25 and 30, this has been only partially addressed to date.

Finally, let us turn to a practical question—namely, how can one learn more about cognitive therapy for depression and for the other disorders discussed in the preceding chapters? Cognitive therapy, unlike many other therapeutic approaches, has developed from an academic/empirical base. Thus, there are few training or certifying institutes for this type of approach. While there are several "centers" for cognitive therapy in the United States, few are as yet fully equipped to train would-be practitioners. Should the reader have an interest in this approach, we would suggest that you write to Aaron T. Beck, M.D., Director, Center for Cognitive Therapy, University of Pennsylvania, 133 South 36th Street, Philadelphia, Pennsylvania 19104, to locate a potential training center in your locale.

REFERENCES

Altshuler KA, Rush AJ: Psychoanalytic and cognitive therapies: a comparison of theory and tactics. Am J Psychotherapy 1984; 37:4-16

Beck AT, Hollon SD, Young J, et al: Combined cognitive–pharmacotherapy versus cognitive therapy in the treatment of depressed outpatients. Arch Gen Psychiatry 1985; 42:142-148

Beck AT, Rush AJ, Shaw BF, et al: Cognitive Therapy for Depression. New York, Guilford Press, 1979

Blackburn IM, Bishop S, Glenn AIM, et al: The efficacy of cognitive therapy in depression: a treatment trial using cognitive therapy and pharmacotherapy, each alone and in combination. Br J Psychiatry 1981; 139:181-189

Rush AJ: Psychotherapy of the affective psychoses. Am J Psychoanal 1980; 40:99-123

Rush AJ: The therapeutic alliance in short-term directive therapies, in Psychiatry Update: The American Psychiatric Association Annual Review, volume 4. Edited by Francis AJ, Hales RE. Washington, DC, American Psychiatric Press, 1985

Rush AJ, Shaw BF: Failures in treating depression by cognitive behavioral therapy, in Failures in Behavior Therapy. Edited by Foa EB, Emmelkamp PMG. New York, John Wiley & Sons, 1983

Afterword

Afterword

by Allen J. Frances, M.D., and Robert E. Hales, M.D.

Undoubtedly this has been a long and a demanding book, both for you and for us. We have learned a great deal in preparing it and hope that we have provided you with a good return for your considerable efforts in reading it. We are spared the need for providing a summary here since each section had its own Afterword and no summary of such a vast canvas could be meaningful. However, several themes to do emerge. Psychiatry is clearly advancing rapidly in its scientific underpinnings and in its clinical effectiveness. There is no need for devotion to reductionistic models, and we are likely to see increasing efforts to integrate biological, psychodynamic, cognitive, behavioral, interpersonal, and social systems to understand psychiatric disorders and to develop methods for treating them. Knowledge in psychiatry is growing at a rate that prevents any of us from being really up to date, but we are fortunate to practice at a time when new scientific discoveries are directly influencing the scope and quality of the care that we can deliver.

Volume 8 of the *Review of Psychiatry* promises to be one of the most exciting books yet. The senior editorship of Volume 8 will pass to the new Scientific Program Committee Chairman, Allan Tasman, M.D., an Associate Professor of Psychiatry at the University of Connecticut and the Director of Psychiatry Residency Training. Jerry Wiener, M.D., and James Egan, M.D., will be editing a section on child psychiatry. Advances occurring in this psychiatric subspecialty the last few years have been enormous. Paul Appelbaum, M.D., will serve as a section editor on the law and psychiatry. This topic has not been reviewed since Volume 1 was published in 1982. Roger E. Meyer, M.D., will be providing an update on alcoholism. This field continues to expand and to be of great clinical relevance for psychiatrists. John G. Gunderson, M.D., will be providing a review on the borderline personality disorder. Patients with this disorder constitute an important area for research and present significant problems for the clinician. Finally, William Sledge, M.D., will be organizing a section on a number of difficult situations in clinical practice. This section will explore particularly important and challenging circumstances that occur in the professional life of practitioners.

We are grateful to the many people who have labored on this volume as section editors, contributors, and readers. We hope you have enjoyed your role as much as we have enjoyed ours. We'll look forward to meeting you again in these pages next year, when Allan Tasman, M.D., takes over the senior editorship and we assist him as junior editors.

Index

Abuse
  child, 395-396
  substance, *see* Alcoholism; Substance
    abuse
Acetylcholine (Ach), abnormalities in
  depression, 182-184
ACQ, *see* Agoraphobic Cognitions
  Questionnaire
Acquired immunodeficiency syndrome
  (AIDS), 268-269
  suicide risk, 423
Acute confusional state, resulting from
  ECT, 498-500
Acute Panic Inventory, 81
Addison's disease, depression in, 264
Adherence, *see* Compliance
Adherence interview, 635-638
ADIS, *see* Anxiety Disorders Schedule
Adolescents
  cognitive therapy with, 584-604
  ECT use in, 471-472
  familial and extrafamilial exposure to
    suicide, 357-358
  familial loading for psychiatric illness,
    395
  girls, suicidality in, 362-363
  methods of suicide, 387-388
  nonfatal suicidality, 390-394
  substance abuse by, 205, 363
  suicidal, 206, 288, 354, 356-358, 362-363,
    386-399, 602-603
  unipolar depression in, 204-206
Adoption studies
  Danish, 154
  of depression, 149, 153-154, 275
  of schizophrenia, 154, 275
  substance use disorders, 153
  of suicidality, 394-395
Adrenocorticotropin hormone (ACTH),
  associated depressive syndromes, 265
Affect, encouragement of, 237
  See also Emotion
Affective disorders
  among Amish, 151, 315
  catatonia as, 468
  catecholamine hypotheses of, 177
  and Cushing's syndrome, 269
  inclusion of anxiety states within, 199
  liability scale, 159
  produced by HIV, 268-269, 423
  as risk factor for suicide, 361-363,
    408-409
  schizoaffective disorder as, 469-470
  seasonal (SAD), 172
  single-locus hypotheses, 160
  sleep–wake changes in, 171
  subsequent malignancies, 359-360
  unipolar depression in, 155-159
  use of term, 147-148, 188-189

Age
  birth cohort effects, *see* Birth cohort
    effects
  and ECT use, 471-472
  of onset, 62, 73-74, 152, 155, 157, 159,
    228, 256, 274
  risk of depression and, 149, 153, 158,
    164
  of secondary depressives, 256, 258
  suicide rates by, 288, 291-294, 307, 309,
    314-316, 327-329, 369, 386-399, 416,
    417, 422-423
Agenda, therapeutic session, to reduce
  hopelessness, 560
Aggressivity, and suicidality, 288, 296-298,
  324, 334, 339-340, 346, 356, 359, 423-424
Agoraphobia
  age of onset, 73-74
  alcohol abuse and, 77
  comorbidity with panic disorder, 58-61,
    63
  and depression, 140
  epidemiology of, 8, 54-64
  imipramine for, 92
  involving family in treatment, 123
  and panic, 58-61, 63, 72, 125-126,
    138-139
  panic attacks as central disturbance in, 67
  rates and risks, 5-6, 56-57, 59, 67
  treatment enhancement and relapse
    prevention, 121
  tripartite assessment of fear, 82
  in vivo exposure, 121-125
  See also Panic disorder; Phobia
Agoraphobic Cognitions Questionnaire
  (ACQ), 80-81
AIDS, *see* Acquired immunodeficiency
  syndrome
Akathisia, and suicide, 364
Albany study, of panic disorder, 131-132
Alcohol
  abuse, 58, 61, 77, 359
  agoraphobics and, 61
  avoidance, by panic patients, 90
  blood content (BAC), in suicides, 316-
    319, 322, 324
  digestive organ cancers and, 359
  effect on monoamines and metabolites,
    337, 339
  and panic disorder, 58, 61, 77, 90
  self-medication with, 6-7, 54, 63, 77,
    198, 324
  and suicidal behavior, 316-325, 327-330
  See also Alcoholism; Substance abuse
Alcoholism
  and agoraphobia and/or social phobia,
    6-7
  birth cohort effects, 152
  CNS monoamines and metabolites, and
    suicidality, 339-340

communication of suicidal intent, 324,
330, 417
as complication of anxiety disorder, 6
definitions used in suicide studies, 317-
323
and depression, 74, 156, 157, 165, 198-
200, 205, 265, 301, 364
disruption of close relationship, and
suicidality, 301, 325, 329, 354-355,
417, 418
family history of, 74
and gender, 162
low MAO and risk of, 163
and panic disorder, 63, 74
and race, 304
as risk factor for suicide, 316, 318-320,
323-325, 327-330, 354, 403, 409, 418
secondary depression and, 256
and suicidality, 301, 303, 324, 330, 339-
340, 373-374
suicide as late sequela of, 324, 330, 363-
364
treatment of suicidality, 373-374
and unipolar depression, 74, 156, 157,
165, 198-200, 205
Alkalosis, panicogenicity, 44-45
Allergies, history of, and MAOIs, 91-92
Alpha$_2$ receptors, 11, 37
Alprazolam
discontinuation and follow-up, 107
dosage and course of treatment, 106-107
for panic, 104-108, 113
side effects, 107
Ambulatory monitoring
ordinary-day, for panic, 35-36, 41, 82,
125
Vitalog MC-2 monitor, 36
Amish
frequency of depression in, 151
suicides and affective disorders among,
315
Amitriptyline, for unipolar depression,
216
Amnesia, iatrogenic, from ECT, 438-440,
500-505
Amozapine, for unipolar depression, 216
Amphetamines
associated depressive syndrome, 265
transient mood improvement, in
depression, 179
Amygdala, cholinergic activity in, 182
Anergia, 189
and hypothyroidism, 175-176
Anesthesia, as setting event for first
panic, 14-15
Anger
expressing, consequences of, 576
mistaken for depression, 263
as panic trigger, 133, 573, 576

Anorexia
and affective disorder, 155-156
comorbidity with depression, 199
Anoxia
as cause of depressive symptoms, 264
cerebral, and suicide risk, 326
Antibodies
antithyroid, 176
HIV, 265
Antidepressants
advent of, 147
available in the U.S., 216
benefit/risk ratio, 366
for medically ill depressed, 270
predicting response to, 178-179
REM sleep effects, 170-171
for secondary depression, 259
sleep deprivation as, 170-171
tricyclic, see Tricyclic antidepressants
tryptophan, 181, 461
Antihypertensives, associated depressive
syndrome, 265
Anti-mental illness bias, 260-261, 491
Antipsychotics, compared with ECT, 467
Antisocial behavior, and subsequent
suicide, 388, 389, 391, 412
Antisocial personality, family history of,
and unipolar depression, 156, 195
Anxiety
alcoholism, depression, and suicide as
consequence of, 6
anticipatory, 112-115, 138
association between caffeine and, 31
cognitive model of, 128-129, 571-573
and depression, 199-200, 217-219
generalized, distinction between panic
and, 73
managing, 112-115, 123-125
nature of, 20-21
separation, 18-19, 236
substance abuse, and panic, 6-7
treatment of anticipatory, 112-115
See also Fear
Anxiety disorders
comparison of DSM-III and DSM-III-R
categories, 68
secondary depression and, 256
and unipolar disorder, 58, 61, 156, 157
See also Panic disorder
Anxiety Disorders Interview Schedule
(ADIS), 78, 79
Aphasia, and depression, 266
Aprosodia, 266-267
Arthritis, juvenile, in suicidal youngsters,
391
Assertion training
gains in social skills from, 245
for panic, 126
Assessment
of drug effect, for panic, 90-91

Calcium
  lab screens, for all psychiatric patients,
    360
  metabolism, and panic, 44-45
Cancer
  pancreatic, 265, 359
  suicide risk, 325, 330, 359-360
Carbon dioxide (CO_2) inhalation
  heightened central sensitivity, 11
  panicogenic mechanism, 44
  provocation of panic by, 30, 32-34, 36,
    42-44, 139
Catatonia, 264
  as atypical subtype of mood disorder,
    468
  ECT for, 468, 470-471, 483, 515, 526
Catharsis
  analytical, 121
  suicidal behavior as, 362
Causal attributions, 542-543, 557, 599
Center for Stress and Anxiety, 131
Cerebrospinal fluid (CSF) monoamine
    metabolites
  5-HIAA, and depression, aggression,
    and suicide, 163-165, 181, 334-342,
    356, 423-424
  HVA, and depression subtypes, L-dopa
    response, 163-165, 180, 181
  serotonergic studies, and suicidality,
    338-340
Change process, CT model of, 643-644
Cheerfulness, inappropriate, and
  apathetic, indifferent state, 266
Childbirth, panic after, 17
Children
  abused, 395-396
  of affectively disordered parents, 156,
    275
  anxiety in, and panic disorder,
    agoraphobia, 63
  cognitive therapy with, 584-604
  ECT use in, 471-472
  familial loading for psychiatric illness,
    395
  loss or death of parent, and suicidality,
    355
  separation anxiety in, and adult
    anxiety, 18-19
  substance abuse by, 205
  suicidality in, 206, 288, 353-375, 602-603
  unipolar disorder in, 204-206
  See also Adolescents
Chlordiazepoxide, for panic, 110
Churchill, Winston, depression in, 147
Cholinergic function
  defects in, and bipolar illness, 164
  and depression, 182-184
  and ECT, 446
Cimetidine, associated depressive
    syndrome, 265

Circadian rhythms
  and depression, 171-172, 176, 180-181
  hyposerotonergic hypothesis of
    depression and, 180-181
  phase-advanced, and depression, 172
  reversed diurnal variation, 100
Clomipramine, for panic, 99-100
Clonazepam, for panic, 108-109
Cocaine
  associated depressive syndrome, 265
  in setting event for first panic, 14-15
  and panic, 14-15, 77
Cognition
  assessment of, in panic, 80-81
  cognitive model of panic, 11-12, 41
  defined, 540
  disordered, in depression, 236, 244,
    556-557
  dysfunctional, and suicide, 355
  effects of ECT on, 438-441, 450-453,
    498-509
  negative cognitive triad, 236, 534-535,
    543, 546, 556
  panic, and catastrophic
    misinterpretation of sensations, 11-12,
    14-15, 24, 44, 46-47, 96-97, 127-129,
    544-545
  reattribution, for panic, 128-129, 131
  style of, and suicidality, 358-359
Cognitive theory, introduction to, 538-545
Cognitive therapy (CT), 553-669
  behavioral techniques, 566-567
  case selection, 558-559
  with children and adolescents, 584-604
  of depression, 235, 236, 246-247, 534-535
  empirical studies on, 643-659
  format, 560-561
  future directions, 547-550
  in groups, 608-623
  growth-directed forms, 565-566
  history of development, 533-534
  introduction to, 538-550
  of panic disorder, 571-582
  for relapse or recurrence of depression,
    246-247
  techniques, 558-567
  for unipolar depression, description of,
    235, 236
Cohort, birth, see Birth cohort effects
Collaborative empiricism, in cognitive
    therapy, 561
Collaborative Study on the Psychobiology
    of Depression, NIMH, 203, 316
Comorbidity, 371
  affective disorders with any other, and
    suicide risk, 363
alcoholism, with other disorders, 6-7, 63,
  74, 156, 157, 165, 198-200, 205, 256, 265,
  301, 364

in the medical setting, 259-260
SCID, 78-79
Diagnostic Interview Schedule (DIS), 70
Diet, effect on monoamines and
metabolites, 337
See also Tyramine; Vitamins
Differential diagnosis
of the confusion/delirium/dementia/
coma complex, 264
DSM-III-R changes, for panic disorder,
67-69
hierarchical rules concerning panic
disorder, 69, 74
organic from panic disorders, 8, 67-82
structured and semistructured
interviews, 78-79
unipolar disorder, 195-198, 205
use of sleep abnormalities in, 170
See also Comorbidity
DIS, *see* Diagnostic Interview Schedule
Disability
and depression, 258
and suicide, 325
Discharge, from hospital, suicide soon
after, 315-316, 329, 364, 416
Disciplinary crisis, as suicide precipitant,
355-356
Diversion/distraction, to cope with
anxiety, 576
Dizziness, between panic attacks, 76
DNA, *see* Deoxyribonucleic acid
Dopamine (DA)
abnormalities in depression, 180
and ECT, 445
HVA, 163-165, 180, 181, 335
Double depression, 362
natural course of, 203
Doxepine, for unipolar depression, 216
Dream analysis, psychoanalytic, for panic,
126
Drugs
advantages and disadvantages of
antipanic medications, 113
antidepressant, available in U.S., 216
avoidance, by panic patients, 90
choosing among, for panic, 111-112
combined with ECT, 461, 467-468,
484-485
combined with psychotherapy, for
depression, 247-251
compared to psychotherapy, for
depression, 238-241
commonly producing depressive
syndrome, 264-265
effect on monoamines and metabolites,
337
memory-enhancing, 505
for panic disorder, 8, 88-115
panic provocation by, 14-15, 30-34, 90

restricting prescription quantity, 356,
366, 415
for situational depression, 220
unfavorable experience with, panic
disorder and, 14-15
in unipolar depression treatment,
213-230
used in ECT, 439, 484-485, 505, 509
See also Side effects; Substance abuse
*DSM-III, see Diagnostic and Statistical
Manual of Mental Disorders, Third Edition*
*DSM-III-R, see Diagnostic and Statistical
Manual of Mental Disorders, Third Edition,
Revised*
DST, *see* Dexamethasone suppression test
Durkheim, E., 287
conclusions, ecological analyses of
suicide, 295-296
Dysfunctional Attitude Scale (DAS), 546
Dysthymic disorder
DSM-III-R criteria, 190-191, 227-228
natural course of, 202-203
somatic treatment, 228-229

Eating disorders, comorbidity with
affective disorders, 156, 199
ECA, *see* Epidemiologic Catchment Area
Survey
Ecological analyses, of suicide, 289-290,
295-296, 303-304
Economic factors, in depression and
suicide, 149, 153, 301, 309
increase in suicides during Great
Depression, 297
Edema, peripheral, 102
Efficacy, of psychosocial treatments,
238-241
Electroconvulsive Therapy, APA Task Force
Report, 515
Electroconvulsive therapy (ECT)
versus active and inactive treatment,
459-461, 466-467
acute confusional state resulting from,
498-500
adverse effects of, 433, 438-441, 450-453,
498-511, 527
anticonvulsant properties, 449-450
versus antipsychotics, 467
appropriate guidelines, 432, 434-435,
526-528
biochemical effects of, 452-453
brain damage from, 505-507
for catatonia, 468, 470-471, 483, 515, 526
cardiac side effects, 509, 510, 527
coercive use of, 432-434
cognitive side effects, 438-441, 450-453,
498-509, 527
combined with drugs, 461, 467-468,
484-485
conditions effective for, 470

consent, 483, 494-495
deaths related to, 509, 527
in depressive disorders, 100, 147, 215, 219-220, 270, 370, 458-465
drugs used in, 439, 484-485, 505, 509
effects on memory, 438-440
electrode placement, 439, 474-476, 485-486, 488, 498, 503-504
ethical concerns, 433-434, 513, 522-524
facilities and staffing for, 482, 490-492
frequency and number of seizures, 477, 490, 498
GAP report of 1947 criticisms, 433, 513-515
indications for use of, 458-478, 482-483
legal regulations, 513, 515-522, 526
maintenance, 464, 469, 490
in mania, 465-466, 476, 483, 515, 526
manual of practice, 482-492
mechanisms of action, 436-453
medical examinations before, 483-484
for medically ill with severe depression, 270
medical supplies and equipment, 497
memory impairment from, 500-505
multiple-monitored (MMECT), 477, 490
nature of efficacy, 437-438, 441-450
neuropathology of cognitive effects, 451
neurophysiological correlates, of cognitive effects, 451-452
organic brain syndrome from, 439, 441
for Parkinson's, 267
poor response, in depression, 100
for potential suicide, 222
predictors of response to, 462-464, 468-469
pretreatment procedures, 482-485, 498, 505
problems with use of, 431-434, 438-441, 450-453, 498-511, 513, 526-528
professional ambivalence about, 431, 513, 526-528
psychiatric self-regulation, 513-515, 526
for psychotic depression, 219-220
record keeping, 491, 497
and reserpine, 485
in schizophrenia, 466-469, 476, 483, 515, 526
seizure induction and monitoring, 477-478, 487-490, 498
for severe melancholic or endogenous depression, 215
spontaneous seizures following, 507-509
stimulus waveform, 476-477, 498, 504-505
systemic adverse effects, 509-510
technique, and efficacy, 474-478, 485-490, 498
for unipolar disorder, 370

use in children and adolescents, 471-472
use in elderly, 472
Electrodes, ECT, placement, 439, 474-476, 485-486, 488, 498, 503-504
Electroencephalogram (EEG), sleep recordings, in depression, 169
Emotion
cognitive theories of, 553
evolutionary purpose, 13, 15, 21-22
expression and recognition of, 237, 263, 266-267, 576
strong, avoidance of, for fear of panic, 133, 573, 576
Emotion theory, view of panic disorder, 7, 10, 20-22, 139
Emotional disorders, cognitive models of, 540-545
Employment, instability in, and suicide, 197, 301-303, 309, 325, 327, 355, 364
Endocrine system
abnormalities, and depression, 172-177, 180-181, 264
neuroendocrine function and ECT, 447-450
serotonergic system and suicidality, 288, 334, 345-346, 359-361
Entrapment, fear of, 21, 72, 572, 576
and phobias, 13-15
Environment
effect on suicidality, 356-358, 394-397
risk factors for suicide, 287
See also Family
Epidemiologic Catchment Area (ECA) Survey, 55-56, 58-61
DIS, 79
Epidemiology
association between MS and bipolar disorder, 268
defined, 54
of depression secondary to medical illness, 257-259
of panic disorder and agoraphobia, 8, 54-64
sources of data, 54-56
suicide studies, 287, 289-304, 386
of unipolar disorder, 148, 151-153
Epilepsy
depressive symptoms, 270
and panic, 76, 91
and suicide, 359-361
Ethics, concerning ECT use, 513, 522-524
Eutonyl, for panic, 100
Exercise, and panic, 35, 36, 44, 128, 132, 133
Expectations, defined, 542
Exposure, to phobic stimuli, 35, 41-42, 121-126
graduated self-directed, 122-123, 125
interoceptive, 127-128, 131, 135
in vivo, 35, 41-42, 121-126, 132, 135

Helplessness
  feelings of, anxiety, and panic, 19-20, 124
  learned, depression model, 182, 543
Hemispheres, brain
  ECT electrode placement, 439, 474-476, 485-486, 488, 503-504
  stroke in right, 266
Hemodialysis, and suicide, 326, 330, 423-424
Hereditary effects
  in affective illness, 183
  genetic risk for suicide, 288, 394-395, 423-424
  in panic disorder, 6, 15, 23-25, 61-63, 67-68, 74, 140
  in psychiatric disorders, familial and not Mendelian, 160
  in unipolar disorder, 6, 149-165, 275
  See also Family studies
Hereditary pancreatitis, depression in, 266
Heredity
  genetic markers for depression, 160-161
  mode of inheritance of depressive illness, 148, 149, 158-162, 275
  multifactorial or polygenic inheritance, 159, 275
Hierarchical rules, concerning panic disorder diagnosis, 69, 74, 140
High-contact psychotherapy, 245
Hippocampus, cholinergic activity in, 182
Hippocrates, black bile theory, 147
Homicide, and suicide, 296-297
Homo symbolicus, 567
Homovanillic acid (HVA), 335
  and depression subtypes, 163-165, 181
  favorable response to L-dopa and, 180
Hopelessness
  decreasing, 558, 560
  and depression and suicide, 390-391
  improvement in, 244
  as predictor of suicide, 314, 316
  provision of hope, 365-366
  as risk factor for suicide, 354, 358, 364, 390, 393, 411, 417, 418
Hospitalization
  for suicidality, 366-367, 398, 414-416
  suicide during, or after discharge, 315-316, 329, 364, 416
HPA, see Hypothalamic-pituitary-adrenal axis
Human immunodeficiency virus (HIV), major affective disorder in, 268-269
Huntington's chorea, depression in, 267-268
  and suicide, 359, 360
  TCA anticholinergic side effects sensitivity, 268
HVA, see Homovanillic acid

Hyperparathyroidism
  mood disturbance in, 360
  as source of organic anxiety syndrome, 77
Hypersomnia, and youth suicidality, 393
Hypertension
  drugs for, depression associated with, 265
  in ECT, 485
  medication for, and suicidality, 359, 361
  and white matter lesions, 268
Hypertensive crisis, with MAOIs, 102, 223
Hyperthermic crisis, on switching MAOIs, 104, 223
Hyperthyroidism
  anxiety as symptom of, 76, 91
  depression with, 175, 264, 360
Hyperventilation
  to activate respiratory panic symptoms, 128, 132
  and anxiety or panic, 30, 32-34, 36, 42-45
  and breathing training, 129, 575
  chronic, 42-44
Hypnotherapy, for panic, 126
Hypnotics, restricting quantity of prescriptions for, 356, 366, 415
Hypoactivity model, of depression, 182
Hypochondriasis, and panic disorder, differential diagnosis, 74-75
  See also Depression, masked
Hypoglycemia, 471
  depression and, 264
  and panic, 45, 76
Hypomania, 148
Hypoparathyroidism, as source of organic anxiety syndrome, 77
Hypotension, salt self-restriction, and MAOIs, 102
Hypothalamic-pituitary-adrenal (HPA) axis
  dysregulation of, 172, 176
  function, and suicidality, 345
Hypothalamus
  cholinergic activity in, 182
  suprachiasmic nucleus of, as biological clock, 172
Hypothyroidism, 471
  association with anxiety, 76, 91
  depression with, 175
  due to lithium, 372
  Grade II or III, 175-176
  mood disturbance in, 360
  psychomotor retardation in, 261
Hysteria, secondary depression and, 256, 264

Iatrogenic amnestic syndromes, from ECT, 438-440, 500-505

Ideation, suicidal, 261, 307, 314, 353-354, 388, 404-405, 414, 463
Illness
  medical, depression and suicidality in, 256-270, 299, 325, 359, 391, 483-484
  mental, 7-8, 10, 22-25, 138-139, 260-261, 491
Imagery
  cognitive therapy techniques, 562-563
  modifying, 577
  phobic, 36, 41-42, 46-47, 125, 132, 577
  positive, 127
Imipramine
  anticholinergic response, specific to panic patients, 96
  course of treatment, 95-97
  hypersensitivity response, 95-96
  versus MAOIs, for panic, 93, 111-112
  for panic, 92-99, 111-113
  specific panic-blocking action, 94
  for unipolar disorder, 216
Immune system, 176, 259
  HIV and AIDS, 268
  lithium induction of antithyroid antibodies, 176
Impulsivity
  alcohol, and suicide, 328
  serotonergic system, and suicidality, 339-340, 346, 358-359
  hostile, modulating, 395
  youth suicidality and, 388, 389, 398
Incarceration, threat of, 355
Indoleamines
  serotonin, 42, 180-182, 288, 334-342, 345-346, 356, 423-424, 445-446
  tryptophan, 181, 461
Information processing
  in depression, 557, 560
  studies of, in anxiety patients, 39-47
  See also Learning; Memory
Insomnia, in depression, 169
  hyposerotonergic hypothesis of, 180-181
Intelligence, high, and suicide, 325
Intentionality, suicidal, 307-308, 324, 354-356, 393
Interoceptive cues, in panic disorder, 14-15, 90, 96-97, 127-129
Interpersonal therapy, for depression, 235
  description of, 237
Interviews
  adherence, 635-638
  family study method, 150, 158
  structured and semistructured, 78-79
  of suicide victim's survivors, 289, 300
  See also Questioning
Intoxication
  alcohol, and suicide, 317-323
  depressive symptoms, 264
  and suicidality, 363-364
Introversion, in unipolar patients, 204

Inventories, self-statement, 80-81
  limitations of, 81
Isocarboxazid
  for panic, 100
  for unipolar depression, 216
Isoproterenol, panicogenic effects, 32, 41

Kindling, ECT, 449-450, 508
Kraepelin, E., 147

Law, concerning ECT use, 513, 515-522, 526
Learning
  impairment, in depression, 557, 560-561
  learned-helplessness model of depression, 182, 543
Lethality, of suicide attempt, 354, 356
Leukoaraiosis, 268
Liability scale, of affective disorders, 159
Life events, negative
  in depression spectrum disease patients, 157, 543
  preceding first panic, 15-18, 139
  and suicide, 309, 325, 328, 329, 354-355, 394
Light, effect on depression, 172
Limbic system, 177
  cholinergic activity in, 182
  dopamine pathways, 180
Lincoln, Abraham, depression in, 147
Linkage studies, in unipolar families, 160-162, 275
Lithium
  antithyroid antibody induction, 176
  and ECT, 485
  hypothyroidism due to, 372
  REM sleep effects, 170-171
  and serotonergic mechanisms in depression, 181
  soft bipolar spectrum, responsive to, 222
  for unipolar depression, 216
Liver, MAOI side effects, 102
Locus coeruleus, 177
  abnormalities in, 11
  cholinergic activity in, 182
  panic pathogenesis of, 31-32, 39, 40
Loss, of key person, and suicide, 301, 309, 325, 328, 329, 354-355, 363
Low-contact psychotherapy, 245
Lymphocytes, defective function in depression, 176, 259

Madden, John, 5
Major depression, DSM-III-R criteria, 189-190
  See also Unipolar depression
Mania, 148
  adrenergic predominance, 182

birth cohort effects, 152
ECT in, 465-469, 476, 483, 515, 526
Manual, treatment
ECT, 482-492
for time-limited psychodynamic
approaches, 237
MAO, see Monoamine oxidase
MAOIs, see Monoamine oxidase inhibitors
Maprotiline, for unipolar depression, 216
Marijuana
and panic, 14-15, 77
schizophrenia, and suicide, 364
Markers
biological, 256, 275
genetic, for depression, 149, 160-162
Marriage
satisfaction, and exposure therapy, 123
and suicide, 301, 309, 325, 327-329, 354-
355, 363
MC-2 panic, 36, 41
Media, effect on youth suicide, 396-397
Medical illness
depression secondary to, 256-270
and ECT, 473-474, 483-484
failure to treat depression in, 259
and suicidality, 299, 325, 359, 391
Medical workup
in depression, 175-176
before ECT, 483-484
for depressed medical inpatient, 265
for panic patients, 75, 77, 91-92, 140,
141
psychiatric patients, 360-363
Medication, fears of, in panic patients,
89-90
See also Drugs
Melancholia, 192, 215, 287
era of, 275-276
Melatonin, delayed secretion onset, in
depression, 172
Memory
anterograde, deficits after ECT, 438-440,
500-501, 505
autobiographical, and ECT, 503
impairment, from ECT, 438-440, 500-505
and learning function, in depression,
557, 560
retrograde deficits, after ECT, 438, 440,
500-502, 505
Menstrual cycles
abnormal, in depression, 171, 276
associated suicidality, 362-363
PMS, 362
pregnancy, 17, 472
Mental illness
bias against, 260-261
integration of biological, psychological,
and social approaches to, 7-8, 10, 22-
25, 138-139

Mental retardation, mistaken for
depression, 263
Metabolism, derangement of, in panic,
44-45
Method, of suicide, 293, 326, 356, 417-418
by gender, 298
prescription drugs, quantity restriction,
356, 366
violent, 336-337, 356, 366, 386-388, 423
Metoclopramide, associated depressive
syndrome, 265
Mitral valve prolapse (MVP)
differential diagnosis, with panic
disorder, 75-76
in panic disorder patients, 45-46
MMECT, see ECT, multiple-monitored
Monitoring, ambulatory
ordinary-day, for panic, 35-36, 41, 82,
125
Vitalog MC-2 monitor, 36
Monoamine metabolites
CSF, 42, 163-165, 180-182, 288, 334-342,
345-346, 356, 423-424, 445-446
and depression subtypes, 163-165, 181
studies of suicides, 334-345
Monoamine oxidase (MAO)
studies in affectively disordered, 163,
165
in suicides and attempters, 335-340
Monoamine oxidase inhibitors (MAOIs)
depression response to, 191
discontinuation and follow-up, 104, 223
and ECT, 485
foods, beverages, and medications to
avoid, 103
and history of asthma or allergy, 91-92
incompatibility with each other, 104,
223
nonresponders, 223
for panic, 100-104, 111-113
REM sleep effects, 170
side effects, 91-92, 100-104, 111-113, 223
switching, 104, 223
for unipolar depression, 216
Mood disorders, 244
catatonia as atypical subtype of, 468
and hyposerotonergic hypothesis of
depression, 180-181
use of term, 147-148
Mortality rates
in panic disorder, 6
in unipolar depression, 202
See also Death
Mothers
depressed, suicidality and child abuse,
395-396
of female adoptees with depression, 154
See also Parents
Motivation, for suicide, 354, 355
MS, see Multiple sclerosis (MS)

Multiple sclerosis (MS)
depressive symptoms, 268
specific HLA antigens associated with, 161
suicidality, 359
MVP, *see* Mitral valve prolapse

National Center for Health Statistics (NCHS), U.S. suicide statistics, 308
National Death Register, 296
National Institute of Mental Health (NIMH)
Collaborative Study on the Psychobiology of Depression, 203, 316
Consensus Conference on ECT, 431-432, 470, 491, 515
Epidemiologic Catchment Area Survey, 55-56, 58-61
Treatment of Depression Collaborative Research Program, 203, 239, 244-246
National Institutes of Health (NIH), OMAR, Consensus Conference on ECT, 431-432, 470, 491, 515
National Survey of Psychotherapeutic Drug Use, 55
Native Americans, suicide in, 388
NCHS, *see* National Center for Health Statistics
NE, *see* Norepinephrine
Nebuchadnezzar, depression in, 147
Negative cognitive triad, 236, 534, 543, 546, 556
Nervous system, 269
underlying instability, in panic, 37, 41
Network against Psychiatric Assault (NAPA), 433
Neurocirculatory asthenia, 44
Neuroleptics, catatonia from, 470-471
Neuropeptide Y, 161, 162
Neurotransmitter function
abnormalities, and panic, 37, 40, 42
depression abnormalities, 177-184
and ECT, 444-447
New Haven survey, of anxiety states, 55, 58
Newfoundland, low suicide rate, 295
Niacin, deficiency of, and depression, 264
NIH, *see* National Institutes of Health
NIMH, *see* National Institute of Mental Health
Nomenclature
cognitive therapy, 540-543
concerning depression, 147-151, 188-189, 213
suicidality, 307-308, 353-354
Nonresponders, treatment strategies for, 222-223, 235
Norepinephrine (NE)
abnormalities in depression, 177-180

and ECT, 444-445
MHPG, 335
Nortriptyline, for unipolar depression, 216
Note taking, by patient and therapist, 560-561

Office of Medical Applications of Research (OMAR), of NIH, Consensus Conference on ECT, 431-432, 470, 491
One Flew over the Cuckoo's Nest, 433
Onset, age of
agoraphobia, 62, 73-74
depression, 256, 274
dysthymic disorder, 228
panic disorder, 62, 73-74
unipolar disorder, 152, 155, 157, 159
Organic anxiety syndrome, and panic disorder, differential diagnosis, 75-77
Organic mental syndrome
from ECT, 439, 441, 485
use of ECT in, 470-471
Overbreathing, and chronic hyperventilation, 43

Pacemaker, or biological clock, 171-172
Pancreas, carcinoma of, depressive symptoms, 265-266, 359
Pain, and suicide, 325
Panic, 11-12, 14-15, 24, 44, 46-47
and agoraphobia, 125-126, 138-139
ambulatory monitoring, ordinary day, 35-36, 41, 82, 125
and anxiety, 73, 88-90
in atypical depression, 218
central noradrenergic activation, 39-40
cognitive–behavioral treatments for, 8, 114, 121-134
cognitive factors in, 11-15, 41, 128-129, 571-573
as consequence of caffeinism, 31
current models of, 7-8, 10-25, 128-129, 138-139, 571-573
and depression, 6, 58
dimensional approaches to assessment, 79-82
eliciting, 29-36, 46-47
exacerbation of symptoms, on clomipramine, 99
expression, observational measures, 81
first, 15
and generalized anxiety, drug effects, 88
hyperventilatory symptoms, and respiratory-control treatment, 130
infrequent, 138-140
lactate-provoked psychological factors in, 46-47
metabolic imbalance, 44-45
multicomponent treatment, 126-132

neurotransmitter abnormalities, 37, 40, 42
nonpharmacological induction of, 34-36
pathogenic mechanisms of, research on, 29-39
pathogenesis, leading hypotheses, 39-47
peripheral nervous hypersensitivity, 40-42
pharmacological provocative testing, 30-34
prevalence of, 5, 22-23, 56-57
provocation by CO_2 inhalation, 32-34
psychoanalytic model, 19-20
psychological aspects, 138-139
respiratory dysfunction, 42-44
self-evaluative attention to interoceptive cues, 90, 96-97, 127-129
sensations of vertigo or movement, 76
separation anxiety model, 18-19
specific organ pathology in, 45-46
spontaneous, studies of, 34-36
stress-diathesis model, 15-18
substance abuse, and anxiety, 6-7
symptoms, rates and risks, 56
treatment developments, 7, 8, 114, 121-134
triggered by sensations other than anxiety, 132-133, 572-573
underlying autonomic instability, 37, 41
in vivo exposure, 35, 41-42, 121-126
vulnerability to, 17-18, 30, 36-39
Panic disorder, 5-142
age of onset, 62, 73-74
with agoraphobia, 58-61, 63, 72
assessment, 8, 67-82
avoidance component, 133-134
breathing training for, 126, 129-131
catastrophic misinterpretations, 128
choosing among drugs for, 111-112
comorbidity, 58-61, 63, 72, 139-140
conditioning and, 14-15
and depression, 58, 61, 63, 100-101, 140, 157, 165
developing terminology for patient's symptoms, 89
diagnostic criteria in *DSM-III* and *DSM-III-R*, 67-71
differential diagnosis, 69-77
drug treatment strategy, 88-90
epidemiology of, 8, 54-64
familial aggregation, 23-25, 61-63, 67-68, 74
family history of narrow angle glaucoma, 91
increased risk for medical disorders, 75, 77, 91
instructions to patients on MAOIs, 103
medical workup, 75, 77, 91-92
and panic attacks, 138

particular sensitivity to clomipramine, 99
prevalence and risk of, 5, 22, 23, 56-57, 59, 67, 410
principles and techniques of CT, 573-581
relatives with depression, anxiety, and alcoholism, 157
self-treated, with alcohol, 54, 58, 63, 77, 141
somatic side effects, of medication, 90
specific anticholinergic response to imipramine, 96
and substance abuse, 54, 58, 63, 77, 141
as suicide risk factor, 410
supportive psychotherapy for, 114
test-retest reliability and concordance, DIS, 79
those who *don't* develop, 22
treatment of, 8, 82-134, 571-582
24-hour telephone availability, 90
vestibular function in, 45, 76
Paradigm, psychotherapeutic, shift in, 538-539
Paradoxical intention, 124
Paradoxical responses
desynchrony, 82
to relaxation instruction, 34-35, 82
stimulant effect of alprazolam, 107
Parathyroid dysfunction, 77, 264, 360
Parents
affectively disordered, 156, 395
early loss, and suicidality, 328, 329, 354
of suicidal youngsters, 394-397
Parkinson's disease
depression in, 267
psychomotor retardation in, 261
Patients
agitated medical, psychiatric consultation, 326
aggressive ECT use on, 433-434
psychosocial profile of those who attempt or complete suicide, 287, 327-328
selection criteria, for short-term psychodynamic approaches, 238
SMR in women, 30-49, 314-315
suicidality in, 299-301, 307-330, 353-364, 403
Pellagra, and depression, 264
Peptides
and ECT, 447-450
neuroactive, 161
Perfectionism, 244
and youth suicide, 389
Personality
affiliative or achievement-oriented, and depression, 549
depressed premorbid, leading to alcoholism, 198

and depression, 203-204, 274, 395, 549, 559
development of, effects of depressive parent on, 395
and suicidality, 328, 358-359
Personality disorders
and panic, 39, 133
as risk factor in suicide, 410
and unipolar depression, 196-197
Pessimism, *see* Hopelessness
Phase delay, in depression, resettling, 171-172
Phenelzine
for panic, 100-104, 113
pyridoxine deficiency from, 102
for unipolar depression, 216
Phobia
avoidance, after initial panic attack, 67
behavior therapy techniques for, 114
evolutionary purpose, 13, 15, 21-22
as false alarm reaction, 11-15, 17, 18, 24, 44, 46-47, 127-129, 139, 571-573
genesis of, 12-14
imipramine for, 92
self-evaluative attention to interoceptive cues and, 11-12, 14-15, 24, 44, 46-47, 96-97, 127-129
simple, 73
social, 69, 73, 115
in vivo exposure, 35, 41-42, 121-126
See also Agoraphobia; Panic
Phosphorus, lab screens for all psychiatric patients, 360
Pilowsky Illness Behavior Questionnaire, 75
PMS, *see* Premenstrual syndrome
Precipitants, for suicidality, 354-355, 417
Prediction
of response to ECT, 462-464, 468-469
of suicide, 301-303, 316, 405-408, 422
Predisposition, to panic proneness, 75
Pregnancy
ECT use during, 472
panic beginning during, 17
Premenstrual syndrome (PMS), 171, 276, 362-363
Prescriptions, limiting quantities, as suicide preventive, 356, 366, 415
Prevalence rates
of agoraphobia, 5-6, 56-57, 59, 67
of depression secondary to medical illness, 257-259
of panic, 5, 22-23, 56-57
of panic disorder, 5, 22, 23, 56-57, 59, 67
of psychiatric disorders, 160
of suicide, in various countries over time, 290-291
unipolar depression, 151
of suicide, 299, 397-399, 403-418

crisis centers, 354, 403
steps to, 414-416
Problem solving, interpersonal, deficits in, and suicide, 355, 358
Prolactin (PRL), 181
in suicidal patients, 346
tumors secreting, 263
Pro-opiomelanocortin (POMC), 161
Propranolol
associated depressive syndrome, 265
for panic, 111
Prosody, lack of, 266-267
Protriptyline, for unipolar depression, 216
Provocation studies, of panic, 29-36
Psychoanalysis
for agoraphobia and panic, 19-20, 121-122, 126, 133
for depression, 147
Psychobiology, of unipolar depression, 148
Psychodynamic therapy, for depression, description of, 147, 235-238
Psychomotor retardation, 261
Psychosocial treatments, for unipolar depression, suicidality, 369-370
Psychostimulants, responsiveness of depressive medically ill to, 262
Psychotherapy
high- and low-contact, 245
and pharmacotherapy for depression, 247-251
Punishment
feelings of, 261
self-administered, 237
Purkinje cells, cerebellar, loss of, 508
Pyridoxine, *see* Vitamins, B$_6$

Questioning, depressed patient
CT technique, 561-562
about suicidality, 404-405, 414
See also Interviews

Race
agoraphobia rates by, 57
ECT administration, 435
older white men, compared with black, 304
suicide rates by, 291-294, 296-297, 304, 314, 321, 329, 369, 388-389
Rapid eye movement (REM) sleep, 164, 169-172
cholinergic induction, and affective illness, 164
effects of cholinergic agonists, 164, 183
hyposerotonergic hypothesis of depression, and short latency, 180
short latency, 164, 170, 180-181, 183
RDC, *see* Research Diagnostic Criteria
Receptors
adrenergic, and depression, 179

treatment of suicidality, 373-374
and youth suicide, 388-390, 412
See also Alcoholism
SUDS, *see* Subjective Units of Distress
Scale
Suffocation alarm mechanism,
hypersensitive, CO_2-responsive, 44
Suicidal Intent Scale, 356
Suicidality
abnormality in serotonergic function
and, 334-347
adolescent, and depression, 389, 390,
395
and alcohol, 316-325, 327-330
availability of lethal agents, 366
in bipolar disorder, treatment, 372
child abuse and, 395-396
communication of, 324, 330, 393, 417
definitions and terminology, 307-308,
353-354
and low CSF 5-HIAA, 163
pharmacologic treatment, 371-372
physician's questions about, 404-405,
414
in schizophrenia, treatment of, 373
spectrum of, definitions, 307, 353-354
suicidal ideation, 261, 307, 314, 353-354,
388, 404-405, 414, 463
violent, reduced serotonergic function
and, 288, 334, 345-346
in youngsters, CT for, 602-603
Suicide
by age, 288, 291-294, 300, 304, 307, 309,
314-316, 327-329, 369, 386-399, 416,
417, 422-423
alcoholism as risk factor for, 301, 303,
316, 318-320, 323-325, 327-330, 354,
403, 409, 418
among Amish, 315
ascertainment artifacts, 291, 294-295,
307-308, 324
attempters versus completers, 287, 302,
327-328
attempts, *see* Suicidality
atypicality of, 290
availability of lethal agent, 298, 356
biological factors associated with, 334-
347, 397, 423
birth cohort effects, 152, 288, 291-293,
387
causal factors, 300
changes in rates with opportunity
shifts, 297-299, 356
by children and adolescents, 206, 288,
386-399
comparison of U.S. natives with
emigrants, 294-295
completions, among psychiatric
patients, 309-316
death certificate studies, 289-300, 308

demographic risk factors, 386-388
and depression, 258, 301, 309, 314, 316,
325, 327, 329, 330, 354, 356, 365-366,
403, 417
after discharge, 315-316, 329, 364, 416
Durkheim's ecological analysis, 287,
295-296
early loss and, 328, 329, 354
ecological analyses, 289-290, 295-296,
303-304
epidemiological approach, 287, 289-304
family risk factors, 357-358, 394-396, 423
fertility, rates of, 291
follow-up studies, on suicidal behavior,
391-394
genetic risk for, 288, 394-395
help-seeking previous to, 324, 330, 393,
417
during hospitalization, 315, 329, 364
HPA function and, 345
identification of patients at risk for, 258,
287-288, 307-347
imitative, 396-397
influence of local culture and historical
events, 290, 296-299
among medical and surgical patients,
258, 309, 325-327, 330
methods of, 293, 298, 326, 336-337, 356,
366, 387-388, 417-418, 423
muscarinic receptor binding activity,
183
negative life events preceding, 301, 309,
325, 328, 329, 354-355
nonserious attempts, 157
note, 308
number of attempts, 307
in patients with anxiety and panic, 7
physician's role in preventing, 404
potential for, and ECT, 222
predicting, 301-303, 316
prevention of, 299, 301, 346-347, 397-
399, 403-418
previous suicidality, 391-394, 412-414
prospective studies, 289, 301-303, 308
provision of hope, 365-366
psychiatric illness at time of death, 300-
301, 307, 309-316, 353-364, 403-404,
422
psychological risk factors, 388-391, 423
rate, for all ages, 307
rates in 15–24-year-olds, 152, 288, 291-
293, 387
rates in various countries and over
time, 290-291, 295-296
reconstructing events preceding, 289,
300-301
retrospective studies, 300-303, 308
risk factors, *see* Risk factors, for suicide
and schizophrenia, 339

desipramine, for panic, 100
discontinuation and follow-up, 98-99
and ECT, 437-438, 485
for Huntington's, 268
imipramine, for panic, 92-99
for nonresponders, 222-223
for panic, 91-100, 111-113
REM sleep effects, 170
side effects, 92, 95-100, 113
for unipolar depression, 216
Trimipramine, for unipolar depression, 216
Tryptophan, as antidepressant, 181, 461
Twin studies
of anxiety disorders, 61-62
for heritability of CSF 5-HIAA or HVA, 164
panic disorder, 140
of suicidality, 394-395
unipolar depression, 149, 153
Tyramine, dietary, and MAOIs, 102-103

Uncontrollability
of false alarm, fear of, 139
feelings of, and anxiety, panic, 19-21, 24, 90, 124, 128, 575-576
Unemployment, and suicide, 297, 301, 302, 309, 325, 327, 355, 364
Unipolar depression, 147-281
acute therapy, 213-223
adoption studies, 149, 153-154
affective spectrum, 155-159
age of onset, 152, 155, 157, 159
alcoholism, and drug dependence, 160, 363
and anxiety disorders, 156, 157
biological rhythm abnormalities, 276
birth cohort effects, 152-153, 155, 159
in children and adolescents, 204-206
chronic, treatment of, 214, 227-229
classification of, 191-195
clinical course, 200-203
cognitive model, 543-546
common genetic liability with bipolar, 149, 165, 171, 275
comorbidity with other nonaffective disorders, 198-200, 205
continuation therapy, 213-214, 223-225
depressive spectrum disease, 156-158, 160, 162, 163, 165, 195
differential diagnosis, 195-198, 205
distinction between bipolar and, 149, 150, 153, 165, 171, 188, 196, 275
DSM-III-R criteria, 147, 150
endogenous depression, 192-193
family studies, 149-151, 154-158
gender effects, 151-152, 154, 155, 158, 164
genetic epidemiology of, 149-165, 275

heterogeneity within category of, 188, 191, 213
liability scale, 159
lithium-responsive soft bipolar spectrum, 222
major depression defined, 189-190
mode of transmission, 148, 149, 158-162
in MS, 268
natural course of, 200-206
and panic disorder, 58, 61, 63, 74, 157
personality factors related to, 203-204
prevalence estimates, 151
preventive therapy, 214, 225-227, 235
primary/secondary distinction, 192, 256
psychotic depression, 194-195
rates in female relatives, 155
rediagnosis, as bipolar, 150
relapse/recurrence, 214
reliability and stability of diagnosis, 150, 200
situational depression, 193-194
somatic treatment of, 213-230, 370-371, 459-462
substance abuse and suicidality, 363
subtypes of, 156-158, 163-165, 275
suicide and mortality, 202, 206, 363, 369-371
symptoms of, 260-263
terminology concerning, 188-189, 213, 221
treatment, psychotherapeutic, 213-214, 225-229, 235-252, 369-370
twin studies, 149, 153
United States, suicide rates in, 290-294
Unpredictability, fear of, 90
Urbanization
and agoraphobia and panic disorder, 57, 62
risk of depression and, 149, 153
and suicide, 293

Vertigo, 76
Vestibular dysfunction, in panic, 45, 76, 132
Videotape, postperformance reconstruction, 80-81
Violence
and alcohol, 324
suicidal, and reduced serotonergic function, 288, 334, 339, 345-346, 423-424
war, homicide, and suicidal behavior, 296-298, 324, 356, 359
Vitalog MC-2 ambulatory monitor, 36
Vitamins
B_1, deficiencies of, 264, 265
B_3, deficiency of, 264
B_6, deficiency, and phenelzine, 102
B_{12}, deficiency of, 264, 265
folic acid, 265

Vulnerability, to panic
    approaches to understanding, 36-39
    cognitive disturbances leading to, 46
    fears of, 572
    negative life events and stress, 17-18,
        139
    psychological component, 38
    and responses to everyday stimuli, 41
    specific, of panic patients, to sodium
        lactate, 30, 76

Weeping, discriminating depressive
    severity by, 261-262

White matter, rarefication, 268
Withdrawal syndrome, alprazolam, 107-
    108
World Health Organization (WHO),
    comparison of European suicide rates,
    1975-1980, 290
Wyatt v. Hardin, 518-520

Yohimbine, 461
    to provoke panic attacks, 31-32, 39, 40

Zurich study, of anxiety states, 55, 58-59